BMA

D1324549

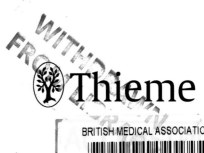

Top Score for the Radiology Boards

Q&A Review for the Core and Certifying Exams

Alan F. Weissman
Senior Staff Diagnostic Radiologist
Desert Radiology
Las Vegas, Nevada

924 illustrations

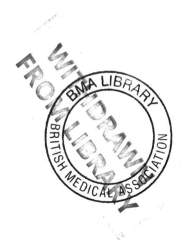

Thieme
New York • Stuttgart • Delhi • Rio de Janeiro

Executive Editor: William Lamsback
Managing Editor: Kenneth Schubach
Director, Editorial Services: Mary Jo Casey
In-house Production Editor: Torsten Scheihagen
Production Editor: Heidi Grauel
International Production Director: Andreas Schabert
Editorial Director: Sue Hodgson
International Marketing Director: Fiona Henderson
International Sales Director: Louisa Turrell
Director of Institutional Sales: Adam Bernacki
Senior Vice President and Chief Operating Officer: Sarah Vanderbilt
President: Brian D. Scanlan

Library of Congress Cataloging-in-Publication Data

Data is on file with the publisher and available upon request.

© 2018 Thieme Medical Publishers, Inc.
Thieme Publishers New York
333 Seventh Avenue, New York, NY 10001 USA
+1 800 782 3488, customerservice@thieme.com

Thieme Publishers Stuttgart
Rüdigerstrasse 14, 70469 Stuttgart, Germany
+49 [0]711 8931 421, customerservice@thieme.de

Thieme Publishers Delhi
A-12, Second Floor, Sector-2, Noida-201301
Uttar Pradesh, India
+91 120 45 566 00, customerservice@thieme.in

Thieme Publishers Rio, Thieme Publicações Ltda.
Edifício Rodolpho de Paoli, 25º andar
Av. Nilo Peçanha, 50 – Sala 2508,
Rio de Janeiro 20020-906 Brasil
+55 21 3172-2297 / +55 21 3172-1896

Cover design: Thieme Publishing Group
Typesetting by The Grauel Group

Printed in India by Replika Press Pvt. Ltd. 5 4 3 2 1

ISBN 978-1-62623-409-3

Also available as an ebook:
eISBN 978-1-62623-410-9

Dedicated to the past masters of radiology
who have brought us so elegantly to this point,
and to the future masters of radiology,
who will take the field to unimaginable places.

Dedicated with love to Nicole, my wife,
without whom this book would not be possible,
and to Josh and Blake, my children,
who provide my inspiration.

Contents

Acknowledgments ix

Foreword xi

Preface xiii

Contributors xv

Section I Breast Imaging 2
    Essentials Cases 2
    Details Cases 22
    Image-Rich Cases 34
    More Challenging Cases 44

Section II Cardiac Imaging 52
    Essentials Cases 52
    Image-Rich Cases 82
    More Challenging Cases 92

Section III Diagnostic Radiology Imaging 102
    Essentials Cases 102
    Details Cases 122
    Image-Rich Cases 132
    More Challenging Cases 142

Section IV Gastrointestinal Imaging 152
    Essentials Cases 152
    Details Cases 172
    Image-Rich Cases 182
    More Challenging Cases 192

Section V Genitourinary Imaging 202
    Essentials Cases 202
    Details Cases 222
    Image-Rich Cases 232
    More Challenging Cases 242

Section VI Interventional Imaging 252
    Essentials Cases 252

Section VII Musculoskeletal Imaging 302
  Essentials Cases 302
  Details Cases 322
  Image-Rich Cases 332
  More Challenging Cases 342

Section VIII Neuroradiology Imaging 352
  Essentials Cases 352
  Details Cases 372
  Image-Rich Cases 382
  More Challenging Cases 392

Section IX Nuclear Medicine Imaging 402
  Essentials Cases 402
  Details Cases 422
  Image-Rich Cases 432
  More Challenging Cases 442

Section X Pediatric Imaging 452
  Essentials Cases 452
  Details Cases 472
  Image-Rich Cases 482
  More Challenging Cases 492

Section XI Thoracic Imaging 502
  Essentials Cases 502
  Details Cases 522
  Image-Rich Cases 532
  More Challenging Cases 542

Section XII Ultrasound/Reproductive/Endocrinology Imaging 552
  Essentials Cases 552
  Details Cases 572
  Image-Rich Cases 582
  More Challenging Cases 592

Section XIII Vascular Imaging 602
  Essentials Cases 602

Section XIV Physics Safety 652
  Essentials Cases 652
  Details Cases 678
  Image-Rich Cases 688
  More Challenging Cases 690

Section XV Artifacts in Imaging 700

Section XVI General Radiology Imaging 716
  Essentials Cases 716

Section XVII Noninterpretive Skills - Available online

Acknowledgments

I am extremely grateful to the world-class organization at Thieme for its belief in the project and its subsequent invaluable guidance and skilled coordination of the manuscript. In particular, Kenn Schubach, Heidi Grauel, Torsten Scheihagen, and Bill Lamsback each deserve a very special thank you.

I am indebted to the numerous experts who have contributed so capably to this book. You are all extremely busy in your own daily practices, and your efforts in creating a text worthy of board preparation is tremendously appreciated. It is my hope that the final product justifies your dedication and commitment to the project.

A special acknowledgment to Drs. Twyla Bartel and Tracey Yarborough, who provided me critical assistance with the editing of this book. To both of you, your experience is apparent and your diligence is commendable.

I'd like to single out one teacher from my own radiology residency, Dr. William Eyler. As an ABR examiner, he liked to say that he was a "tough examiner, but an easy grader." That line has always stuck with me, and I agree that tough on the front end is a good strategy.

Finally, thanks to the talented residents and fellows who are at the very precipice of practice. To reach this point, you must have overcome formidable obstacles. Take solace in understanding that the hardest battles are reserved for the strongest soldiers, and trust yourselves as you enter your practice. You probably know more than you think.

Foreword

All of us who have sat for the American Board of Radiology examination or the overseas equivalents—including the respective Royal Colleges of Radiology examinations—know what a stressful time this is. For six months to a year, we are focused on passing the Radiology Boards, and the stress increases as the exam inexorably comes closer and closer. All we finally care about is passing this examination. Differential diagnoses are memorized again and again, particular attention is paid to difficult and rare diagnoses, and discussion is had as to what cases were shown previously. Consultant radiologists, going about their lawful duties in academic and other departments, are tormented with difficult questions about this or that possible diagnosis by anxious trainees, who then disagree with their staff and each other!

Dr. Weissman and his coauthors are to be congratulated on producing an excellent textbook to help radiology residents prepare for the American Board of Radiology and other similar radiology examinations. All of the subspecialty areas of radiology have their own chapters, and each is divided into four subsets. Essentials and Details sections present board-standard cases along with a thorough discussion on the differential diagnoses given. These cases involve one or more high-quality images. Multiple-choice questions in the subspecialty are also given and the answers discussed. Image-rich sections present multiple high-quality images of specific diagnoses, which the reader must identify. The diagnoses and imaging findings are then discussed. The final part of each chapter presents More Challenging cases with image-based and multiple-choice questions. The diagnoses and imaging findings are then discussed. Finally, key top tips and a suggested reading list are included.

I am certain this book will be extremely useful in helping radiology residents prepare for the Radiology Boards and beyond. As we all know, after we pass the examination and become consultant radiologists, we do not suddenly know everything. Our education is a lifelong learning process. This book will also be very helpful for practicing radiologists wishing to review their skills in subspecialty areas.

I wholeheartedly recommend this book to you and offer appreciation and thanks to Alan and his coauthors.

Joseph G. Craig, MB, ChB
Clinical Professor of Radiology
Wayne State University School of Medicine
Consultant Radiologist
Henry Ford Hospital
Detroit, Michigan

Preface

An investment in knowledge pays the best interest.
-Ben Franklin

Who doesn't love a good quiz? From game shows to board games, the challenge of a quiz is an enticing hook. And by the way, it is no accident that both of these examples have "game" in their title. The very best quizzes employ a game component, to engage the participant in the action of education.

Every single one of you preparing for an American Board of Radiology (ABR) examination has faced an astonishingly large number of quizzes (practice and actual) over the years. Just try to add up your lifetime number of quizzes—first, you literally can't, and second, it would be a colossal number.

I confess that I love quizzes. I recall my nervous delight when I was first introduced to noon conference and hot seat test cases. That pressure cooker stimulated us trainees to routinely create our own memory aids, some of which remain extremely effective to this day, yet are absolutely unsuitable for printing! Recently, inspired by my teenage son and his college-board preparation, I decided to study for and retake the SAT. I reviewed a number of SAT preparation books and in doing so, gained serendipitous insight into various methods of test preparation.

This Q and A prep is designed to systematically cover the major topics that can be typically expected on the ABR boards. Through a series of four different case types, each with its own unique purpose, the book aims to continually reinforce topics that will provide both rapid and lasting mastery. While a book like this may also have great value for the practicing physician, its primary focus is the test, and the objective throughout is to ready the student for the ABR Core and Certifying exams.

The stakes are high. From your perspective, you have worked extremely hard for a very long time, and this is the final hurdle as you prepare to actually practice medicine. From everyone else on the planet's perspective, you better darned well know your craft cold.

My friends and I used to joke early on in our practice, shortly after training:

"Hey! Remember last year at noon conference when our attendings would grill us with quiz cases and then correct us when we were wrong?"

"Yeah. Good thing now that we are board-certified, we never make mistakes anymore!"

The truth is that in addition to vigilance, confidence, and effort, radiology requires just enough humility to spur on lifelong education. We are fortunate, as most careers don't.

This upcoming test is an opportunity, not a problem. So, take this time to thoroughly review. Best of luck on the test, and please contact me with any comments.

Alan F. Weissman, MD

Contributors

Raag Airan, MD, PhD
Assistant Professor of Radiology
Division of Neuroimaging and Neurointervention
Stanford University
Stanford, California

Sindhura Alapati, MD
Practicing Radiologist
Choctaw Regional Medical Clinic
Diagnostic Imaging Associates
Durant, Oklahoma

Teresita L. Angtuaco, MD
Diagnostic Radiology
University of Arkansas for Medical Sciences
Little Rock, Arkansas

Anil Attili, MD
Associate Professor
Cardiothoracic Radiology
University of Michigan
Ann Arbor, Michigan

Twyla B. Bartel, DO, MBA, FACNM
Co-Owner
Global Advanced Imaging, PLLC
Little Rock, Arkansas

Pooja Doshi, MD
Body Radiologist
Northside Radiology Associates
Atlanta, Georgia

Nikhil Goyal, MD
Diagnostic Radiology
Emory School of Medicine
Atlanta, Georgia

Michael Iv, MD
Clinical Assistant Professor of Radiology (Neuroradiology)
Stanford University
Stanford, California

Frederick Johnson, MD
Practicing Interventional Radiologist
Jackson Radiology Associates
Jackson, Tennessee

Diana L. Lam, MD
Assistant Professor of Radiology, Breast Imaging Section
Breast Imaging Fellowship Program Director
Associate Director, Diagnostic Radiology Residency
University of Washington School of Medicine, Seattle
    Cancer Care Alliance
Seattle, Washington

Douglas G. Larson, MD
Roseburg Radiologists
Roseburg, Oregon

Archana Laroia, MD
Associate Professor of Radiology
University of Iowa Hospitals and Clinics
Carver College of Medicine
Iowa City, Iowa

Scott Lenobel, MD
Assistant Professor
Musculoskeletal Imaging
Department of Radiology
The Ohio State University Wexner Medical Center
Columbus, Ohio

Kiran K. Maddu, MD
Assistant Professor Radiology
Division of Emergency and Trauma Imaging
Emory University Hospital
Atlanta, Georgia

Srikanth Medarametla, MD
Intereventional Radiology Fellow
University of Miami
Miami, Florida

David J. Murphy, MB BCh BAO, FRCR
Fellow in Thoracic Imaging
Brigham and Women's Hospital and
    Harvard Medical School
Boston, Massachusetts

Lee A. Myers, MD
Assistant Professor of Clinical Radiology
Program Director, Emergency and Trauma Radiology
    Fellowship
Keck School of Medicine of USC
LAC+USC Medical Center
Los Angeles, California

Anh-Vu Ngo, MD
Assistant Professor
University of Washington
Department of Radiology
Seattle Children's Hospital
Seattle, Washington

O. Kenechi Nwawka, MD
Assistant Professor of Radiology
Weill Medical College of Cornell University
Attending Radiologist
Radiology and Imaging
Hospital for Special Surgery
New York, New York

D. Michael Plunkett, MD
Desert Radiology
Las Vegas, Nevada

Chad Poopat, MD
Cardiothoracic Imaging
Desert Radiology
Las Vegas, Nevada

Diamanto Rigas
Staff Radiologist
VA Palo Alto
Stanford University
Santa Clara, California

Stephen G. Routon, MD
Radiology Consultants of Little Rock
Little Rock, Arkansas

Michael Schunk, MD
Desert Radiology
Las Vegas, Nevada

Maria C. Shiau, MD, MA
Associate Professor in Radiology
Director of Medical Student Education in Radiology
NYU Langone School of Medicine
Department of Radiology
NYU Langone Health
New York, New York

Eric Tranvinh, MD
Clinical Instructor of Radiology (Neuroradiology)
Stanford University
Stanford, California

Jennifer W. Uyeda, MD
Assistant Professor of Radiology
Harvard Medical School
Brigham and Women's Hospital
Boston, Massachusetts

Elizabeth Valencia, MD, JD
Clinical Instructor
Mayo Clinic College of Medicine
Senior Associate Consultant
Department of Radiology
Mayo Clinic
Rochester, Minnesota

Jeffrey L. Weinstein, MD
Instructor in Radiology
Harvard Medical School
Staff Radiologist
Vascular and Interventional Radiology
Beth Israel Deaconess Medical Center
Boston, Massachusetts

Alan F. Weissman
Senior Staff Diagnostic Radiologist
Desert Radiology
Las Vegas, Nevada

Tracy L. Yarbrough, MD, PhD, MAEd
Co-Owner
Global Advanced Imaging, PLLC
Associate Professor of Physiology
California Northstate University College of Medicine
Elk Grove, California

Top Score for the Radiology Boards

Q&A Review for the Core and Certifying Exams

Essentials 1

■ Case

A 52-year-old asymptomatic woman presents for a screening mammogram.

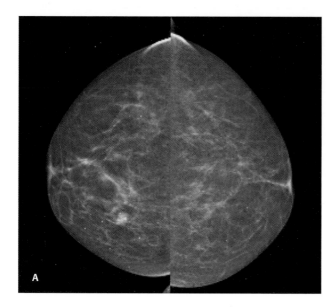
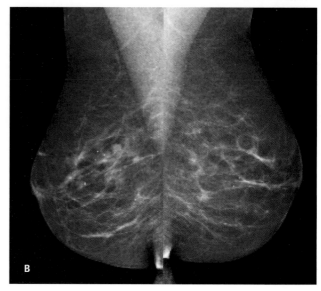

■ Questions

1. Which of the following is the appropriate overall Breast Imaging Reporting and Data System (BI-RADS) category for this screening mammogram?
   A. BI-RADS category 0
   B. BI-RADS category 1
   C. BI-RADS category 2
   D. BI-RADS category 3
   E. BI-RADS category 4

2. Regarding screening guidelines, which of the following are the current recommendations for screening mammography for the average-risk woman, according to the American Cancer Society in 2015?
   A. Annual screening mammography for women aged 45 to 54 years with the option of beginning annual screening between ages 40 to 44. Biennial mammography screening starting at age 55 with the option to continue annual screening.
   B. Annual screening mammogram starting at age 40.
   C. Annual screening mammogram and whole breast ultrasound starting at age 40.
   D. Biennial screening mammography for women aged 50 to 74 years with an individual decision to start screening prior to 50 years old.
   E. Alternating biennial screening mammography and breast magnetic resonance imaging starting at age 45.

3. Regarding breast cancer risk factors and high-risk patients, which ONE of the following is correct?
   A. Women who are characterized as "high-risk" have a > 30% lifetime risk of developing breast cancer.
   B. Women who have had previous chest irradiation between the ages of 10 and 30 years old should begin screening mammography at age 30.
   C. Women who have a first-degree relative with breast cancer should begin screening mammography at an age 10 years earlier than the age of the affected relative at time of diagnosis, or between 25 and 30 years old, whichever is later.
   D. In women with "dense breasts" as their sole breast cancer risk factor, supplemental screening breast ultrasound and breast magnetic resonance imaging are indicated.
   E. In women who have had a previous diagnosis of atypical ductal hyperplasia on excisional biopsy with no other known risk factors, breast magnetic resonance imaging is indicated.

■ Answers and Explanations

Question 1

A. Correct! BI-RADS category 0. Each BI-RADS category is paired with an assessment and recommendation. There is a mass present in the upper inner quadrant of the right breast, and additional imaging is needed to evaluate this mass. Therefore, this is BI-RADS category 0—additional imaging is needed.

Other choices and discussion

B. BI-RADS category 1 assessment means that there are no abnormalities on the mammogram. It is "negative," with a management recommendation of routine mammography screening.

C. BI-RADS category 2 assessment means that there is a benign finding (history of excisional biopsy, lumpectomy, bilateral benign masses, etc.), and there are no suspicious abnormalities. The management recommendation is the same as a BI-RADS category 1 assessment.

D. BI-RADS category 3 assessment means that the finding is probably benign (>0% but ≤ 2% likelihood of malignancy). The only BI-RADS categories permitted after a screening exam are 0, 1, and 2. A diagnostic workup needs to be completed before a BI-RADS category 3 can be given.

E. BI-RADS category 4 assessment represents a suspicious abnormality. This category can be rendered after diagnostic workup and should not be used as an assessment on screening mammogram.

Question 2

A. Correct! Annual screening mammography for women aged 45 to 54 years with the option of beginning annual screening between ages 40 and 44. Biennial screening mammography starting at age 55 with the option to continue annual screening. These are the most recent 2015 American Cancer Society recommendations. Women should continue screening as long as they have good overall health and a life expectancy of ≥ 10 years.

Other choices and discussion

B. Annual screening mammogram starting at age 40 is the American College of Radiology and Society of Breast Imaging's recommendation.

C. There are no guidelines that currently recommend both mammography and whole breast screening ultrasound for the average-risk woman.

D. Biennial screening mammography for women aged 50 to 74 years with an individual decision to start screening prior to 50 years old is the 2016 recommendation from the United States Preventative Services Task Force. The task force also concludes that there is insufficient evidence to assess the balance of benefits and harm for women > 75 years old.

E. Screening breast magnetic resonance imaging is not recommended in women of average risk for breast cancer.

Question 3

C. Correct! Women who have a first-degree relative with breast cancer should begin screening mammography at an age 10 years earlier than the age of the affected relative at time of diagnosis, or between 25 and 30 years old, whichever is later. This is according to the American College of Radiology's appropriateness criteria.

Other choices and discussion

A. High-risk women include women with a > 20% lifetime risk, *BRCA* gene mutation carrier, women who has a first-degree relative with a BRCA gene mutation but themselves are untested, history of chest irradiation between ages 10 and 30, and other genetic mutations that lead to an increased incidence of breast cancer such as Li-Fraumeni syndrome.

B. According to the American College of Radiology's appropriateness criteria, women who have had chest irradiation between the ages of 10 and 30 should begin screening mammography 8 years after radiation therapy, starting the earliest at age 25.

D. Woman with "dense breasts" do have a small increased risk of developing breast cancer compared to those who do not. However, there is currently insufficient evidence for adjunctive screening with other modalities.

E. A diagnosis of atypia (atypical ductal hyperplasia, atypical lobular hyperplasia) by itself does not put a woman at high enough risk to warrant supplemental screening with a breast magnetic resonance imaging.

■ Suggested Readings

D'Orsi CJ SE, Mendelson EB, Morris EA, et al. ACR BI-RADS® Atlas, Breast Imaging Reporting and Data System. 5th ed. Reston, VA: American College of Radiology

Nainiero MB, Lourenco A, Mahoney MC, et al. ACR Appropriateness Criteria® Breast Cancer Screening. Available at https://acsearch.acr.org/docs/70910/Narrative/. American College of Radiology. Accessed February 18, 2016

Oeffinger KC, Fontham EH, Etzioni R, et al. Breast cancer screening for women at average risk: 2015 guideline update from the american cancer society. JAMA 2015;314:1599–1614

Siu AL. Screening for Breast Cancer: U.S. Preventive Services Task Force Recommendation Statement Screening for Breast Cancer. Ann Intern Med 2016;164:279–296

Top Tips

- On screening mammography, only a BI-RADS category of 0, 1, or 2 can be given.

- The current recommendations on when to initiate screening mammography differ between different organizations. In general, all organizations agree that initiation of screening mammography at age 40 saves the most lives; however, there needs to be a balance between the benefits and harms of screening.

- According to the American College of Radiology, supplemental screening with bilateral breast MRI is indicated in women with a > 20% lifetime risk of developing breast cancer, *BRCA* gene mutation carrier and untested first-degree relative, history of chest irradiation between ages 10 and 30, and other genetic mutations that lead to an increased incidence of breast cancer such as Li-Fraumeni syndrome.

Essentials 2

■ Case

A 52-year-old woman presents with a right breast, subareolar, palpable abnormality. Craniocaudal and mediolateral oblique spot magnification views are shown.

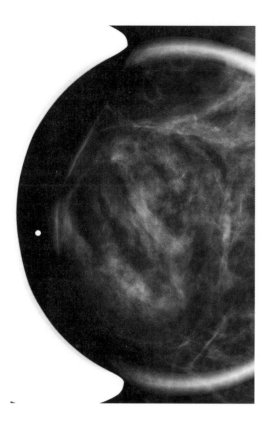 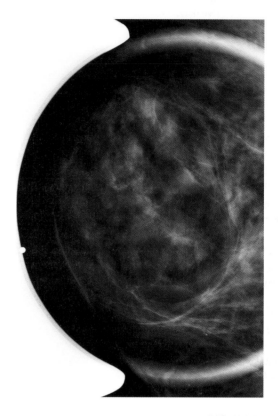

■ Questions

1. Regarding the imaging findings, which ONE of the following is the *best* answer?
   A. Oval mass with circumscribed margins and complex internal architecture. Recommend targeted ultrasound.
   B. A targeted ultrasound would show a complex solid and cystic mass.
   C. Biopsy of this lesion will reveal "benign, normal glandular tissue." This is radiologic-pathologic concordant.
   D. On a baseline screening mammogram, this mass would be categorized as BI-RADS category 0—additional imaging is needed.
   E. Fat-containing mass. Benign. There is absolutely no risk of cancer development within this lesion.

2. Regarding a fat-containing mass, which ONE of the following is the *best* answer?
   A. Most oval, circumscribed, fat-containing masses on routine screening mammography are benign and require no additional workup.

   B. A slowly growing, painful, fat-containing mass is benign, and no additional workup is needed.
   C. Two-dimensional mammography is the most sensitive modality to evaluate for fat within a breast lesion.
   D. Evaluation of questionable fat content within a lesion seen on ultrasound is an appropriate indication for breast magnetic resonance imaging.
   E. On ultrasound, lipomas are hypoechoic to the surrounding fat.

3. Which of the following can be included in the differential diagnosis for a malignant fat-containing lesion of the breast? (Select ALL that apply.)
   A. Liposarcoma
   B. Phyllodes tumor
   C. Invasive ductal carcinoma
   D. Invasive lobular carcinoma
   E. Radial scar

■ Answers and Explanations

Question 1

C. Correct! Biopsy of this lesion will reveal "benign, normal glandular tissue." This is radiologic-pathologic concordant. This is a hamartoma. On pathology, a hamartoma cannot be differentiated from normal breast tissue, since they are the same glandular elements. Therefore, core biopsy may not be helpful for making the definitive diagnosis of a hamartoma.

Other choices and discussion

A. There is an oval, fat-containing mass with circumscribed margins at the site of the palpable abnormality. Findings are characteristic for a hamartoma, and no additional imaging (including ultrasound) is needed. Hamartomas are masses within the breast composed of both glandular tissue and fat and are described as having a "breast within a breast" appearance.

B. On ultrasound, hamartomas can appear as oval, circumscribed masses with heterogeneous internal echotexture similar to normal breast tissue.

D. If the typical appearance of a hamartoma is present on a screening mammogram, no additional imaging is needed.

E. As hamartomas contain normal glandular elements, cancer can arise within a hamartoma. Thus, any suspicious finding (calcifications, suspicious mass, etc.) within a hamartoma should be worked up and biopsied to evaluate for malignancy.

Question 2

A. Correct! Most oval, circumscribed, fat-containing masses on routine screening mammography are benign and require no additional workup. Differential diagnosis of these benign entities includes lipoma, hamartoma, fat necrosis, galactocele, and lymph node.

Other choices and discussion

B. A painful, enlarging, fat-containing mass may need surgical excision, as this would be atypical for the presentation of a benign lipoma or hamartoma.

C. With the advanced technology of digital breast tomosynthesis, the ability to detect fat within masses has improved, and it is possible to visualize fat within a breast cancer. The cancer can engulf fat as it grows.

D. Mammography is currently the standard modality for the evaluation of fat within a mass originally seen on ultrasound. A bilateral breast magnetic resonance imaging is generally not used for problem solving mammographic- or ultrasound-detected lesions.

E. On ultrasound, lipomas are typically oval, circumscribed masses that range from slightly hypoechoic to hyperechoic relative to the surrounding fat. They are usually found superficially, but can appear within the deeper breast tissue.

Question 3

A–D. All of these choices are correct! Although rare, there are malignant, fat-containing lesions. These include primary liposarcoma of the breast, phyllodes tumors, and invasive cancers such as invasive ductal carcinoma and invasive lobular carcinoma. The belief is that tumors can incorporate fat within the breast as they grow.

Other choice and discussion

E. Radial scars are benign sclerosing lesions with a central fibroelastic core and radiating spiculations. In general, radial scars cause architectural distortion that is seen on mammography. Occasionally, they may centrally contain fat. A radial scar is viewed as a "high-risk lesion," and surgical excision is recommended for core needle biopsy revealing this pathology.

■ Suggested Readings

Ayyappan AP, Crystal P, Torabi A, Foley BJ, Fornage BD. Imaging of fat-containing lesions of the breast: A pictorial essay. J Clin Ultrasound 2013;41:424–433

Freer PE, Wang JL, Rafferty EA. Digital breast tomosynthesis in the analysis of fat-containing lesions. Radiographics 2014;34:343–358

Yang Wei Tse. Fibroadenolipoma (Hamartoma). Statdx. http://www.statdx.com. Accessed December 29, 2015

Top Tips

◆ Fat-containing, oval, circumscribed masses without suspicious findings are benign and do not need further workup.

◆ Differential diagnosis of benign fat-containing masses includes lipoma, hamartoma, fat necrosis, galactocele, and lymph node.

◆ Hamartomas have the classic appearance of a "breast within a breast" on screening mammography and do not need further diagnostic workup.

Essentials 3

■ Case

Screening mammogram on a 57-year-old woman. No comparisons are available.

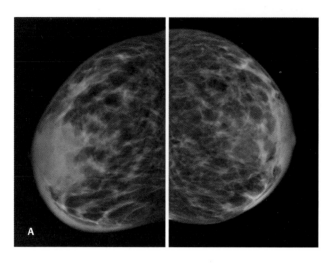

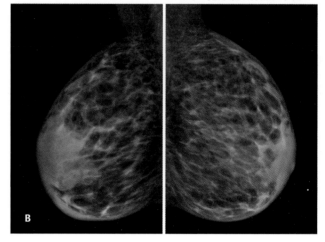

■ Questions

1. Which of the following is the *least* likely reason for the imaging findings?
   A. Inflammatory breast cancer
   B. Renal failure on dialysis
   C. Venous obstruction due to superior vena cava thrombosis
   D. Congestive heart failure

2. A 35-year-old woman presents with unilateral breast enlargement, erythema, and edema for 2 days. Which ONE of the following is the *best* answer?
   A. If there is unilateral focal skin and trabecular thickening on mammography, then her clinical and imaging findings are pathognomonic for inflammatory breast cancer, and a referral to tumor board should be made.
   B. If her mammogram and ultrasound are both negative, magnetic resonance imaging should be performed.
   C. If her mammogram and ultrasound show skin thickening without underlying suspicious abnormality, a trial of antibiotics and clinical follow up is recommended.
   D. If a targeted ultrasound shows a fluid collection with surrounding hyperemia, a biopsy should be performed, with all samples submitted in formalin.

3. Regarding inflammatory breast cancer, which ONE of the following is the *best* answer?
   A. The clinical presentation usually involves a slow progression of redness and skin thickening over a period of months to years.
   B. A skin punch biopsy can differentiate inflammatory breast cancer from locally advanced breast cancer.
   C. In a patient with newly diagnosed inflammatory breast cancer, positron emission tomography/computed tomography is indicated.
   D. Inflammatory breast cancer has a good prognosis, with a 5-year survival rate of 80 to 90%.
   E. Treatment of inflammatory breast cancer usually includes mastectomy followed by radiation therapy. Chemotherapy has not demonstrated survival benefit.

■ Answers and Explanations

Question 1

A. Correct! There is diffuse bilateral trabecular and skin thickening on the mammogram. Inflammatory breast cancer usually presents as *unilateral* breast enlargement with increased density, trabecular thickening, and skin thickening on imaging. In rare cases, the findings may be bilateral secondary to severe locally advanced disease. Axillary adenopathy is present in about 50% of cases of inflammatory breast cancer.

Other choices and discussion

B. The differential for bilateral trabecular and skin thickening include systemic causes of volume overload, such as congestive heart failure, hepatic failure, and renal failure. Of note, edema resulting from these etiologies may be asymmetric due to the patient preference of positioning when in the supine position.

C. Central venous obstruction (as in superior vena cava thrombosis) can cause bilateral edema, manifested by trabecular and skin thickening. Vascular causes of unilateral breast edema include subclavian or axillary vein thrombosis.

D. In this specific case, the woman had a history of corrected tetralogy of Fallot and current severe heart and liver failure.

Question 2

C. Correct! The differential with this clinical presentation is mastitis versus inflammatory breast cancer. The clinical history, mammography, and ultrasound are collectively useful in differentiating underlying malignancy from abscess. A trial of antibiotics should first be attempted, and if findings do not completely improve after adequate antibiotic therapy, a skin punch biopsy would be advised.

Other choices and discussion

A. Inflammatory breast cancer is a clinical diagnosis. However, there must be a *pathologic* diagnosis of cancer coupled with an appropriate clinical presentation to make the diagnosis.

B. Magnetic resonance imaging is not indicated prior to a trial of antibiotics or before a definitive diagnosis of inflammatory breast cancer is made.

D. If the clinical history and imaging findings are concerning for abscess, an abscess drainage should be performed, with fluid sent to microbiology for culture. If no fluid can be aspirated, or if there is concern for a malignant mass, a subsequent biopsy could be performed with samples sent in formalin.

Question 3

C. Correct! Positron emission tomography/computed tomography is beneficial in newly diagnosed inflammatory breast cancer to evaluate for distant metastasis. Bone is the most common site of distant metastasis.

Other choices and discussion

A. The clinical presentation of inflammatory breast cancer is usually that of rapidly progressive breast erythema, edema, and tenderness, developing over a period of weeks to a few months. There is a lack of response to a trial of antibiotics. A commonly seen clinical finding is peau d'orange, meaning "skin of an orange" in French, caused by dermal lymphatic obstruction from tumor emboli.

B. Locally advanced breast cancer is cancer that progresses and directly invades the skin. The timeline of symptoms is the key feature that differentiates inflammatory breast cancer from locally advanced breast cancer (the latter with a slower progression and longer onset of symptoms, without the erythema or edema).

D. Inflammatory breast cancer has a highly aggressive course, with a 5-year survival rate of 25 to 50%. It accounts for approximately 2 to 5% of all breast cancers. About 20 to 40% of patients present with distant metastasis at the time of diagnosis.

E. Neoadjuvant chemotherapy followed by mastectomy and radiation therapy is the standard of care for inflammatory breast cancer. Neoadjuvant chemotherapy can shrink the existing tumor burden, helping with both locoregional control and systemic disease.

■ Suggested Readings

Berg, Wendie A. Trabecular Thickening, Edema (Mammography). Statdx. Accessed December 28, 2015

Yeh ED, Jacene HA, Bellon JR, et al. What radiologists need to know about diagnosis and treatment of inflammatory breast cancer: a multidisciplinary approach. RadioGraphics 2013;33:2003–2017

Top Tips

- For bilateral trabecular and skin thickening, think systemic causes such as fluid overload.

- The main differential for an erythematous, edematous breast is mastitis versus inflammatory breast cancer. The first step in the management is an initial trial of antibiotics and, if symptoms do not resolve, a skin punch biopsy.

- Imaging is integral in the evaluation of inflammatory breast cancer, directing biopsy, staging, and pretherapy planning.

Essentials 4

■ Case

A 29-year-old lactating woman presents with a palpable abnormality in the left breast. A targeted ultrasound was initially performed. Subsequently, a diagnostic mammogram was performed. Spot magnification views are shown.

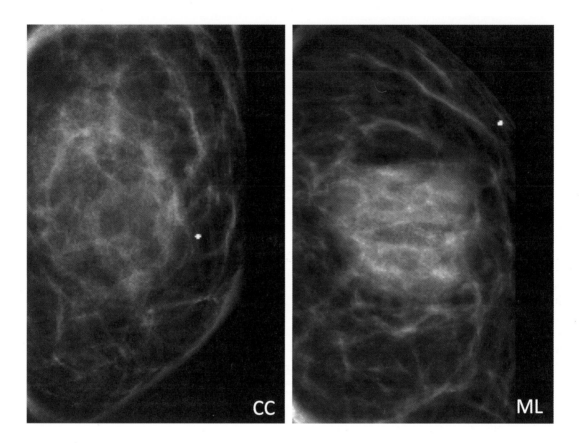

■ Questions

1. Regarding the imaging finding above, which ONE of the following is the best answer?
   A. A mammogram should have been performed first to avoid a targeted ultrasound.
   B. This is a suspicious abnormality, and an ultrasound-guided biopsy should be performed.
   C. This is compatible with the most common benign breast mass in a lactating woman.
   D. Aspiration of this finding would result in foul-smelling, serosanguinous fluid.
   E. During informed consent for biopsy, no special or unusual procedural complication discussion is needed.

2. Regarding imaging of the pregnant or lactating patient, which ONE of the following is the best answer?
   A. Mammography is contraindicated for the pregnant patient due to potential radiation-induced carcinogenic and teratogenic effects.

B. Bilateral breast magnetic resonance imaging is a safe imaging modality for the fetus during pregnancy and for the infant during lactation.
   C. Lactating patients should pump or nurse prior to having a mammogram performed.
   D. Pregnancy-associated breast cancer most commonly presents as a painful lump.
   E. The prognosis of women with pregnancy-associated breast cancer is worse than those with age- and stage-matched controls.

3. Which of the following should be included in the differential diagnosis of a breast mass in a pregnant or lactating patient? (Select ALL that apply.)
   A. Pregnancy-associated breast cancer
   B. Fibroadenoma
   C. Lactating adenoma
   D. Galactocele
   E. Breast abscess

■ Answers and Explanations

Question 1

C. Correct! This is compatible with a galactocele, which is the most common benign breast mass in a lactating woman. These form as a result of duct dilation and inflammation. A fat-fluid level is considered pathognomonic for a galactocele; however, this may also be seen in fat necrosis.

Other choices and discussion

A. The initial imaging workup for a woman < 30 years old with a palpable abnormality should be a targeted ultrasound. Ultrasound is also the first-line imaging modality in the workup of a palpable breast mass for a pregnant or lactating patient. This is because of ultrasound's lack of ionizing radiation and its high sensitivity for detecting cancer in this patient population. In cases where sonographic findings are equivocal for a galactocele, a mammogram can aid in the diagnosis. The mammographic images shown in this case are consistent with a galactocele. Therefore, no ultrasound is needed.

B. This is not a suspicious abnormality, and biopsy is not indicated. Mammogram reveals an oval mass with obscured margins and a fat-fluid level on the mediolateral view. These findings, in addition to the clinical context of lactation, are consistent with a galactocele.

D. Galactoceles are cysts that contain milk and often contain necrotic or inflammatory debris. Aspiration would result in milky-colored fluid (not foul-smelling, serosanguineous fluid).

E. Additional potential complications following breast biopsy of a lactating woman include a milk-duct fistula (which is extremely rare) and blood within the breast milk. These risks should be discussed prior to the procedure.

Question 2

C. Correct! The milk may increase breast density and obscure important findings. Thus, prior to mammography, lactating patients are asked to pump or nurse to decrease the volume of milk.

Other choices and discussion

A. The low levels of scatter radiation do not support delaying mammography during pregnancy, when clinically indicated.

B. Bilateral breast magnetic resonance imaging requires intravenous gadolinium-based contrast. These contrast agents are NOT recommended during pregnancy because of the possible harmful effects to the developing fetus. However, there is a negligible excretion of this contrast in breast milk (a rate of 0.0004% of the maternal dose), and breast MRI can be safely performed in the lactating patient.

D. Pregnancy-associated breast cancer most commonly presents as a painless lump. It may also present as a unilateral enlarging breast with skin thickening, focal pain, and suspicious nipple discharge.

E. Traditionally, it was thought that women with pregnancy-associated breast cancer had a worse prognosis than those who did not. This may be explained by a delay in diagnosis (with larger tumor size at presentation). However, compared to age- and stage-matched controls, there are actually similar survival rates between woman with pregnancy and non-pregnancy-related breast cancers.

Question 3

All are correct!

A. Pregnancy-associated breast cancer represents approximately 10% of all newly diagnosed breast cancer cases in women < 40 years old. The mean age at diagnosis is between 32 and 34 years. The most common histology is high-grade, estrogen and progesterone receptor negative, invasive ductal carcinoma.

B. Growth of fibroadenomas can occur during pregnancy, as these are hormone-sensitive masses.

C. Lactating adenomas are benign lesions thought to be a fibroadenoma variant, tubular adenoma, or lobular hyperplasia due to the physiologic changes of pregnancy. In general, these may regress after pregnancy.

D. Galactoceles are the most common benign lesions in lactating woman. They are cysts that contain milk and inflammatory debris.

E. Disruption of the nipple-areolar complex and milk stasis places lactating women at risk for infection. If abscess is suspected, a clinical exam and ultrasound are recommended as the best initial workup.

■ Suggested Readings

American College of Radiology. ACR manual on contrast media v10.1. From: http://www.acr.org/quality-safety/resources/contrast-manual. Published 2015. Accessed February 12, 2015

Barnes DM, Newman LA. Pregnancy-associated breast cancer: a literature review. Surg Clin North Am 2007;87:417–430, x

Chetlen AL, Brown KL, King SH, et al. JOURNAL CLUB: scatter radiation dose from digital screening mammography measured in a representative patient population. Am J Roentgenol 2016;206:359–365

Sabate JM, Clotet M, Torrubia S, et al. Radiologic evaluation of breast disorders related to pregnancy and lactation. RadioGraphics 2007;27:S101–S124

Vashi R, Hooley R, Butler R, Geisel J, Philpotts L. Breast imaging of the pregnant and lactating patient: imaging modalities and pregnancy-associated breast cancer. Am J Roentgenol 2013;200:321–328

Top Tips

◆ Although mammography is safe to the fetus during pregnancy, ultrasound is the BEST initial imaging modality when evaluating a palpable abnormality in the pregnant or lactating patient.

◆ A fat-fluid level seen within a mass on mammography in a lactating patient is consistent with a galactocele.

◆ Pregnancy-associated breast cancer accounts for approximately 10% of breast cancers in woman < 40 years old.

Essentials 5

■ Case

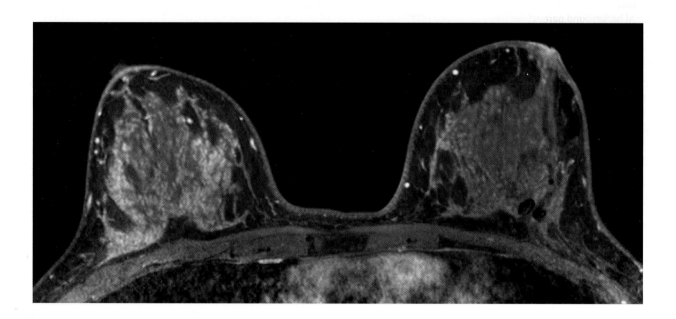

■ Questions

1. Which of the following is the *best* possible reason for this finding on magnetic resonance imaging?
   A. A history of radiation therapy on the left
   B. Inflammatory breast cancer on the right
   C. Exogenous hormones
   D. The patient was imaged on day 23 of her menstrual cycle
   E. Injection of gadolinium on the right

2. Which of the following are generally accepted indications for bilateral breast magnetic resonance imaging? (Select ALL that apply.)
   A. Screening for a patient with > 10% lifetime risk and no additional risk factors
   B. Evaluation of a woman with newly diagnosed breast cancer
   C. Evaluation of a patient with metastatic axillary adenocarcinoma and an unknown primary
   D. Evaluation of saline implant integrity
   E. Evaluation of breast cancer response to neoadjuvant chemotherapy

3. Regarding dynamic kinetic enhancement characteristics of magnetic resonance imaging findings, which ONE of the following is the best answer?
   A. The first postcontrast phase of the exam should be acquired within the first 2 minutes postinjection.
   B. There are three main phases of the time-intensity curve: initial, peak, and delayed.
   C. A lesion with rapid initial phase enhancement and washout on delayed phase enhancement is suspicious and should be biopsied.
   D. A lesion with medium initial phase enhancement and persistent delayed phase enhancement is benign.
   E. A lesion that does not meet the 50% enhancement threshold kinetics is benign.

■ Answers and Explanations

Question 1

A. Correct! A history of radiation therapy on the left. Susceptibility artifact from surgical clips is present in the posterolateral left breast in this patient with a history of left lumpectomy and radiation therapy. The enhancement on the right corresponds to normal background parenchymal enhancement (BPE). Radiation therapy is known to decrease the amount of BPE.

Other choices and discussion

B. Although inflammatory breast cancer can present as asymmetric trabecular thickening and enhancement, there is no evidence of breast enlargement or skin enhancement in this patient.

C. BPE is dependent on several factors, one of which is hormones. Although the presence of exogenous hormones can increase the BPE, this typically results in bilateral and symmetric variation.

D. Similar to the influence of exogenous hormones, timing of the menstrual cycle can affect the amount of BPE. However, this fluctuation would typically be symmetric. The ideal imaging time with the least amount of BPE is during the follicular phase of the cycle (days 7 to 15).

E. There are no studies to show that laterality of contrast injection affects the amount of enhancement in the breast.

Question 2

B. Correct! Current National Comprehensive Cancer Network practice guidelines recommend that a breast magnetic resonance imaging (MRI) can be considered to evaluate the extent of disease in a patient with newly diagnosed breast cancer.

C. Correct! In patients with mammographically occult breast cancer and biopsy-proven axillary metastatic adenocarcinoma, a bilateral breast MRI can discover the primary lesion in approximately 60 to 70% of cases.

E. Correct! Results from the American College of Radiology Imaging Network (ACRIN 6657) study showed that MRI findings are a stronger predictor of pathologic response from neoadjuvant chemotherapy and residual cancer burden than is the clinical assessment.

Other choices and discussion

A. The American Cancer Society currently recommends the use of screening breast MRI for patients with a > 20% lifetime risk of breast cancer. In a high-risk patient population, combined MRI and mammography have a higher sensitivity (92.7%) than combined ultrasound and mammography (52%).

D. Bilateral breast MRI can evaluate for *silicone* implant integrity. Saline implant complications are usually apparent on clinical exam, and the saline is reabsorbed within the body.

Question 3

A. Correct! The first postcontrast phase of the exam should be acquired within the first 2 minutes postinjection. Imaging after this time will result in missing the peak enhancement of the lesion.

Other choices and discussion

B. The time intensity curves are divided into two phases: the "initial phase," with images acquired within the first 2 minutes after injection, and the "delayed phase," with images acquired after the first 2 minutes or peak enhancement. In general, peak enhancement usually occurs after 2 to 3 minutes of injection.

C. Although the most suspicious type of kinetic enhancement is initial rapid enhancement with washout on delayed images, there are benign findings (e.g., lymph nodes) that have the same enhancement characteristics. Thus, morphologic characteristics should be examined before a biopsy recommendation is made.

D. Kinetics are useful in the evaluation of any lesion (focus, mass, non-mass enhancement). However, a benign kinetic enhancement profile should not dissuade further workup for a morphologically suspicious mass or non-mass enhancement.

E. The enhancement threshold for computer-aided analysis tools can be selected by the interpreting radiologist and is usually set between a 50 and 100% increase in signal intensity from baseline to the first postcontrast study. Absence of a morphologically suspicious finding to meet threshold kinetic features does not prove benignity.

■ Suggested Readings

Berg WA. Tailored supplemental screening for breast cancer: what now and what next? Am J Roentgenol 2009;192:390–399

Brenner RJ. Evaluation of breast silicone implants. Magn Reson Imaging Clin N Am 2013;21:547–560

de Bresser J, de Vos B, van der Ent F, Hulsewé K. Breast MRI in clinically and mammographically occult breast cancer presenting with an axillary metastasis: a systematic review. Eur J Surg Oncol 2010;36:114–119

Hylton NM, Blume JD, Bernreuter WK, et al. Locally advanced breast cancer: MR imaging for prediction of response to neoadjuvant chemotherapy—results from ACRIN 6657/I-SPY TRIAL. Radiology 2012;263:663–672

Top Tips

- The American Cancer Society currently recommends the use of screening breast MRI for patients with a > 20% lifetime risk of breast cancer.

- The amount of BPE is influenced by hormonal factors and can fluctuate depending upon menstrual cycle and exogenous estrogens.

- A benign kinetic enhancement curve is reassuring. However, these features do not override suspicious morphologic features when evaluating a lesion.

Essentials 6

■ Case

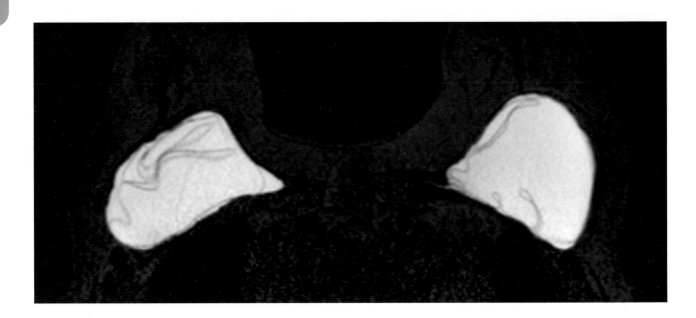

■ Questions

1. Regarding the bilateral breast magnetic resonance imaging performed for silicone implant evaluation, which ONE of the following is shown?
   A. Normal intact implants with bilateral complex radial folds
   B. Intracapsular rupture on the left and extracapsular rupture on the right
   C. Bilateral intracapsular rupture
   D. Bilateral extracapsular rupture without intracapsular rupture
   E. Bilateral intracapsular and extracapsular rupture

2. Regarding silicone breast implants, which ONE of the following is the *best* answer?
   A. Silicone implants are harmful and increase the risk of developing breast cancer.
   B. Mammography is useful in the evaluation of intracapsular silicone implant rupture.
   C. Breast magnetic resonance imaging is the second-line imaging modality to evaluate for a silicone implant complication.

   D. The presence of breast implants decreases mammographic sensitivity for detecting breast cancer.
   E. A standard T2-weighted sequence should be used to evaluate for silicone implant complication.

3. Regarding silicone implant complications, which ONE of the following is the best answer?
   A. A breast magnetic resonance imaging should be performed annually to evaluate for silicone implant complication in asymptomatic patients.
   B. Extracapsular rupture can only occur when the implant capsule is fully collapsed.
   C. Implant herniation implies underlying intracapsular rupture.
   D. Radial folds can generally be traced back to the implant capsule, whereas folds from a collapsed rupture are separated from the capsule.
   E. Silicone granulomas have the same T2 signal intensity on water-suppressed images as the silicone gel within the implants.

■ Answers and Explanations

Question 1

C. Correct! There is bilateral intracapsular rupture. There is a "linguine" sign on the right, which indicates complete collapse of the silicone implant shell, and both a "linguine" (medially) and "keyhole" or "teardrop" (posteriorly) sign on the left. The keyhole sign indicates silicone gel outside of the implant shell but still contained within the fibrous capsule.

Other choices and discussion

A. Radial folds are normal infoldings of the implant shell, and they may mimic intracapsular rupture when complex. However, in this case, there is discontinuity of the implant capsule bilaterally (with partial collapse of the right implant).

B. There is no evidence of extracapsular rupture (silicone within the surrounding breast tissue) or silicone within lymph nodes on this image.

C. There must be intracapsular rupture (defect in the silicone implant shell) for extracapsular rupture to be present (rent in the fibrous capsule surrounding the implant).

D. There is no evidence of extracapsular rupture.

Question 2

D. Correct! In a study evaluating the effect of breast augmentation on the accuracy of mammography and cancer characteristics, the sensitivity of screening mammography was lower in women who had breast augmentation than in those who did not. However, the prognostic factors (tumor stage, nodal status, and estrogen-receptor status) were similar.

Other choices and discussion

A. There is no evidence that shows a cause or effect relationship between silicone breast implants and the development of breast cancer.

B. With intracapsular rupture, the implant shell (or envelope) is defective. However, the fibrous capsule that the body creates and surrounds the implant with is still intact. Thus, if there is an intracapsular silicone implant rupture, magnetic resonance imaging is superior to mammography for detection.

C. Manufacturer recommendations approved by the U.S. Food and Drug Administration support magnetic resonance imaging as the first-line imaging modality in the evaluation of a silicone implant complication.

E. Silicone gel has a T2-signal intensity that is higher than fat but lower than water. Thus, to truly evaluate for silicone extravasation either surrounding the implant shell or into the breast, it is best to use a T2-weighted sequence that suppresses both fat and water.

Question 3

D. Correct! Radial folds can generally be traced back to the implant capsule, whereas folds from a collapsed rupture are separated from the capsule. Tracing the origin of radial folds to the inner surface of the implant capsule is the key to distinguishing complex radial folds from intracapsular rupture.

Other choices and discussion

A. Asymptomatic women with implants are advised to have an MRI to check for implant rupture 3 years after placement and every 2 years thereafter, although some authors believe this may be too frequent and suggest every 10 years for patients without a breast cancer history.

B. Intracapsular rupture can be staged based upon the extent of deflation, ranging from not collapsed to fully collapsed. Extracapsular rupture can occur during any of these stages.

C. The term herniation is used when the implant shell is extruded through the fibrous capsule that surrounds the implant. Implants with herniation may not necessarily have a rupture, but herniation does imply a focal weakening/defect in that area.

E. Both silicone granulomas and silicone within lymph nodes have lower signal intensity on T2 water-suppressed sequences than does pure silicone gel. This is due to tissue ingrowth and the ratio of lymph node to silicone within nodes, respectively.

■ Suggested Readings

Middleton MS. MR evaluation of breast implants. Radiol Clin North Am 2014;52:591–608

Miglioretti DL, Rutter CM, Geller BM, et al. Effect of breast augmentation on the accuracy of mammography and cancer characteristics. JAMA 2004;291:442–450

Wiedenhoefer JF, Shahid H, Dornbluth C, Otto P, Kist K. MR imaging of breast implants: useful information for the interpreting radiologist. Appl Radiol 2015;44(10):18–24

Top Tips

- *Saline* implant rupture is a clinical diagnosis.

- There are two major types of silicone implant rupture: intracapsular, which describes a break in the silicone implant shell, and extracapsular, which occurs when there is both a break in the implant shell and in the fibrous capsule.

- Complex radial folds can mimic intracapsular rupture. Tracing the folds back to the implant capsule helps to differentiate the two.

Essentials 7

■ Case

A 40-year-old woman presents for a baseline screening mammogram.

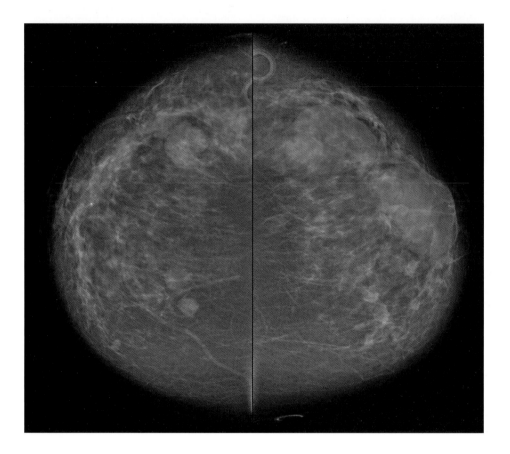

■ Questions

1. Regarding the imaging findings, which ONE of the following is the BEST answer?
   A. BI-RADS 6. The imaging findings are consistent with multicentric breast cancer.
   B. BI-RADS 0. Recommend spot compression views and ultrasound for confirmation.
   C. BI-RADS 4. Recommend biopsy of the most suspicious appearing mass.
   D. BI-RADS 3. Probably benign masses. Recommend short interval follow up.
   E. BI-RADS 2. The imaging findings are benign. Recommend normal interval follow up.

2. Regarding bilateral benign-appearing masses, which ONE of the following is correct?
   A. Diagnosis requires at least two masses, with one located in each breast.
   B. A round or oval mass with indistinct margins meets diagnostic criteria.

   C. Imaging findings are still considered benign even in the setting of a palpable lump.
   D. A mass appearing distinctly different from the others warrants diagnostic workup.
   E. There is an associated increased risk of breast cancer.

3. A baseline screening mammogram demonstrates bilateral calcifications. Regarding calcifications, which ONE of the following is correct?
   A. Tram-track calcifications are suspicious.
   B. Large rod-like calcifications radiating toward the nipple are suspicious.
   C. Similar appearing groups of bilateral coarse heterogeneous calcifications are considered suspicious.
   D. Diffuse punctate and round calcifications are benign.
   E. Rim calcifications are suspicious.

■ Answers and Explanations

Question 1

E. Correct! BI-RADS 2. The mammographic findings are classic for bilateral benign-appearing masses. Normal interval follow up is recommended.

Other choices and discussion

The imaging findings are most consistent with bilateral benign-appearing masses. There is no mammographic evidence of malignancy. No further imaging is required, short-term follow up imaging is not needed, and biopsy is not indicated.

Question 2

D. Correct! Overall, the bilateral benign-appearing masses should appear similar. A mass appearing distinctly different from the others warrants diagnostic workup.

Other choices and discussion

A. Diagnosis requires at least three masses, with at least one located in each breast.

B. A round or oval mass with circumscribed margins meets diagnostic criteria. A mass with indistinct margins warrants diagnostic workup.

C. A palpable lump requires dedicated diagnostic workup, even if there are bilateral benign-appearing masses.

E. There is no increased risk of malignancy.

Question 3

D. Correct! Diffuse punctate and round calcifications are considered benign. These often represent fibrocystic change. BI-RADS 2.

The other choices are all benign calcifications. Vascular calcifications are known for their tram-track appearance. Secretory calcifications appear large and rod-like, with extension toward the nipple. Groups of coarse heterogeneous calcifications that appear similar bilaterally often represent fibroadenomatoid change. Oil cysts demonstrate classic rim calcification.

■ Suggested Readings

Berg WA. Multiple bilateral similar findings. Statdx. http://www.statdx.com. Accessed February 2016

Leung JW, Sickles EA. Multiple bilateral masses detected on screening mammography: assessment of need for recall imaging. Am J Roentgenol 2000;175(1):23–29

Top Tips

◆ Bilateral benign-appearing masses most commonly represent cysts and/or fibroadenomas.

◆ Bilateral benign-appearing masses are known to fluctuate in size (wax and wane) due to the development and regression of cysts over time.

◆ A benign assessment for bilateral benign-appearing masses can be rendered on a baseline screening mammogram.

Essentials 8

■ Case

A 38-year-old man presents with a left breast lump.

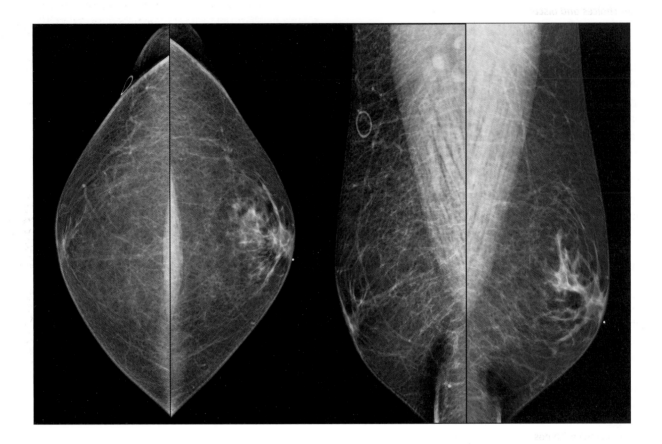

■ Questions

1. Regarding the imaging findings, which ONE of the following is the BEST answer?
   A. There is an irregular spiculated mass in the left retroareolar region.
   B. A targeted ultrasound is required to confirm the diagnosis.
   C. Palpable gynecomastia is highly suspicious for malignancy. Recommend biopsy.
   D. Unilateral gynecomastia is probably benign. Recommend 6-month follow up.
   E. Standard imaging workup begins with a bilateral diagnostic mammogram.

2. Regarding gynecomastia, which ONE of the following is correct?
   A. Pseudogynecomastia refers to asymptomatic gynecomastia.
   B. Physiologic gynecomastia has a trimodal age distribution.
   C. Dendritic gynecomastia is the earliest pattern and is reversible.
   D. Atypical gynecomastia occurs eccentric to the retroareolar region.
   E. Nodular gynecomastia has a circumscribed convex margin posteriorly.

3. Regarding male breast cancer, which ONE of the following is correct?
   A. A total of 15% of all breast cancer occurs in men.
   B. Male breast cancer is usually asymptomatic.
   C. Male breast cancer often presents at an early stage.
   D. The most common male breast cancer is ductal carcinoma in situ.
   E. An increased risk of male breast cancer is associated with BRCA 2 and Klinefelter syndrome.

■ Answers and Explanations

Question 1

E. Correct! Although the area of clinical of concern may be unilateral, a diagnostic bilateral mammogram is recommended to allow comparison with the contralateral side.

Other choices and discussion

A. This is a retroareolar flame-shaped density, consistent with gynecomastia. There is no irregular spiculated mass.

B. Mammographic findings clinch the diagnosis. Ultrasound is unnecessary.

C. Gynecomastia has no risk for malignancy even if it is symptomatic.

D. Both unilateral and bilateral gynecomastia are benign. No further imaging is needed.

Question 2

B. Correct! Physiologic gynecomastia has a trimodal age distribution. Neonates may develop gynecomastia from high maternal hormones, whereas prepuberty and elderly patients may develop gynecomastia from hormonal imbalances.

Other choices and discussion

A. Pseudogynecomastia refers to breast enlargement due to extra fat deposition. In contrast, gynecomastia is caused by benign ductal hyperplasia and stromal proliferation.

C. Nodular gynecomastia is the reversible early pattern (duration < 1 year). Dendritic gynecomastia is an irreversible chronic pattern (duration > 1 year). Diffuse gynecomastia results from exogenous estrogen.

D. Gynecomastia *only* occurs in the retroareolar region. Any finding eccentric to the nipple is suspicious and warrants additional imaging with possible biopsy to exclude malignancy.

E. Nodular gynecomastia should still have flame-shaped tissue posteriorly that fades into the adjacent fat. A posterior convex margin is suspicious and warrants additional imaging with possible biopsy to exclude malignancy.

Question 3

E. Correct! An increased risk of male breast cancer is associated with BRCA 2 and Klinefelter syndrome.

The other choices are all incorrect. Male breast cancer accounts for 1% of all breast cancer, usually presents with a breast lump, and most often presents at an advanced stage. The most common male breast cancer is invasive ductal carcinoma.

■ Suggested Readings

Appelbaum AH, Evans GF, Levy KR, et al. Mammographic appearances of male breast disease. Radiographics 1999;19:559

Yang Wei Tse. Gynecomastia. Statdx. http://www.statdx.com. Accessed January 2016

Top Tips

◆ Gynecomastia can clinically present with a retroareolar breast lump or pain.

◆ Imaging workup for gynecomastia begins with a bilateral diagnostic mammogram.

◆ In adult men, ultrasound is indicated if mammographic findings are indeterminate or suspicious.

Essentials 9

■ Case

A 68-year-old woman presents with a new left breast lump. A targeted ultrasound was performed.

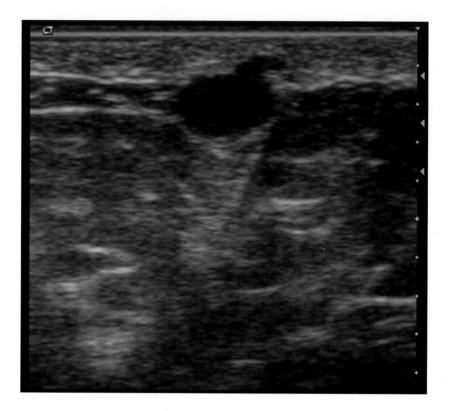

■ Questions

1. Which assessment and recommendation is correct?
   A. Fluid collection concerning for abscess. BI-RADS 4. Recommend aspiration.
   B. Complex solid mass. BI-RADS 5. Recommend ultrasound biopsy.
   C. Evolving hematoma. BI-RADS 3. Probably benign. Recommend follow up.
   D. New palpable solid mass. BI-RADS 4. Recommend an ultrasound biopsy.
   E. Benign skin mass. BI-RADS 2. Return to routine screening schedule.

2. Regarding the imaging findings, which ONE of the following is correct?
   A. A skin mass should appear anechoic to be considered benign.
   B. A benign skin mass can present with a margin that is not circumscribed.
   C. A skin tail detected on ultrasound confirms an epidermoid or sebaceous cyst.
   D. A dermal claw sign, if present, suggests the mass has caused skin retraction.
   E. Biopsy of epidermoid cysts should be avoided due to high discordance rates.

3. Regarding skin findings on mammography, which ONE of the following correct?
   A. Skin findings are not reliably detected on tomosynthesis.
   B. Tangential images are special views to determine if a finding is in the skin.
   C. A benign skin mass on mammography should not demonstrate calcifications.
   D. A halo sign on mammography suggests a mass has surrounding edema.
   E. Dermal calcifications should layer on a diagnostic true lateral view.

■ Answers and Explanations

Question 1

E. Correct! BI-RADS 2. Imaging findings are consistent with a sebaceous or epidermoid inclusion cyst. These are indistinguishable on imaging and are referred to as benign skin masses. The appropriate recommendation is return to screening.

Other choices and discussion

A. There is no abscess. Aspiration is unnecessary.

B. There is no complex or solid component. Biopsy is not indicated

C. There is no hematoma. Follow up imaging is unwarranted.

D. This is a benign skin mass. Ultrasound biopsy is unnecessary.

Question 2

C. Correct! Occasionally, an epidermoid or sebaceous cyst will demonstrate a skin tail on ultrasound. A skin tail is an obstructed hair follicle that extends from the epidermis to the mass and is indicative of an epidermoid or sebaceous cyst. High frequency transducers, standoff pads, or a mound of gel can improve detection.

Other choices and discussion

A. A benign skin mass can have variable echogenicity (appearing echogenic, hypoechoic, or anechoic) depending on its internal contents.

B. A benign skin mass should have circumscribed margins. A margin that is not circumscribed is suspicious and warrants additional imaging or biopsy.

C. A dermal claw sign indicates a mass is of dermal origin. When seen, the posterior dermal line will wrap around the posterior margin of the skin mass.

D. Biopsy of epidermoid cysts is generally avoided because of the risk for a complicated inflammatory reaction. If removal is desired, then a dermatology or surgical consultation is advised.

Question 3

B. Correct! An alphanumeric grid is used to place a BB over the finding. Then tangential magnification views are done to determine if the finding is within the skin.

Other choices and discussion

A. Tomosynthesis reliably demonstrates skin findings either in tangent within the skin itself or shows them in the skin on the initial or last image slices.

B. A total of 20% of epidermoid or sebaceous cysts demonstrate calcifications.

C. A halo sign is a skin finding (i.e., skin mole) surrounded by air.

D. Dermal calcifications are lucent centered and often located in the parasternal, axillary tail, and inframammary fold areas. Milk of calcium calcifications layer on diagnostic true lateral views.

■ Suggested Readings

Berg, WA. Skin localization, breast. Statdx. http://www.statdx.com. Accessed January 2016

Giess, CS, Raza S, Birdwell RL. Distinguishing breast skin lesions from superficial breast parenchymal lesions: diagnostic criteria, imaging characteristics and pitfalls. Radiographics 2011;31(7):1959–1972

Top Tips

- A skin mass in a patient with a history of cancer warrants greater suspicion because it may represent metastatic disease to the skin or local recurrence.

- An indeterminate skin mass should be not be followed with imaging surveillance, but rather biopsied for definitive histology.

- An infected or inflamed, sebaceous or epidermoid cyst has increased peripheral vascularity on ultrasound. Management includes clinical follow-up and if indicated, oral antibiotic therapy.

Essentials 10

■ Case

A 45-year-old woman presents for a screening mammogram.

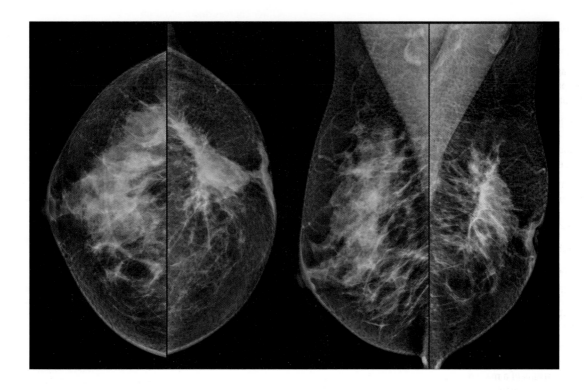

■ Questions

1. Which ONE of the following is the correct assessment and recommendation?
   A. BI-RADS 0. Recommend comparison with prior imaging.
   B. BI-RADS 0. Recommend diagnostic spot magnification views and ultrasound.
   C. BI-RADS 5. Findings are highly suspicious. Recommend ultrasound biopsy.
   D. BI-RADS 0. Recommend diagnostic spot compression views and ultrasound.
   E. BI-RADS 0. Recommend an extent of disease breast magnetic resonance imaging.

2. According to the 2013 BI-RADS lexicon, when describing a mass on mammography, which ONE of the following descriptors is correct?
   A. *Circumscribed* requires at least 75% of the margin to be sharply defined.
   B. *Obscured* indicates more than 50% of the margin is not well seen.

   C. *Ill-defined* is used when the majority of the margin is not clearly delineated.
   D. *Density* of a mass can be described as hypodense, isodense, or hyperdense.
   E. *Nodule* is an appropriate descriptor to describe the shape of a small mass.

3. According to the 2013 BI-RADS lexicon, when describing a mass on ultrasound, which ONE of the following descriptors is correct?
   A. An *indistinct* shape describes a mass that is neither round nor oval.
   B. Margins on ultrasound are either *circumscribed* or not circumscribed.
   C. *Circumscribed* indicates at least 75% of the margin is well defined.
   D. A margin that is not circumscribed, can be further described as lobulated.
   E. Mass echogenicity is described relative to fibroglandular tissue.

■ Answers and Explanations

Question 1

D. Correct! BI-RADS 0. Recommend diagnostic spot compression views and ultrasound. A mass detected on screening warrants a diagnostic mammogram with spot compression views followed by a diagnostic ultrasound.

Other choices and discussion

A. Prior imaging is irrelevant given the suspicious finding.

B. Spot magnification views are used to evaluate calcifications. Spot compression views are used to evaluate a mass, architectural distortion, focal asymmetry, and an asymmetry.

C. An abnormal screening exam should be rendered a BI-RADS 0 because additional imaging allows for complete assessment prior to intervention. A BI-RADS 5 should not be rendered on a screening exam.

E. An extent of disease breast magnetic resonance imaging is indicated once there is a biopsy-proven malignancy.

Question 2

A. Correct! A circumscribed margin on mammography requires at least 75% of the margin be sharply defined.

Other choices and discussion

B. An obscured margin on mammography indicates more than 25% of the margin is not well seen.

C. Ill-defined is not a BI-RADS lexicon term. Indistinct is the appropriate term. There are five BI-RADS lexicon terms used to describe the margins of a mass on mammography: circumscribed, obscured, microlobulated, indistinct, and spiculated.

D. There are four BI-RADS lexicon terms used to describe the density of a mass on mammography: fat-density, low-density, equal-density, and high-density.

E. Nodule is not a BI-RADS lexicon term. There are three BI-RADS lexicon terms used to describe the shape of a mass on mammography: oval, round, and irregular.

Question 3

B. Correct! Margins on ultrasound are described as either circumscribed or not circumscribed.

Other choices and discussion

A. An irregular shape describes a mass that is neither round nor oval. Margins on ultrasound are described as either circumscribed or not circumscribed.

C. On ultrasound, a circumscribed margin indicates 100% of the margin is well defined. On mammography, only 75% must be well defined.

D. Lobulated is not a BI-RADS lexicon term. There are four BI-RADS lexicon terms, which can be used to further describe a margin that is not circumscribed on ultrasound: microlobulated, angular, indistinct, and spiculated.

E. Mass echogenicity is described relative to mammary fat.

■ Suggested Readings

Ikeda, DM. The Requisites Breast Imaging. Philadelphia, PA: Elsevier; 2004

Mendelson EB, Bohm-Velez M, Berg WA, et al. ACR BIRADS® ultrasound. In: ACR BIRADS® Atlas, Breast Imaging Reporting and Data System. Reston, VA: American College of Radiology; 2013

Sickles, EA, D'Orsi CJ. ACR BIRADS® follow-up and outcome monitoring. In: ACR BIRADS® Atlas, Breast Imaging Reporting and Data System. Reston, VA: American College of Radiology; 2013

Sickles, EA, D'Orsi CJ, Bassett LW, et al. ACR BIRADS® mammography. In: ACR BIRADS® Atlas, Breast Imaging Reporting and Data System. Reston, VA: American College of Radiology; 2013

Top Tips

- Differential diagnosis for a benign spiculated mass: postsurgical scar, fat necrosis, radial scar, sclerosing adenosis, fibromatosis, and granular cell tumor.

- Differential diagnosis for a malignant spiculated mass: invasive ductal, invasive lobular, and tubular carcinoma.

- Differential diagnosis for a malignant round mass: high-grade invasive ductal carcinoma, mucinous carcinoma, medullary carcinoma, metastases, and papillary carcinoma.

Details 1

■ **Case**

What is this test and how often does it need to be performed?

A. Phantom image quality, daily

B. Phantom image quality, weekly

C. Processor quality control, daily

D. Processer quality control, weekly

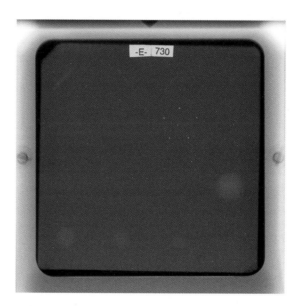

■ **The following questions pertain to physics concepts for mammography.**

1. To pass the phantom image quality test, what is the minimum number of fibers, speck groups, and masses that must been seen on the ACR phantom?

2. The average glandular dose delivered by a single craniocaudal view of a 4.2-cm thick, compressed breast consisting of 50% glandular and 50% adipose tissue must not exceed _____.

3. Motion blurring can be minimized by _____ (increasing or decreasing) compression, _____ (increasing or decreasing) exposure time, and _____ (increasing or decreasing) kVp.

4. With the same kVp, increasing the mAs will _____ tissue contrast.

5. With the same mAs, increasing kVp will _____ tissue contrast.

6. The target and filter combination that provides better image contrast for thinner breasts (2 to 5 cm compression) is _____. The target and filter combination that provides better image contrast for thicker breasts (5 to 7 cm) is _____.

7. The best target and filter combination for dense breasts is _____.

8. True or False. For adequate positioning on mammography, the measurement difference of the posterior nipple line between a craniocaudal view and a mediolateral view should be 1 cm or less.

9. Under the Mammography Quality Standards Act, a written and signed report must be provided to the healthcare provider within _____ days of the exam; and, if the lesion is Breast Imaging Reporting and Data System (BI-RADS) category 4 or 5, reasonable attempts to communicate with the healthcare provider must be made within _____ business days.

10. True or False. Under the ACR Practice Parameters for Image Quality in Digital Mammography, the amount of ambient light (illuminance) should be approximately equal to the level of the average luminance of a clinical image being displayed, generally in the 20 to 45 lux range.

■ Answers and Explanations

B. This is an image of the American College of Radiology (ACR) phantom. Phantom image quality must be checked weekly.

Question 1

To pass the phantom image quality test, the minimum number of fibers, speck groups, and masses that must been seen on the ACR phantom is four fibers, three speck groups, and three masses.

Question 2

The average glandular dose delivered by a single craniocaudal view of a 4.2-cm thick, compressed breast consisting of 50% glandular and 50% adipose tissue must not exceed 0.3 rad (3 mGy).

Question 3

Motion blurring can be minimized by increasing compression, decreasing exposure time, and increasing kVp.

Question 4

With the same kVp, increasing the mAs will increase tissue contrast.

Question 5

With the same mAs, increasing kVp will decrease tissue contrast.

Question 6

The target and filter combination that provides better image contrast for thinner breasts (2 to 5 cm compression) is Mo/Mo. The target and filter combination that provides better image contrast for thicker breasts (5 to 7 cm) is Mo/Mo or Mo/Rh.

Question 7

The best target and filter combination for dense breasts is Rh/Rh.

Question 8

True. The length of the posterior nipple line on the craniocaudal view should be no more than 1 cm shorter than the posterior nipple line on the mediolateral oblique view.

Question 9

Under the Mammography Quality Standards Act, a written and signed report must be provided to the healthcare provider within 30 days of the exam days of the exam; and, if the lesion is BI-RADS category 4 or 5, reasonable attempts to communicate with the healthcare provider must be made within 3 business days.

Question 10

True. Under the ACR Practice Parameters for Image Quality in Digital Mammography, the amount of ambient light (illuminance) should be approximately equal to the level of the average luminance of a clinical image being displayed, generally in the 20 to 45 lux range.

■ Suggested Readings

American College of Radiology. ACR-AAPM-SIIM Practice Parameter for Determinants of Imaging Quality in Digital Mammography. http://www.acr.org/~/media/ACR/Documents/PGTS/guidelines/Image_Quality_Digital_Mammo.pdf. Accessed December 23, 2015

American College of Radiology. ACR Practice Parameter for the Performance of Screening and Diagnostic Mammography. http://www.acr.org/~/media/ACR/Documents/PGTS/guidelines/Screening_Mammography.pdf. Accessed December 23, 2015

Top Tips

- For the ACR Phantom Image Quality, remember 4, 3, 3—fibers, specks, masses (**F**our **F**ibers).

- The average glandular dose on the ACR phantom per view is 3 mGy.

- Adequate mammography positioning includes nipple in profile on at least one view of each breast and the pectoralis musculature extending at or below the posterior nipple line.

Details 2

■ Case

A 45-year-old woman has a stereotactic biopsy of the following calcifications. Pathology reveals atypical ductal hyperplasia (ADH). Which of the following is correct regarding radiologic-pathologic concordance and recommendation?

A. Concordant, recommend routine screening mammography
B. Concordant, recommend surgical excisional biopsy
C. Discordant, recommend surgical excisional biopsy
D. Discordant, recommend bilateral breast magnetic resonance imaging

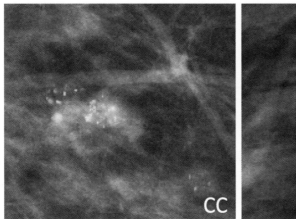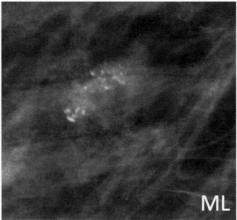

■ The following questions pertain to the radiologic-pathologic concordance of high-risk lesions.

1. True or False. The sensitivity of core needle biopsy for a breast lesion depends on both the type of device and lesion sampling.
2. Lesions considered "high-risk" in breast imaging include: _____.
3. True or False. All "high-risk" lesions found on core needle biopsy should undergo surgical excision due to the risk of underlying malignancy.
4. True or False. There are variants of lobular carcinoma in situ (LCIS) that may have more aggressive behavior than classic atypical lobular hyperplasia or LCIS.
5. True or False. Papillomas with atypia on core biopsy should undergo surgical excisional biopsy.
6. True or False. Radial scar and complex sclerosing lesion have the same histology, differing only by size.

7. True or False. A core needle biopsy revealing columnar cell changes without atypia necessitates surgical excisional biopsy.
8. Two different groups of calcifications were biopsied, revealing high-risk lesions: a group of amorphous calcifications and a group of fine linear calcifications. Which is more likely to upgrade to ductal carcinoma in situ upon excisional biopsy?
9. Traditionally, radial scars (or complex sclerosing lesions) found on core needle biopsy subsequently have surgical excisional biopsy due to their imaging resemblance to _____.
10. True or False. Stereotactic biopsy of coarse heterogeneous calcifications reveals fibroadenomatoid change. This is concordant.

■ Answers and Explanations

B. Images show a group of amorphous and coarse heterogeneous calcifications. The underestimation of concurrent malignancy for ADH at core biopsy is well known, and most institutions would recommend surgical excisional biopsy.

Question 1

True. The sensitivity of core needle biopsy for a breast lesion depends on the type of device (spring loaded versus vacuum-assisted), needle gauge, and extent of sampling. Additional considerations include specimen processing and pathologic evaluation.

Question 2

High-risk lesions in breast imaging include ADH, atypical lobular hyperplasia, lobular carcinoma in situ (LCIS), flat epithelial atypia, radial scar, and papilloma.

Question 3

False. There is controversy over whether all lesions characterized as "high-risk," such as papillomas, after concordant radiologic-pathologic correlation, should be surgically excised.

Question 4

True. Both LCIS with central necrosis and pleomorphic-type LCIS may behave more aggressively than classic LCIS. Thus, surgical excisional biopsy is recommended when these variants are present on core biopsy.

Question 5

True. There is a general consensus that papillomas with atypia or multiple papillomas on core biopsy should be excised. However, it is controversial whether benign intraductal papillomas should undergo surgical excision in asymptomatic patients.

Question 6

True. Both radial scar and complex sclerosing lesion are used to describe the same histology (central stromal area with glands radiating from the central stellate lesion). However, radial scars measure < 1 cm, whereas complex sclerosing lesions measure > 1 cm.

Question 7

False. Columnar cell changes without evidence of atypia are benign and do not need additional surgical intervention. However, if there is associated flat epithelial atypia, some breast experts recommend surgical excision.

Question 8

Fine linear and branching calcifications have a higher predictive value of upgrading to ductal carcinoma in situ than do amorphous calcifications upon excisional biopsy.

Question 9

Radial scars (or complex sclerosing lesions) on core needle biopsy subsequently have surgical excisional biopsy due to their imaging resemblance to tubular carcinoma.

Question 10

True. Stereotactic biopsy of coarse heterogeneous calcifications revealing fibroadenomatoid change is concordant.

■ Suggested Readings

Georgian-Smith D, Lawton TJ. Controversies on the management of high-risk lesions at core biopsy from a radiology/pathology perspective. Radiol Clin North Am 2010;48:999–1012

Krishnamurthy S, Bevers T, Kuerer H, Yang WT. Multidisciplinary considerations in the management of high-risk breast lesions. Am J Roentgenol 2012;198:W132–140

Top Tips

◆ Recommendations for management of high-risk lesions at core needle biopsy are institution dependent, particularly for papillomas without atypia.

◆ Most institutions recommend surgical excisional biopsy for any core biopsy revealing atypia.

◆ Radial scars and complex sclerosing lesions have the same histology, differing only by size.

Details 3

■ Case

The images are provided for a negative bilateral screening hand-held ultrasound. Are this exam and documentation complete based on what was performed during the American College of Radiology Imaging Network (ACRIN) 6666 trial?

A. Yes. This is a complete exam.
B. No. There should be four images per breast.
C. No. There should be five images per breast.
D. No. There should be nine images per breast.

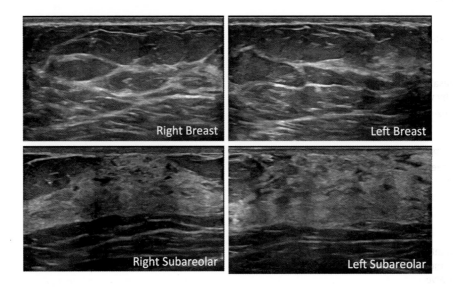

■ The following questions pertain to important studies regarding mammography, whole breast ultrasound, and tomosynthesis.

1. The Digital Mammography Imaging Screening Trial (DMIST) compared film-screening mammography to _____.

2. DMIST showed that full field digital mammography had greater diagnostic accuracy in which three specific subgroups?

3. The _____ was the first breast cancer screening trial in the United States. It was initiated in 1963 to investigate efficacy of screening mammography. The intervention group had _____ (25, 50, 75)% lower breast cancer mortality in women aged 40 to 49 and 50 to 59 than control.

4. The Swedish Two County Trial demonstrated an absolute reduction in breast cancer mortality with screening mammography, with about _____ prevented breast cancer deaths per 1000 women aged 40 to 69 years old screened every 2 years.

5. The Canadian National Breast Screening Study (CNBSS) showed that the 25-year *survival* was _____ (higher, lower, the same) in women with breast cancer detected with mammography and physical exam versus physical exam alone.

6. The CNBSS showed that the cumulative mortality over 25 years in woman diagnosed with breast cancer over

the screening period was _____ (higher, lower, similar) between women detected with mammography and physical exam versus physical exam alone.

7. Simulation modeling for radiation-induced breast cancer incidence and mortality shows that annual screening of 100,000 women aged 40 to 74 was projected to induce about _____ (25, 125, 225, 325) breast cancer cases leading to 16 deaths, relative to about _____ (70, 370, 670, 970) breast cancer deaths prevented from screening.

8. True or False. The ACRIN 6666 study evaluated hand-held whole breast screening ultrasound and mammography versus mammography alone in women at high risk of breast cancer. Although more cancers were detected with the addition of hand-held ultrasound, there was an increased number of false-positive findings.

9. Breast cancer screening using breast tomosynthesis in combination with digital mammography, compared to digital mammography alone, _____ (increases, decreases, no change) recall rates, _____ (increases, decreases, no change) breast cancer detection, and _____ (increases, decreases, no change) in false-negative rates.

10. True or False. There is an association between increasing breast density and breast cancer risk.

■ Answers and Explanations

C. Correct! No. There should be five images per breast. There is currently no standard for documenting a negative screening ultrasound examination. However, ACRIN 6666 did document the need for one image in one plane (usually radial) per quadrant, the same distance from the nipple, in addition to one image of the subareolar region. This means five images per breast: one per quadrant and one in the subareolar position.

Question 1

The DMIST compared film-screening mammography to full field digital mammography.

Question 2

For the entire population, digital mammography performed similarly to film-screen mammography. However, in patients <50 years old, those with heterogeneous or dense breasts, and pre- or perimenopausal woman, the diagnostic accuracy of digital mammography was significantly higher than that of film-screen mammography.

Question 3

The Health Insurance Plan Randomized Control Trial was the first breast cancer screening trial in the United States. It was initiated in 1963 to investigate efficacy of screening mammography. The intervention group had **25%** lower breast cancer mortality in women aged 40 to 49 and 50 to 59 than control.

Question 4

The Swedish Two County Trial demonstrated an absolute reduction in breast cancer mortality with screening mammography, with about **8 to 11** prevented breast cancer deaths per 1000 women aged 40 to 69 years old screened every 2 years.

Question 5

The CNBSS showed that the 25-year *survival* was **higher** in women with breast cancer detected with mammography and physical exam versus physical exam alone. The 25-year survival was 70.6% for women with breast cancer detected via mammography and clinical breast exam versus 62.8% in those detected with clinical breast exam alone.

Question 6

The CNBSS showed that the cumulative mortality over 25 years in woman diagnosed with breast cancer over the screening period was **similar** between women detected with mammography and physical exam versus physical exam alone.

Question 7

Simulation modeling for radiation-induced breast cancer incidence and mortality shows that annual screening of 100,000 women aged 40 to 74 was projected to induce about **125** breast cancer cases leading to 16 deaths, relative to about **970** breast cancer deaths prevented from screening.

Question 8

True. In the ACRIN 6666 study, there were 4.2 per 1000 additional cancers detected. However, there was also a significant number of false-positive findings, with a 9% positive predictive value of biopsy in ultrasound-only findings compared to 23% in mammography-only findings.

Question 9

Breast tomosynthesis in conjunction with digital mammography **decreases** recall rates (8.7 vs. 10.4%), **increases** cancer detection (5.9 vs. 4.4/1000 women screened), and results in **no significant** change in false-negative rates (0.46 vs. 0.60/1000 women screened), when compared to digital mammography alone.

Question 10

True. There is an association between increasing breast density and breast cancer risk.

■ Suggested Readings

Berg WA, Blume JD, Cormack JB, et al. Combined screening with ultrasound and mammography vs mammography alone in women at elevated risk of breast cancer. JAMA 2008;299:2151–2163

Conant EF, Beaber EF, Sprague BL, et al. Breast cancer screening using tomosynthesis in combination with digital mammography compared to digital mammography alone: a cohort study within the PROSPR consortium. Breast Cancer Res Treat 2016;156:109–116

Miglioretti DL, Lange J, van den Broek JJ, et al. Radiation-induced breast cancer incidence and mortality from digital mammography screening: a modeling study. Ann Intern Med 2016;164:205–214

Miller AB, Wall C, Baines CJ, Sun P, To T, Narod SA. Twenty five year follow-up for breast cancer incidence and mortality of the Canadian National Breast Screening Study: randomised screening trial. BMJ 2014;348

Pisano ED, Gatsonis C, Hendrick E, et al. Diagnostic performance of digital versus film mammography for breast-cancer screening. N Engl J Med 2005;353: 1773–1783

Shapiro S. Periodic screening for breast cancer: the HIP Randomized Controlled Trial. Health Insurance Plan. J Natl Cancer Inst Monogr 1997:27–30

Tabar L, Vitak B, Chen TH, et al. Swedish two-county trial: impact of mammographic screening on breast cancer mortality during 3 decades. Radiology 2011;260:658–663

Top Tips

- ◆ Whole breast screening ultrasound, in addition to mammography, increases cancer detection rate when compared to mammography alone. However, there are more false-positive findings in the cohort with whole breast ultrasound screening.

- ◆ For a negative hand-held ultrasound screening breast exam, a minimum of five images should be documented (based on the ACRIN 6666 trial).

- ◆ Breast tomosynthesis decreases recall rates and increases cancer detection rates (notably for invasive cancers), when compared to digital mammography alone.

Details 4

■ **Case**

The following represents a 2 × 2 table comparing test results with the actual presence of disease. Which of the following is true? (Select ALL that apply.)

Disease

	$\oplus$	$\ominus$
Test $\oplus$	A	B
$\ominus$	C	D

A. Box A represents true-positive results.
B. Box B represents true-negative results.
C. Box C represents false-positive results.
D. Box D represents false-negative results.

■ **The following questions pertain to statistics and breast imaging.**

1. Using the 2 × 2 table above, which ONE of the following calculations represents the negative predictive value?
   A. a / (a + b)
   B. b / (a + b)
   C. c / (c + d)
   D. d / (c + d)
2. True or False. Screening for a disease is useful if there is a high prevalence of the disease, the disease causes significant morbidity and mortality, there is benefit for asymptomatic detection, and there is available and effective treatment which can improve outcomes.
3. True or False. A test with a high sensitivity means that a patient with a positive result has a high likelihood of having the disease.
4. A test with a high sensitivity is most useful for ruling _____ (in or out) disease.
5. A test with a high specificity is most useful for ruling _____ (in or out) disease.
6. If the prevalence of disease in the population increases, this affects a test's _____ (sensitivity, specificity, positive predictive value, and/or negative predictive value).

7. True or False. A diagnostic examination in breast imaging can be performed to evaluate clinical signs or symptoms, evaluate an abnormal screen-detected finding, or to follow up a previous Breast Imaging Reporting and Data System (BI-RADS) 3 or BI-RADS 6 lesion.
8. True or False. The breast cancer detection rate should be the same at each institution regardless of patient population.
9. In an American College of Radiology breast imaging audit, a false-negative occurs if there is a tissue diagnosis of cancer within 1 year of a negative examination, which includes BI-RADS category 1, 2, or 3 for a diagnostic examination.
10. True or False. In an American College of Radiology breast imaging audit, the positive predictive value 2 (PPV2) refers to the percent of diagnostic examinations for which a tissue diagnosis is recommended that results in the diagnosis of cancer within 1 year.

■ Answers and Explanations

A. Box A represents true-positive results, Box B represents false-positive results, Box C represents false-negative results, and Box D represents true-negative results.

Question 1

D. d / (c + d). The negative predictive value represents the percent of test results that are true-negatives.

Question 2

True. Screening for a disease is useful if there is a high prevalence of the disease, the disease causes significant morbidity and mortality, there is benefit for asymptomatic detection, and there is available and effective treatment that can improve outcomes. In addition, the test must be readily available, have both good sensitivity and specificity, and have low risk to the patient.

Question 3

False. A test with a high *positive predictive value* means that a patient with a positive result has a high likelihood of having the disease.

Question 4

A test with a high sensitivity is most useful for ruling **out** disease. The sensitivity of the test is the proportion of people who have the disease in question and test positive for it.

Question 5

A test with a high specificity is most useful for ruling **in** disease. The specificity of the test is the proportion of the people who do not have the disease who do not test positive for the disease.

Question 6

If the prevalence of disease in the population increases, this affects a test's positive and negative predictive value. The sensitivity and specificity are characteristics of a test and do not change based upon the patient population. However, the positive and negative predictive values do depend on the prevalence of disease in the population.

Question 7

True. A diagnostic examination in breast imaging can be performed to evaluate clinical signs or symptoms, to evaluate an abnormal screen-detected finding, or to follow up a previous BI-RADS 3 or BI-RADS 6 lesion. A screening examination is used in asymptomatic patients to detect clinically unsuspected cancer.

Question 8

False. The cancer detection rate is the number of cancers detected at screening mammogram per 1000 patients. This can vary depending on the prevalence of cancer in the population.

Question 9

True. In an American College of Radiology breast imaging audit, a false-negative occurs if there is a tissue diagnosis of cancer within 1 year of a negative examination, which includes BI-RADS category 1, 2, or 3 for a diagnostic examination.

Question 10

True. In an American College of Radiology breast imaging audit, the PPV2 refers to the percent of diagnostic examinations for which a tissue diagnosis is recommended that results in a diagnosis of cancer within 1 year. PPV2 = True positives/(number of examinations recommended for tissue diagnosis)

■ Suggested Readings

American Board of Radiology. Noninterpretive skills domain specification and resource guide. http://www.theabr.org/sites/all/themes/abr-media/pdf/Noninterpretive_Skills_Domain_Specification_and_Resource_Guide.pdf. Accessed February 27, 2016

D'Orsi CJ SE, Mendelson EB, Morris EA, et al. ACR BI-RADS® Atlas, Breast Imaging Reporting and Data System. 5th ed. Reston, VA: American College of Radiology; 2013

Top Tips

◆ Sensitivity and specificity are characteristics of a particular test (e.g., a screening mammogram) and do not depend on the patient population.

◆ Positive and negative predictive values can change depending on disease prevalence.

◆ **SeN**sitivity is useful for ruling **OUT** disease (SNOUT), while **SP**ecificity is useful for ruling **IN** disease (SPIN).

Details 5

■ Case

A 40-year-old woman was diagnosed with invasive ductal carcinoma in the left breast. The following breast magnetic resonance imaging (MRI) was performed to evaluate the extent of disease.

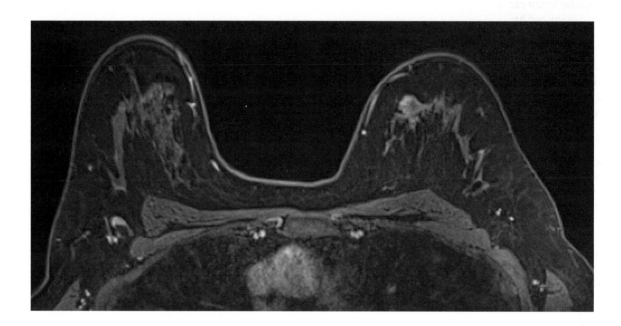

■ Questions

1. Preoperative breast MRI detects ipsilateral malignancy in ____% and contralateral malignancy in ____% of cases.
2. Triple _____ breast cancer most commonly occurs in BRCA _____ mutation carriers and has poor survival rates.
3. Herceptin is used for _____ receptor positive breast cancer and _____ is used for estrogen receptor positive breast cancer.
4. Imaging workup begins with _____ for a palpable at the mastectomy site.
5. Although post-lumpectomy imaging protocols are variable, most institutions recommend a mammogram every ____ months for ____years.
6. On mammography, breast conservation therapy changes are most prominent in the ____ year and stabilize or subside after the ____ year.

7. According to the 2013 American College of Radiology BI-RADS Atlas, which one of the following is considered a breast cancer?
   a. Medullary carcinoma
   b. Metastatic lymphoma/leukemia
   c. Metastatic melanoma
   d. Malignant phyllodes
   e. Sarcoma
8. A patient with known lymphoma has a screening mammogram that demonstrates only axillary lymphadenopathy and no other mammographic abnormality. The correct BI-RADS assessment is _____.
9. The most common cause of a metastasis to the breast is due to cancer of the _____.
10. Regarding extramammary metastases to the breast, the most common cause is _____ and the second most common cause is _____.

■ Answers and Explanations

Question 1

Preoperative breast MRI detects additional ipsilateral malignancy in **15%** and contralateral malignancy in **4%** of cases.

Question 2

Triple **negative** breast cancer most commonly occurs in **BRCA 1** mutation carriers and has poor survival rates.

Question 3

Herceptin is used for **HER2** receptor positive breast cancer and **tamoxifen** is used for estrogen receptor positive breast cancer. Of note, aromatase inhibitors can also be used for estrogen positive receptor breast cancer.

Question 4

Imaging workup begins with a **ultrasound** for a palpable at the mastectomy site. Although total-mastectomy patients undergo clinical surveillance (rather than imaging), the unaffected breast should still have an annual screening mammogram.

Question 5

Although postlumpectomy imaging protocols are variable, many institutions recommend a mammogram every 6 months for 2–3 years (or every 12 months for 5 years). A routine annual mammogram is recommended for the unaffected breast.

Question 6

On mammography, breast conservation therapy changes are most prominent in the **first** year and stabilize or subside after the **third** year.

Question 7

A. Medullary carcinoma is a breast cancer (an invasive ductal carcinoma subtype). The American College of Radiology BI-RADS Atlas defines breast cancer as ductal carcinoma in situ or invasive cancer arising from the breast. Malignant phyllodes, sarcoma, and extramammary metastases to the breast (lymphoma, leukemia, and melanoma) are technically not considered breast cancer.

Question 8

Lymphadenopathy due to known lymphoma is not a breast cancer. This is a BI-RADS category 2 with a recommendation of routine mammographic follow up.

Question 9

The most common metastasis to the breast is due to cancer of the **contralateral breast**.

Question 10

Regarding extramammary metastases to the breast, the most common cause is **melanoma** and the second most common cause is **lymphoma**.

■ Suggested Readings

ACR Practice Parameters for the performance of contrast enhancing magnetic resonance imaging (MRI) of the breast. www.acr.org. Accessed April 2016

Black DM, Kuerer HM. Mastectomy. Statdx. http://www.statdx.com. Accessed April 2016

Sickles, EA, D'Orsi CJ. ACR BI-RADS ® follow-up and outcome monitoring. In: ACR BI-RADS ® Atlas, Breast Imaging Reporting & Data System. Reston, VA: American College of Radiology; 2013.

Yang WT. Metastases to breast. Statdx. http://www.statdx.com. Accessed March 2016

Yang WT, Berg WA. Post breast-conserving surgery. Statdx. http://www.statdx.com. Accessed April 2016

Top Tips

◆ Breast MRI has high sensitivity for the detection of invasive lobular carcinoma.

◆ The correct assessment for a biopsy proven malignancy arising from the breast is a BI-RADS category 6.

◆ The correct assessment for an extramammary malignancy is a BI-RADS category 2.

Details 6

■ Case

A 58 year-old woman had a screening mammogram and the following mediolateral (MLO) views are shown.

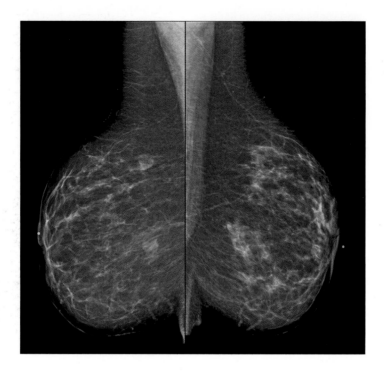

■ Questions

1. A technical repeat Breast Imaging Reporting and Data System (BI-RADS) category 0 was rendered due to inadequate positioning of the right breast. The posterior nipple line must be perpendicular to the _____ on the MLO view to ensure adequate coverage of the posterior tissue.
2. The posterior nipple line on the craniocaudal (CC) view must be within _____ cm of the posterior nipple line measured on the MLO view to ensure adequate coverage of the posterior tissue.
3. The _____ must be seen in profile on at least one view for each breast.
4. Blur detected on a mammogram is designated a BI-RADS _____.
5. Punctate high density in the axilla on the MLO view, that is presumed to be deodorant artifact is a BI-RADS _____.

6. In breast ultrasound, adjust the field of view (depth) to show _____ in the far field.
7. A high-resolution _____ transducer is used in breast ultrasound with a center of frequency of at least _____ MHz.
8. In breast ultrasound, set the _____ at the level of interest to optimize lateral resolution.
9. In breast ultrasound, the orientation of a mass is in reference to the _____.
10. In breast ultrasound, avoid setting the _____ too low or too high because that can lead to misdiagnosis.

■ Answers and Explanations

Question 1

The posterior nipple line must be perpendicular to the **pectoralis** on MLO view to ensure adequate coverage of the posterior tissue.

Question 2

The posterior nipple line on the CC view must be within **1 cm** of the posterior nipple line measured on the MLO view to ensure adequate coverage of the posterior tissue on the CC view.

Question 3

The **nipple** must be seen in profile on at least one view for each breast.

Question 4

Blur detected on a mammogram is designated a **BI-RADS 0** (Technical Repeat). Blur is motion artifact, and views with motion should be repeated to avoid missing subtle findings such as calcifications.

Question 5

Punctate high density in the axilla on the MLO view, that is presumed to be deodorant artifact is a **BI-RADS 0**. Use a wipe to remove any residual deodorant and repeat the MLO projection to distinguish artifact from calcifications.

Question 6

On ultrasound, adjust the field of view (depth) to show **the pectoralis** in the far field.

Question 7

A high-resolution **linear** transducer is used in breast ultrasound with a center of frequency of at least **10 MHz**. High-resolution images are obtained at the high frequency range (between 12 MHz and 18 MHz). In particular, a frequency of 18 MHz provides high-resolution images of findings within or near the skin. At the lower frequency ranges, tissue penetration of 5 cm can be achieved, which can improve resolution of findings deeper with the breast.

Question 8

On breast ultrasound, set the **focal zone** at the level of interest to optimize lateral resolution.

Question 9

In breast ultrasound, the orientation of a mass is in reference to **the skin**.

Question 10

In breast ultrasound, avoid setting **the gain** too low or too high because that can lead to misdiagnosis. A gain too low makes the background appear black, and a solid mass can falsely appear as a cyst. A gain set too high makes the background appear white, and a cyst can falsely appear as a solid mass.

■ Suggested Readings

American College of Radiology. ACR practice parameter for the performance of a breast ultrasound examination. Reston, VA: ACR; Amended in 2014

Berg WA. Breast-artifacts: ultrasound. Statdx. http://www.statdx.com. Accessed January 2016

Berg WA. Mammography: positioning. Statdx. http://www.statdx.com. Accessed February 2016

Top Tips

◆ The pectoralis muscle is seen on the CC view in only 30% of exams.

◆ The inframammary fold should be well visualized on the MLO view.

◆ Use harmonics to reduce artifact within a cyst.

Image Rich 1

■ Case

Selected breast magnetic resonance imaging (MRI) in four different patients highlighting four different findings are shown below. Match the images with the correct finding.

A. Cyst
B. Fibroadenoma
C. Lymph node
D. Invasive ductal carcinoma

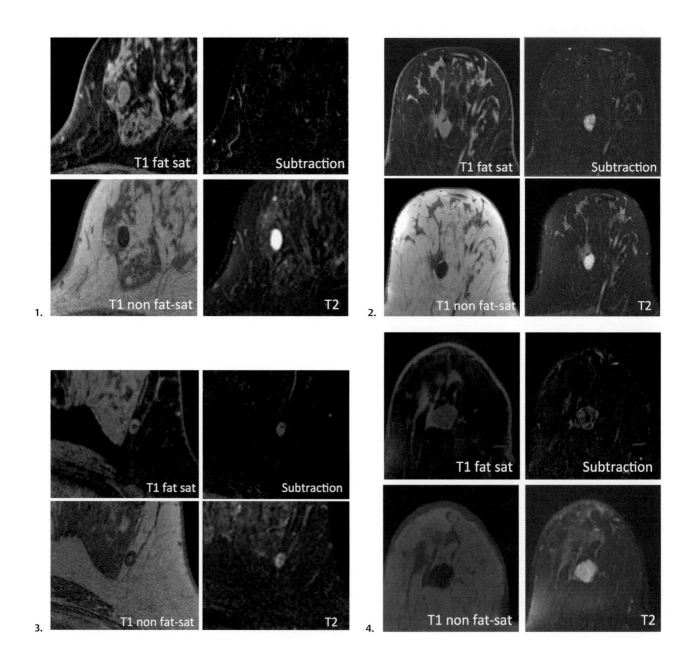

■ Answers and Explanations

The purpose of this case is to discuss the differential diagnosis and imaging characteristics of the most common masses with high T2 signal intensity. By far, most masses that have high T2 signal intensity are benign. However, certain types of intraductal carcinoma are also T2 hyperintense.

1. A. Cyst. On MRI, cysts are oval or round circumscribed masses with no internal enhancement. Inflamed cysts may have a thin rim of uniform enhancement. A cyst may have varying levels of T2 signal hyperintensity depending upon internal protein content.

2. B. Fibroadenoma. On MRI, fibroadenomas are oval, circumscribed masses that may or may not enhance. The level of enhancement as well as the T2 signal intensity depends upon the stage of the fibroadenoma. Fibroadenomas can have nonenhancing internal septations on MRI. Involuting fibroadenomas, which dessicate and calcify over time, may lose their T2 hyperintensity. Internal calcification may result in areas of signal void.

3. C. Lymph node. On MRI, lymph nodes are oval or round circumscribed masses. The cortex of a lymph node typically exhibits T2 hyperintensity. However, the fatty hilum is not bright on T2-weighted images. It is important to note that the kinetic enhancement profile of a lymph node (a rapid rise during the initial phase and washout during the delayed phase) is similar to that of more suspicious lesions.

4. D. Invasive ductal carcinoma. Certain types of invasive ductal carcinoma, particularly high grade, triple-negative cancers, may exhibit high T2 signal intensity due to necrosis within the tumor. Mucinous and intracystic papillary carcinomas can also have T2 signal hyperintensity because of mucinous or cystic components, respectively. Evaluation of other morphologic characteristics (shape, margin, and kinetic features) can differentiate between these suspicious lesions and benign masses.

■ Suggested Reading

Berg, WA. T2 hyperintensity (MR). StatDx. Accessed March 10, 2016

Top Tips

- ◆ The differential for masses with high T2 signal intensity includes cyst, fibroadenoma, lymph node, and mucinous carcinoma.

- ◆ Breast Imaging Reporting and Data System (BI-RADS) assessment should be based on the most suspicious morphologic characteristic.

- ◆ Dynamic kinetic enhancement profiles can be helpful but should not be used as the sole indicator in differentiating benign from suspicious lesions.

Image Rich 2

■ Case

Selected breast magnetic resonance imaging (MRI) in four different patients highlighting four different findings are shown below. Match the images with the correct finding.

    A. Inflamed cyst
    B. Fat necrosis
    C. Mucinous breast cancer
    D. Postoperative seroma

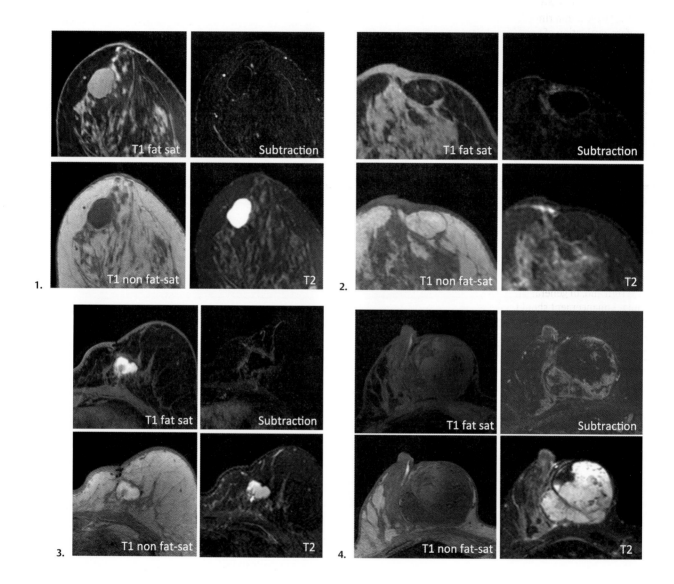

■ Answers and Explanations

The purpose of this case is to discuss the differential diagnosis and imaging characteristics of the most common causes of rim enhancement. It is important to understand that rim enhancement is a morphologic characteristic of a mass. There is a separate descriptor, "clustered ring enhancement," which is used to described non-mass enhancement.

1. A. Inflamed cyst. Cysts are round or oval circumscribed masses that can have varied internal appearances on T1- and T2-weighted sequences, depending upon the internal protein content. They may also have fluid-fluid levels. In general, cysts do not have postcontrast enhancement. However, inflamed cysts may have a thin rim of uniform, peripheral enhancement. Therefore, evaluation of the T1- and T2-weighted sequences to confirm that these lesions are inflamed cysts is key to avoid further workup or possible intervention.

2. B. Fat necrosis. There are various MRI appearances of fat necrosis based on the evolution of the histologic process. Initially, there is inflammation and hemorrhage, followed by liquefaction and necrosis of the fat cells. Subsequently, histiocytes will wall off the necrotic debris while fibrosis develops, which can give the mass irregular or spiculated margins. On MRI, fat necrosis may demonstrate thin rim enhancement. The key to the evaluation is assessing the T1 non-fat and fat-saturated images to identify fat within the mass. When available, comparison with mammogram is also useful to potentially detect rim or dystrophic calcifications, which may not be visible on MRI.

3. D. Postoperative seroma. On MRI, postoperative seromas usually appear as round or oval masses with a thin rim of smooth peripheral enhancement. These contain a mixture of blood and serum and, in general, are T1 hyperintense. Irregular or nodular enhancement should raise suspicion for residual malignancy, and correlation with the pathologic margins should be performed.

4. C. Mucinous breast cancer. Rim enhancement is considered suspicious for malignancy unless there are other features to explain the enhancement, such as an inflamed cyst or fat necrosis. Mucinous cancers are known to have high signal intensity on T2-weighted images in both pure and mixed forms. They can also have peripheral rim enhancement, which is generally thick and irregular.

■ Suggested Readings

Chala LF, de Barros N, de Camargo Moraes P, et al. Fat necrosis of the breast: mammographic, sonographic, computed tomography, and magnetic resonance imaging findings. Curr Probl Diagn Radiol 2004;33:106–126

Daly CP, Jaeger B, Sill DS. Variable appearances of fat necrosis on breast MRI. Am J Roentgenol 2008;191:1374–1380

Drukteinis JS, Gombos EC, Raza S, Chikarmane SA, Swami A, Birdwell RL. MR imaging assessment of the breast after breast conservation therapy: distinguishing benign from malignant lesions. RadioGraphics 2012;32:219–234

Monzawa S, Yokokawa M, Sakuma T, et al. Mucinous carcinoma of the breast: MRI features of pure and mixed forms with histopathologic correlation. Am J Roentgenol 2009;192:W125–131

Top Tips

♦ Differential diagnosis of a rim-enhancing mass on MRI includes necrotic or mucinous breast cancer, inflamed cyst, fat necrosis, and postoperative seroma.

♦ Use the T1 non-fat-saturated sequence for fat necrosis, and the T1 and T2 sequences for cysts.

♦ Fat necrosis may avidly enhance and may not always demonstrate internal fat-signal intensity on MRI. Correlative imaging with mammography in these cases may be helpful.

Image Rich 3

■ Case

Selected breast magnetic resonance imaging (MRI) (subtraction sequence) in four different patients highlighting four different findings are shown below. Which of the following best matches the description for distribution of non-mass enhancement (NME)?

A. Linear
B. Focal
C. Segmental
D. Regional

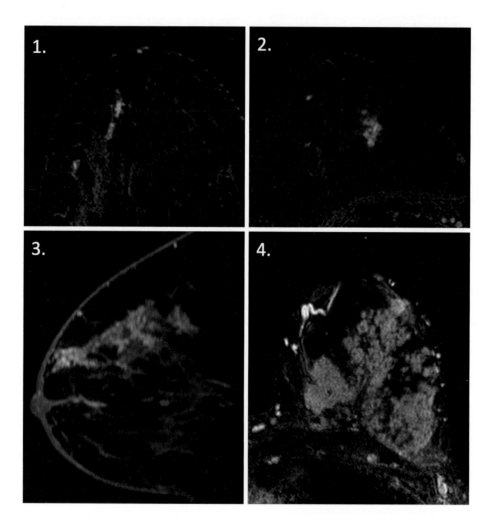

■ Answers and Explanations

NME is the term used to describe areas of enhancement that are discrete from the surrounding fibroglandular tissue but do not meet the criteria for a mass or focus. It is characterized by its internal enhancement pattern in addition to its distribution. The purpose of this question is to understand the different distributions of NME.

1. A. Linear NME. Linear NME corresponds to enhancement distributed in a line or in a line that branches. This line does not necessarily need to be straight. In general, linear NME is a suspicious finding as, pathologically, this represents enhancement within or around a duct.

2. B. Focal NME. Focal NME is a confined area that is less than one quadrant. Pathologically, it represents enhancement of a single ductal system.

3. C. Segmental NME. Segmental NME corresponds to a conical distribution (may look triangular on a single two-dimensional image), with the apex of the cone directed toward the nipple. This is a suspicious finding, as it suggests enhancement within or around the duct and its branches, and may represent more extensive or multifocal cancer in a segment or lobe of the breast.

4. D. Regional NME. A regional distribution of NME suggests enhancement that spans a large area of breast tissue and involves more than one quadrant. Pathologically, this represents enhancement of more than one ductal system.

Other distributions of NME (not shown) include multiple regions NME and diffuse NME, with the latter describing enhancement distributed randomly throughout the breast.

■ Suggested Readings

D'Orsi CJ, Sickles EA, Mendelson EB, Morris EA, et al. ACR BI-RADS® Atlas, Breast Imaging Reporting and Data System. Fifth edition. Reston, VA: American College of Radiology; 2013

Giess CS, Raza S, Birdwell RL. Patterns of nonmasslike enhancement at screening breast MR imaging of high-risk premenopausal women. RadioGraphics 2013;33(5):1343–1360

Top Tips

◆ NME is described by its internal enhancement pattern and distribution.

◆ MRI Breast Imaging Reporting and Data System (BI-RADS) descriptors for internal enhancement of NME: homogeneous, heterogeneous, clumped, and clustered ring.

◆ MRI BI-RADS descriptors for distribution of NME: focal, linear, segmental, regional, multiple regions, and diffuse.

Image Rich 4

■ Case

The following are classic key cases. What is the finding or diagnosis for each case?

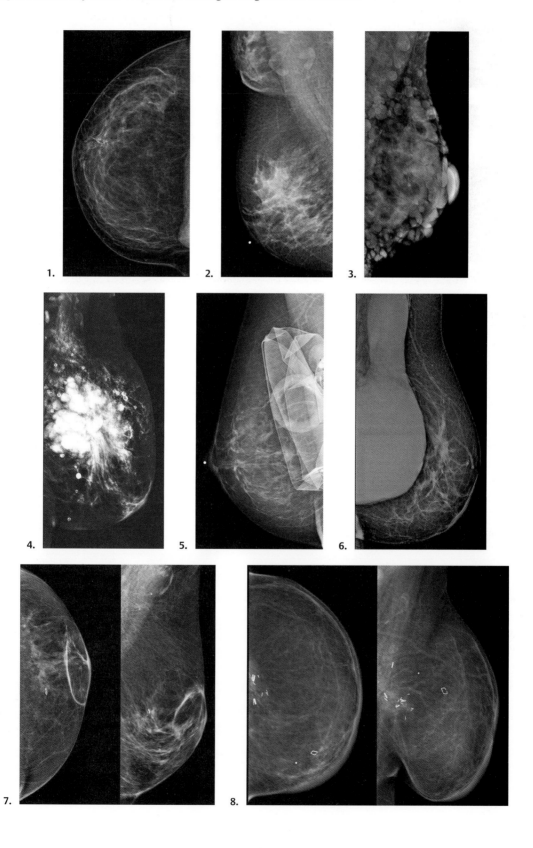

1.

2.

3.

4.

5.

6.

7.

8.

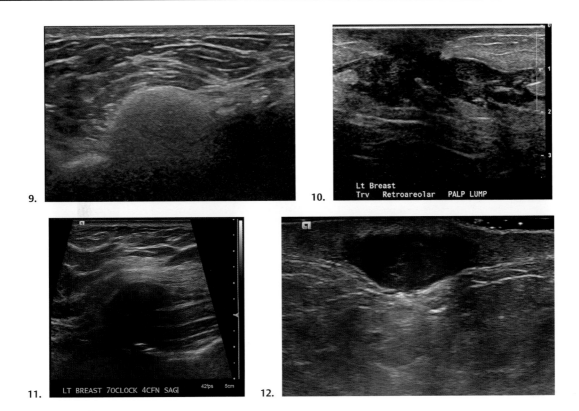

9.

10.
Lt Breast
Trv   Retroareolar   PALP LUMP

11.   LT BREAST 7OCLOCK 4CFN SAGI   42fps   5cm

12.

■ Answers and Explanations

1. Sternalis: normal variant parasternal muscle seen medially on the craniocaudal view

2. Accessory breast tissue: separate island of fibroglandular tissue in the axilla

3. Neurofibromatosis: neurofibromas in the skin often demonstrate a halo sign, which means there is air between the compression paddle and the periphery of the skin finding.

4. Silicone injections: appear as extremely dense masses on mammography

5. Saline implant rupture: clinical diagnosis; imaging confirmation unnecessary

6. Silicone implant rupture: mammography can detect extracapsular rupture

7. Reduction mammoplasty: tissue is shifted to the inferior breast, retroareolar fibrotic band, periareolar and inframammary fold, skin thickening, and areas of fat necrosis

8. Autologous reconstruction: transverse rectus abdominis myocutaneous and deep inferior epigastric perforator are most common flap techniques.

9. Silicone granuloma: "snowstorm" echogenic area with posterior acoustic shadowing.

10. Gynecomastia: appears as retroareolar flame-shaped tissue on ultrasound

11. Rib: oval anechoic with posterior acoustic shadowing, located posterior to the pectoralis muscle

12. Dermal claw sign: indicates a mass is of dermal origin. When seen the posterior dermal line will wrap around the posterior margin of the skin mass.

■ Suggested Readings

Anello M. Implant, saline. Statdx. http://www.statdx.com. Accessed February 2016

Anello M, Berg WA. Implant, silicone. Statdx. http://www.statdx.com. Accessed February 2016

Cao MM, Hoyt AC, Bassett LW. Mammographic signs of systemic disease. RadioGraphics 2011;31(4):1085–1100.

Venkataraman S, Hines N, Slanetz P. Challenges in mammography: part 2, multimodality review of breast augmentation-imaging findings and complications. Am J Roentgenol 2011;197(6):W1031–W1045

Top Tips

◆ A breast MRI (with silicone selective sequences) can evaluate for both intracapsular and extracapsular rupture.

◆ Similar to the linguine sign on MRI, the stepladder sign on ultrasound confirms intracapsular rupture. Specifically, the stepladder sign refers to multiple, parallel, echogenic lines within the implant lumen, which indicate the implant shell has collapsed.

◆ A silicone granuloma indicates current or prior history of extracapsular rupture. Correlate with clinical history for prior implant rupture or explantation.

Image Rich 5

■ Case

What is the correct Breast Imaging Reporting and Data System (BI-RADS) assessment for each case?

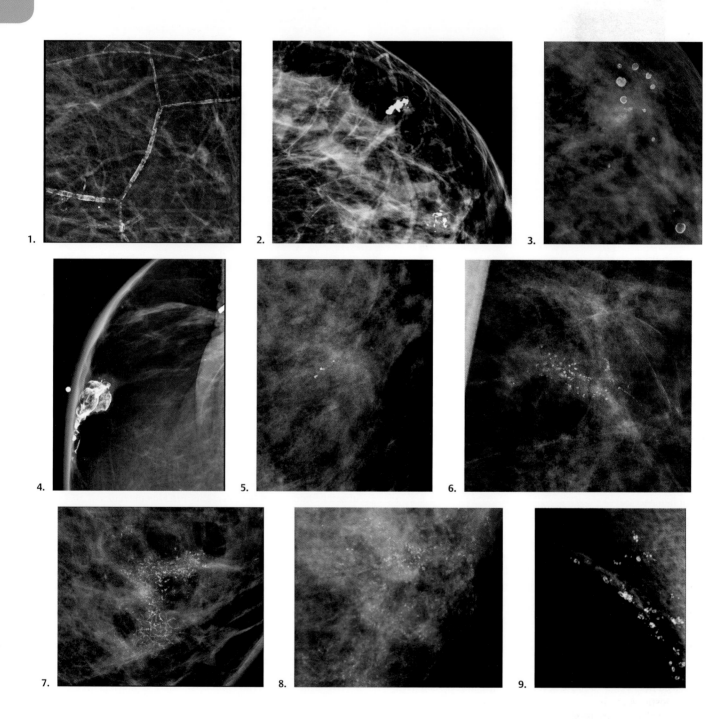

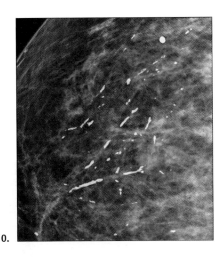

10.

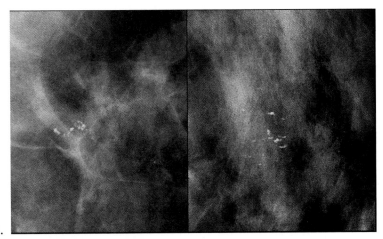

11.

Craniocaudal magnification view   True lateral magnification view

■ Answers and Explanations

1. BI-RADS 2. Benign vascular calcifications

2. BI-RADS 2. Benign popcorn calcifications (degenerating fibro-adenoma)

3. BI-RADS 2. Benign rim calcifications (oil cysts)

4. BI-RADS 2. Benign dystrophic calcifications

5. BI-RADS 4. Punctate calcifications in a linear distribution

6. BI-RADS 4. Fine pleomorphic calcifications in a grouped distribution

7. BI-RADS 4. Fine linear branching calcifications in a segmental distribution

8. BI-RADS 4. Fine pleomorphic calcifications in a segmental distribution

9. BI-RADS 2. Benign milk of calcium (smudgy on craniocaudal view and layer on mediolateral view)

10. BI-RADS 2. Benign secretory calcifications (large rod-like)

11. BI-RADS 2. Benign skin calcifications

■ Suggested Reading

D'Orsi CJ, Sickles EA, Mendelson EB, Morris EA, et al. ACR BI-RADS® Atlas, Breast Imaging Reporting and Data System. Reston VA, American College of Radiology; 20131. 2. 3. 4.

■ Discussions

Additional diagnostic imaging (BI-RADS 0) is required for calcifications that do not meet strict criteria for classically benign calcifications.

Diagnostic workup of calcifications includes spot magnification views and a true lateral view. The morphology and distribution of calcifications is best characterized on the spot magnification views. Calcifications that layer, consistent with benign milk of calcium, are best demonstrated on the true lateral views.

In addition, consider tangential views, which are special diagnostic views that use an alphanumeric grid, to confirm if calcifications are in the skin.

Top Tips

◆ Both morphology and distribution are used to determine the overall likelihood of malignancy.

◆ The positive predictive value of calcification morphology ranges from fine linear branching (70%), fine pleomorphic (29%), amorphous (21%), and coarse heterogeneous (13%).

◆ The positive predictive value of calcification distribution ranges from segmental (62%), linear (60%), grouped (31%), regional (26%), and diffuse (0%).

More Challenging 1

■ Case

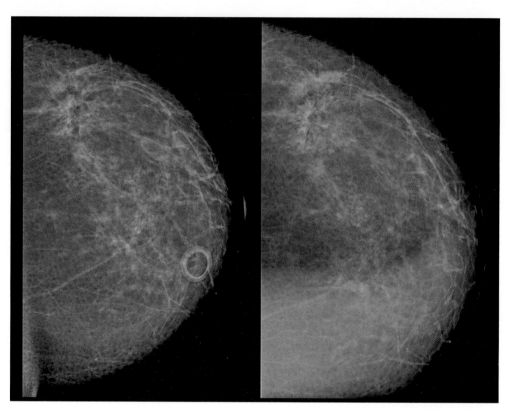

Right craniocaudal view   Spot Compression craniocaudal view

■ Questions

1. Which ONE of the following best describes the abnormal imaging finding in the lateral breast?
   A. Focal asymmetry
   B. Spiculated mass
   C. Architectural distortion
   D. Superimposition of normal fibroglandular tissue
   E. Ill-defined density

2. Regarding architectural distortion, which ONE of the following is correct?
   A. Architectural distortion must be seen on two views.
   B. Architectural distortion is usually too subtle to detect on ultrasound.
   C. Architectural distortion can be associated with skin or nipple retraction.
   D. Spot compression views are not needed to evaluate architectural distortion.
   E. Tomosynthesis does not detect subtle architectural distortion.

3. Regarding architectural distortion, which ONE of the following is correct?
   A. Asymptomatic architectural distortion is rarely associated with malignancy.
   B. Architectural distortion on mammography without a sonographic correlate is considered benign.
   C. If pathology reveals radial scar, then excisional biopsy is unwarranted.
   D. Benign causes of architectural distortion include postsurgical scarring, radial scar, and complex sclerosing lesion.
   E. Malignant causes of architectural distortion include medullary carcinoma and breast metastases.

■ Answers and Explanations

Question 1

C. Correct! Architectural distortion. Architectural distortion on mammography most commonly appears as distorted breast parenchyma with lines radiating from a central point.

Other choices and discussion

A. A focal asymmetry lacks architectural distortion, mass, or calcifications.

B. This is not a mass. It lacks central density and convex margins.

C. This is not superimposition. The abnormality persists on spot compression.

E. An "ill-defined density" is not a Breast Imaging Reporting and Data System (BI-RADS) lexicon term.

Question 2

C. Correct! Architectural distortion can be associated with skin or nipple retraction.

Other choices and discussion

A. Architectural distortion can present as a one-view finding.

B. On ultrasound, architectural distortion can present as a mass, distorted tissue, or abnormal Cooper's ligaments that appear straight, thickened, or tethered.

D. Spot compression views can reveal other associating findings such as an underlying mass or occult calcifications.

E. Tomosynthesis can detect even subtle architectural distortion that is not apparent on two-dimensional images.

Question 3

D. Correct! Benign causes of architectural distortion include postsurgical scarring, radial scar, and complex sclerosing lesion. Other benign causes include postbiopsy change, fat necrosis, sclerosing adenosis, and focal fibrosis.

Other choices and discussion

A. Architectural distortion is the third most common presentation of breast cancer.

B. Architectural distortion on mammography without a sonographic correlate is still suspicious and warrants stereotactic-guided biopsy.

C. If pathology yields radial scar, then an excisional biopsy is warranted. Although radial scars and complex sclerosing lesions are benign, management is surgical excision because of the risk that some will upgrade to malignancy.

E. Malignant causes of architectural distortion include invasive ductal carcinoma, invasive lobular carcinoma, and tubular carcinoma. Medullary carcinoma and breast metastases present as round masses.

■ Suggested Readings

Gaur S, Dialani V, Slanetz PJ, Eisenberg RL. Architectural distortion of the breast. Am J Roentgenol 2013;201:W662–670

Yang WT, Berge WA. Architectural distortion (mammography). Statdx. www.statdx.com. Accessed February 2016

Top Tips

◆ Architectural distortion imaging protocol includes diagnostic spot compression views and ultrasound.

◆ Correlate with prior interventional history for a possible benign etiology. In the absence thereof, proceed to biopsy to exclude malignancy.

◆ When architectural distortion is detected, evaluate for associated suspicious findings, such as nipple retraction, skin thickening or retraction, and lymphadenopathy.

More Challenging 2

■ Case

A 35-year-old presents with suspicious nipple discharge.

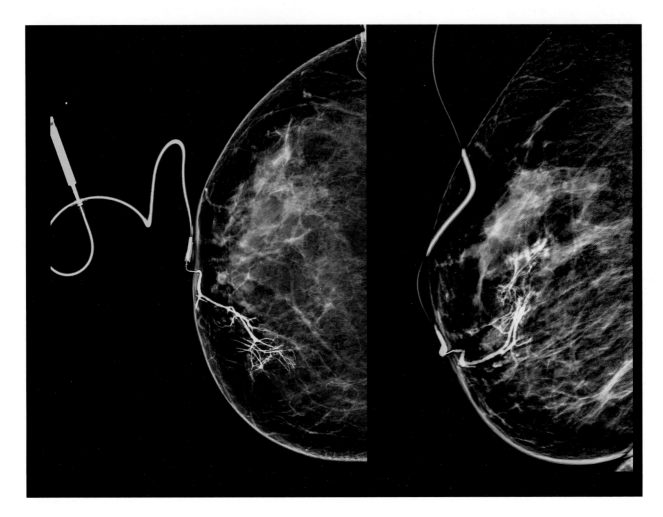

■ Questions

1. Regarding the procedure performed in this case, which ONE of the following is correct?
   A. Cannulation of any ductal orifice in the affected breast will suffice.
   B. A filling defect may be due either to an air bubble artifact or an intraductal lesion.
   C. Imaging workup for nipple discharge should begin with this exam.
   D. There are no significant contraindications.
   E. A total of 10 mL of contrast is gently instilled into the duct.

2. Regarding nipple discharge, which ONE of the following clinical features is considered suspicious?
   A. White color
   B. Nonspontaneous
   C. Multiductal
   D. Clear color
   E. Bilateral

3. Regarding nipple discharge etiologies, which ONE of the following statements is correct?
   A. The most common benign etiology is ductal ectasia.
   B. The most common malignant etiology is papillary carcinoma.
   C. Papillary carcinoma occurs in young women and has a poor prognosis.
   D. Papillomatosis refers to a solitary intraductal papilloma within a central duct.
   E. Paget's disease of the breast can present with nipple discharge.

■ Answers and Explanations

Question 1

B. Correct! A filling defect may be due either to an air bubble artifact or an intraductal lesion. These are distinguished on the orthogonal views. An air bubble artifact will change position, whereas an intraductal lesion remains fixed.

Other choices and discussion

A. A ductal orifice expressing discharge at time of exam should be cannulated.

C. The workup for nipple discharge is as follows: In patients > 30 years, imaging begins with diagnostic mammogram and ultrasound. In patients < 30 years, imaging begins with ultrasound. If conventional imaging is negative, then suspicious nipple discharge can be further evaluated with a breast magnetic resonance imaging (MRI) or a ductogram.

D. Contraindications include infection or severe contrast allergy.

E. Only 0.2 to 0.3 mL of contrast is used, to avoid extravasation.

Question 2

Correct! Suspicious nipple discharge can be bloody, serous, or clear in color.

Other choices and discussion

A. White, green, or yellow nipple discharge is benign.

B. Nonspontaneous nipple discharge is benign. Spontaneous nipple discharge is suspicious.

C. Multiductal nipple discharge is benign. Uniductal nipple discharge is suspicious.

E. Bilateral nipple discharge is benign. Unilateral nipple discharge is suspicious.

Question 3

Correct! Paget's disease of the breast is a malignancy that can present with nipple discharge, nipple eczema, or a subareolar mass.

Other choices and discussion

A. Intraductal papilloma is the most common benign cause of nipple discharge.

B. Ductal carcinoma in situ is the most common malignant etiology.

C. Papillary carcinoma often presents as a complex cystic and solid mass in women over the age of 60 years and has an overall good prognosis.

D. Papillomatosis refers to multiple papillomas predominately located within the peripheral ducts of the breast.

■ Suggested Readings

Berg WA. Ductography of breast. Statdx. http://www.statdx .com. Accessed March 2016

Ferris-James DM, Iuanow E, Mehta TS, Shaheen RM, Slanetz PJ. Imaging approaches to diagnosis and management of common ductal abnormalities. Radiographics 2012;32(4):1009–1030

Sobolewski R, Berg WA. Nipple discharge. Statdx. http://www .statdx.com. Accessed March 2016

Top Tips

- Suspicious nipple discharge is spontaneous, unilateral, and uniductal, with a bloody, serous, or clear color.
- Benign nipple discharge differential diagnosis: papilloma, ductal ectasia, fibrocystic change.
- Malignant nipple discharge differential diagnosis: papillary carcinoma, ductal carcinoma in situ, invasive cancer.

More Challenging 3

■ Case

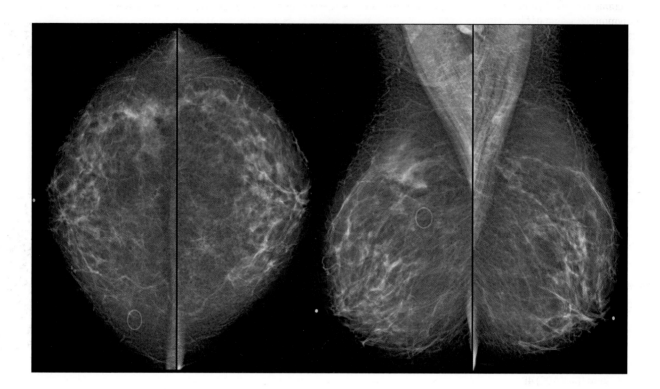

■ Questions

1. A 54-year-old woman presents for a screening mam-mogram. Which ONE of the following is present in the right breast?
   A. Architectural distortion in the upper outer quadrant
   B. Spiculated mass in the upper outer quadrant
   C. An asymmetry in the superior breast, on the mediolateral oblique (MLO) view
   D. Focal asymmetry in the upper outer quadrant
   E. Skin thickening in the upper outer quadrant

2. Regarding focal asymmetry imaging features, which ONE of the following is correct?
   A. Global asymmetry is an focal asymmetry that in-volves the skin.
   B. A developing asymmetry is a new focal asymmetry compared to prior exams.
   C. A developing asymmetry is probably benign, with a < 2% risk of malignancy.

D. A focal asymmetry that demonstrates at least one year of stability is benign.
   E. A developing asymmetry without a sonographic cor-relate is benign.

3. Regarding the diagnostic workup of an asymmetry or focal asymmetry, which ONE of the following is correct?
   A. Rolled views are used to localize a focal asymmetry.
   B. Nipple triangulation is used to localize an asymmetry.
   C. Screening recalls for focal asymmetries increases with tomosynthesis.
   D. A focal asymmetry that does not persist on diagnos-tic views is due to superimposition.
   E. A baseline screen-detected focal asymmetry, that is not suspicious on the subsequent diagnostic views is deemed benign.

■ Answers and Explanations

Question 1

D. Correct! There is a focal asymmetry in the upper outer quadrant. A focal asymmetry is a two-view finding (seen on both craniocaudal [CC] and MLO views) that is comprised of an asymmetric island of fibroglandular tissue when compared to the contralateral breast. It lacks mass-like features, calcifications, or distortion.

Other choices and discussion

A. There are no lines radiating from a central point to suggest architectural distortion.

B. There is no mammographic evidence of a mass in the right breast.

C. An asymmetry is a one-view finding. In this case, there is a two-view finding.

E. There is no skin thickening. The finding is in the breast parenchyma.

Question 2

B. Correct! A developing asymmetry is a focal asymmetry that is new, denser, or larger, when compared to prior mammograms.

Other choices and discussion

A. A global asymmetry is a large focal asymmetry occupying more than one breast quadrant.

C. A developing asymmetry is a Breast Imaging Reporting and Data System (BI-RADS) 4B, with a 13-27% risk of malignancy.

D. A focal asymmetry with at least two years of stability is considered benign.

E. A developing asymmetry without a sonographic correlate is still suspicious and should be biopsied under stereotactic guidance.

Question 3

D. Correct! A focal asymmetry that does not persist on diagnostic views is due to superimposition. Superimposition is summation artifact from overlapping breast tissue.

Other choices and discussion

A. Rolled views are diagnostic views used to localize a one-view finding (asymmetry) that is only seen on a CC view. An asymmetry that moves in the direction of the rolled view is located in the superior breast. An asymmetry that moves in the opposite direction is located in the inferior breast.

B. Nipple triangulation localizes a two-view finding on a third view. First place the MLO between the CC and true lateral views at the nipple level. Then draw a line to connect the finding seen on two views. The line should intersect the finding on the third view.

C. Tomosynthesis actually decreases recalls because the additional image slices improve distinction between a true focal asymmetry and summation artifact.

E. A baseline screen-detected focal asymmetry that is not suspicious on subsequent diagnostic views is probably benign (BI-RADS 3). It can be deemed benign (BI-RADS 2) after 2 years of stability.

■ Suggested Readings

Berg WA. Asymmetries (mammography). Statdx. http://www.statdx.com. Accessed January 2016

Price ER, Joe BN, Sickles EA. The developing asymmetry: revisiting a perceptual and diagnostic challenge. Radiology 2015;274:642–651

Top Tips

- The majority of asymmetries are due to superimposition of normal tissue.

- Invasive lobular carcinoma frequently presents as an asymmetry that is most often detected on the CC view.

- A palpable focal, global, or developing asymmetry is suspicious for malignancy and warrants diagnostic workup.

More Challenging 4

■ Case

A 28-year-old presents with a breast lump. A targeted ultrasound was performed.

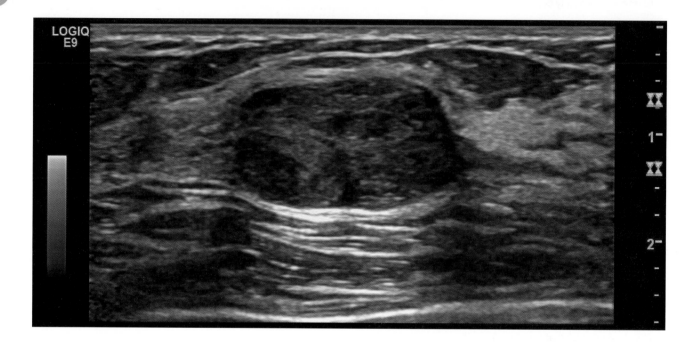

■ Questions

1. Which ONE of the following is the correct assessment and recommendation?
   A. Fibroadenoma. Breast Imaging Reporting and Data System (BI-RADS) 2. Recommend clinical follow up.
   B. Indeterminate mass. BI-RADS 0. Recommend spot compression views.
   C. Solid mass with some indistinct margins. BI-RADS 4. Recommend biopsy.
   D. Probable benign mass. BI-RADS 3. Recommend imaging surveillance.
   E. Probable complicated cyst. BI-RADS 4. Recommend cyst aspiration.

2. After diagnostic workup, which ONE of the following could correctly be given a probably benign BI-RADS 3 assessment?
   A. Complex cystic and solid mass
   B. Solid oval mass with some angular margins

   C. Focal asymmetry that is increasing in density compared to prior mammograms
   D. Solitary group of amorphous calcifications
   E. Probable microcysts

3. Regarding BI-RADS 3 follow up, which ONE of the following is correct?
   A. Even if the finding completely resolves, a 6-month follow up is still recommended to be cautious.
   B. Even if a finding markedly decreases in size, continued imaging surveillance is still recommended.
   C. If the finding increases in size by 10% in 6 months, then biopsy is indicated.
   D. If the finding develops suspicious features, then biopsy is indicated.
   E. If the mass demonstrates 1 year of stability, then it is benign.

■ Answers and Explanations

Question 1

D. Correct! This is a probably benign mass, most likely representing a fibroadenoma in a patient of this age. BI-RADS 3. Imaging surveillance recommended. A BI-RADS 3 assessment means that there is a < 2% risk of malignancy. Imaging surveillance intervals typically occur at 6, 12, and 24 months.

Discussion

This is a probably benign mass and spot views are unnecessary. The mass is solid and has circumscribed margins. Biopsy is not indicated. These imaging findings could be considered benign if this mass was a biopsy-proven fibroadenoma or if prior imaging demonstrated 2 years of stability.

Question 2

E. Correct! Simple microcysts are benign. However, microcysts that are too small to characterize or located at a far posterior depth on ultrasound can be given a BI-RADS 3.

Other choices and discussion

A. A complex cystic and solid mass is a suspicious finding (BI-RADS 4). A solitary complicated cyst can be considered probably benign (BI-RADS 3).

B. Angular margins are a suspicious finding (BI-RADS 4). A solid oval mass with circumscribed margins is considered probably benign (BI-RADS 3).

C. A focal asymmetry that is increasing in density compared to prior mammograms is called a developing asymmetry and is considered a suspicious finding (BI-RADS 4). A baseline screen-detected focal asymmetry that is not suspicious on subsequent diagnostic views is probably benign (BI-RADS 3).

D. A solitary group of amorphous calcifications is a suspicious finding (BI-RADS 4). A solitary group of punctate calcifications is probably benign (BI-RADS 3).

Question 3

D. Correct! If the finding develops suspicious features, then biopsy is indicated.

Other choices and discussion

A. If the mass resolves, then it becomes a BI-RADS 1 negative.

B. If the finding markedly decreases in size, then it becomes a BI-RADS 2 benign.

C. An increased size of 20% in 6 months warrants biopsy, BI-RADS 4 suspicious. In the setting of a very rapidly growing mass, consider phyllodes tumor.

E. If 2 years of stability are shown, then it becomes BI-RADS 2 benign.

■ Suggested Readings

Berg, WA. Probably benign lesions. Statdx. www.statdx.com. Accessed March 2016

D'Orsi CJ, Sickles EA, Mendelson EB, Morris EA, et al. ACR BIRADS Atlas®, Breast Imaging Reporting and Data System. Reston, VA: American College of Radiology; 2013

Top Tips

Imaging workup of a palpable abnormality begins with the following:

◆ Diagnostic mammogram in women age ≥ 40

◆ Diagnostic mammogram or ultrasound in women age 30 to 39

◆ Ultrasound in women < 30

Essentials 1

■ Case

A 35-year-old male patient presents for a cardiac magnetic resonance (CMR) examination and is found to have a left ventricle (LV) end-diastolic volume (EDV) 90 mL/m², left ventricular ejection fraction 58%, right ventricle (RV) EDV 85 mL/m², and right ventricular ejection fraction 56%.

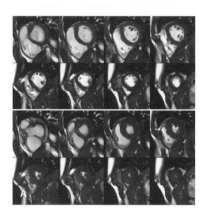 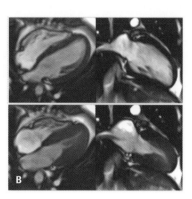

■ Questions

1. Regarding the CMR images shown, which ONE of the following is TRUE? See videos for cines.*
   A. Cine images of this nature to evaluate morphology and function require contrast administration.
   B. Imaging was performed using a spin echo technique.
   C. The RV and LV are dilated.
   D. A two-chamber imaging plane is shown in A, and three-chamber and left ventricular outflow tract imaging planes are shown in B.
   E. Quantification of LV and RV size and function is performed using the images in A.

2. Which ONE of the following is NOT an advantage of cardiac CMR?
   A. Higher spatial and contrast resolution compared to echocardiography
   B. Imaging is not affected by patient body habitus.
   C. It is the test of choice for detection of diastolic dysfunction.
   D. Allows accurate noninvasive quantification of large vessel flow
   E. Provides superior evaluation of biventricular size and systolic function compared to echocardiography

3. Which ONE of the following is NOT a contraindication for CMR?
   A. Implantable cardioverter defibrillator (ICD)
   B. Pacemaker
   C. Cochlear implant
   D. Coronary stent
   E. Intracranial shrapnel

---

* Videos in this chapter can be accessed at MediaCenter.Thieme.com. Please follow the instructions found on the MediaCenter page at the front of this book.

■ Answers and Explanations

Question 1

E. Correct! Ventricular volumes and function are calculated from sequential short axis cine images covering the entire ventricle by contour tracing.

Other choices and discussion

A. Cine CMR is performed using a gradient echo sequence (GRE), which provides a "bright blood effect" without the need for intravenous contrast. Cine CMR uses a special form of GRE imaging called steady state free precession (SSFP), a family of sequences that are currently the backbone of cine CMR imaging. Members of the SSFP family include balanced fast field echo, fast imaging employing steady-state acquisition, and true fast imaging with SSFP. SSFP produces bright blood images with excellent contrast between myocardium and blood within the heart (blood pool).

B. Spin echo imaging produces static black blood images that are used for evaluation of cardiac anatomy and morphology.

C. The LV and RV volumes are within normal limits. Normal limits for LV EDV in a 35-year-old male are 53 to 97 mL/m^2 and 67 to 111 mL/m^2 for RV EDV.

D. A short-axis view of the heart is shown in A, and four- and two-chamber views of the heart are shown in B.

Question 2

C. Correct! Echocardiography is the test of choice for detection of diastolic dysfunction due to its higher temporal resolution and real-time nature as compared to cardiac CMR.

Other choices and discussion

A. Image quality of CMR is superior to echocardiography with notably higher spatial resolution and contrast resolution.

B. Unlike echocardiography, a large body habitus is not a disadvantage for cardiac CMR.

D. CMR, using the phase contrast technique, allows accurate noninvasive determination of flow in large vessels.

E. CMR measures of ventricular size and function do not depend on geometric assumptions, are unaffected by body habitus, and are accurate and reproducible. CMR is the reference standard for biventricular size and systolic function.

Question 3

D. Correct! CMR can be safely performed with coronary stents. Most coronary stents are non-ferromagnetic and labeled as "magnetic resonance (MR) safe." The remainder have been labeled as "MR conditional."

Other choices and discussion

A. ICD is a relative contraindication to CMR. Potential hazards include device dislodgement, programming changes, asynchronous pacing, activation of anti-tachycardiac therapies, inhibition of pacing output, and induced lead currents. An increasing number of patients have an implanted "MR-conditional" device, allowing them to safely undergo MR scanning (provided the manufacturer's guidance is adhered to). In addition, some patients with non-MR-conditional devices may undergo MR scanning if no other imaging modality is deemed suitable and there is a clear clinical indication for scanning that outweighs the potential risk.

B. A pacemaker is a relative contraindication to CMR. Potential hazards are similar to ICDs. MR imaging may be performed under specific circumstances in nonconditional devices if benefits outweigh the risks. MR-conditional pacemakers are now available.

C. Cochlear implants are electronically activated devices. Consequently, an MR procedure may be contraindicated for a patient with this type of implant because of the possibility of injuring the patient and/or altering or damaging the function of the device. Recently, some cochlear implants have received approval designating them as "MR conditional."

E. Intracranial shrapnel is a contraindication to CMR.

■ Suggested Reading

Herzog B, Greenwood J, Plein S. Cardiovascular Magnetic Resonance Pocket Guide. Version 1.2. Updated 2016. http://www.cmr-guide.com

---

Top Tips

◆ Cine CMR is performed using a special form of GRE imaging called SSFP imaging.

◆ CMR is the reference standard for LV and RV size and systolic function, which are calculated by planimetry of a series of short axis slices.

◆ Major indications for CMR in clinical practice include evaluation of myocardial viability in ischemic heart disease, assessment of cardiomyopathies, comprehensive evaluation of adult congenital heart disease, and identification and characterization of cardiac masses including thrombi.

Essentials 2

■ Case

A 50-year-old man presents with chest pain.

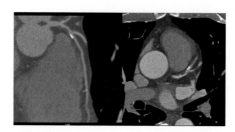

■ Questions

1. What is the abnormality present on the coronary computed tomography angiography (CCTA) images shown?
   A. Minimal (< 25%) non-flow-limiting disease in the left anterior descending coronary artery
   B. Mild (25 to 49%) non-flow-limiting disease in the left anterior descending coronary artery
   C. Moderate (50 to 69%) possible flow-limiting disease in the left anterior descending coronary artery
   D. Left anterior descending coronary artery occlusion
   E. Moderate (50 to 69%) possible flow-limiting disease in the left circumflex artery

2. Mark the FALSE statement regarding the benefits and applications of CCTA.
   A. Coronary artery calcium (CAC) scoring may be used for risk stratification and reclassification in asymptomatic patients with intermediate probability of coronary artery disease (CAD).
   B. The use of CCTA is appropriate for detection of obstructive CAD in symptomatic patients when functional stress testing cannot be performed or is nondiagnostic.
   C. The use of CCTA in the emergency department in patients with chest pain and negative cardiac enzymes allows safe discharge, reduces length of stay, and is cost saving.
   D. The use of CCTA is appropriate for preoperative evaluation in patients undergoing heart surgery for noncoronary indications when the risk of CAD is low to intermediate.
   E. A major advantage of CCTA is its high positive predictive value for detection of obstructive CAD.

3. Which of the following methods is NOT a radiation dose-lowering method in CCTA?
   A. Lowering the heart rate with beta blockers
   B. Use of prospective ECG triggering
   C. 100 kvp tube potential
   D. Use of an iterative reconstruction method
   E. Use of a high spatial frequency reconstruction filter

■ Answers and Explanations

Question 1

C. Correct! The CCTA images show moderate (50 to 69%) possible flow-limiting disease in the LAD. The LAD arises from the left main coronary artery and travels in the anterior interventricular groove, giving rise to diagonal branches and septal perforators. The left circumflex artery arises from the left main coronary artery and travels posteriorly into the left atrioventricular groove. CCTA quantification of lesion severity in clinical practice is visually evaluated and reported in terms of percent maximal diameter stenosis using the stenosis grading scheme below:

0—Normal: absence of plaque and no luminal stenosis
1—Minimal: plaque with < 25% stenosis
2—Mild: 25 to 49% stenosis
3—Moderate: 50 to 69% stenosis
4—Severe: 70 to 99% stenosis
5—Occluded

Question 2

E. Correct! CCTA is an excellent test to rule out CAD in selected low- to intermediate-risk patients due to its high negative predictive value for exclusion of obstructive CAD (90–99%). The positive predictive value of CCTA for obstructive CAD is moderate, and it should be a rule-out test rather than a rule-in test for obstructive CAD.

Other choices and discussion

A. CAC scoring is most useful for risk stratification of asymptomatic patients with an intermediate Framingham risk of future cardiovascular events (10 to 20%, 10-year risk), in whom a high-risk CAC score may prompt an increase in aggressive medical therapy.

B. The use of CCTA is appropriate and guideline-supported for detection of obstructive CAD in symptomatic patients with intermediate probability of CAD when functional stress testing such as stress electrocardiogram (ECG), myocardial perfusion scintigraphy, or dobutamine stress echo cannot be performed or is nondiagnostic.

C. Multiple studies have shown that the use of CCTA in the emergency department in patients with chest pain and negative cardiac enzymes allows safe discharge, reduces length of stay, and is a cost-saving measure compared to the usual standard of care, including functional testing for detection of CAD.

D. As part of the preoperative evaluation, CCTA is viewed as a potential option among patients undergoing heart surgery for noncoronary indications (e.g., valve replacement surgery or atrial septal defect closure) when the pretest CAD risk is intermediate.

Question 3

E. Correct! A high spatial resolution reconstruction filter can be used to decrease blooming artifact from stents and calcium in CCTA and DOES NOT lead to a reduction in radiation dose.

Other choices and discussion

A. Vigorous heart rate-lowering ($\leq$ 60 bpm) with beta blockers will allow the use of prospective ECG triggering, which leads to substantial radiation dose reduction ($\sim$40 to 50%) as compared to retrospective ECG gating needed at higher heart rates.

B. Prospective ECG-gated CCTA acquisition mode refers to an acquisition triggered by the ECG signal. The table moves periodically in "steps," and the X-ray tube is on intermittent ("shoot")—the so-called step-and-shoot mode. The user selects the phase in which to acquire the images (usually diastole). The major advantage of this technique is substantial radiation dose reduction, as the X-ray tube is on for only 20 to 25% of the cardiac cycle in diastole and is completely off for the majority of the remaining cardiac cycle.

C. A relatively small change in peak voltage of 20 kVp (from 120 to 100 kVp) results in a decrease in radiation dose of 30 to 40%. Multiple studies support 100-kV imaging for patients weighing up to 90 kg or with a body mass index of up to 30 kg/m^2.

D. Iterative reconstruction methods can reduce the impact of X-ray quantum noise on computed tomography images and allow a lower radiation dose while preserving clinical diagnostic utility.

■ Suggested Readings

Litmanovich DE, Tack DM, Shahrzad M, et al. Dose reduction in cardiothoracic CT: review of currently available methods. RadioGraphics 2014;34:1469–1489

Taylor AJ, Cerqueira M, Hodgson J, et al. ACCF/SCCT/ACR/AHA/ASE/ASNC/NASCI/SCAI/SCMR 2010 appropriate use criteria for cardiac computed tomography. J Cardiovasc Comput Tomogr 2010;4:e1–407.e33

Top Tips

- CCTA is appropriate for detection of obstructive CAD in low- to intermediate-risk symptomatic patients.
- The negative predictive value of CCTA for obstructive CAD is high ($\sim$90 to 99%).
- With proper attention to technique, including lowering of heart rate with beta blockers, prospective ECG triggering, optimization of imaging parameters (including kVp and scan range), and use of modern computed tomography scanners, the radiation dose of CCTA is low (in the range of 1 to 3 mSv with sub-mSv doses possible in select cases).

Essentials 3

■ Case

A 25-year-old male patient presents with chest pain. Physical examination is remarkable for ectopia lentis.

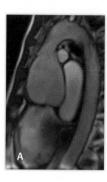
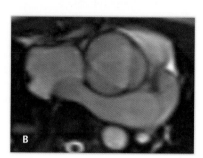

■ Questions

1. The CORRECT diagnosis is:
   A. Marfan syndrome
   B. Bicuspid aortic valve disease
   C. Loeys-Deitz syndrome
   D. Turner syndrome
   E. Noonan syndrome

2. Which of the following statements is FALSE regarding prophylactic surgical repair of thoracic aortic aneurysms?
   A. Surgical repair in Marfan syndrome is recommended when the aorta reaches 5.0 cm (unless there is a family history of aortic dissection), a rapidly expanding aneurysm, or the presence of significant aortic valve regurgitation.
   B. In Loeys-Dietz syndrome, surgical repair is recommended at an aortic diameter of 4.4 to 4.6 cm by computed tomography and/or magnetic resonance imaging.
   C. Surgical treatment of asymptomatic patients with degenerative ascending aortic aneurysms should be considered when the diameter ≥ 5.5 cm.
   D. Patients undergoing aortic valve repair or replacement and who have an ascending aorta or aortic root > 4.5 cm should be considered for concomitant repair of the aortic root or replacement of the ascending aorta.
   E. Operative intervention to repair the aortic sinuses or replace the ascending aorta is indicated in patients with a bicuspid aortic valve if the diameter of the aortic sinuses or ascending aorta is ≥ 4.5 cm.

3. All of the following genetic conditions are associated with thoracic aortic aneurysms and/or dissection EXCEPT:
   A. Loeys-Dietz syndrome
   B. Autosomal dominant polycystic kidney disease
   C. Bicuspid aortic valve
   D. Ehlers-Danlos syndrome
   E. Williams syndrome

---

* Videos in this chapter can be accessed at MediaCenter.Thieme.com. Please follow the instructions found on the MediaCenter page at the front of this book.

■ Answers and Explanations

Question 1

A. Correct! Marfan syndrome is an inheritable disorder of the connective tissue with a prevalence of 1 in 3000 to 5000 individuals. The condition is inherited in an autosomal dominant manner and results from mutations in the *FBN1* gene. The ocular manifestation that is both sensitive and fairly specific for Marfan syndrome is ectopia lentis (lens displacement). The most common cardiovascular complication is progressive aortic root enlargement initially occurring at the sinuses of Valsalva and leading to effacement of the sinotubular junction. Note the dilatation of the aortic root at the sinuses (annulo-aortic ectasia), effacement of the sinotubular junction, mitral valve prolapse, and regurgitation in this case.

Other choices and discussion

B. The aortic valve is tricuspid in this case as shown on the short axis enface view. The most common pattern of aortic dilatation in bicuspid aortic valves is a tubular dilatation of the ascending aorta followed by dilatation of the sinuses of Valsalva.

C. Loeys-Deitz syndrome is characterized by the triad of arterial tortuosity and aneurysms, hypertelorism, and bifid uvula or cleft palate (or a uvula with a wide base or prominent ridge on it). Although Loeys-Dietz syndrome and Marfan syndrome have some overlapping features, the presence of ectopia lentis is distinct for Marfan syndrome.

D. Cardiovascular manifestations of Turner syndrome include aortic dilatation, bicuspid aortic valves, aortic coarctation, and aortic dissection.

E. The most common cardiovascular lesions in Noonan syndrome are pulmonic valve stenosis and hypertrophic cardiomyopathy.

Question 2

E. Correct! This statement is FALSE. Operative intervention to repair the aortic sinuses or replace the ascending aorta is indicated in patients with a bicuspid aortic valve if the diameter of the aortic sinuses or ascending aorta is > 5.5 cm. Replacement of the ascending aorta is reasonable in patients with a bicuspid aortic valve if the diameter of the ascending aorta is > 4.5 cm only if they are undergoing aortic valve surgery because of severe AS or AR.

Other choices and discussion

A. Surgical repair is recommended in Marfan syndrome when the diameter of the aortic root or other parts of the thoracic aorta is 5.0 cm or more.

B. There is a higher risk of dissection in patients with Loeys-Dietz syndrome, and hence, thresholds for surgical replacement are lower: > 4.2 cm by time of flight and 4.4 to 4.6 cm by computed tomography or magnetic resonance imaging.

C. Surgical or endovascular treatment of degenerative ascending aortic aneurysms in the absence of genetic syndromes and valve disease is recommended when the diameter exceeds 5.5 cm or when the growth rate exceeds 0.5 cm/year.

D. Patients undergoing aortic valve repair or replacement and who have an ascending aorta or aortic root > 4.5 cm should be considered for concomitant repair of the aortic root or replacement of the ascending aorta.

Question 3

E. Correct! Williams syndrome is a congenital, multisystem disorder involving the cardiovascular, connective tissue, and central nervous systems. Supravalvular aortic stenosis, either in the form of an hourglass discrete narrowing at the sinotubular junction or long segment stenosis of the thoracic aorta, is the most common cardiovascular lesion followed by pulmonary arterial stenosis.

Other choices and discussion

A. Loeys-Dietz syndrome is an autosomal dominant aortic aneurysm syndrome with involvement of many other systems. The vascular disease in these patients is particularly aggressive, and most patients have aortic root aneurysms (98%) that lead to aortic dissection.

B. There is an association of arterial dissections, including thoracic aortic dissections, in patients with autosomal dominant polycystic kidney disease.

C. Aortic aneurysms are found in 20% of patients undergoing surgery for a bicuspid aortic valve, and 15% of patients with acute aortic dissection have bicuspid valves.

D. Most of the fatal complications in the Ehlers-Danlos syndrome are caused by arterial rupture with most deaths attributable to arterial dissections or ruptures involving primarily the thoracic or abdominal arteries.

> ### Top Tips
>
> ◆ Marfan syndrome is an inherited (autosomal dominant) connective tissue disorder with the most common cardiovascular complication being progressive aortic root enlargement initially occurring at the sinuses of Valsalva and leading to effacement of the sinotubular junction (annulo-aortic ectasia).
>
> ◆ Surgical repair is recommended when the diameter of the aortic root or other parts of the thoracic aorta is 5.0 cm. A lower diameter of 4.5 to 5 cm is considered for surgical repair in the presence of a family history of aortic dissection, rapid diameter change (> 0.5 cm/year), significant valvular regurgitation, or a desire for pregnancy.
>
> ◆ Surgical treatment of degenerative ascending aortic aneurysms in the absence of genetic syndromes and valve disease is recommended when the diameter exceeds 5.5 cm or when the growth rate exceeds 0.5 cm/year.

Essentials 4

■ Case

A 55-year-old man is admitted with acute chest pain.

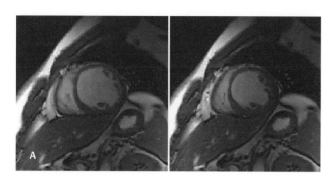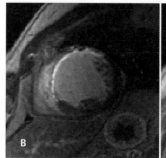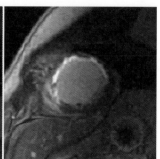

■ Questions

1. Based on the provided cardiac magnetic resonance (CMR) images, which ONE of the following statements is CORRECT?
   A. The patient has had a myocardial infarction in the right coronary artery distribution and will likely improve function by revascularization.
   B. The patient has had a myocardial infarction in the left anterior descending coronary artery distribution and is best managed medically.
   C. The patient has had a myocardial infarction in the left circumflex artery distribution and is best managed medically.
   D. Images indicate acute myocarditis, and treatment should be supportive.
   E. If the measured left ventricular ejection fraction (LVEF) is 30%, implantable cardioverter defibrillator placement is recommended before discharge from the hospital.

2. Which of the following sequences is used for viability imaging in routine clinical practice?
   A. T1-weighted postcontrast turbo spin echo
   B. T2-weighted noncontrast turbo spin echo
   C. T1-weighted postcontrast inversion recovery gradient echo
   D. T1 mapping precontrast
   E. Steady state free precession noncontrast cine

3. Which of the following statements is FALSE regarding the applications of CMR in ischemic heart disease (IHD)?
   A. Late gadolinium enhancement (LGE) has a higher spatial resolution and accuracy than cardiac single-photon emission computed tomography (SPECT) for detection of MI and viability.
   B. CMR myocardial stress perfusion imaging has a higher sensitivity and specificity than cardiac SPECT for detection of obstructive coronary artery disease.
   C. CMR is appropriate for evaluation of ventricular size and function in IHD when echo windows are unsatisfactory.
   D. CMR is the test of choice for direct anatomical evaluation of coronary stenosis.
   E. The identification of microvascular obstruction on CMR is an adverse prognostic finding in IHD.

---

* Videos in this chapter can be accessed at MediaCenter.Thieme.com. Please follow the instructions found on the MediaCenter page at the front of this book.

■ Answers and Explanations

Question 1

B. Correct! The left anterior descending coronary artery (LAD) supplies the anterior wall, anterior septum, and anterior lateral wall of the left ventricle. The delayed enhancement (right image) is in the LAD territory affecting the subendocardium and is nearly transmural ($>$ 75% thickness of myocardium enhanced). The transmural extent of delayed enhancement is a marker of myocardial viability. Myocardium with $>$ 50% enhancement is considered nonviable and unlikely to improve function following revascularization. Such patients are best managed medically.

Other choices and discussion

A. The right coronary artery supplies the inferior septum and inferior wall of the left ventricle.

C. The left circumflex artery supplies the inferior lateral wall of the left ventricle.

D. Myocarditis causes subepicardial or mid-wall enhancement in a noncoronary distribution.

E. In patients with ischemic heart disease, an implantable cardioverter defibrillator should be considered if indications (LVEF $\leq$ 35%, New York Heart Association II/III, or LVEF $\leq$ 30%, New York Heart Association I or asymptomatic) exist at least 40 days after MI. A possible exception to this rule is in post-MI patients ($>$ 48 hours) who develop sustained ventricular tachycardia/ventricular fibrillation not due to transient or reversible causes.

Question 2

C. Correct! Viability imaging uses a segmented (imaging performed over multiple heart beats) T1-weighted inversion recovery (180-degree inversion pulse to increase conspicuity between normal and contrast-enhanced abnormal myocardium) fast gradient echo sequence 10 to 15 minutes post gadolinium administration.

Other choices and discussion

A. T1-weighted postcontrast turbo spin echo imaging may be used for tissue characterization such as in the evaluation of cardiac masses. However, it does not provide adequate contrast resolution to accurately detect MI.

B. T2-weighted noncontrast spin echo imaging may be used for detection of myocardial edema and inflammation. However, it is does not provide adequate contrast for detection of MI and viability.

D. T1 mapping of the myocardium is a novel and expanding application of CMR imaging and has the potential to depict diffuse interstitial fibrosis in a variety of cardiac diseases. Precontrast T1 mapping can detect MI without intravenous contrast. However, further validation of the technique is required, and it is not a routine clinical application at this time.

E. Steady state free precession noncontrast cine imaging is used for evaluation of cardiac anatomy and function.

Question 3

D. Correct! This statement is FALSE. CMR for direct anatomic evaluation of coronary stenosis is limited by spatial resolution and long imaging times. Computed tomography and direct catheter angiography are the preferred modalities for direct visualization of coronary stenosis.

Other choices and discussion

A. The in-plane spatial resolution of LGE CMR is in the range of 1.4 $\times$ 1.8 mm and allows detection of MI including small subendocardial infarctions with higher accuracy than SPECT.

B. Myocardial vasodilator stress perfusion magnetic resonance imaging allows detection of obstructive coronary artery disease with higher accuracy than SPECT due to superior image quality independent of body habitus and higher spatial resolution.

C. The use of CMR is considered appropriate for evaluation of ventricular function in IHD when echo windows are unsatisfactory, such as due to obesity.

E. Microvascular obstruction in acute MI identified as low-signal intensity regions with hyperenhancing myocardium is an indicator of adverse prognosis including negative remodeling and arrhythmias.

■ Suggested Reading

Hundley WG, Bluemke DA, Finn JP, et al. ACCF/ACR/AHA/NASCI/SCMR 2010 expert consensus document on cardiovascular magnetic resonance: a report of the American College of Cardiology Foundation task force on expert consensus documents. J Am Coll Cardiol 2010;55:2614–2662

Top Tips

- ◆ Late gadolinium imaging is appropriate for determining the extent of myocardial necrosis and viability in ischemic heart disease.

- ◆ LGE in a coronary artery distribution involving the subendocardium is indicative of MI.

- ◆ The transmural extent of LGE is a marker of myocardial viability: subendocardial to $<$ 25% enhancement = viable; 25 to 50% = mixed and likely viable; 50 to 75% = mixed and likely nonviable; $>$ 75% enhancement = nonviable.

Essentials 5

■ Case

A 54-year-old man has increasing shortness of breath for which a cardiac magnetic resonance (CMR) examination was performed.

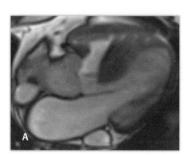
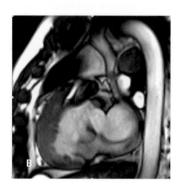

■ Questions

1. In conjunction with the provided images, the CORRECT diagnosis is:
   A. Double outlet right ventricle
   B. D-Transposition of the great arteries
   C. Isolated pulmonary valve stenosis
   D. Truncus arteriosus
   E. Tetralogy of Fallot

2. Following primary anatomic repair of the condition presented, the most common/major hemodynamic complication is which of the following?
   A. Residual pulmonic stenosis
   B. Tricuspid insufficiency
   C. Residual VSD
   D. Pulmonary regurgitation
   E. Aortic root dilatation

3. Pulmonic valve replacement (PVR) in repaired tetralogy of Fallot is generally performed when the magnetic resonance–measured RV end-diastolic volume (EDV) reaches which of the following values?
   A. 90 to 110 mL/m^2
   B. 110 to 130 mL/m^2
   C. 150 to 170 mL/m^2
   D. 170 to 200 mL/m^2
   E. 200 to 250 mL/m^2

---

* Videos in this chapter can be accessed at MediaCenter.Thieme.com. Please follow the instructions found on the MediaCenter page at the front of this book.

■ Answers and Explanations

Question 1

E. Correct! TOF is characterized by ventricular septal defect (VSD), overriding aorta, right ventricular outflow tract (RVOT) obstruction, and right ventricular hypertrophy (RVH). Note the aorta overriding the right ventricle (RV) and the subaortic VSD in A. In the RVOT view (B), a dephasing jet from subpulmonic stenosis in systole is shown along with RVH (and incidental note of a left superior vena cava draining to the coronary sinus).

Other choices and discussion

A. Double outlet RV is a type of abnormal ventriculo-arterial connection where both the aorta (> 50% of circumference) and the pulmonary artery arise entirely or predominantly from the RV.

B. In D-transposition of the great arteries, the aorta arises entirely from the RV and the pulmonary artery from the left ventricle. There is atrioventricular concordance and ventriculo-arterial discordance.

C. Isolated pulmonary valve stenosis can be due to a dome-shaped valve with commissural fusion or a dysplastic valve. There are other associated anomalies in this case.

D. Truncus arteriosus consists of a single arterial trunk giving origin to the pulmonary arteries, the coronary arteries, and the aorta.

Question 2

D. Correct! Pulmonic regurgitation is the most common/major complication following anatomic repair. Complete anatomic repair of TOF consists of closure of the VSD and relief of RVOT obstruction by resection of obstructing muscle bundles and pulmonary valvotomy (with or without an annular or RVOT patch). Relief of RVOT obstruction in TOF often involves disruption of pulmonary valve integrity, which leads to PR in the majority of patients. Without intervention, PR results in RV dilation and may lead to a cascade of other complications, including biventricular dysfunction, tachyarrhythmias, exercise intolerance, heart failure, and death.

Other choices and discussion

A. Residual pulmonic stenosis may exist at the subvalvular, valvular, or supravalvular level in repaired TOF. However, it is not the most common residual defect.

B. Tricuspid insufficiency is usually secondary to annular dilatation from RV dilatation and PR. While it has been associated with supraventricular arrhythmias, it is not the most common hemodynamic abnormality.

C. Residual VSD may be present in repaired TOF leading to a left-to-right shunt. However, it is not the most common or major hemodynamic lesion.

E. Aortic root dilation is seen in approximately 15% of adults late after repair and relates to both intrinsic abnormalities of the aorta (cystic medial necrosis) and increased flow (i.e., patients with pulmonary atresia). It may lead to aortic regurgitation, and rarely, to aortic dissection.

Question 3

C. Correct! PVR in survivors of primary TOF repair with PVR improves symptoms, the New York Heart Association class, and can lead to reduction and normalization of RV volumes when properly timed. Normalization of RV dimensions have been documented when preoperative CMR-measured RV EDVs are in the range of 150 170 mL/m^2, and this number is usually used as a guide in conjunction with patient symptoms, electrocardiogram, and exercise testing when deciding on PVR.

Other choices and discussion

A. The upper limits of normal for RV size is 90 to 110 mL/m^2, and PVR is not performed at this value. Annual echocardiography and CMR at three-year intervals is generally performed for surveillance.

B. An RV EDV in the 110 to 130 mL/m^2 range indicates a mildly dilated RV. In the absence of other significant lesions and symptoms, CMR should be repeated in three years in a stable patient.

D and E. An RV EDV > 170 mL/m^2 indicates a severely dilated RV that may not normalize in volume after PVR. PVR is recommended before the RV dilates to this value.

■ Suggested Reading

Bhatt AB, Foster E, Kuehl K, et al. Congenital heart disease in the older adult. A scientific statement from the American Heart Association. Circulation 2015;131:1884–1931

Top Tips

◆ TOF: VSD, overriding aorta, right ventricular outflow obstruction, RVH

◆ Anatomic repair of TOF consists of VSD patch repair and relief of RVOT obstruction. The primary hemodynamic defect/complication in adult survivors after repair is residual PVR.

◆ CMR is used to guide the timing of PVR, which is performed before the RV is severely dilated to a value of > 150 mL/m^2 for EDV, as larger RVs may not return to a normal size following PVR.

Essentials 6

■ Case

A 45-year-old woman presents with syncope.

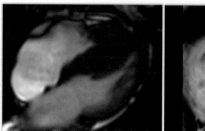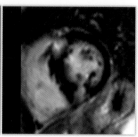

■ Questions

1. The CORRECT diagnosis is:
   A. Hypertrophic cardiomyopathy
   B. Hypertensive cardiomyopathy
   C. Athlete's heart
   D. Cardiac amyloidosis
   E. Fabry disease

2. The following are advantages of cardiac magnetic resonance (CMR) in the evaluation of the diagnosis in the case EXCEPT:
   A. Accurate measurement of wall thickness and LV mass
   B. Accurate evaluation of the LV apex and basal segments
   C. Detection of myocardial fibrosis
   D. Differentiation of HCM from phenocopies
   E. Measurement of outflow tract gradients

3. Which ONE of the following is NOT a major risk factor for sudden cardiac death (SCD) in HCM?
   A. Wall thickness > 30 mm
   B. Family history of SCD
   C. Sustained VT/resuscitated VF
   D. Unexplained syncope
   E. Atrial fibrillation

---

* Videos in this chapter can be accessed at MediaCenter.Thieme.com. Please follow the instructions found on the MediaCenter page at the front of this book.

■ Answers and Explanations

Question 1

A. Correct! There is asymmetric septal hypertrophy, which represents the most common form of hypertrophic cardiomyopathy (HCM). Patchy mid-wall enhancement is seen in the septum at the junction points of the right ventricle and left ventricle (LV) and is a typical enhancement pattern in HCM.

Other choices and discussion

B. Hypertensive cardiomyopathy may lead to cardiac hypertrophy, which is usually concentric and rarely asymmetric with greater involvement of the septum. Usually the hypertrophy does not exceed 15 mm.

C. Athlete's heart may lead to concentric hypertrophy that usually does not exceed 13 mm and may be accompanied by LV dilatation. Delayed enhancement is negative.

D. Cardiac amyloidosis manifests as concentric LV hypertrophy with diffuse global subendocardial myocardial enhancement.

E. Fabry disease may present with concentric hypertrophy or asymmetric hypertrophy and is characteristically associated with mid-wall enhancement in the inferior lateral wall of the LV.

Question 2

E. Correct! Magnetic resonance imaging does not accurately determine left ventricular outflow tract gradients in obstructive HCM, due to its lower temporal resolution and lack of real-time data compared with echocardiography.

Other choices and discussion

A. This is an advantage. Compared with echocardiography, CMR allows more accurate estimation of wall thickness and LV mass.

B. Evaluation of the LV apex and basal segments (particularly the basal anterior wall) may challenging with echocardiography, but is straightforward with CMR.

C. Using the late gadolinium enhancement (LGE) technique with magnetic resonance imaging can detect myocardial fibrosis.

D. Phenocopies (including hypertensive cardiomyopathy, infiltrative pathology, storage diseases, and athlete's heart) can be differentiated from HCM by magnetic resonance imaging, using a combination of morphologic features and tissue characterization by LGE.

Question 3

E. Correct! Atrial fibrillation may be a finding in HCM. However, it is NOT considered a major risk factor for SCD. The fifth major risk factor for SCD in HCM, in addition to those mentioned above, is a hypotensive response to exercise.

Other choices and discussion

A. This is a risk factor. Massive hypertrophy defined as wall thickness > 30 mm is a major risk factor for SCD in HCM.

B. A family history of SCD, known or presumed to be due to HCM, is a major risk factor.

C. Sustained VT or resuscitated VF is a risk factor for SCD in HCM.

D. Unexplained syncope, presumed to be due to non-neurohumoral causes, is a major risk factor for SCD.

■ Suggested Reading

Baxi AJ, Restrepo CS, Vargas D, et al. Hypertrophic cardiomyopathy from A to Z: genetics, pathophysiology, imaging, and management. Radiographics 2016;36(2):335–354

Top Tips

◆ HCM is characterized by thickening of the LV wall involving one or more segments ≥ 15 mm in the absence of LV loading conditions or other causes of hypertrophy.

◆ The asymmetric septal form is the most common phenotype of HCM.

◆ LGE CMR detects fibrosis in HCM and is useful for risk stratification for SCD. HCM is the most common cause of SCD in young people. Major risk factors for SCD in HCM include family history of SCD, syncope, massive wall thickness > 30 mm, nonsustained ventricular tachycardia, and an abnormal hypotensive response to exercise. Implantable cardioverter defibrillator placement by current guideline is recommended when one or more major risk factors are present. LGE on CMR, which appears to reflect fibrosis, is being proposed as a possible risk factor for SCD in HCM. LGE has shown to be predictive of arrhythmias, SCD, and heart failure in HCM. Extensive LGE may be used as an arbitrator for implantable cardioverter defibrillator placement in HCM when risk stratification by conventional methods using the major risk factors is unclear.

Essentials 7

■ Case

A 30-year-old man with acute chest pain presents for cardiac magnetic resonance (CMR).

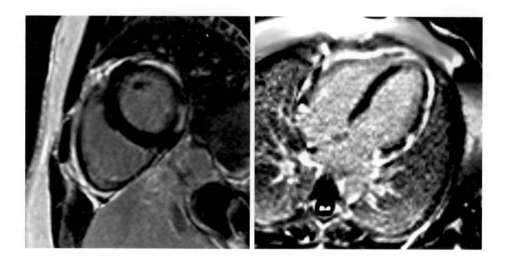

■ Questions

1. The CORRECT diagnosis is:
   A. Acute myocardial infarction
   B. Acute myocarditis
   C. Hypertrophic cardiomyopathy
   D. Stress cardiomyopathy
   E. Idiopathic dilated cardiomyopathy

2. The MOST COMMON etiology in patients presenting with chest pain, elevated troponin, and normal coronary arteries is which of the following?
   A. Acute myocardial infarction
   B. Acute myocarditis

C. Hypertrophic cardiomyopathy
D. Stress cardiomyopathy
E. Kawasaki disease

3. Linear mid-wall enhancement in the septum is a feature of which of the following conditions?
   A. Idiopathic dilated cardiomyopathy
   B. Hypertrophic cardiomyopathy
   C. Ischemic cardiomyopathy
   D. Cardiac amyloidosis
   E. Eosinophilic myocarditis

■ Answers and Explanations

Question 1

B. Correct! There is subepicardial enhancement in the lateral wall. There is corresponding mild hypokinesis in this segment in the midventricular level (see cine images). These are features of acute myocarditis.

Other choices and discussion

A. Myocardial infarction is characterized by enhancement in a coronary artery distribution involving the subendocardium.

C. HCM is characterized by hypertrophy involving one or more segment > 15 mm. Late gadolinium enhancement typically shows enhancement in a patchy mid-wall distribution at the junction points of the right ventricle and left ventricle (LV) and elsewhere in a thickened myocardium.

D. Stress cardiomyopathy is characterized by apical wall motion abnormality, myocardial edema, and no delayed enhancement.

E. Idiopathic DCM shows LV dilatation and reduced global wall motion. The majority of patients do not show delayed enhancement.

Question 2

B. Correct! Acute myocarditis is usually due to a viral infection of the myocardium with normal coronary arteries. Several studies have shown that the most common underlying etiology of patients presenting with suspected acute coronary syndrome and unobstructed coronary arteries is myocarditis.

Other choices and discussion

A. AMI is usually due to rupture of an unstable plaque in the presence of preexisting coronary artery disease. A total of 7 to 10% of patients presenting with ST-elevation myocardial infarction and 10 to 15% of patients presenting with non-ST-elevation myocardial infarction have unobstructed coronary artery disease on urgent angiography. AMI with unobstructed coronary arteries is the second most common etiology in this cohort of patients. Several different pathophysiologic mechanisms have been proposed to explain this phenomenon (e.g., rupture or erosion of a vulnerable plaque causing transitory occlusion that resolves spontaneously without leaving any residual visible intracoronary lesion) and distal vessel or small-caliber side-branch disease. Other mechanisms include distal embolization, coronary vasospasm, and inflammation.

C. HCM may present with acute chest pain, elevated troponins, and normal large epicardial coronary arteries, due to a mismatch between oxygen demands of the hypertrophied myocardium and blood supply in the presence of small vessel disease. However, this is a rare presentation of the disease and an uncommon diagnosis in this cohort of patients.

D. Stress cardiomyopathy is the third most common cause of chest pain, elevated troponins, and normal coronary arteries. It is characterized by reversible wall motion abnormalities involving the LV apex in the presence of unobstructed large epicardial coronary arteries.

E. Chest pain in Kawasaki disease is due to coronary aneurysms, thromboembolic disease, and myocardial infarction. Overall, it is an uncommon cause of chest pain in this cohort of patients.

Question 3

A. Correct! The majority of patients with idiopathic DCM do not show enhancement. However, approximately 40% can show mid-wall linear enhancement in the septum.

Other choices and discussion

B. The majority of patients with HCM show patchy mid-wall enhancement in the hypertrophied segments.

C. Ischemic cardiomyopathy is characterized by subendocardial enhancement in a coronary artery distribution.

D. In cardiac amyloidosis, there is global subendocardial enhancement or diffuse enhancement throughout the myocardium.

E. Eosinophilic myocarditis is characterized by global subendocardial enhancement in the apical regions, and apical LV thrombus may also be present.

■ Suggested Reading

Dastidar AG, Rodrigues JCL, Ahmed N, et al. The role of cardiac MRI in patients with troponin-positive chest pain and unobstructed coronary arteries. Curr Cardiovasc Imaging Rep 2015;8:28

Top Tips

- ◆ Acute myocarditis is usually due to a viral infection of the myocardium and may present with acute chest pain in the presence of normal coronary arteries.

- ◆ CMR is useful for noninvasive diagnosis and risk stratification in acute myocarditis.

- ◆ CMR features of acute myocarditis include wall motion abnormalities, pericardial effusion, myocardial edema, and typically subepicardial delayed enhancement, particularly in the lateral wall of the LV.

Essentials 8

■ Case

A 35-year-old woman presents with heart failure and monocular blindness.

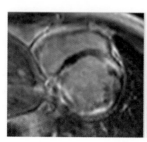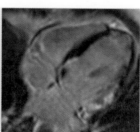

■ Questions

1. The CORRECT diagnosis is:
   A. Multivessel coronary artery disease
   B. Cardiac sarcoidosis
   C. Arrhythmogenic right ventricular dysplasia/ cardiomyopathy
   D. Idiopathic dilated cardiomyopathy
   E. Hypertrophic cardiomyopathy

2. Which of the following statements BEST characterizes the case diagnosis?
   A. A majority of patients are symptomatic.
   B. Histologic confirmation is needed before treatment.
   C. Conduction disturbances may be evident on electrocardiogram.
   D. Corticosteroid treatment is contraindicated.
   E. Pathognomonic findings are seen on echocardiography.

3. The most common area of scarring/late gadolinium enhancement in cardiac sarcoidosis is:
   A. Basal interventricular septum
   B. Inferior left ventricle
   C. Lateral left ventricle
   D. Anterior left ventricle
   E. Anterior right ventricle

---

* Videos in this chapter can be accessed at MediaCenter.Thieme.com. Please follow the instructions found on the MediaCenter page at the front of this book.

■ Answers and Explanations

Question 1

B. Correct! Multiple patchy areas of delayed enhancement, including mid-wall and subepicardial enhancement, and involvement of the interventricular septum, are features of CS. The blindness from optic neuropathy favors a multisystem disorder. The left ventricle (LV) is dilated with global hypokinesis and a severely depressed ejection fraction (see cine movies).

Other choices and discussion

A. In cardiomyopathy due to coronary artery disease, enhancement always involves the subendocardium in a coronary artery distribution.

C. Arrhythmogenic right ventricular dysplasia/cardiomyopathy is characterized primarily by right ventricle segmental wall motion abnormalities, dilatation, and dysfunction. LV abnormalities may also occur, and delayed enhancement may involve either ventricle in a non-ischemic pattern.

D. Idiopathic dilated cardiomyopathy is characterized by no delayed enhancement or linear mid-wall enhancement in a dilated and poorly functioning LV.

E. Hypertrophic cardiomyopathy is characterized by LV hypertrophy > 15 mm in one or more segments. There may be patchy mid-wall enhancement in the hypertrophied segments.

Question 2

C. Correct! The primary clinical manifestations of CS, in order of frequency, include conduction abnormalities and arrhythmias, congestive heart failure, and sudden death. Conduction abnormalities in CS vary from isolated bundle branch block to complete heart block, which can be detected in 23 to 30% of cases. Electrocardiogram conduction abnormalities of second- or third-degree heart block are one of the diagnostic criteria for CS.

Other choices and discussion

A. Clinical findings of myocardial involvement are evident in only about 5% of patients with sarcoidosis. However, autopsy studies have revealed a relatively greater prevalence of subclinical myocardial involvement, ranging from 20 to 60%.

B. Endomyocardial biopsy is an invasive technique with low sensitivity due to patchy involvement of the myocardium. Therefore, the decision to initiate treatment is based largely on the patient's clinical symptoms, imaging findings, and the course of the disease, rather than by histologic confirmation.

D. Immunosuppressive therapy with systemic corticosteroids and other immunomodulators is the current standard treatment for CS. Because of the critical nature of re-entrant arrhythmias and the increased risk for sudden cardiac death, some experts advocate early use of implantable cardiac devices, particularly defibrillators, in patients with biopsy-proven systemic sarcoidosis and positive cardiac imaging results.

E. Echocardiography has no pathognomonic finding for CS but will often be the first imaging test ordered for patients clinically suspected of having this entity. Echocardiographic findings may include regional wall motion abnormalities, aneurysms, thinning of the basal septum, a dilated LV, and impaired right or left ventricular systolic or diastolic function.

Question 3

A. Correct! The basal interventricular septum is the most common area of involvement and LGE in cardiac sarcoidosis. Subepicardial scars are most common, followed by mid myocardial and subendocardial scars.

■ Suggested Reading

Jeudy J, Burke AP, White CS, et al. Cardiac sarcoidosis: the challenge of radiologic-pathologic correlation: from the radiologic pathology archives. Radiographics 2015;35:657–679

Top Tips

◆ The spectrum of findings in CS includes conduction abnormalities, ventricular or supraventricular arrhythmias, heart failure, and sudden death.

◆ LGE in the basal septum in a subepicardial or mid-wall pattern is the most common cardiac magnetic resonance finding in CS.

◆ Studies investigating the usefulness of cardiac magnetic resonance and, in particular, the LGE sequence for the diagnosis of CS, report a sensitivity of 75 to 100% and specificity of up to 78%.

Essentials 9

■ Case

A 70-year-old man presents with heart failure.

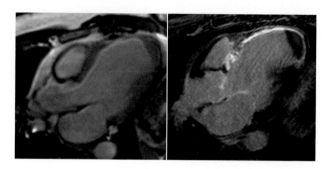

■ Questions

1. Based upon these images provided (still images from a cine three-chamber view and late gadolinium enhancement [LGE]), the MOST likely diagnosis is:
   A. Amyloid heart disease
   B. Ischemic cardiomyopathy
   C. Idiopathic dilated cardiomyopathy
   D. Hemochromatosis
   E. Cardiac sarcoidosis

2. Which of the following sequences for delayed enhancement would be preferable for infarct detection in a patient with heart failure requiring rapid imaging because of difficulty with breath holding?
   A. Segmented inversion recovery (IR)-GRE
   B. Single shot IR steady state free precession (SSFP)
   C. Three-dimensional (3D) IR with navigator gating
   D. 3D IR sequence in a single breath hold
   E. T1 mapping

3. The MOST sensitive technique for cardiac thrombus detection is:
   A. Transthoracic echocardiography (TTE)
   B. Cine SSFP
   C. LGE with a 250- to 300-ms inversion time 10 minutes after gadolinium administration
   D. LGE with a 600- to 800-ms inversion time 10 minutes after gadolinium administration
   E. Contrast ventriculography

---

* Videos in this chapter can be accessed at MediaCenter.Thieme.com. Please follow the instructions found on the MediaCenter page at the front of this book.

◼ Answers and Explanations

Question 1

B. Correct! The most likely diagnosis is ischemic cardiomyopathy. Ischemic cardiomyopathy due to coronary artery disease is characterized by enhancement involving the subendocardium in a coronary distribution. Note extensive enhancement that is near transmural, with subendocardial involvement in the anterior wall, apex, and septum in the left anterior descending coronary artery distribution. There is also a low-signal intensity structure attached to the left ventricle apex, representing a thrombus.

Other choices and discussion

A. Cardiac amyloidosis features include left ventricle hypertrophy and diffuse myocardial or global subendocardial enhancement.

C. Idiopathic dilated cardiomyopathy shows none or mid-wall enhancement.

D. Hemochromatosis may present as a dilated cardiomyopathy. T2* decay signal is characteristically reduced. LGE is not a specific finding.

E. Cardiac sarcoidosis typically demonstrates a patchy non-ischemic heart disease pattern of enhancement in the sub-epicardium or mid-wall of the myocardium, most often with involvement of the basal septum.

Question 2

B. Correct! A single-shot IR SSFP delayed enhancement sequence is the preferred option in patients requiring rapid imaging and who are unable to perform multiple breath holds such as in heart failure. The entire ventricle is covered in a short single breath hold of approximately 16 seconds. The sequence can also be performed during shallow breathing with little motion artifact.

Other choices and discussion

A. A segmented IR-GRE sequence is the reference standard for delayed enhancement. Here, each slice is performed with a single breath hold, with the entire ventricle covered in 8 to 10 breath holds and a mean imaging time of 5 to 8 minutes. This sequence has higher signal-to-noise ratio and carrier-to-noise ratio.

C. A 3D IR-GRE sequence performed during free breathing with a navigator beam placed on the diaphragm for respiratory gating is an option in patients unable to breath hold for LGE. However, the examination times are long, in the range of 10 to 15 minutes.

D. A 3D IR-GRE sequence can be used to cover the left ventricle in single or multiple breath holds. However, acquisition times are longer compared to a single shot IR-SSFP sequence.

E. T1 mapping techniques are emerging noncontrast sequences for myocardial tissue characterization, particularly for diffuse diseases involving the myocardium, and have the advantage of not requiring intravenous gadolinium. T1 mapping is not a standard sequence at this time for delayed enhancement and infarct detection, and breath holding is required.

Question 3

D. Correct! Thrombus (avascular tissue) typically lacks contrast enhancement. Viable myocardium also has a lower degree of contrast enhancement as compared to infarcted myocardium (note that scar tissue has the greatest enhancement). A tailored delayed enhancement cardiac magnetic resonance (CMR) sequence in which the inversion time is increased from that needed to null viable myocardium (250 to 350 msec) to a fixed time (600 msec) needed to selectively null avascular tissue such as thrombus optimizes thrombus detection. With this "long inversion time" (long-TI) sequence, regions with contrast uptake (i.e., left ventricle [LV] cavity and myocardium) appear bright, thrombus appears homogeneously black, and there is improved thrombus delineation.

Other choices and discussion

A. TTE remains the imaging modality most widely used to screen for LV thrombi, as it is cost-effective, accessible, and noninvasive. Despite the widespread use of TTE, diagnostic performance is suboptimal, with a sensitivity of only 33% and a specificity of 91%. Contrast echocardiography has been shown to significantly improve detection of an LV thrombus, enhancing endocardial border definitions, and overall, improve image quality.

B. Cine SSFP may miss thrombi which have isointense signal relative to myocardium or small adherent thrombi.

C. Delayed enhancement (DE)-CMR can establish LV thrombus based on avascular tissue characteristics, an approach that has been shown to be highly accurate in multiple validation studies. On standard DE-CMR, a thrombus typically has an etched appearance, whereas viable myocardium is black and infarcted myocardium is white. The diagnosis of thrombus by standard DE-CMR can sometimes be challenging, as both viable myocardium and thrombus appear relatively dark and are difficult to distinguish from one another.

E. Contrast ventriculography is not a technique specifically used for thrombus detection.

Top Tips

- ◆ Ischemic heart disease is characterized by subendocardial enhancement in a coronary artery distribution.

- ◆ Left ventricular thrombus is a frequent complication after anterior myocardial infarction with systolic dysfunction. Large infarcts, aneurysms, and a low ejection fraction are risk factors for cardiac thrombi.

- ◆ Comparative studies have demonstrated CMR with the LGE technique improves thrombus detection as compared to echocardiography. LGE using a fixed long inversion time of 600 to 800 ms optimizes thrombus detection.

Essentials 10

■ Case

An 8-year-old boy presents with chest pain.

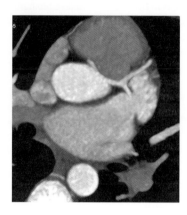

■ Questions

1. The computed tomography angiography (CTA) shows which ONE of the following abnormalities?
   A. Anomalous left main coronary artery from the right sinus with an interarterial course
   B. Anomalous right coronary artery from the left sinus with an interarterial course
   C. Normal coronary origins and proximal course
   D. Single coronary artery
   E. Circumflex coronary artery from the right sinus with a retroaortic course

2. The MOST common cause of sudden cardiac death (SCD) in young athletes is
   A. Hypertrophic cardiomyopathy
   B. Coronary anomalies of the wrong sinus with an interarterial course
   C. Arrhythmogenic right ventricular dysplasia
   D. Myocardial infarction
   E. Myocarditis

3. Which of the following is NOT an appropriate indication for coronary CTA (CCTA)?
   A. Suspected coronary anomaly
   B. Asymptomatic patient with a strong family history of coronary artery disease (CAD) and risk factors
   C. Ischemic symptoms, low to intermediate probability of CAD, and unable to exercise
   D. Persistent chest pain with a prior normal exercise stress test
   E. Acute chest pain low to intermediate probability of CAD with negative electrocardiogram and cardiac enzymes

■ Answers and Explanations

Question 1

B. Correct! The right coronary artery arises from the left sinus and has an interarterial course between the aorta and the main pulmonary artery.

Other choices and discussion

A. The left main coronary artery arises from the left coronary sinus.

C. In a normal person, the left main coronary artery arises from the left-facing sinus and the right coronary artery from the right-facing sinus.

D. There are two separate coronary arteries and two ostia.

E. The left circumflex artery arises normally from the left main coronary artery

Question 2

A. Correct! HCM is the most common cause of SCD in young athletes.

Other choices and discussion

B. Coronary artery anomalies of the wrong sinus with an interarterial course are the second most common cause of SCD in young athletes.

C, D, and E. Arrhythmogenic right ventricular dysplasia, myocardial infarction, and myocarditis are also recognized causes of sudden death. However, they are relatively uncommon compared to HCM and coronary anomalies.

Question 3

B. Correct! CCTA is considered inappropriate or uncertain for use in asymptomatic patients with risk factors. The use of a noncontrast calcium computed tomography scan is appropriate for risk stratification in such cases.

Other choices and discussion

A. CCTA is appropriate for evaluation of coronary anomalies.

C. The use of CCTA is appropriate in patients with ischemic symptoms, low to intermediate probability of CAD, and inability to exercise.

D. Persistent chest pain with a prior normal exercise stress test is an appropriate indication for CCTA.

E. Acute chest pain, low to intermediate probability of CAD, and negative electrocardiogram and cardiac enzymes are appropriate indications for CCTA.

■ Suggested Reading

Shriki JE, Shinbane JS, Rashid MA, et al. Identifying, characterizing, and classifying congenital anomalies of the coronary arteries. Radiographics 2012;32(2):453–468

Top Tips

- Coronary anomalies with origin from the opposite sinus and an interarterial course are the second most common cause of SCD in young patients after HCM.

- CCTA is a widely available, provides rapid examination, and is capable of depicting three-dimensional anatomy of the coronary arteries with a high spatial resolution. It is considered appropriate for use in the investigation of coronary artery anomalies.

- Other appropriate indications for CCTA include:

  ◇ Nonacute ischemic symptoms, low to intermediate probability of CAD, and inability to exercise

  ◇ Persistent chest pain with a prior normal stress test

  ◇ Acute chest pain, low to intermediate probability of CAD with a negative electrocardiogram, and cardiac enzymes

Essentials 11

■ Case

A 25-year-old woman presents with progressive shortness of breath.

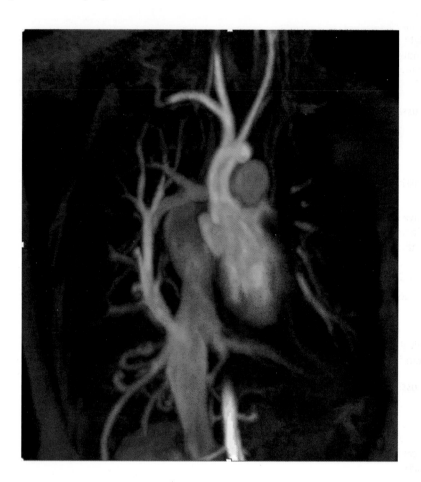

■ Questions

1. Based on review of the magnetic resonance angiogram (MRA), the CORRECT diagnosis is:
   A. Coarctation of the aorta
   B. Scimitar syndrome
   C. Congenital hypoplastic right lung
   D. Isolated pulmonic valve stenosis
   E. Total anomalous pulmonary venous return

2. MRA of the chest in routine clinical practice uses which ONE of the following sequences?
   A. Three-dimensional (3D) T1-weighted postcontrast spoiled gradient echo imaging
   B. 3D isotropic precontrast electrocardiogram-synchronized steady state free precession imaging
   C. Two-dimensional (2D) cine gradient echo noncontrast imaging
   D. 2D time-of-flight (TOF) imaging
   E. T1-weighted double inversion recovery turbo spin imaging

3. Which ONE of the following statements is INCORRECT regarding scimitar syndrome?
   A. Almost always occurs on the right side
   B. Associated congenital heart disease occurs in approximately 25%, with the most common associated lesion being a ventricular septal defect
   C. Recurrent respiratory symptoms and dyspnea are the most common presentations in adults
   D. May present in infancy with tachypnea, heart failure, and pulmonary hypertension
   E. Residual scimitar vein stenosis after repair is seen at follow up in approximately 15% of patients

■ Answers and Explanations

Question 1

B. Correct! Scimitar syndrome is characterized by (1) anomalous pulmonary venous return from all or a part of the right lung to the inferior vena cava (IVC), (2) hypoplasia of the right lung with abnormal segmental or lobar anatomy, (3) hypoplasia of the ipsilateral pulmonary artery, and (4) anomalous systemic arterial supply to the right lower lobe. Patients may exhibit some features of the syndrome, but others may not. The main feature is anomalous pulmonary venous return of all or a part of the right lung to the IVC.

Other choices and discussion

A. Coarctation of the aorta is a discrete obstructive lesion in the thoracic aorta usually located just distal to the origin of the left subclavian artery.

C. In congenital hypoplastic right lung, pulmonary venous return is usually normal.

D. Isolated pulmonic valve stenosis may lead to preferential enlargement of the main and left pulmonary arteries. However, there are other abnormalities in this case.

E. In total anomalous pulmonary venous return, all four pulmonary veins join the systemic veins. Left-sided pulmonary veins can be seen draining toward the left atrium in this case (see video).

Question 2

A. Correct! MRA in clinical practice routinely uses a 3D T1-weighted postgadolinium fast spoiled gradient echo technique.

Other choices and discussion

B. Electrocardiogram and respiratory (navigator) motion-corrected isotropic 3D steady state free precession imaging is an option for noncontrast MRA. However, it requires a longer acquisition time and greater operator skill, and is not utilized routinely in clinical practice.

C. MRA images are typically 3D acquisitions enabling multiplanar reformations. 2D cine imaging is performed without contrast for evaluation of intra- and extracardiac anatomy, morphology, and cardiac function, though it can also be performed after contrast administration to shorten examination times.

D. TOF technique relies on inflow enhancement to generate images of blood flow. 2D TOF imaging can be used to image the thoracic vessels. However, it has been replaced by 3D contrast-enhanced MRA owing to shorter acquisition times, greater anatomic coverage, and decreased pulsatility and flow artifacts.

E. T1-weighted double inversion recovery turbo spin imaging produces static 2D "black blood" images useful for evaluation of intra- and extracardiac anatomy and tissue characterization.

Question 3

B. Correct! This statement is false. Overall, 19 to 31% of patients with scimitar syndrome have associated cardiac anomalies. About 70% of these patients have an associated atrial septal defect. The syndrome also has been described less commonly in association with other cardiac malformations including tetralogy of Fallot, ventricular septal defect, coarctation of the aorta, hypoplastic left heart syndrome, total anomalous pulmonary venous connection, patent ductus arteriosus, cor triatriatum, bicuspid aortic valve, and subaortic stenosis.

Other choices and discussion

A. Scimitar syndrome almost always occurs on the right, though rare left-sided cases have been described.

C. In older children and adults, scimitar syndrome may present with dyspnea, fatigue, and recurrent respiratory infections, or may be an incidental finding on chest radiography.

D. The infantile form generally presents within the first 2 months of life with tachypnea, recurrent pneumonia, failure to thrive, and signs of heart failure. Pulmonary hypertension may be present.

E. The surgical repair of scimitar syndrome consists of redirecting the pulmonary venous drainage into the left atrium, either baffling the anomalous drainage into the left atrium via a tunnel or transecting the "scimitar drainage" near its entrance into the IVC and then re-implanting it directly into the left atrium. The majority of patients are asymptomatic at follow up. However, there is a relatively high incidence of residual scimitar drainage stenosis (15.5%) requiring reoperation or hemodynamic re-intervention (which is similar in the two reported surgical techniques).

■ Suggested Reading

Vida VL, Padalino MA, Boccuzzo G, et al. Scimitar syndrome: a European Congenital Heart Surgeons Association (ECHSA) multicentric study. Circulation 2010;122:1159–1166

Top Tips

◆ Scimitar syndrome is characterized by (1) anomalous pulmonic valve replacement from all or a part of the right lung to the IVC (this is the main feature); (2) right lung hypoplasia with abnormal segmental or lobar anatomy; (3) hypoplasia of the ipsilateral pulmonary artery; and (4) anomalous systemic arterial supply to the right lower lobe.

◆ Characteristic findings on chest X-ray include right lung hypoplasia, dextroversion of the heart, and an arcuate structure representing the scimitar vein coursing toward the right hemidiaphragm.

◆ Magnetic resonance imaging and computed tomography are useful for confirmation of the diagnosis and for surgical planning. Computed tomography provides high spatial resolution rapid imaging of cardiac and extracardiac anatomy. Cardiac magnetic resonance imaging has the added advantages of being nonionizing and able to accurately quantify right ventricular size and function, and quantify Qp/Qs as a measure of the degree of left-to-right shunt caused by the anomalous pulmonary venous drainage.

Essentials 12

■ Case

A 50-year-old woman presents with increasing shortness of breath on activity.

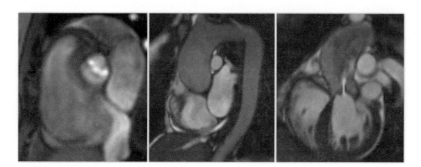

■ Questions

1. Which ONE of the following is the CORRECT diagnosis?
   A. Supravalvular left ventricular outflow tract obstruction
   B. Bicuspid aortic valve disease
   C. Subvalvular left ventricular outflow tract obstruction
   D. Degenerative tricuspid aortic valve stenosis
   E. Marfan syndrome

2. The magnetic resonance imaging technique used to measure flow and velocity is known as:
   A. Double inversion recovery spin echo imaging
   B. Steady state free precession cine imaging
   C. Phase contrast imaging
   D. Time-of-flight imaging
   E. Myocardial tagging

3. Which ONE of the following statements regarding aortic stenosis (AS) is TRUE?
   A. The normal aortic valve in an adult has an area of 4 to 5 cm².
   B. Severe AS is defined by an open valve area < 1 cm² or < 0.6 cm²/m² body surface area.
   C. In severe AS, the maximum velocity should exceed 3 m/s.
   D. Repair of the ascending aorta in bicuspid valve disease is indicated when the maximum dimension reaches 5 cm.
   E. Dilatation of the ascending aorta in BAV disease is dependent of the severity of AS.

---

* Videos in this chapter can be accessed at MediaCenter.Thieme.com. Please follow the instructions found on the MediaCenter page at the front of this book.

■ Answers and Explanations

Question 1

B. Correct! The aortic valve is bicuspid with two leaflets. There is aortic stenosis (dephasing jet originating at the aortic valvular level). The ascending aorta is dilated.

Other choices and discussion

A. Supravalvular LVOTO may occur rarely in isolation as an hourglass deformity or more often as a diffuse abnormality involving the entire aorta. Usually, supravalvular LVOTO is a part of Williams syndrome.

C. Subvalvular LVOTO is usually either a discrete fibromuscular ridge or a long fibromuscular narrowing beneath the base of the aortic valve.

D. The aortic valve is bicuspid.

E. Marfan syndrome is characterized by dilatation of the aortic root, including the annulus region, the sinuses, and efface-ment of the sinotubular junction. The aortic valve is typically tricuspid in Marfan syndrome.

Question 2

C. Correct! Phase contrast imaging is used to measure flow and velocity in the great vessels and in the heart.

Other choices and discussion

A. Double inversion recovery spin echo imaging produces black blood static images and is used to evaluate cardiac and great vessel morphology.

B. Steady state free precession imaging is a special form of cine gradient echo imaging and is the standard pulse sequence for evaluation of dynamic cardiac anatomy and function.

D. Time-of-flight imaging is a gradient echo imaging technique that uses the effect of inflowing nonsaturated blood to provide a magnetic resonance angiographic picture.

E. Myocardial tagging applies grid lines over the heart to quantify strain and deformation.

Question 3

B. Correct! In severe AS, the aortic valve open area is $< 1 \text{ cm}^2$ or $< 0.6 \text{ cm}^2/\text{m}^2$ body surface area.

Other choices and discussion

A. The normal aortic valve in an adult has an area of 3 to 4 cm^2.

C. In severe AS, the maximum velocity across the valve should be $\geq 4\text{m/s}$.

D. Repair of the ascending aorta in bicuspid valve disease is recommended when it reaches 5.5 cm or earlier at 4.5 to 5 cm if there is coexistent severe AS, progressive aortic dilatation, or a family history of sudden death due to aortic disease.

E. An aortopathy is believed to be present with BAVs and the dilatation of the ascending aorta is independent of the degree of AS.

■ Suggested Reading

Hiratzka LF, Bakris GL, Beckman JA, et al. ACCF/AHA/AATS/ACR/ASA/SCA/SCAI/SIR/STS/SVM guidelines for the diagnosis and management of patients with Thoracic Aortic Disease: a report of the American College of Cardiology Foundation/American Heart Association Task Force on Practice Guidelines, American Association for Thoracic Surgery, American College of Radiology, American Stroke Association, Society of Cardiovascular Anesthesiologists, Society for Cardiovascular Angiography and Interventions, Society of Interventional Radiology, Society of Thoracic Surgeons, and Society for Vascular Medicine. Circulation 2010;121:e266–369

Top Tips

◆ BAV is the most common congenital cardiac anomaly, occurring in 1 to 2% of the population with a male predominance.

◆ AS is the most common complication in patients with a BAV and occurs at an earlier age and a higher rate of progression compared to patients with tricuspid aortic valve disease.

◆ Dilatation of the ascending aorta is a frequent finding in BAV disease and is independent of the severity of valve dysfunction.

Essentials 13

■ Case

A young female patient presents with arrhythmia. Cine magnetic resonance (MR) still image in diastolic short axis plane is presented. Delayed enhancement images (not shown) were negative for late gadolinium enhancement.

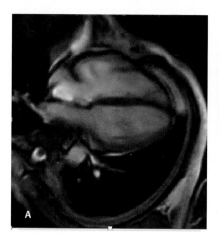
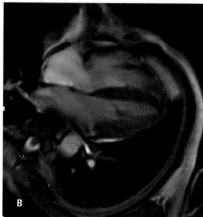
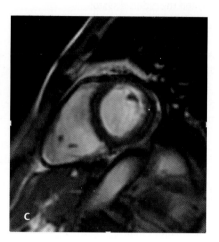

■ Questions

1. The CORRECT diagnosis is:
   A. Idiopathic dilated cardiomyopathy
   B. Hypertrophic cardiomyopathy
   C. Myocarditis
   D. Arrhythmogenic right ventricular dysplasia/ cardiomyopathy
   E. Cardiac sarcoidosis

2. Which of the following abnormalities is a prerequisite for cardiac MR (CMR) fulfillment of diagnostic criteria for the case syndrome?
   A. RV akinesia, dyskinesia, or dyssynchronous contraction
   B. Dilated RV

   C. Depressed RV ejection fraction
   D. Fat in the free wall of the RV
   E. Delayed enhancement of the RV wall

3. Which of the following statements is INCORRECT regarding ARVD/C?
   A. Familial cardiomyopathy with an autosomal dominant inheritance
   B. Affected individuals are usually in the second and third decades
   C. A normal CMR excludes the diagnosis of ARVD/C
   D. The abnormality is due to defect in desmosomes
   E. Recognized as a major cause of sudden cardiac death

---

* Videos in this chapter can be accessed at MediaCenter.Thieme.com. Please follow the instructions found on the MediaCenter page at the front of this book.

■ Answers and Explanations

Question 1

D. Correct! Akinesia, dyskinesia, or dyssynchronous right ventricle (RV) wall contraction in association with a dilated RV and reduced systolic function are features of arrhythmogenic right ventricular dysplasia/cardiomyopathy (ARVD). Note the aneurysmal segments in the anterior wall of the RV, the dilated RV, and the reduced systolic function.

Other choices and discussion

A. DCM is characterized by biventricular dilatation and global systolic dysfunction. Mid-wall delayed enhancement may occur in the septum.

B. Hypertrophic cardiomyopathy is characterized by hypertrophy involving one or more segments of the left ventricle ≥ 15 mm.

C. In myocarditis, the ventricles may be normal in size or dilated with regional or global dysfunction. Subepicardial or mid-wall delayed enhancement is a classic feature.

E. Cardiac sarcoidosis may present with features of DCM or restrictive cardiomyopathy. Global or segmental wall motion abnormalities may affect either ventricle. Typically, there is patchy mid-wall enhancement in the LV affecting the basal interventricular septum.

Question 2

A. Correct! RV akinesia, dyskinesia, or dyssynchronous RV contractions are essential criteria for the diagnosis of ARVD as per the current 2010 task force criteria for diagnosis of ARVD.

Other choices and discussion

B. The RV may be dilated in ARVD. However, it is not a prerequisite for the diagnosis and fulfills diagnostic criteria only when RV akinesia, dyskinesia, or dyssynchronous RV contraction is also present.

C. The RV ejection fraction may be depressed in ARVD. However, it is not a prerequisite for the diagnosis and fulfills diagnostic criteria only when RV akinesia, dyskinesia, or dyssynchronous RV contraction are also present.

D. Fat in the free wall of the RV is not required for CMR fulfillment of ARVD (per 2010 ARVD task force guidelines). Fat in the RV wall is a histologic criterion.

E. Delayed enhancement in the RV or the left ventricle may be present in ARVD reflecting fibrosis. However, it is not a diagnostic criterion.

Question 3

C. Correct! This statement about ARVD/C is incorrect. A definite diagnosis of ARVD is made on the basis of the presence of major and minor criteria encompassing structural, histologic, electrocardiographic, arrhythmic, and family history criteria, as proposed by the task force in 2010. A normal CMR does not exclude the diagnosis if other criteria are met.

Other choices and discussion

A. ARVD is a familial cardiomyopathy inherited as an autosomal dominant trait.

B. An affected individual typically presents in the second or third decade of life.

D. ARVD is associated with mutations in genes encoding proteins that are involved in the desmosome apparatus.

E. ARVD is recognized as a major cause of sudden cardiac death, particularly in the young and athletes.

■ Suggested Reading

Rastegar N, Burt JR, Corona-Villalobos CP, et al. Cardiac MR findings and potential diagnostic pitfalls in patients evaluated for arrhythmogenic right ventricular cardiomyopathy. Radiographics 2014;6:1553–1570

Top Tips

◆ ARVD/C is a familial cardiomyopathy resulting in progressive RV dysfunction and malignant ventricular arrhythmia. Affected individuals typically present in the second to fourth decade of life with arrhythmias originating from the RV.

◆ The diagnosis of ARVD/C is currently based on fulfilling a combination of clinical, imaging, pathologic, and/or genetic criteria set forth by the 2010 modified task force criteria.

◆ CMR is included in these criteria and plays an important role in the management of ARVD/C.

CMR major criteria for diagnosis of ARVD:

◆ Regional RV akinesia or dyskinesia or dyssynchronous RV contraction and one of the following:

  ◇ Ratio of RV end-diastolic volume to body surface area ≥ 110 mL/m² (male) or ≥ 100 mL/m² female)

  ◇ RV ejection fraction ≤ 40%

CMR minor criteria for diagnosis of ARVD:

◆ Regional RV akinesia or dyskinesia or dyssynchronous RV contraction and one of the following:

  ◇ Ratio of RV end-diastolic volume to body surface area ≥ 100 to < 110 mL/m² (male) or ≥ 90 to < 100 mL/m² (female)

  ◇ RV ejection fraction > 40% to ≤ 45%

Essentials 14

■ Case

A 65-year-old woman presents with heart failure.

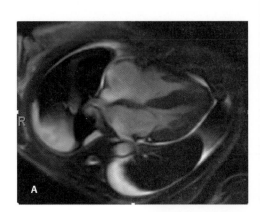

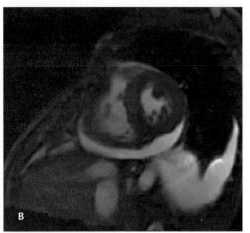

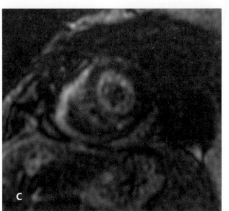

■ Questions

1. With the history and images provided, the CORRECT diagnosis is:
   A. Hypertrophic cardiomyopathy
   B. Arrhythmogenic right ventricle cardiomyopathy
   C. Dilated cardiomyopathy
   D. Cardiac amyloidosis
   E. Fabry disease

2. The MOST COMMON clinical presentation of the case diagnosis is:
   A. Atrial fibrillation
   B. Mitral insufficiency
   C. Aortic stenosis
   D. Restrictive cardiomyopathy
   E. Pericardial effusion and tamponade

3. Regarding imaging findings in cardiac amyloidosis, which ONE of the following statements is FALSE?
   A. Morphologic features include ventricular wall thickening, atrial enlargement, and pericardial effusion.
   B. Diffuse global myocardial enhancement or circumferential subendocardial enhancement are characteristic LGE patterns.
   C. On the inversion time scout, the blood pool crosses the null time before the myocardium.
   D. Impaired diastolic functional parameters are seen on echocardiography.
   E. Cardiac magnetic resonance imaging may detect abnormalities in suspected amyloid when echocardiography is normal.

■ Answers and Explanations

Question 1

D. Correct! Concentric thickening of the left ventricle (LV), bi-atrial dilatation, pericardial effusion, and global subendocardial delayed enhancement are typical magnetic resonance imaging (MRI) features of cardiac amyloidosis.

Other choices and discussion

A. Hypertrophic cardiomyopathy is characterized by hypertrophy involving one or more heart segments > 15 mm. Late gadolinium enhancement (LGE) typically shows atchy mid-wall enhancement at the junction points of the RV and LV in the septum and elsewhere in hypertrophied myocardium in a nonischemic distribution.

B. Arrhythmogenic RV cardiomyopathy is characterized by RV dyskinesia, akinesia, or dyssynchronous contraction, RV dilatation, and reduced RV ejection fraction.

C. In dilated cardiomyopathy, there is biventricular dilatation and thinning of the walls. Mid-wall delayed enhancement may occur in the septum.

E. Fabry disease may present with concentric LV hypertrophy. LGE typically involves the inferior lateral wall in a nonischemic distribution sparing the subendocardium.

Question 2

D. Correct! The most common clinical presentation of cardiac amyloidosis is diastolic dysfunction and restrictive cardiomyopathy.

Other choices and discussion

A. Atrial fibrillation may occur in cardiac amyloid. However, it is not the most common clinical presentation.

B. Atrioventricular valve regurgitation may occur in amyloidosis. However, it is not the most common clinical presentation.

C. The aortic valve may be thickened in cardiac amyloidosis. However, the presentation as aortic stenosis is rare.

E. Pericardial effusion is a common associated finding in cardiac amyloidosis. However, it is not usually a presenting feature.

Question 3

C. Correct! This statement is FALSE. Generally, the blood pool contains a higher concentration of gadolinium and passes through the null point before the myocardium. In cardiac amyloidosis, however, this normal blood-pool-to-myocardium relationship is reversed, and as such, the myocardium reaches the null point before the blood pool.

Other choices and explanations

A. Morphologic features of cardiac amyloidosis do include thickening of the walls of the ventricles, bi-atrial dilatation, thickening of the interatrial septum, and pericardial effusion.

B. Characteristic LGE patterns in amyloidosis include circumferential global subendocardial enhancement and diffuse myocardial enhancement.

D. Impaired diastolic function detected by echocardiography is a characteristic finding in cardiac amyloidosis.

E. Cardiac magnetic resonance imaging using the LGE technique can detect cardiac amyloidosis even when wall thickness is normal on echocardiography.

■ Suggested Reading

Cummings KW, Bhalla S, Javidan-Nejad C. A pattern-based approach to assessment of delayed enhancement in non-ischemic cardiomyopathy at MR imaging. Radiographics 2009;29:89–103

Top Tips

◆ Cardiac amyloidosis is a common cause and important differential diagnosis for diastolic dysfunction and restrictive cardiomyopathy, particularly in the elderly.

◆ Cardiac amyloidosis is characterized morphologically by thickened ventricular walls (in particular, concentric LV hypertrophy), atrial enlargement, valvular dysfunction, interatrial septal thickening, and pericardial effusions.

◆ LGE typically shows global subendocardial enhancement, diffuse myocardial enhancement, or inability to null the myocardium.

Essentials 15

■ Case

Cardiac magnetic resonance (CMR) in a patient with right heart failure is shown. Still images from a real-time acquisition are in Figure A. Please see cine clips.

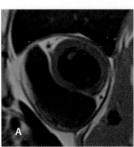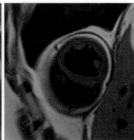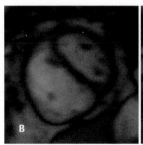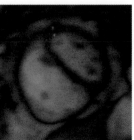

■ Questions

1. Which is the CORRECT diagnosis?
   A. Pulmonary hypertension
   B. Tricuspid insufficiency
   C. Ebstein anomaly
   D. Constrictive pericarditis
   E. Restrictive cardiomyopathy

2. The basic difference between a spin echo and gradient echo sequence is:
   A. Spin echo sequences are faster than gradient echo sequences.
   B. Spin echo sequences have T1 and T2 weighting, whereas gradient echo sequences have only T2-weighting.
   C. Fat is bright on spin echo sequences but not on gradient echo sequences.
   D. Gradient echo sequences deposit more energy into tissues.
   E. Spin echo sequences require a refocusing pulse to restore spin magnetization.

3. A patient undergoing CMR has a heart rate of 60 bpm. The duration of the cardiac cycle for the patient (R-R interval) is 1000 ms. To assess ventricular function, 25 phases are acquired per cardiac cycle. What is the temporal resolution of the sequence?
   A. 25 ms
   B. 40 ms
   C. 50 ms
   D. 60 ms
   E. 80 ms

---

* Videos in this chapter can be accessed at MediaCenter.Thieme.com. Please follow the instructions found on the MediaCenter page at the front of this book.

■ Answers and Explanations

Question 1

D. Correct! There is circumferential pericardial thickening > 4 mm. With inspiration, there is diastolic septal bounce and paradoxical motion toward the left ventricle. Note flattening of the septum on the real-time capture images in B and cine clips. These are features of constrictive pericarditis and help to differentiate it from restrictive cardiomyopathy, the most important differential.

Other choices and discussion

A. Pulmonary hypertension may also result in paradoxical septal motion. However, pericardial thickening and accentuation on real-time inspiratory imaging are not features.

B, C. Tricuspid insufficiency and Ebstein anomaly may lead to right heart failure. However, a regurgitant jet or morphologic abnormalities in the tricuspid valve will be seen.

E. See answer explanation for D.

Question 2

E. Correct! Spin echo sequences require 180-degree refocusing pulses to restore spin magnetization.

Other choices and discussion

A. In general, spin echo sequences take longer than gradient echo sequences.

B. Both spin echo and gradient echo sequences can have T1 and T2 weighting.

C. Fat is bright on both T1- and T2-weighted spin echo and gradient echo sequences

D. Energy deposited is a function of repetition time, flip angles, magnetic and gradient field strength, among others.

Question 3

B. Correct! The cardiac cycle is divided into 25 phases. Thus, each phase spans 40 ms (1000/25), which is the temporal resolution of the acquisition.

■ Suggested Reading

Verhaert D, Gabriel RS, Johnston D, et al. The role of multimodality imaging in the management of pericardial disease. Circ Cardiovasc Imaging 2010;3:333–343

Top Tips

- Pericardial thickening > 4 mm, diastolic septal bounce, and paradoxical septal motion toward the left ventricle are features of constrictive pericarditis. Other features include abnormalities in the contour of the pericardium, conical deformity ("tubing") of the ventricles, right atrial (sometimes bi-atrial) enlargement, and inferior vena cava plethora. Morphologic and physiologic abnormalities are well evaluated with CMR, but computed tomography is far superior in detecting any pericardial calcification.

- Spin echo sequences require a 180-degree refocusing pulse, and they provide a black blood effect in the cardiovascular system, especially when combined with a double inversion recovery prepulse to suppress blood signal. They are particularly useful in evaluation of cardiac anatomy and morphology, such as pericardial thickening.

- Rapid dynamic real-time cine cardiac images (one cardiac cycle or one R-R interval) may compromise temporal and spatial resolution. However, they provide a quick visual evaluation of cardiac function and septal motion (as in the presence of arrhythmia and constrictive pericarditis).

Image Rich 1

■ Case

Match the cardiac magnetic resonance images to the correct diagnosis.
- A. Apical hypertrophic cardiomyopathy
- B. Eosinophilic endomyocarditis
- C. Apical infarction and thrombus
- D. Left ventricular noncompaction

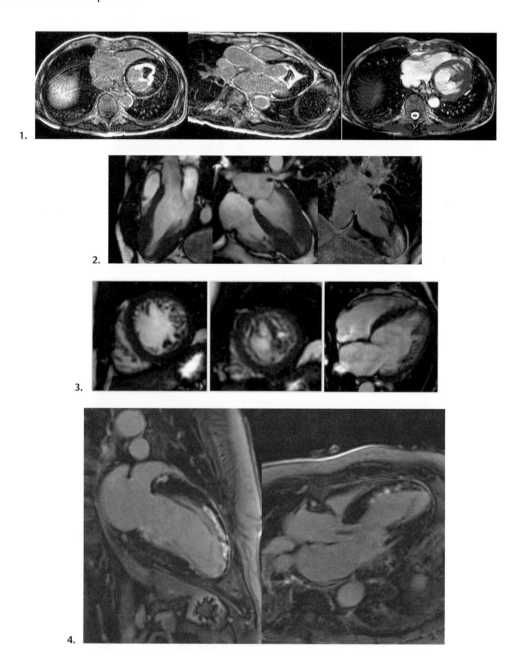

■ Answers and Explanations

1. B. Eosinophilic endomyocarditis. There is thickening of the left ventricle (LV) apex, diffuse subendocardial enhancement in the apical segments extending into the myocardium, and a nonenhancing low signal intensity structure representing a thrombus attached to the LV apex.

2. A. Apical hypertrophic cardiomyopathy. The muscle of the LV apex is disproportionately thickened compared to the base, and the apex-to-base-thickness ratio is > 1.5. The LV cavity has a spade-like shape. Diffuse enhancement is present in the LV apical myocardium.

3. D. Left ventricular noncompaction. Hypertrabeculated noncompacted myocardium is seen at the LV apex with a ratio of noncompacted to compacted myocardium > 2.3.

4. C. LV apical infarction. There is enhancement in the left anterior descending artery distribution involving the apical anterior wall, apical cap, and apical septum, affecting the subendocardium.

■ Suggested Reading

Cummings KW, Bhalla S, Javidan-Nejad C. A pattern-based approach to assessment of delayed enhancement in nonischemic cardiomyopathy at MR imaging. Radiographics 2009;29:89–103

Herzog B, Greenwood J, Plein S. Cardiovascular Magnetic Resonance Pocket Guide. Version 1.2. Updated 2016. http://www.cmr-guide.com

SECTION II
CARDIAC IMAGING

Top Tips

- The apical region of the LV can be difficult to visualize by echocardiography, and pathology affecting the apex is a common reason for cardiac magnetic resonance referral.

- Infarction in the LV apex is due to left anterior descending coronary artery disease and is recognized by enhancement involving the subendocardium with variable extent into the myocardium. It is important to search for and exclude an apical thrombus, for which magnetic resonance imaging is superior to echocardiography.

- Eosinophilic endomyocarditis can be seen in the setting of eosinophilia (either idiopathic, associated with neoplasms or other cause such as parasitic infection, and drugs). It is characterized by thickening of the LV apex due to eosinophilic infiltration, subendocardial enhancement extending to varying degrees into the myocardium, and often an associated apical thrombus.

- LV noncompaction is a genetic cardiomyopathy showing a two-layered myocardial structure with hypertrabeculated noncompacted myocardium and a thinner compacted layer. For diagnosis, the ratio of noncompacted to compacted myocardium should exceed 2.3 in diastole.

- Apical hypertrophic cardiomyopathy is a specific phenotype of hypertrophic cardiomyopathy preferentially affecting the apex of the LV, producing a spade-like left ventricular cavity. The thickness of the apical segments typically exceeds 13 mm, with a ratio of apical to basal segmental thickness > 1.5. Delayed enhancement may be seen within the muscle of the thickened LV apex and the apex may be aneurysmal.

Image Rich 2

■ **Case**

Match the atrial septal defects (ASDs) to the correct diagnosis.
   A. Sinus venosus ASD
   B. Secundum ASD
   C. Atrioventricular septal defect
   D. Unroofed coronary sinus/coronary sinus ASD

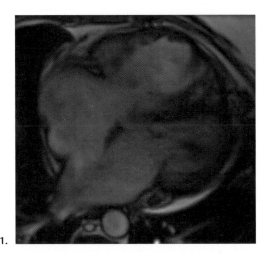

1.

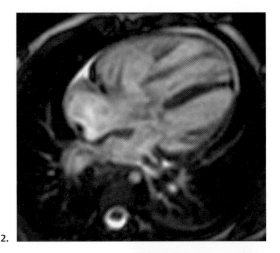

2.

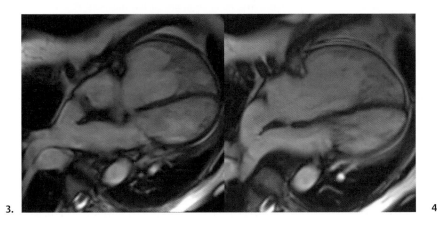

3.

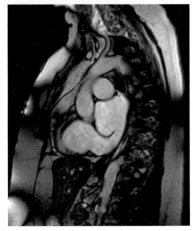

4.

■ Answers and Explanations

1. B. An ostium secundum ASD is present and located at the fossa ovalis region.

2. C. Atrioventricular septal defect. During embryologic development, the endocardial cushions form the medial aspects of the mitral and tricuspid valves, the portion of the atrial septum adjacent to the atrioventricular valves, and the inlet portion of the ventricular septum. An ostium primum ASD (located immediately posterior to the atrioventricular valves) associated with abnormal development of the atrioventricular valves or ventricular septum is known as an endocardial cushion defect.

3. A. There is a superior sinus venosus ASD defect located high in the interatrial septum communicating the right atrium–superior vena cava (SVC) junction with the left atrium.

4. D. A coronary sinus ASD results from a lack of septation between the inferior left atrium and the roof of the coronary sinus, allowing communication between the left and right atria.

■ Suggested Reading

Rojas CA, El-Sherief A, Medina HN, Chung JH, Choy G, Ghoshhajra BB, Abbara S. Embryology and Developmental Defects of the Interatrial Septum. Am J Roentgenol 2010 195:5, 1100–1104

Top Tips

◆ ASDs are classified according to their location along the atrial septum.

◆ Ostium primum ASDs are immediately posterior to the atrioventricular valves. Ostium secundum ASDs are located at the fossa ovalis region. During embryologic development, the endocardial cushions form the medial aspects of the mitral and tricuspid valves, the portion of the atrial septum adjacent to the atrioventricular valves, and the inlet portion of the ventricular septum. An ostium primum ASD associated with abnormal development of the atrioventricular valves or ventricular septum is known as endocardial cushion defect. A superior sinus venosus ASD defect communicates the right atrium–SVC junction with the left atrium and is located high up in the interatrial septum. It is associated in more than 90% of cases with partial anomalous pulmonary venous return of the right upper lobe pulmonary vein to the SVC. A coronary sinus ASD results from a lack of septation between the inferior left atrium and the roof of the coronary sinus, allowing communication between the left and right atria.

◆ Cardiac magnetic resonance allows accurate identification of ASDs with respect to location and size, associated partial anomalous pulmonary venous return, and a measurement of ventricular volumes, function, and estimation of the Qp/Qs for shunt quantification.

Image Rich 3

■ Case

Match the cardiac magnetic resonance images to the correct postoperative adult congenital heart disease.
   A. Repaired tetralogy of Fallot
   B. D-Transposition of the great arteries postarterial switch
   C. D-TGA postatrial switch
   D. Fontan procedure

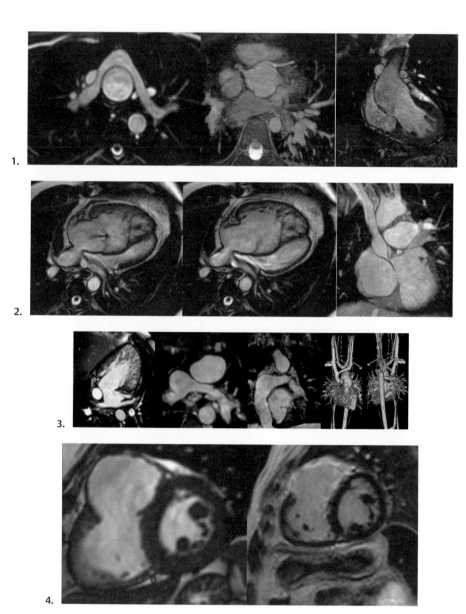

1.

2.

3.

4.

■ Answers and Explanations

1. B. D-TGA postarterial switch. The main pulmonary artery and its branching, located immediately anterior to the aorta and behind the sternum, is a characteristic configuration of the great vessel postarterial switch operation. The aortic root is dilated, which is a recognized complication of postarterial switch. There is narrowing of the ostial left main coronary artery.

2. C. D-TGA postatrial switch. The left-sided pulmonary veins can be seen routed into the right atrium and draining into the right ventricle. The right ventricle is dilated, hypertrophied, and has a markedly reduced systolic function, as it is the systemic ventricle connected to the aorta. There is tricuspid regurgitation. The SVC can be seen baffled to the left-sided atrium, and the lower aspect of the baffle is narrowed.

3. D. Fontan procedure. There is a single functional ventricle in this patient with hypoplastic left heart syndrome. The defect has been palliated with a total cavopulmonary connection, with the superior vena cava and inferior vena cava directly connected to the pulmonary arteries. This constitutes the Fontan procedure.

4. A. Postoperative tetralogy of Fallot. The right ventricle is markedly dilated. The outflow tract region is thin, aneurysmal, and shows delayed enhancement. The most common postoperative complications in treated tetralogy of Fallot is pulmonary insufficiency leading to progressive RV dilatation and dysfunction. The outflow tract region replaced by a patch may be aneurysmal and scarred.

■ Suggested Reading

Gaca AM, Jaggers JJ, Dudley LT, Bisset III GS. Repair of Congenital Heart Disease: A Primer–Part 1. Radiology 2008 247:3, 617–631

Gaca AM, Jaggers JJ, Dudley LT, Bisset III GS. Repair of Congenital Heart Disease: A Primer—Part 2. Radiology 2008 248:1:44–60

Top Tips

- ◆ Cardiac magnetic resonance imaging allows comprehensive evaluation of intracardiac and extracardiac anatomy, and ventricular function and flow in adult congenital heart disease. It is the test of choice for follow up of these patients.

- ◆ The most common complication in adult tetralogy of Fallot survivors post repair is pulmonic insufficiency and right ventricular enlargement. If right ventricular outflow tract patch reconstruction was performed, the outflow tract region may be aneurysmal and delayed enhancement may be present. Both findings are considered risk factors for adverse events, including arrhythmias in adult survivors of tetralogy of Fallot repair.

- ◆ D-TGA (atrioventricular concordance and ventricular great artery discordance) is corrected anatomically and physiologically in the current era with an arterial switch procedure. First, the left and right coronary arteries are transferred to the posterior artery (the main pulmonary artery, now the "neo-aorta") and then the gaps in the aorta are patched. The supravalvular ascending aorta and supravalvular main pulmonary are then transected and switched. This redirects blood flow in the normal way. The neo-aorta is positioned posteriorly to the main pulmonary artery bifurcation after an arterial switch operation. Major complications after an arterial switch procedure are coronary artery obstruction, right ventricular outflow tract obstruction, and neo-aortic root dilatation.

- ◆ Atrial switch operations for D-TGA were performed until the late 20th century. Venous blood is redirected to the opposite ventricle either using native atrial (Sennings procedure) or pericardial or synthetic patches (Mustard procedure). After an atrial level switch, the right ventricle remains as the systemic ventricle pumping blood into the aorta, with the left ventricle as the subpulmonic ventricle pumping blood to the lungs. Complications in adult survivors after an atrial level switch include baffle obstruction or leak, systemic right ventricular failure, outflow tract obstruction, and arrhythmias.

- ◆ The Fontan procedure or total cavopulmonary connection is performed to treat several complex congenital heart abnormalities with a single functioning ventricle, including tricuspid atresia, pulmonary atresia with intact ventricular septum, hypoplastic left heart syndrome, and double-inlet ventricle. Modern total cavopulmonary circulation is achieved with direct anastomosis of the superior vena cava to the pulmonary arteries (a hemi-Fontan procedure) and construction of an intra-arterial tunnel or extracardiac conduit to direct flow from the inferior vena cava to the pulmonary arteries. Cardiac magnetic resonance imaging is the test of choice for comprehensive evaluation of the Fontan patient, and the examination should be focused on patency of the Fontan pathway, pulmonary veins, branch pulmonary arteries, single ventricle function, atrioventricular valve and aortic valve function, size of the thoracic aorta including the arch, and an assessment for collateral vessels.

Image Rich 4

■ Case

Match the cardiac magnetic resonance images and delayed enhancement patterns to the correct diagnosis.
- A. Infarction
- B. Cardiac amyloidosis
- C. Myocarditis
- D. Cardiac sarcoidosis

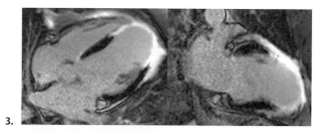

1.

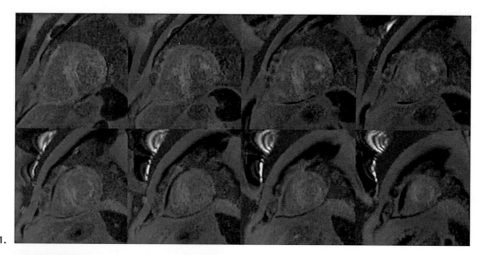

2.

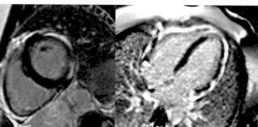

3.

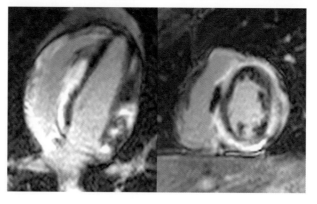

4.

■ Answers and Explanations

1. B. Cardiac amyloidosis. There is diffuse hyperenhancement throughout the left ventricle myocardium and an inability to null the myocardium. The blood pool appears unusually dark.

2. C. Myocarditis. There is subepicardial enhancement in the lateral wall, which is a typical finding.

3. A. Myocardial infarction. There is full-thickness transmural enhancement seen involving the subendocardium in the distal left anterior descending artery distribution: distal anterior wall, anterior septum, apical cap, and apical inferior wall.

4. D. Cardiac sarcoidosis. There is extensive enhancement in the left ventricular myocardium sparing the subendocardium in a nonischemic pattern. Enhancement is present in the basal interventricular septum, a typical location involved in cardiac sarcoidosis. The free wall of the right ventricle also enhances.

■ Suggested Reading

Cummings KW, Bhalla S, Javidan-Nejad C. A pattern-based approach to assessment of delayed enhancement in nonischemic cardiomyopathy at MR imaging. Radiographics 2009;29:89–103

SECTION II
CARDIAC IMAGING

Top Tips

Late gadolinium enhancement cardiac magnetic resonance imaging allows identification of etiology in cardiomyopathy patients with diverse presentations, including chest pain, heart failure, and arrhythmias. An important distinction is between ischemic and nonischemic cardiomyopathies. Late gadolinium enhancement in ischemic cardiomyopathy will involve the subendocardium and is in a coronary distribution. Cardiac amyloidosis causes diffuse hyperenhancement throughout the myocardium or global subendocardial enhancement. An inability to achieve proper nulling of the myocardium and an unusually dark appearance of the blood pool are also features of cardiac amyloidosis. Cardiac sarcoidosis is characterized by patchy nonischemic distribution of enhancement, and the basal interventricular septum is a typical location for involvement. Subepicardial enhancement in the lateral wall is a classical location for acute myocarditis, which may also produce a mid-wall pattern of enhancement. Dilated cardiomyopathy exhibits an enlarged globally hypokinetic ventricle with no enhancement or mid-wall enhancement in the interventricular septum.

Image Rich 5

■ Case

Match the chest X-ray findings to the correct diagnosis.
- A. Tetralogy of Fallot
- B. Constrictive pericarditis
- C. Atrial septal defect
- D. Mitral stenosis

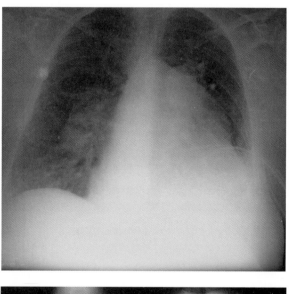

1.

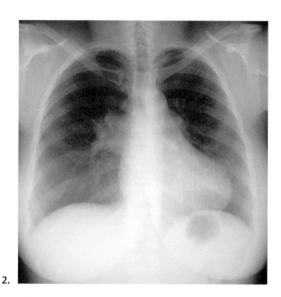

2.

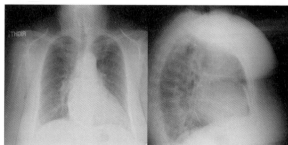

3.

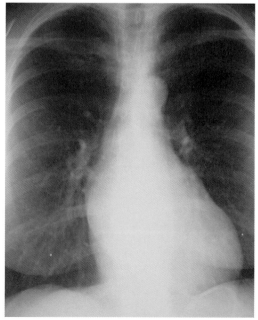

4.

■ Answers and Explanations

1. C. Atrial septal defect. The pulmonary arteries are markedly enlarged and there is increased pulmonary vascularity in the lungs indicating that a left to right shunt may be present. The heart is enlarged. An atrial septal defect is the most common cause of a left-to-right shunt in an adult and causes volume overloading of the right heart.

2. A. Tetralogy of Fallot. There is a typical boot-shaped configuration to the cardiac silhouette due to an upturned apex caused by right ventricle enlargement. The lung fields are oligemic due to reduced vascularity from right ventricular outflow tract obstruction.

3. B. Constrictive pericarditis. There is linear high density along the pericardium representing calcification. This is best seen on the lateral view. Such a finding is almost pathognomonic for the presence of constrictive pericarditis in a patient with typical symptoms.

4. D. Mitral stenosis. The left atrium (LA) is enlarged, causing a double density on the frontal view. There is enlargement of the left atrial appendage seen as a convexity of the left heart border below the left pulmonary artery.

■ Suggested Reading

Webb RW, Higgins CB. Thoracic Imaging: Pulmonary and Cardiovascular Radiology. Radiography of Heart Diseases: 768–818

Top Tips

◆ Several cardiac diseases are associated with pathognomonic chest X-ray findings allowing recognition.

◆ Among the congenital heart diseases, tetralogy of Fallot causes a typical boot-shaped cardiac silhouette, due to right ventricle enlargement, and an upturned cardiac apex. The lung fields are typically oligemic from reduced pulmonary blood flow due to right ventricular outflow tract obstruction. A right-sided aortic arch may be present in up to 25% of patients.

◆ Atrial septal defect is the most common shunt lesion in adults, causing a left-to-right shunt, dilated pulmonary arteries, right atrium and right ventricle enlargement, and pulmonary plethora.

◆ Pericardial calcification is often best appreciated on lateral radiographs as high density outlining the cardiac border. This allows a confident diagnosis of constrictive pericarditis on chest X-ray in patients with right heart symptoms and signs.

◆ Mitral stenosis is recognized by LA and LA appendage enlargement, right ventricle enlargement, and upper lung blood diversion.

More Challenging 1

■ Case

An 8-year-old girl presents with chest pain with exertion.

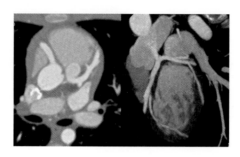

■ Questions

1. The CORRECT diagnosis is:
   A. Anomalous left main from the right sinus with an interarterial course
   B. Anomalous right coronary artery from the left sinus with a interarterial course
   C. Coronary artery fistula
   D. Anomalous left main coronary artery from the pulmonary artery
   E. Coronary arteriovenous malformation

2. Which ONE of the following is a *nonmalignant* coronary anomaly?
   A. Anomalous left main coronary artery from the right sinus with an interarterial course
   B. Anomalous right coronary artery from the left sinus with an interarterial course
   C. ALCAPA
   D. Right coronary artery to right atrial fistula
   E. Anomalous circumflex coronary artery from the right sinus with a retro-aortic course

3. All the following statements regarding ALCAPA are true EXCEPT:
   A. It presents in infancy with congestive heart failure and dilated cardiomyopathy.
   B. Mitral insufficiency and echogenic papillary muscles on echocardiography are recognized findings.
   C. Chest pain and myocardial ischemia are recognized presentations in older children and adults.
   D. The anomaly causes a right-to-left extracardiac shunt.
   E. The preferred treatment in the newborn and infants consists of a coronary button transfer.

■ Answers and Explanations

Question 1

D. Correct! The left main coronary artery arises from the main pulmonary artery (ALCAPA syndrome).

Other choices and discussion

A. The left main coronary artery does not arise from the right sinus.

B. The right coronary artery arises from the right sinus.

C. A coronary artery fistula is a direct communication from a coronary artery opening into a cardiac chamber.

E. Coronary arteriovenous malformations consist of an abnormal communication between a coronary artery and a cardiac chamber or adjacent vessel. The origins of the coronary arteries are normal.

Question 2

E. Correct! A retro-aortic course of an anomalous coronary artery is a benign (*nonmalignant*) abnormality, without risk of sudden death.

Other choices and discussion

A. Interarterial course of an anomalous coronary artery, particularly the left main coronary artery, is considered a dangerous or *malignant* anomaly, due to the risk of sudden death.

B. Interarterial course of the right coronary artery arising from the left sinus is also considered a dangerous or *malignant* anomaly, due to the risk of sudden death.

C. ALCAPA syndrome is a malignant or dangerous coronary anomaly, as it may be associated with arrhythmias, myocardial infarction, and sudden death.

D. Coronary artery fistula may be associated with myocardial ischemia, arrhythmias, and sudden death.

Question 3

D. Correct! This statement regarding ALCAPA is FALSE. In the ALCAPA syndrome, an extracardiac *left-to-right* shunt from the aorta via the right coronary artery and into the left coronary artery through coronary anastomosis and the low pressure pulmonary circulation occurs. Retrograde flow of contrast into the main pulmonary artery can be seen on image B (a contrast blush at the ostium of the left main coronary artery).

Other choices and discussion

A. This statement is true. ALCAPA is a consideration in infants presenting with congestive heart failure and a dilated heart.

B. Inadequate blood supply to the left ventricle myocardium may lead to myocardial infarction, including papillary muscle infarction, mitral insufficiency, and an echogenic appearance to the papillary muscles on echocardiography.

C. Chest pain and myocardial ischemia are recognized presentations in older adults.

E. The treatment of choice in newborns and infants is surgical repair using the coronary button transfer technique. This involves re-implantation of the anomalous left coronary artery along with a button of adjacent pulmonary artery tissue into the aorta.

■ Suggested Reading

Peña E, Nguyen ET, Merchant N, et al. ALCAPA syndrome: not just a pediatric disease. Radiographics 2009;29:553–565

Top Tips

◆ ALCAPA syndrome is a rare congenital anomaly in which the left coronary artery originates from the main pulmonary artery.

◆ There are two types: infant and adult types, each of which has different clinical manifestations and carries a different prognosis. The anomaly causes a left-to-right extracardiac shunt. It may present in infancy with congestive heart failure and dilated cardiomyopathy. Chest pain and myocardial ischemia are recognized presentations in older children and adults.

◆ On electrocardiogram-gated multidetector computed tomography and magnetic resonance angiographic images, direct visualization of the left coronary artery originating from the main pulmonary artery is a primary imaging feature of ALCAPA syndrome. Another important imaging feature is retrograde flow from the left coronary artery into the main pulmonary artery.

More Challenging 2

■ Case

Cardiac magnetic resonance (CMR) sequences, including resting cine and vasodilator stress perfusion images, from a 55-year-old man with stable chest pain on exertion are presented. The still image is a capture from the stress perfusion examination. See cine clips.

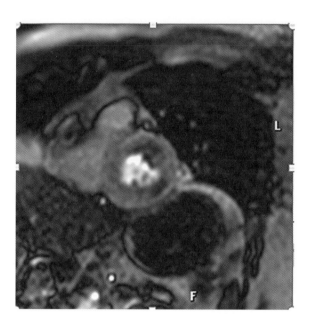

■ Questions

1. Choose the ONE best answer, based upon the information provided.
   A. Perfusion defects in the LAD and RCA distributions
   B. Perfusion defects in the LCX and RCA distributions
   C. Perfusion defects in the LAD and LCX distributions
   D. Susceptibility artifacts
   E. Hibernating myocardium in the LAD and LCX distributions

2. Choose the ONE correct statement regarding vasodilator stress perfusion CMR.
   A. The pharmacologic agent most commonly used is dobutamine.
   B. A fast T2-weighted sequence is used.
   C. CMR has higher spatial resolution than single photo emission computed tomography and is a better predictor of adverse events.

D. CMR requires administration of gadolinium contrast material at the rate of 2 to 3 mL/min.
   E. A reversible stress-induced area of myocardial perfusion in the presence of delayed enhancement is indicative of ischemia.

3. Which ONE of the following will increase the temporal resolution of a segmented cine gradient echo CMR acquisition?
   A. Decreasing the phase-encoding matrix from 160 to 128
   B. Decreasing the number of views per segment from 25 to 16
   C. Increasing the flip angle from 40 to 70 degrees
   D. Increasing the number of reconstructed phases from 25 to 30
   E. Increasing the pulse repetition time (TR)

---

* Videos in this chapter can be accessed at MediaCenter.Thieme.com. Please follow the instructions found on the MediaCenter page at the front of this book.

■ Answers and Explanations

Question 1

A. Correct! There are low signal intensity perfusion defects in the anterior wall and the inferior lateral wall of the left ventricle. The LAD supplies the anterior wall, anterior septum, anterior lateral wall, and the apical regions of the left ventricle. The LCX supplies the inferior lateral wall of the left ventricle.

Other choices and discussion

A. The RCA supplies the inferior septum and the inferior wall of the left ventricle, which shows normal perfusion on vasodilator stress.

B. The RCA supplies the inferior septum and the inferior wall of the left ventricle, which shows normal perfusion on vasodilator stress.

D. Susceptibility artifacts may appear as dark rim low signal intensity areas in the subendocardial region on perfusion CMR, although they are usually not persistent and do not confirm a coronary artery distribution.

E. Hibernating myocardium is characterized by reversible contractile dysfunction (hypokinetic myocardium at rest, with improvement in wall motion upon the administration of inotropes such as dobutamine) and downregulation of blood flow (perfusion defects on vasodilator stress MR) in the presence of chronic ischemia. Resting wall motion is normal in the test case.

Question 2

C. Correct! Stress perfusion CMR has a higher spatial resolution and image quality compared to SPECT and is a better predictor of major adverse cardiac events.

Other choices and discussion

A. The usual pharmacologic agent for vasodilator stress perfusion CMR is either adenosine or regadenoson (Lexiscan; Astellas US LLC, Northbrook, IL). Dobutamine is a positive ionotropic agent that may be used to induce wall motion abnormality at high doses as a manifestation of ischemia or to detect hibernating myocardium by improvement in wall motion at low doses.

B. Perfusion CMR uses a fast T1-weighted sequence postgadolinium infusion. A variety of pulse sequences are currently available for CMR perfusion imaging. These include gradient echo, hybrid gradient echo-planar imaging, and steady-state free precession sequences.

D. The recommended infusion rate of gadolinium for stress perfusion imaging is 4 to 5 mL/min.

E. Hypoperfused myocardium is generally identified as a hypointense area compared to normal myocardium. A reversible stress-induced area (perfusion defect at stress and not at rest) of hypoperfused myocardium in a coronary artery distribution that lasts eight heartbeats or longer in the absence of late gadolinium enhancement (LGE) is consistent with underlying coronary ischemia. An area of irreversible myocardial hypoperfusion (perfusion defect present at rest and stress) in a coronary distribution with matched LGE is seen in the setting of myocardial infarction or scarring.

Question 3

B. Correct! The temporal resolution of a segmented cine acquisition (i.e., the time between successive cine phases) is the product of the views per segment and the TR. Decreasing the number of views per segment will increase the temporal resolution.

Other choices and discussion

A. For a given heart rate, decreasing the number of phase-encoding steps will decrease the imaging time and spatial resolution. However, it will not affect the temporal resolution.

C. Increasing or decreasing the flip angle will affect signal and tissue weighting, but not the temporal resolution.

D. Increasing the number of reconstructed phases postacquisition will not affect the temporal resolution.

E. Increasing the TR will decrease the temporal resolution of a cine gradient echo acquisition.

■ Suggested Reading

Shehata ML, Basha TA, Hayeri MR, et al. MR myocardial perfusion imaging: insights on techniques, analysis, interpretation, and findings. Radiographics 2014;34:1636–1657

Top Tips

- CMR stress perfusion imaging has evolved to become a reliable and robust tool, providing accurate visual and quantitative assessment of regional myocardial perfusion. Owing to its high spatial resolution, noninvasive nature, and absence of ionizing radiation, CMR perfusion imaging has improved the detection of clinically relevant coronary artery disease when compared to SPECT.

- Reversible stress-induced area of hypoperfused myocardium involving the subendocardium and lasting more than eight heartbeats in a coronary artery distribution in the absence of LGE = ischemia.

- Irreversible hypoperfused myocardium with matched LGE = infarction/scarring.

- The usual pharmacologic agent used for CMR stress perfusion imaging is either adenosine or regadenoson. A fast T1-weighted gradient echo sequence is used, and the technique can be combined with cine imaging and delayed enhancement imaging to provide comprehensive assessment of cardiac function, ischemia detection, and viability in a single examination.

More Challenging 3

■ Case

An 18-year-old woman presents with fatigue and increasing shortness of breath on exertion.

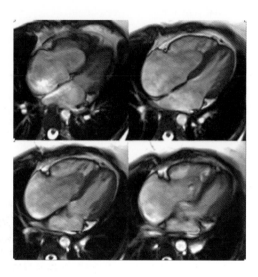

■ Questions

1. Which of the following is the CORRECT diagnosis?
   A. Arrhythmogenic right ventricular dysplasia
   B. Ebstein anomaly
   C. Uhl anomaly
   D. Tricuspid atresia
   E. Tetralogy of Fallot

2. Which ONE of the following is the most common lesion associated with the diagnosis above?
   A. Ventricular septal defect
   B. Patent foramen ovale
   C. Aortic coarctation
   D. Bicuspid aortic valve
   E. Patent ductus arteriosus

3. Which ONE of the following statements is FALSE regarding Ebstein anomaly?
   A. Ebstein anomaly is a rare congenital heart disorder occurring in ~1 per 200,000 live births and accounting for < 1% of all cases of congenital heart disease.
   B. Maternal lithium therapy can rarely lead to Ebstein anomaly in the offspring.
   C. Cardinal symptoms in Ebstein anomaly include cyanosis, right-sided heart failure, arrhythmias, and sudden cardiac death.
   D. Echocardiography is the diagnostic test of choice for Ebstein anomaly.
   E. The principal feature of Ebstein anomaly is apical displacement of the septal leaflet of the tricuspid valve from the insertion of the anterior leaflet of the mitral valve by at least 20 mm/m² body surface area.

---

* Videos in this chapter can be accessed at MediaCenter.Thieme.com. Please follow the instructions found on the MediaCenter page at the front of this book.

■ Answers and Explanations

Question 1

B. Correct! This patient has Ebstein anomaly. There is apical displacement of the attachment of the septal leaflet of the tricuspid valve. The anterior leaflet of the tricuspid valve is elongated, sail-like, and tethered. Tricuspid regurgitation is present. A portion of the RV is atrialized. These findings are all seen with Ebstein anomaly.

Other choices and discussion

A. Arrhythmogenic RV dysplasia is characterized by segmental RV wall motion abnormalities, RV dilatation, and reduced systolic function. Tricuspid valve morphology is normal in arrhythmogenic RV dysplasia.

C. Uhl anomaly of the RV is an unusual cardiac disorder with almost complete absence of RV myocardium, a normal tricuspid valve, and preserved septal and left ventricle myocardium.

D. Tricuspid atresia is defined as congenital absence or agenesis of the tricuspid valve. The RV is small and hypoplastic, and the right atrium is large.

E. Tetralogy of Fallot is characterized by an aorta overriding the RV, pulmonic stenosis, ventricular septal defect (VSD), and RV hypertrophy.

Question 2

B. Correct! An interatrial communication is present in 80 to 94% of patients with Ebstein anomaly. An atrial septal defect is present in more than one-third of cases, and most of the remainder have a patent foramen ovale, accounting for a right-to-left shunt. Additional less commonly associated anomalies include bicuspid or atretic aortic valves, pulmonary atresia or hypoplastic pulmonary artery, subaortic stenosis, coarctation, mitral valve prolapse, accessory mitral valve tissue, or muscle bands of the left ventricle, VSD, patent ductus arteriosus, and pulmonary stenosis.

Question 3

E. Correct! This is not true. The principal feature of Ebstein anomaly is apical displacement of the septal leaflet of the tricuspid valve from the insertion of the anterior leaflet of the mitral valve by at least *8 mm/m^2* body surface area.

Other choices and explanations

A. Ebstein anomaly is a rare congenital heart disorder occurring in ~1 per 200,000 live births and accounting for < 1% of all cases of congenital heart disease.

B. Most cases are sporadic, although there has been a link to maternal lithium therapy.

C. There is a range of clinical presentations, depending upon the severity of the lesion and associated tricuspid regurgitation. Infants with severe forms of the disease may present at birth with cyanosis and heart failure. Older patients may present with arrhythmias, right heart failure, fatigue, and exercise intolerance. Sudden death may occur from arrhythmias.

D. Precise evaluation of the tricuspid valve leaflets, chordal attachments, and the diagnosis of Ebstein anomaly can be made by echocardiography in most cases, due to its superior spatial and temporal resolution compared to cardiac magnetic resonance (CMR). CMR can be used as a complementary technique to assess tricuspid valve morphology and RV size and function, when echocardiographic windows are inadequate.

■ Suggested Reading

Attenhofer Jost CH, Connolly HM, Dearani JA, et al. Congenital heart disease for the adult cardiologist. Ebstein's anomaly. Circulation 2007;115:277–285

Top Tips

◆ The principal feature of Ebstein anomaly is apical displacement of the septal leaflet of the tricuspid valve from the insertion of the anterior leaflet of the mitral valve by at least 8 mm/m^2 body surface area. The anterior tricuspid valve leaflet is elongated, sail-like, and may be tethered to the RV wall. The right atrium is dilated and a portion of the RV is atrialized.

◆ The main hemodynamic abnormality producing symptoms in Ebstein malformation is tricuspid regurgitation.

◆ CMR imaging may be used to assess ventricular size and function as well as tricuspid valve morphology when echocardiographic image quality is inadequate.

More Challenging 4

■ Case

A 43-year-old woman has cardiac masses on echocardiography. A series of images from a cardiac magnetic resonance examination is presented in the following order: steady-state free precession, T1 BB, T1 BB with fat saturation, T2 BB with fat saturation, and late gadolinium enhancement (LGE).

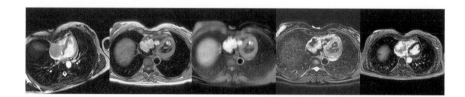

■ Questions

1. The correct diagnosis is MOST likely which of the following?
   A. Cardiac lipomas
   B. Metastases from melanoma
   C. Metastases from breast cancer
   D. Multiple myxomas
   E. Cardiac thrombi

2. Which of the following statements is TRUE regarding the most common location, site of origin, or involvement by cardiac tumors or tumor-like conditions?
   A. Myxoma: right atrium
   B. Papillary fibroelastoma: pulmonary valve
   C. Angiosarcoma: left atrium
   D. Lymphoma: epicardial surfaces of the heart and right atrium
   E. Carcinoid heart disease: left-sided heart valves

3. Which ONE of the following statements is TRUE regarding magnetic resonance signal characteristics of cardiac masses and tumors.
   A. Fibroma: isointense on T1, low on T2, and intense enhancement
   B. Metastases: low to isointense on T1, low on T2, and heterogenous enhancement
   C. Lipoma: low on T1, high on T2, and no enhancement
   D. Myxoma: isointense on T1, high on T2, and no enhancement
   E. Rhabdomyoma: isointense on T1, high on T2, and intense enhancement

SECTION II
CARDIAC IMAGING

■ Answers and Explanations

Question 1

B. Correct! There are masses in the right atrium and left ventricle, which have uniform high signal on T1-weighted imaging (without and with fat saturation), heterogeneous high signal on T2 imaging, and heterogeneous enhancement on LGE. These are features of melanoma metastases (in particular, the T1 hyperintensity). Most other cardiac metastases are low to intermediate signal on T1 imaging, high signal on T2 imaging, and with some enhancement on LGE.

Other choices and discussion

A. Cardiac lipomas will have high signal on T1-weighted imaging and will suppress on fat-suppressed imaging.

C. Most other cardiac metastases, including those due to breast cancer, are low to intermediate signal on T1 imaging, high signal on T2 imaging, and demonstrate some enhancement on LGE.

D. Myxomas are variable in signal intensity, usually low to intermediate on T1 imaging, intermediate to high signal on T2 imaging, and demonstrate some enhancement on LGE.

E. Cardiac thrombi are typically low on T1 and T2 and characteristically do not show enhancement on LGE (appearing dark).

Question 2

D. Correct! A unique feature of cardiac lymphoma is the tendency of the tumor to extend along the epicardial surfaces of the heart, primarily encasing adjacent structures including coronary arteries and the aortic root. Frequently, it also follows along the right atrioventricular groove and involves the base of the heart. When infiltration beyond the myocardium occurs, the right atrium is most commonly involved.

Other choices and discussion

A. The left atrium is the most common location for a myxoma, which typically appears as a pedunculated mass attached to the region of the fossa ovalis.

B. Papillary fibroelastomas are the most common valve tumors and are most often found attached to the aortic valve as small sessile or pedunculated masses.

C. Angiosarcomas are the most common primary malignancies arising in the heart and typically are located in the right atrium. They appear as aggressive, infiltrative masses arising from the atrial wall.

E. The vast majority of patients with cardiac involvement in carcinoid syndrome present with signs of right heart failure secondary to severe dysfunction of the tricuspid and pulmonary valves (regurgitation greater than stenosis). Thickening of the tricuspid valve and pulmonic valve and their subvalvular apparatus, valve dysfunction, and right-sided chamber enlargement may be noted on magnetic resonance imaging or computed tomography.

Question 3

A. Correct! Cardiac fibromas are typically isointense on T1 imaging, characteristically low on T2 imaging, and show intense enhancement postcontrast on LGE.

Other choices and discussion

B. Most cardiac metastases are typically low to isointense on T1, isointense to high on T2, and show heterogeneous enhancement postcontrast on LGE.

C. Lipomas are hyperintense on T1 and T2 imaging and typically show no LGE.

D. The signal characteristics of myxomas are variable depending on their composition. However, most are low to isointense on T1, high on T2, and show a variable degree of LGE.

E. Rhabdomyomas are isointense on T1, isointense to high on T2, and typically show no or minimal LGE.

■ Suggested Reading

Motwani M, Kidambi A, Herzog BA, et al. MR imaging of cardiac tumors and masses: a review of methods and clinical applications. Radiology 2013;268(1):26–43

Top Tips

- Approximately 75% of all primary cardiac tumors are benign, and the most common in the adult population are myxomas (50%), papillary elastomas (20%), lipomas (15–20%), and hemangiomas (5%). The other 25% of primary cardiac tumors are malignant—95% of these are sarcomas and 5% are lymphomas.

- Metastases involving the heart and pericardium (secondary cardiac tumors) from direct invasion or hematologic spread are 20 to 40 times more common than primary cardiac tumors.

- Magnetic resonance imaging can be used to evaluate the signal properties and morphologic characteristics of a cardiac mass and help to determine the nature of the mass lesion. Although cardiac metastases do not have any specific appearances, they generally have low signal intensity on T1-weighted images and high signal intensity on T2-weighted images—with the exception of melanoma metastases, which may appear bright on T1-weighted images because of the melanin pigment. The uptake of contrast material in metastases is usually heterogeneous.

More Challenging 5

■ Case

Cardiac magnetic resonance images of a 60-year-old patient are presented.

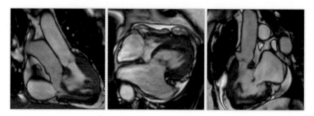

■ Questions

1. Which of the following is the CORRECT diagnosis?
   A. Tetralogy of Fallot
   B. Truncus arteriosus
   C. Double outlet right ventricle
   D. Double outlet left ventricle
   E. Congenitally corrected transposition of the great arteries (CCTGA)

2. The following is a feature of a morphologic LV:
   A. Trabeculated septal surface
   B. Moderator band
   C. Fibrous continuity between the AV and semilunar valve
   D. Thick muscular wall compared to the RV
   E. Origin to the aorta

3. Which ONE of the following statements is INCORRECT regarding the condition presented?
   A. The coronary arteries are inverted along with the ventricles: the morphologic right coronary artery is on the left side, and the morphologic left coronary artery is on the right side.
   B. Approximately 99% of patients with corrected transposition have associated anomalies such as VSD, pulmonary stenosis, or tricuspid valve abnormalities.
   C. A conduction abnormality frequently is present, and complete heart block develops in up to 30% of adolescents and adults with corrected transposition, which often necessitates implantation of an artificial cardiac pacemaker.
   D. The AV valves remain with their respective atria.
   E. Anatomic repair can be carried out by a double switch procedure.

---

* Videos in this chapter can be accessed at MediaCenter.Thieme.com. Please follow the instructions found on the MediaCenter page at the front of this book.

■ Answers and Explanations

Question 1

E. Correct! CCTGA is characterized by atrioventricular (AV) discordance and ventriculoarterial discordance. The right atrium enters the LV, which gives rise to the pulmonary artery, and the left atrium enters the RV, which gives rise to the aorta. It is also called L-transposition because the morphologic RV is in the levoposition on the left side of the LV. The aorta is usually, but not universally, anterior and to the left of the main pulmonary artery. Also, the great arteries may be side by side.

Other choices and discussion

A. Tetralogy of Fallot consists of the combination of pulmonic stenosis, aorta overriding the right ventricle, ventricular septal defect (VSD), and RV hypertrophy.

B. Truncus arteriosus is characterized by a single arterial vessel arising from the heart through a common arterial valve, giving origin directly to the systemic, pulmonary, and coronary arteries.

C. Double outlet RV is a ventriculoarterial connection, where > 50% of both great arteries arise from the RV.

D. Double outlet LV is a ventriculoarterial connection where > 50% of both great arteries arise from the LV.

Question 2

C. Correct! The morphologic LV shows fibrous continuity between the mitral valve and the semilunar valve.

Other choices and discussion

A. The septal surface of the morphologic LV is smooth, whereas the septal surface of the RV is trabeculated with origin to the septal leaflet of the tricuspid valve.

B. The moderator band is a feature of the morphologic RV.

D. The thickness of the ventricular chambers depends on the outflow pressures and is not necessarily a defining morphologic feature.

E. In a congenitally malformed heart, the aorta can arise from either or both ventricles.

Question 3

D. Correct! This statement is incorrect. The AV valves always remain with their respective ventricles (not with the atria) in hearts with abnormal segmental connections. Thus, the tricuspid valve is always connected to the morphologic RV and the mitral valve connected to the morphologic LV.

Other choices and discussion

A. The coronary anatomy is concordant in a CCTGA, and therefore the morphologic RV is perfused by a single right coronary artery on the left side and the morphologic LV is perfused by the left coronary artery on the right side.

B. Most patients have one or more associated cardiac anomalies, and the presence or absence of these markedly alters the natural history. The most common anomalies are VSD (70%), pulmonic stenosis (40%), and tricuspid valve abnormalities (90%), such as an Ebstein malformation or a dysplastic valve.

C. The AV node and His bundle have an unusual position and course, and many patients have dual AV nodes. The second anomalous AV node and bundle are usually anterior, and the long penetrating bundle is vulnerable to fibrosis with advancing age. There is a progressive incidence of complete AV block occurring at ~2% per year. Complete AV block develops in up to 30% of adolescents and adults with corrected transposition, which often necessitates implantation of an artificial cardiac pacemaker.

E. Complete anatomic repair in selected patients with CCTGA can be accomplished by an arterial switch procedure and a venous switch procedure (Mustard or Sennings; i.e., a double switch operation).

■ Suggested Reading

Warnes CA. Transposition of the great arteries. Circulation 2006;114:2699–2709

Top Tips

- CCTGA is characterized by AV discordance and ventriculoarterial discordance. The right atrium enters the LV which gives rise to the pulmonary artery, and the left atrium enters the RV which gives rise to the aorta. Thus, the circulation continues in the appropriate direction but flows through the "wrong" ventricles. The anomaly is also known as L-transposition of the great arteries, L-TGA. The RV is situated to the left of the LV (L-looped ventricles) and gives rise to the aorta usually situated anterior and to the left of the main pulmonary artery (L-configuration of the great vessels).

- The abnormality is compatible with long-term survival and longevity provided no major additional congenital defects are present. However, most patients have one or more associated cardiac anomalies, and the presence or absence of these markedly alters the natural history. The most common anomalies are VSD (70%), pulmonic stenosis (40%), and tricuspid valve abnormalities (90%) such as an Ebstein malformation or a dysplastic valve.

- Failure of the systemic RV and systemic (tricuspid) valve regurgitation are the major hemodynamic problems in long-term survivors.

Essentials 1

■ Case

A 21-year-old woman presents with pelvic pain and a positive pregnancy test.

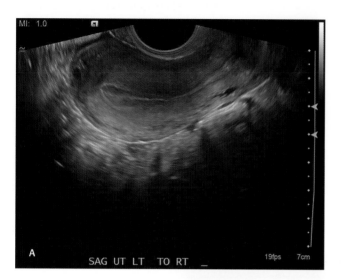

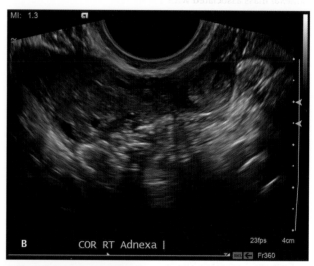

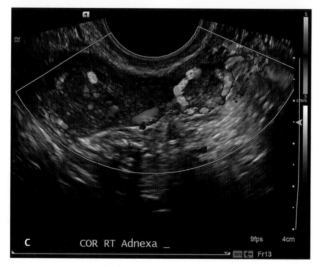

■ Questions

1. Which ONE of the following is the MOST likely diagnosis?
   A. Early intrauterine pregnancy
   B. Ectopic pregnancy
   C. Ruptured ectopic pregnancy
   D. Spontaneous abortion
   E. Molar pregnancy

2. Which ONE of the following is the MOST common location for the case diagnosis?
   A. Ampullary
   B. Isthmic
   C. Fimbrial
   D. Interstitial
   E. Ovarian

3. Which measurement is diagnostic of pregnancy failure?
   A. Crown–rump length ≥ 7 mm and no yolk sac
   B. Crown–rump length ≥ 7 mm and no heartbeat
   C. Mean sac diameter of 16 to 24 mm and no embryo
   D. Enlarged yolk sac > 7 mm
   E. Small gestational sac in relation to the size of the embryo, < 5 mm difference between the mean sac diameter and crown–rump length

■ Answers and Explanations

Question 1

B. Correct! In a patient with a positive pregnancy test, an adnexal mass, and no intrauterine gestational sac, an ectopic pregnancy is the most likely diagnosis. The test case images demonstrate the lack of an intrauterine gestation sac and an adnexal mass associated with a ring of fire.

Other choices and discussion

A. Early intrauterine pregnancy is a diagnostic consideration, but the adnexal mass makes this choice less likely.

C. A ruptured ectopic pregnancy would demonstrate hemorrhagic free fluid, which is not seen in this case.

D. Spontaneous abortion is a diagnostic consideration, but the adnexal mass makes this choice less likely.

E. Abnormal tissue within the uterus would be expected with a hydatidiform molar pregnancy. Hydatidiform moles are a benign form of gestational trophoblastic disease and can either be a complete (absence of an embryo) or partial (abnormal fetus/fetal demise) molar pregnancy.

Question 2

A. Correct! Ampullary. The most common location for an ectopic pregnancy is within the fallopian tube. Within the tube, the most common location is the ampullary portion (75 to 80%). The answer choices are listed in decreasing frequency. Abdominal, cervical, and scar ectopic pregnancies are rare.[1]

Question 3

B. Correct! A crown–rump length $\geq$ 7 mm and no heartbeat is diagnostic of pregnancy failure.

Other choices and discussion

A. This is not a criterion.

C. Mean sac diameter of 16 to 24 mm without an embryo is suspicious but not diagnostic for pregnancy failure.

D. Enlarged yolk sac > 7 mm is suspicious but not diagnostic for pregnancy failure.

E. A small gestational sac relative to the size of the embryo is suspicious but not diagnostic for pregnancy failure.

■ References

1. Levine D. Ectopic pregnancy. Radiology 2007;245(2):385–397

2. Doubilet PM, Benson CB, Bourne T, et al. Diagnostic criteria for nonviable pregnancy early in the first trimester. N Engl J Med 2013;369(15):1443–1451

Top Tips

- "Ring of fire" is not a specific sonographic finding and can be seen in ectopic pregnancy, corpus luteal cyst, or hemorrhagic cyst.

- Methotrexate is the treatment of choice in stable patients with tubal ectopic pregnancy. Surgical treatment is indicated if the ectopic pregnancy has cardiac activity or if the adnexal mass is > 4 cm.

- Findings diagnostic of pregnancy failure include:

  ◇ Crown–rump length $\geq$ 7 mm and no heartbeat

  ◇ Mean sac diameter of $\geq$ 25 mm and no embryo

  ◇ Absence of embryo with heartbeat $\geq$ 2 weeks after a scan that showed a gestational sac without a yolk sac

  ◇ Absence of embryo with heartbeat $\geq$ 11 days after a scan that showed a gestational sac with a yolk sac[2]

Essentials 2

■ Case

A 44-year-old man presents with left flank pain.

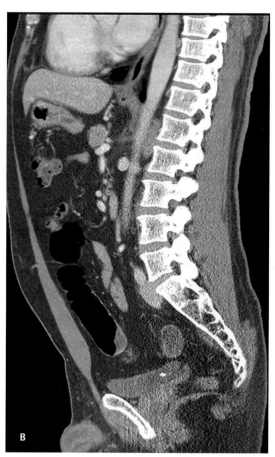

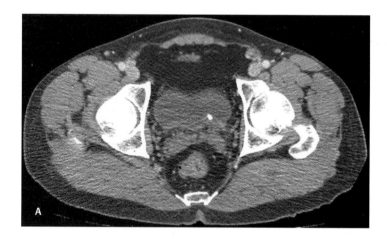

■ Questions

1. Which ONE of the following is the MOST likely diagnosis?
   A. Bladder calculus
   B. Left ureterovesicular junction calculus
   C. Phlebolith
   D. Bladder wall calcification
   E. Calcification of a bladder carcinoma

2. What is the largest sized urinary calculus that will likely (> 50%) pass with medical treatment alone?
   A. 3 mm
   B. 4 mm
   C. 5 mm
   D. 6 mm
   E. 7 mm

3. Which ONE of the following type of urinary calculus is radiolucent on computed tomography?
   A. Calcium oxalate
   B. Cystine
   C. Indinavir
   D. Struvite
   E. Uric acid

■ Answers and Explanations

Question 1

B. Correct! There is a calculus at the UVJ that is impacted or "telescoped" into the bladder. The axial images demonstrate subtle left posterior wall thickening and enhancement that extends to the calculus. The images show a "floating" calculus, signifying that it is held by soft tissue. If desired, prone images could be used to confirm that the calculus is impacted in the UVJ.

Other choices and discussion

A. Bladder calculi are most commonly found in the most dependent portion of the bladder (i.e., the midline or within a diverticulum). Bladder calculi can either form within the urinary bladder from urinary stasis or can represent calculi that move from the proximal collecting system into the bladder.

C. Phleboliths are calcifications within veins and are the most common mimic of urinary calculi in the distal ureter. Phleboliths are not surrounded by ureteral tissue, however, as is seen in this case.

D. Bladder wall calcifications are normally more thin and linear than the depicted ovoid calcification. Causes of bladder wall calcifications include schistosomiasis, tuberculosis, and bladder carcinoma.[1]

E. Calcifications found with bladder carcinoma normally "encrust" the tumor along the intravesicular side.

Question 2

C. Correct! 5 mm. It is generally accepted that calculi that are ≤ 5 mm will spontaneously pass the majority of time (68%), and stones that are between 5 and 10 mm will pass < 50% of the time. Calcium channel blockers and alpha-receptor antagonists can be used to help facilitate passage. When medical therapy fails or if the calculi are too large to pass, shock-wave lithotripsy and ureteroscopy are the next steps in management.[2]

Question 3

C. Correct! Indinavir sulfate is a protease inhibitor used in the treatment of human immunodeficiency virus. These stones form in approximately 20% of patients and are not reliably seen on computed tomography (CT).[3]

Other choices and discussion

The remaining stones can all be seen on CT.
A. Calcium-based stones are the most common type of genitourinary stones (70 to 80%).

B. Cystine stones are associated with cystinuria, which is an autosomal recessive inherited disease that causes impairment in reabsorption of cystine in the proximal tubules.

D. Struvite stones form in the setting of urinary tract infections (urease-producing bacteria) and produce magnesium ammonium phosphate crystals. They can form staghorn calculi.

E. Uric acid stones are not seen on conventional radiography but are seen on CT. These can be treated with urinary alkalinization as first-line therapy.[4]

■ References

1. Shinagare AB, Sadow CA, Sahni VA, Silverman SG. Urinary bladder: normal appearance and mimics of malignancy at CT urography. Cancer Imaging 2011;11:100–108

2. Preminger GM, Tiselius HG, Assimos DG, et al. 2007 guideline for the management of ureteral calculi. J Urol 2007;178(6):2418–2434

3. Schwartz BF, Schenkman N, Armenakas NA, Stoller ML. Imaging characteristics of indinavir calculi. J Urol 1999;161(4):1085–1087

4. Kambadakone AR, Eisner BH, Catalano OA, Sahani DV. New and evolving concepts in the imaging and management of urolithiasis: urologists' perspective. Radiographics 2010;30(3):603–623

Top Tips

- <u>I</u>ndinavir = <u>i</u>nvisible on all imaging
- <u>U</u>ric acid = <u>u</u>ncovered on CT, invisible on radiography
- <u>S</u>truvite = <u>s</u>taghorn
- <u>C</u>alcium <u>o</u>xalate = <u>c</u>ommonly <u>o</u>ccurring
- <u>C</u>ystine = <u>c</u>ongenital
- Calculi ≤ 5 mm = medical treatment (calcium channel blocker and alpha-receptor antagonist)

Essentials 3

■ **Case**

A 52-year-old man presents with costovertebral angle tenderness.

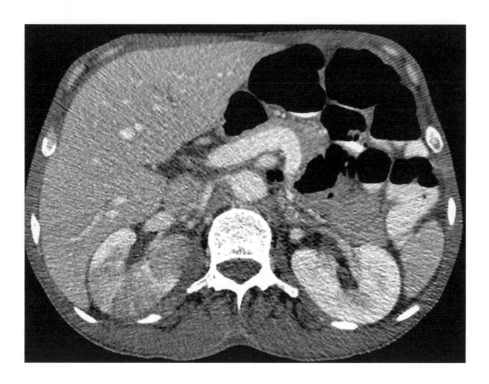

■ **Questions**

1. Which ONE of the following is the MOST likely diagnosis?
   A. Obstructive uropathy
   B. Pyelonephritis
   C. Pyonephrosis
   D. Renal infarction
   E. Lymphoma

2. Which ONE of the following is the BEST management for a young and otherwise healthy female suspected to have an uncomplicated case of the diagnosis shown above?
   A. Computed tomography (CT) to confirm pyelonephritis, outpatient treatment with oral antibiotics
   B. CT to confirm pyelonephritis, inpatient intravenous (IV) antibiotics
   C. CT to confirm pyelonephritis, IV antibiotics in an emergency department, outpatient treatment with oral antibiotics

   D. Ultrasound to confirm pyelonephritis, IV antibiotics in an emergency department, inpatient treatment with IV antibiotics
   E. Clinical assessment to confirm pyelonephritis, IV antibiotics in an emergency department, outpatient treatment with oral antibiotics

3. How does treatment differ between pyelonephritis and pyonephrosis?
   A. No difference
   B. Pyonephrosis needs more aggressive hydration
   C. Antibiotic treatment for pyelonephritis, outpatient treatment for pyonephrosis
   D. Antibiotic treatment for pyelonephritis, urgent percutaneous nephrostomy for pyonephrosis
   E. Antibiotic treatment for pyelonephritis, surgical nephrectomy for pyonephrosis

■ Answers and Explanations

Question 1

B. Correct! The "striated" nephrogram seen in the test case is the classic appearance of pyelonephritis. The areas of low attenuation involve both the cortex and medullary components, and the differentiation between the two is blurred. Areas of normal intervening parenchymal enhancement are commonly seen. This case is slightly atypical, as pyelonephritis is more common in women than in men.

Other choices and discussion

A. Obstructive uropathy can cause asymmetric delayed enhancement of the kidney. However, the process affects the entire kidney, and the corticomedullary differentiation is usually maintained. Obstruction can result from calculi, intrinsic/extrinsic mass, or bladder outlet obstruction.

C. Pyonephrosis refers to infection or pus within the collecting system with an obstructive component. This obstructive component can occur from calculi or a mass, but can also result from the pus alone. Imaging findings show a dilated collecting system, which is not seen in this case. Ultrasound shows debris within the collecting system.

D. Renal infarction can have wedge-shaped areas of nonenhancement, which can look similar to this striated nephrogram. Unless embolic, infarcts are less often multiple (and if embolic and originating from the heart, bilateral disease would be expected). In addition, the "cortical-rim" sign is absent, which is seen in approximately 50% of renal infarcts. The cortical-rim sign refers to normal enhancement along the capsule from the capsular artery. It usually takes at least 8 hours for this sign to develop.[1]

E. Lymphoma could mimic the appearance of the test case. Infiltrative lymphoma often enlarges the kidney, however, which is not seen in this case. In addition, retroperitoneal lymph node involvement is absent.

Question 2

E. Correct! If a young female that is otherwise healthy has clinical signs and symptoms of uncomplicated pyelonephritis, no imaging is needed! The patient should be evaluated in an emergency department and treated with IV fluids and a dose of IV antibiotics. The patient can then be treated as an outpatient with oral antibiotics. If the patient fails outpatient treatment after 72 hours or has suspected complicated pyelonephritis, a CT with contrast is the study of choice. In these cases, renal abscess, pyonephrosis, and source of obstruction should be sought. These patients should also be admitted to the hospital for IV antibiotic therapy.[2,3]

Question 3

D. Correct! Urgent percutaneous nephrostomy or ureteral stent placement for decompression and drainage of the infective debris is the treatment of choice for pyonephrosis.

Discussion

Pyelonephritis should be evaluated in an emergency department with IV antibiotics and aggressive IV hydration.

Pyonephrosis needs urgent decompression of the dilated collecting system and drainage of the pus.

Although pyonephrosis can lead to urosepsis, surgical removal of the kidney is the last resort.

■ References

1. Kamel IR, Berkowitz JF. Assessment of the cortical rim sign in posttraumatic renal infarction. J Comput Assist Tomogr 1996;20(5):803–806

2. Soulen MC, Fishman EK, Goldman SM, Gatewood OM. Bacterial renal infection: role of CT. Radiology 1989;171(3):703–707

3. Nikolaidis P, Casalino DD, Remer EM, et al. ACR Appropriateness Criteria® Acute Pyelonephritis. https://acsearch.acr.org/docs/69489/Narrative/. Accessed February 29, 2016

Top Tips

- Pyonephrosis requires urgent percutaneous catheter drainage or ureteral stent placement

- Cortical-rim sign can be seen in renal vascular compromise (infarct), but this sign is only seen about 50% of the time and only becomes apparent after 8 hours.

- Lymphoma can mimic pyelonephritis on CT.

Essentials 4

■ Case

A 24-year-old man with epigastric pain presents to the emergency department.

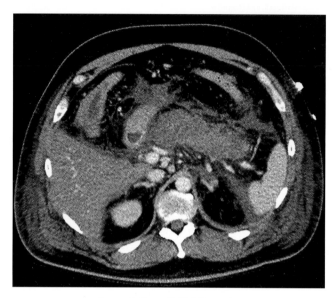

Image A: time of initial diagnosis.

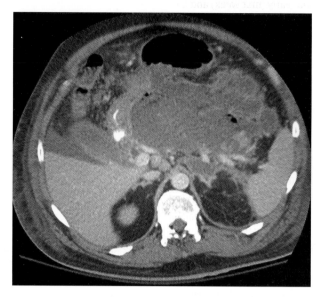

Image B: 5 weeks later.

■ Questions

1. Based only on image A, what is the MOST likely diagnosis?
   A. Acute necrotizing pancreatitis
   B. Acute edematous pancreatitis
   C. Chronic pancreatitis
   D. Duodenitis
   E. Gastritis

2. Follow-up imaging of the same patient 5 weeks later is shown in image B. What does this collection most likely represent?
   A. Acute peripancreatic collection with superimposed infection
   B. Acute necrotic collection with superimposed infection

C. Pseudocyst without superimposed infection
D. Pseudocyst with superimposed infection
E. Walled-off necrosis with superimposed infection

3. Which ONE of the following is a criterion for pseudocyst treatment?
   A. Compression of small vessels
   B. Sterile pseudocyst
   C. Compression of the common bile duct
   D. At least 3 cm in diameter
   E. Pancreaticoduodenal fistula

■ Answers and Explanations

Question 1

A. Correct! On image A, we see decreased enhancement of nearly the entire pancreas, which is a sign of necrotizing pancreatitis. Peripancreatic inflammation as well as peripancreatic and intraperitoneal fluid are present. Acute pancreatitis is classified into early (first week) and late (> 1 week) phases. Acute pancreatitis is also classified into edematous and necrotizing pancreatitis.[1] The severity of pancreatitis is based on the presence or absence of organ failure.

Other choices and discussion

B. Acute edematous pancreatitis usually maintains normal or nearly normal enhancement, unlike this case. There may be mildly decreased attenuation due to pancreatic and peripancreatic edema.

C. Chronic pancreatitis is a recurrent process with the following common associations: pancreatic ductal dilatation, pancreatic atrophy, and parenchymal calcifications.

D. Although the inflammation of duodenitis can extend into the peripancreatic space, the inflammation in the test case is pancreas-centered. The most common cause of duodenitis is secondary inflammation from pancreatitis.

E. Gastritis is normally depicted as gastric wall or submucosal edema. Gastric ulceration may also be present. These findings are not seen in the test case. The most common cause of gastritis is *Helicobacter pylori* infection.

Question 2

E. Correct! This is walled-off necrosis of the pancreas. By definition, this occurs after 4 weeks. Walled-off necrosis is usually *centered* in the space where the pancreas resides. In this case, there are multiple gas bubbles, which are compatible with superimposed infection. This collection should be treated.

Other choices and discussion

A. Acute peripancreatic collection is seen within the first 4 weeks of edematous pancreatitis. It is usually adjacent to the pancreas and has a homogenous fluid density.

B. Acute necrotic collection is seen within the first 4 weeks of necrotizing pancreatitis and is a heterogeneous collection.

C. Pseudocysts occur after 4 weeks and are usually *adjacent* to the pancreas. They have a well-defined wall and are usually homogenous and of fluid density. Pseudocysts may communicate directly with the pancreatic ducts.

D. Although this collection is infected, it is not a pseudocyst.

Question 3

C. Correct! A pseudocyst should be treated if it causes external compression on the common bile duct.

Other choices and discussion

A. A pseudocyst should be treated if there is compression of *large* vessels.

B. *Infected* pseudocysts should be drained.

D. A pseudocyst should be treated if the diameter is > 5 *cm* and size and morphology have not changed for more than 6 weeks.

E. A pseudocyst should be treated if there is a *pancreaticopleural* fistula.[2]

■ References

1. Thoeni RF. The revised Atlanta classification of acute pancreatitis: its importance for the radiologist and its effect on treatment. Radiology 2012;262(3):751–764

2. Aghdassi AA, Mayerle J, Kraft M, Sielenkamper AW, Heidecke CD, Lerch MM. Pancreatic pseudocysts—when and how to treat? HPB (Oxford) 2006;8(6):432–441

Top Tips

◆ Pseudocysts require > 4 weeks to develop in acute pancreatitis by definition (Revised Atlanta classification of acute pancreatitis 2012).

◆ Severity of acute pancreatitis is based on whether organ failure (OF) is present and, if present, for how long. These are separated into mild (no OF), moderate (< 48 hours of OF), and severe (> 48 hours of OF).

◆ Necrotizing pancreatitis demonstrates lack of enhancement on computed tomography imaging.

Essentials 5

■ Case

A 56-year-old man presents with chest pain and shortness of breath.

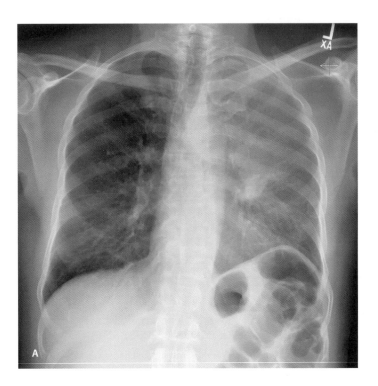
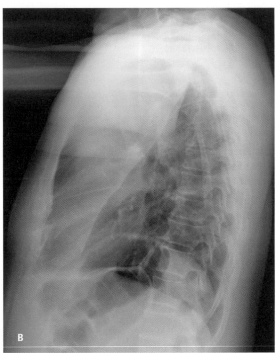

■ Questions

1. Which ONE of the following is the MOST likely diagnosis?
   A. Pulmonary edema
   B. Pneumonia
   C. Pleural effusion
   D. Pneumothorax
   E. Atelectasis

2. Which ONE of the following is a DIRECT sign of the case diagnosis?
   A. Increased lung density
   B. Elevation of the diaphragm
   C. Hilar displacement
   D. Mediastinal shift
   E. Compensatory hyperinflation

3. What is the MOST appropriate next step in the management of this patient?
   A. No further management necessary
   B. Incentive spirometry
   C. Chest computed tomography
   D. Bronchodilator
   E. Antibiotics

■ Answers and Explanations

Question 1

E. Correct! This is a case of atelectasis. There is volume loss of the left lung depicted by elevation of the left hemidiaphragm and leftward shift of the mediastinum. Left upper lobe atelectasis can have varying degrees of volume loss. It typically collapses anteriorly and superiorly, as is shown on the lateral radiograph. This can cause a left lung "veil-like" density on the frontal radiograph. It is important to remember that particularly in an adult, lobar atelectasis should be considered secondary to neoplasm until proven otherwise.

Other choices and discussion

A. Pulmonary edema is typically bilateral and when unilateral, it usually affects the right, not the left, lung.

B. Pneumonia is a differential consideration in this case. Typically, pneumonia should be a space-occupying lesion (pus in the alveoli), not a process that predominantly causes volume loss.

C. Pleural effusions can cause increased density overlying the left hemithorax on the frontal view, but the lateral radiograph shows the opacity along the anterior chest wall. Free-flowing pleural fluid would be expected posteriorly.

D. A tension pneumothorax can shift the mediastinum, but would not cause an anterior opacity on the lateral radiograph. Additionally, a visceral pleural line to confirm a pneumothorax would be expected.

Several named signs of volume loss:

"Golden S" sign—Right upper lobe collapse with minor fissure elevation and a downward bulge in the medial portion of the minor fissure. Caused by a centrally obstructing mass.[1]

"Luftsichel" sign—Hyperinflated superior segment of the left lower lobe outlining the aortic arch. Seen in left upper lobe collapse.[1]

"Flat waist" sign—Left lower lobe collapse with cardiac rotation and subsequent loss of the left heart border concavity.[2]

Question 2

A. Correct! Increased pulmonary density is a direct sign of atelectasis. Other direct signs of atelectasis include displacement of the fissures and crowding of the bronchi.

Other choices and discussion

B. Elevation of the diaphragm is an indirect sign of atelectasis.

C. Hilar displacement is an indirect sign of atelectasis.

D. Mediastinal shift is an indirect sign of atelectasis.

E. Compensatory hyperinflation is an indirect sign of atelectasis.

Note that ipsilateral intercostal space narrowing is also an indirect sign of atelectasis.

Question 3

C. Correct! The use of a chest CT is invaluable for the evaluation of a potential centrally obstructing mass that causes secondary atelectasis.

Other choices and discussion

A. Further management *is* needed. The cause of the left upper lobe atelectasis must be determined.

B. Incentive spirometry is a commonly used tool to help promote healthy lung function following surgery or a respiratory illness, but is not used to diagnose an unknown cause of lobar atelectasis.

D. Mucous plugging (e.g., with asthma) causing atelectasis can be improved with bronchodilator therapy, but a CT chest to exclude an underlying mass is crucial.

E. Antibiotics are used to treat an infectious process, not atelectasis.

■ References

1. Woodring JH, Reed JC. Radiographic manifestations of lobar atelectasis. J Thorac Imaging 1996;11(2):109–144

2. Kattan KR, Wlot JF. Cardiac rotation in left lower lobe collapse. "The flat waist sign." Radiology 1976;118(2):275–279

Top Tips

◆ Direct signs of atelectasis:

◇ Increased density

◇ Displacement of fissures

◇ Crowding of bronchi

◆ Indirect signs of atelectasis:

◇ Mediastinal shift

◇ Elevation of the ipsilateral hemidiaphragm

◇ Ipsilateral intercostal space narrowing

◇ Compensatory hyperinflation of other lobes or the contralateral lung

◆ Where does the collapsed lung go?

◇ Left upper lobe—anteriorly and superiorly

◇ Right upper lobe—superiorly and medially

◇ Right middle lobe—inferiorly and medially

◇ Right lower lobe and left lower lobe—inferiorly, medially, and posteriorly

Essentials 6

■ Case

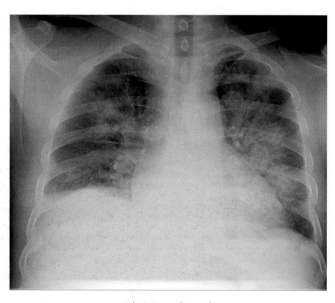

Admission radiograph

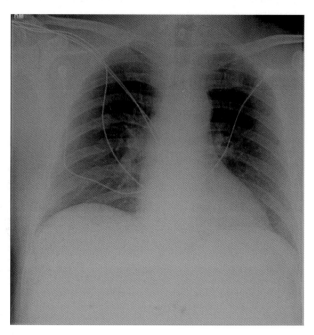

Follow-up: 2 days after admission

■ Questions

1. Which ONE of the following is the MOST likely diagnosis?
   A. Pulmonary edema
   B. Lobar pneumonia
   C. Usual interstitial pneumonia
   D. Sarcoidosis
   E. Pulmonary emboli with pulmonary infarction

2. What pulmonary wedge pressure is MOST commonly seen with an INTERSTITIAL case of the diagnosis above?
   A. 8 to 12 mm Hg
   B. 12 to 17 mm Hg
   C. 17 to 25 mm Hg
   D. > 25 mm Hg

3. Which ONE of the following can cause localized right upper lobe pulmonary edema?
   A. Acute mitral regurgitation
   B. Chronic mitral regurgitation
   C. Mitral stenosis
   D. Low ejection fraction
   E. Dilated cardiomyopathy

■ Answers and Explanations

Question 1

A. Correct! This is pulmonary edema. Bilateral perihilar opacities have a broad differential diagnosis. The key to this diagnosis is the follow up radiograph, which demonstrates resolution of the pulmonary opacities. Given this short time interval, pulmonary edema is the most likely diagnosis.

Other choices and discussion

B. Lobar pneumonia is typically seen in one lobe and often depicted by consolidation with air bronchograms. The test case image could represent bronchopneumonia, which is commonly associated with multifocal patchy opacities, as well as tree-in-bud opacities on computed tomography.

C. Usual interstitial pneumonia is an interstitial lung disease that predominately affects the lung bases. It has a reticular pattern and subpleural involvement with pulmonary fibrosis and associated "honeycombing."

D. Sarcoidosis has five radiographic stages (0 to 4). Stage 0 has a normal chest radiograph. Stage 1 has the classic 1-2-3 sign, which depicts lymph node enlargement of the right paratracheal, right hilar, and left hilar lymph nodes. Stage 2 has nodal enlargement and parenchymal disease. Stage 3 has only parenchymal disease. Stage 4 is end-stage pulmonary sarcoidosis, associated with pulmonary fibrosis. Although the test case could have the appearance of stage 3 pulmonary sarcoidosis, the rapid resolution of the pulmonary opacities would be atypical.

E. Pulmonary emboli with pulmonary infarction may cause consolidative opacity. However, this opacity usually extends to the periphery. Hampton's hump is a radiologic sign of pulmonary infarction, depicted by a wedge-shaped peripheral opacity.

Question 2

C. Correct! Interstitial pulmonary edema is seen at 17 to 25 mm Hg. Kerley lines are present.[1]

Other choices and discussion

A. The normal pulmonary wedge pressure is 8 to 12 mm Hg.

B. Pressures of 12 to 17 mm Hg will demonstrate cephalization (redistribution to the upper lobes).

D. Alveolar pulmonary edema is seen when the pulmonary wedge pressure increases beyond 25 mm Hg.

Question 3

A. Correct! Acute mitral regurgitation can lead to acute right upper lobe pulmonary edema. This can be secondary to myocardial infarction with subsequent papillary muscle rupture or rupture of the chordae tendineae. Mitral valve replacement is the treatment of choice.[2] Other etiologies include infective endocarditis and acute rheumatic fever.

Other choices and discussion

B. Chronic mitral regurgitation will lead to left ventricular enlargement, dilatation of the left atrium, and ultimately, the development of left ventricular failure. This results in diffuse pulmonary edema.[3]

C. Mitral stenosis is commonly associated with an enlarged left atrium, which is seen as the "double density" sign on chest radiography. This condition may lead to diffuse interstitial pulmonary edema.

D. Low ejection fracture may cause diffuse pulmonary edema.

E. Dilated cardiomyopathy is normally depicted as a large left ventricle with associated diffuse pulmonary edema.

■ References

1. Gluecker T, Capasso P, Schnyder P, et al. Clinical and radiologic features of pulmonary edema. Radiographics 1999;19(6):1507–1531; discussion 1532–1503

2. Schnyder PA, Sarraj AM, Duvoisin BE, Kapenberger L, Landry MJ. Pulmonary edema associated with mitral regurgitation: prevalence of predominant involvement of the right upper lobe. Am J Roentgenol 1993;161(1):33–36

3. Woolley K, Stark P. Pulmonary parenchymal manifestations of mitral valve disease. Radiographics 1999;19(4):965–972

> ## Top Tips
>
> - Chest radiographic findings of pulmonary edema wax and wane over hours or days, depending on fluid status.
>
> - Acute mitral valve regurgitation (papillary muscle rupture) can lead to right upper lobe pulmonary edema after myocardial infarction.
>
> - Bronchopneumonia is commonly seen as multifocal patchy pulmonary opacities on chest radiograph and may have tree-in-bud opacities on computed tomography.

Essentials 7

■ Case

A 73-year-old man presents with abdominal pain.

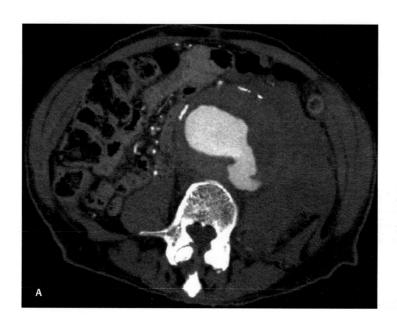
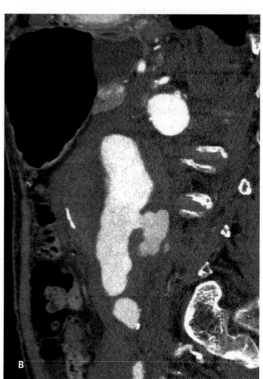

■ Questions

1. Which ONE of the following is the MOST important finding on the test case images?
   A. Aortic dissection
   B. Intramural hematoma
   C. Abdominal aortic aneurysm
   D. Aortic pseudoaneurysm
   E. Aortic rupture

2. Which ONE of the following criteria warrants elective repair of the case diagnosis?
   A. AAA measuring 4.5 cm in a woman
   B. AAA measuring 5 cm in a man
   C. AAA measuring at least 1.5 times the expected diameter of the aorta
   D. AAA expanding at a rate of at least 5 mm/year
   E. AAA expanding at a rate of at least 10 mm/year

3. Which sign is associated with impending AAA rupture?
   A. Aortic nipple sign
   B. Draping aorta sign
   C. Three sign
   D. Hyperattenuating crescent sign
   E. Air crescent sign

■ Answers and Explanations

Question 1

E. Correct! The critical finding on this case is a ruptured abdominal aortic aneurysm (AAA) with a large volume of retroperitoneal hemorrhage. Most unruptured AAAs are asymptomatic. Rupture is associated with a high mortality. The images provided demonstrate a large aortic aneurysm with contrast extending through a posterolateral defect and a large left retroperitoneal hematoma.

Other choices and discussion

A. Aortic dissection is not demonstrated. Aortic dissection is most commonly associated with hypertension.

B. There is intramural hematoma, but this is not the salient finding. Intramural hematoma refers to hemorrhage within the aortic wall from the vaso vasorum.[1]

C. An AAA is absolutely present in this case, but the rupture is the most important finding. AAA is defined as enlargement of the abdominal aorta > 1.5 times the normal adjacent diameter or a measurement of > 3 cm.

D. Aortic pseudoaneurysms are usually posttraumatic and result in focal outpouchings of the aorta. There is disruption of at least one layer of the aortic wall, and these are contained ruptures.

Question 2

E. Correct! An AAA expanding at a rate of at least 10 mm/year is a criterion warranting elective AAA repair.

Other choices and discussion

A. AAA size of > 5 cm in female patients warrants elective AAA repair.

B. AAA size of > 5.5 cm in male patients warrants elective AAA repair.

C. An AAA is defined when the vessel measures at least 1.5 times the expected diameter of the aorta. However, this is not a criterion for elective repair.

D. A *rapidly* expanding AAA is measured as > 5 mm in 6 months or > 10 mm in 1 year, and these criteria warrant elective AAA repair.

Question 3

D. Correct! The hyperattenuating crescent sign on noncontrast computed tomography (CT) can be seen in patients with impending AAA rupture. This sign represents acute hematoma in either the mural thrombus or within the aortic wall. A noncontrast CT examination can help in differentiating between blood pool and aortic wall/mural thrombus.

Other choices and discussion

A. The "aortic nipple" sign is a tiny bump along the aortic arch on plain radiography that correlates with the left superior intercostal vein.

B. The "draping aorta" sign signifies a contained rupture.

C. The "three" sign is seen in coarctation of the aorta. This is comprised of the dilated left subclavian artery, indentation of the coarctation, and the poststenotic aortic dilatation.

E. The "air crescent" sign is seen as a radiolucent pulmonary cavity surrounding a mass. This is classically seen with aspergilloma.

■ References

1. Macura KJ, Corl FM, Fishman EK, Bluemke DA. Pathogenesis in acute aortic syndromes: aortic dissection, intramural hematoma, and penetrating atherosclerotic aortic ulcer. Am J Roentgenol 2003;181(2):309–316

2. Khosa F, Krinsky G, Macari M, Yucel EK, Berland LL. Managing incidental findings on abdominal and pelvic CT and MRI, Part 2: white paper of the ACR Incidental Findings Committee II on vascular findings. J Am Coll Radiol 2013;10(10):789–794

■ Suggested Readings

Restrepo CS, Ocazionez D, Suri R, Vargas D. Aortitis: imaging spectrum of the infectious and inflammatory conditions of the aorta. Radiographics 2011;31(2):435–451

Takayama T, Miyata T, Nagawa H. True abdominal aortic aneurysm in Marfan syndrome. J Vasc Surg 2009;49(5):1162–1165

SECTION III DIAGNOSTIC RADIOLOGY IMAGING

Top Tips

◆ Due to the increasing chance of AAA rupture based on size, as the AAA grows, the imaging follow-up interval should decrease. Recommended guidelines for follow-up include[2]:

Aortic diameter	Imaging interval
2.5–2.9 cm	5 years
3.0–3.4 cm	3 years
3.5–3.9 cm	2 years
4.0–4.4 cm	1 year
4.5–4.9 cm	6 months
5.0–5.5 cm	3–6 months

◆ Atherosclerosis is the most common cause of AAAs. Other risk factors include smoking, male gender, diabetes, hypertension, and hypercholesterolemia.[2]

◆ Acute intramural hematoma can be seen in cases of impending AAA rupture. On noncontrast CT, this manifests as crescentic high attenuation (60 to 70 HU) thickening of the aortic wall.

Essentials 8

■ Case

A 34-year-old woman status post motor vehicle collision.

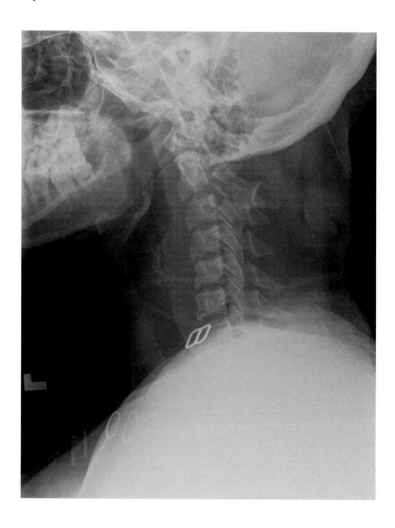

■ Questions

1. Which ONE of the following is the MOST likely diagnosis?
   A. Jefferson burst fracture (C1)
   B. Hangman's fracture (C2)
   C. Flexion teardrop injury
   D. Extension teardrop injury
   E. Rotary subluxation

2. Using the Levine and Edwards classification, how would this injury be classified? (Hint: there is 3.5 mm of anteroposterior translation, and angulation is present.)
   A. Type I
   B. Type II
   C. Type IIA
   D. Type III

3. What is the appropriate treatment for type I traumatic spondylolisthesis of the axis?
   A. Rigid cervical collar for 4 to 6 weeks
   B. Halo immobilization for 6 to 12 weeks
   C. Internal fixation
   D. Reduction using hyperextension, then halo immobilization for 6 to 12 weeks

■ Answers and Explanations

Question 1

B. Correct! This is a hangman's fracture. Traumatic spondylolisthesis of the axis is also known as a hangman's fracture, a name termed after judicial hangings. However, this type of injury is now most commonly seen in motor vehicle collisions and falls. It is defined by bilateral fractures of the pars interarticularis of C2. The mechanism of injury is hyperextension.[1] The test case image demonstrates bilateral fractures of the pars interarticularis of C2 with anterior translation of C2 on C3 and angulation of C2.

Other choices and discussion

A. Jefferson burst fracture involves C1 and is best evaluated on the open-mouth odontoid view.

C. Flexion teardrop injury is considered a distraction-type injury. It usually affects the subaxial cervical spine, with injury starting from the supraspinous ligament and continuing anteriorly with a superimposed compression component. This causes a large fracture fragment of the anteroinferior portion of the affected vertebral body.

D. Extension teardrop injury is considered a distraction-type injury. It usually affects the subaxial cervical spine, with the injury starting from the anterior aspect of the cervical spine. There is an avulsion fracture of the anterior aspect of the inferior endplate.

E. Rotary subluxation involves the C1–C2 articulation.

Question 2

B. Correct! This is type II. Type I fractures have < 3 mm anteroposterior translation without an angulation component. Type II fractures have > 3 mm of anteroposterior translation with angulation (> 11 degrees) and disruption of the posterior longitudinal ligament. Type IIA fractures have a horizontal fracture line instead of a vertical fracture line, with angulation. This injury does not have anteroposterior translation. Type III injuries have unilateral or bilateral facet dislocation with translation and are very unstable. Immediate application of halo traction is used to reduce the facet dislocation.[2]

Question 3

A. Correct! Rigid cervical collar for 4–6 weeks. A type I fracture is stable and will usually heal with a rigid cervical collar.

Other choices and discussion

B, C. These treatments can be used for type II fractures, depending on the amount of displacement. Displacement of > 5 mm will likely need internal fixation.

D. This is usually used for type IIA injures.

■ References

1. Mirvis SE, Young JW, Lim C, Greenberg J. Hangman's fracture: radiologic assessment in 27 cases. Radiology 1987;163(3):713–717

2. Levine AM, Edwards CC. The management of traumatic spondylolisthesis of the axis. J Bone Joint Surg Am 1985;67(2):217–226

**SECTION III
DIAGNOSTIC RADIOLOGY
IMAGING**

Top Tips

◆ Type I injuries are stable injuries, and type III injuries are grossly unstable.[2]

◆ Type I and type II injuries cause widening of the spinal canal, which decreases the chance of neurologic compromise, although neurologic deficits sometimes do occur.

◆ Although not specifically discussed in this case, *dens* fractures and mimics are also important to know. See the following:

Type I	Rare, oblique fracture of the tip of the dens	Evaluate for craniocervical dissociation
Type II	Most common, fracture at the base of the dens	Unstable. Complication: nonunion
Type III	Fracture into the vertebral body	Unstable. Heals well with immobilization
Os odontoideum	Well-corticated ossicle with two subtypes: Orthotopic—Ossicle is in anatomic position Dystopic—Ossicle is not in anatomic position	Both types may be associated with instability

Essentials 9

■ Case

A 67-year-old man presents with neck pain after a fall from 12 feet.

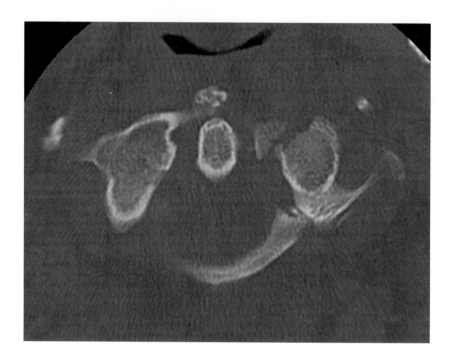

■ Questions

1. What is the most common mechanism for this type of injury?
   A. Axial compression
   B. Anteroposterior flexion
   C. Anteroposterior extension
   D. Rotational
   E. Craniocaudal distraction

2. What is the most important factor in determining stability for the injury in the test case?
   A. Alar ligament integrity
   B. Transverse ligament integrity
   C. Anterior longitudinal ligament integrity
   D. Tectorial membrane integrity
   E. Apical ligament integrity

3. An unstable C1 burst fracture is demonstrated by a sum of the lateral mass displacement of greater than:
   A. 5 mm
   B. 6 mm
   C. 7 mm
   D. 8 mm
   E. 9 mm

■ Answers and Explanations

Question 1

A. Correct! Axial loading from a fall onto the head is the most common mechanism for this injury. Other common causes include motor vehicle collision or heavy object falling onto the head. Due to the angulation of the articular surfaces of the lateral masses, fractures and splaying of the anterior and/or posterior arch commonly occur with this mechanism.[1] In the image provided, there is a fracture of the anterior arch of C1 extending into the left lateral mass. The lateral mass is displaced laterally. There is also a fracture of the posterior arch of C1.

Other choices and discussion

B. Anteroposterior flexion usually leads to distraction injury of the subaxial cervical spine in a step-wise fashion. This includes the supraspinous ligament, interspinous ligament, facet capsular joint, ligamentum flavum, and the posterior longitudinal ligament. If the injury continues, it can cause either a fracture of the vertebral body (e.g., in the case of "flexion teardrop" injury, when a component of compression is present) or it can disrupt the disk and anterior longitudinal ligament.

C. Anteroposterior extension is not the most common mechanism. However, hyperextension can cause fractures of the C1 posterior arch. The first reported case of this type of injury involved Sir Geoffrey Jefferson as the treating physician. On a misty morning in 1919, a pilot crashed into telegraph wires and was thrown from his plane. Dr. Jefferson described the resultant segmental fracture of the posterior arch, and the fracture was later named after him.

D. Rotational injuries are usually described as atlantoaxial rotatory fixation, traumatic isolation of the articular pillar, and unilateral interfacetal dislocation. These patients are unable to return their head from a rotated to a neutral position.[2]

E. Craniocaudal distraction injury may occur at any level, but is most frequently found at the craniocervical junction, with craniocervical dissociation/dislocation and widening of the occipital condyle-C1 articulation.

Question 2

B. Correct! Transverse ligament integrity. Jefferson burst fractures involve C1, with the stability reliant on the function of the lateral masses to provide support of the head and restrict lateral subluxation. If both the anterior and posterior arches are fractured, the transverse ligament is the only structure that can prevent this subluxation.

Other choices and discussion

A. The alar ligament attaches the occipital condyles to the dens. Alar ligament integrity is important in craniocervical injuries.

C. Although the anterior longitudinal ligament offers support for the entire spine, this ligament is not normally injured in a C1 burst fracture.

D. The tectorial membrane is a continuation of the posterior longitudinal ligament and is the strongest ligament at the craniocervical junction.

E. The apical ligament is a weak ligament that extends from the dens to the foramen magnum. It does not play any role in the stability of C1 burst fractures.

Question 3

C. Correct! 7 mm. When the C1 lateral masses overhang the C2 articulations on open-mouth odontoid view or coronal cross-sectional imaging, the sum of the overhang bilaterally (if present) should be calculated. If the combined displacement is > 7 mm, the injury is unstable. The main difference in the treatment of stable versus unstable injuries of the cervical spine is internal fixation or halo for unstable injuries and cervical brace/rigid support for stable injuries.

■ References

1. Jefferson G. Fracture of the atlas vertebra: report of four cases and a review of those previously recorded. Br J Surg 1919;7(27):407–422

2. Rhea JT. Rotational injuries of the cervical spine. Emerg Radiol 2000;7:149–159

Top Tips

◆ The transverse ligament plays a crucial role in the stability of C1 burst fractures, and its integrity can be evaluated by the lateral mass displacement of C1 on C2. Use the open-mouth odontoid view or a coronal CT.

◆ If there is > 7 mm lateral mass displacement (sum of right and left), the transverse ligament is likely torn, indicating an unstable injury and the need for cranial traction.

◆ C1 burst fractures are not normally associated with neurologic deficits.

Essentials 10

■ Case

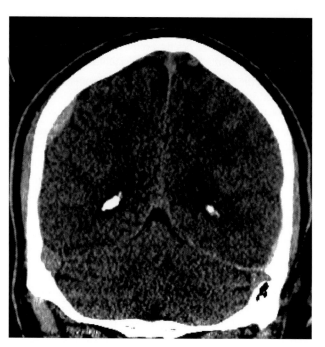

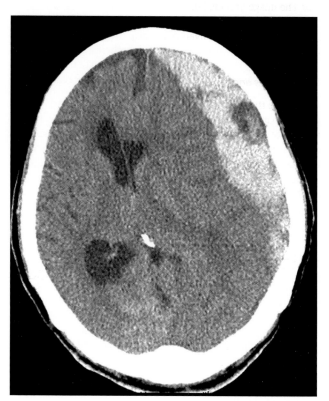

Patient A: Motor vehicle collision with direct blow on the right.

Patient B: Ground level fall

■ Questions

1. Regarding patient A, which ONE of the following is the most common cause of this type of injury?
   A. Injury to the bridging veins, while receiving anticoagulation
   B. Fracture, with injury to the middle meningeal artery
   C. Hemorrhage of a cerebral arteriovenous malformation
   D. Coup contrecoup injury causing intraparenchymal contusion
   E. Ruptured intracranial aneurysm.

2. How is the hemorrhage type (patient A) distinguished from other types of intracranial hemorrhages? This type of hemorrhage:
   A. Can cross the calvarial sutures, but not the midline
   B. Is restricted by the calvarial sutures

   C. Extends directly into the ventricular system via the lateral ventricle
   D. Is confined to the brain parenchyma.
   E. May redistribute into the ventricles, with layering commonly seen in several cisterns

3. What does the low-density material within the high-density subdural hemorrhage signify? (patient B)
   A. Beam hardening artifact due to the thickness of the calvarium
   B. Acute on chronic hemorrhage, with the low attenuating areas representing the chronic component
   C. Active or hyperacute hemorrhage
   D. Neoplasm
   E. Thrombosed aneurysm

■ Answers and Explanations

Question 1

B. Correct! The most common cause of an epidural hemorrhage is a calvarial fracture with injury to the middle meningeal artery. The image provided demonstrates a subgaleal hematoma and enlargement of the temporalis musculature, which suggests a direct injury. A calvarial fracture was also present, but not shown.

Other choices and discussion

A. Injury to the bridging veins is most commonly found in subdural hematoma (patient B). This type of injury is often seen in elderly patients with cerebral atrophy. This patient population also has an increased risk of intracranial hemorrhage, if undergoing anticoagulation treatment.

C. Although cerebral arteriovenous malformations (AVM) can hemorrhage with or without trauma, there is no sign of an intracerebral AVM on the reference image. Additionally, the epidural space would be an uncommon location for an AVM hemorrhage. AVM can hemorrhage into the brain parenchyma, subarachnoid space, or the ventricular system.

D. Although coup contrecoup injuries do commonly cause intraparenchymal contusion, the reference image depicts an extra-axial hemorrhage with mass effect on the brain parenchyma. The coup contrecoup injury can result in epidural, subdural, subarachnoid, and intraparenchymal blood. It is important to evaluate not only the site of scalp soft tissue swelling, but the contrecoup injury with a high index of suspicion.

E. Ruptured aneurysms normally present as subarachnoid, not epidural, hemorrhage on a noncontrast head CT.

Question 2

B. Correct! Epidural hemorrhages occur between the periosteal layer of the dura mater and the calvarium. The periosteal layer is "tacked down" to the calvarium at the sutures and restricts hemorrhage from crossing the sutures. The falx cerebri does not impede the extension of epidural across midline. The classic appearance of an epidural hematoma (patient A) is a biconvex or lentiform shaped extra-axial hemorrhage.

Other choices and discussion

A. Subdural hemorrhage is not restricted by the calvarial sutures. The subdural space is a potential space between the meningeal layer of the dura mater and the arachnoid mater. The dura mater is a component of the falx cerebri and usually restricts subdural hemorrhage from crossing the midline.

C. Large intraparenchymal hemorrhages may extend directly into the lateral ventricles.

D. Cerebral contusions are confined to the brain parenchyma and are commonly associated with subarachnoid hemorrhage.

E. Redistribution of extra-axial hemorrhage into the ventricles and cisterns is normally seen with subarachnoid hemorrhage.

Question 3

C. Correct! Internal hypoattenuation within extra-axial hemorrhage (epidural or subdural) is compatible with hyperacute hemorrhage (i.e., bleeding while being imaged). This represents unclotted blood. In this case (patient B), the extra-axial hemorrhage has a predominately concave shape and crosses the coronal suture, which are features of subdural hemorrhage.

Other choices and discussion

A. When beam hardening artifact causes decreased attenuation, it is normally more linear in appearance and will also cross into other structures.

B. Acute on chronic hemorrhage usually shows a fluid–fluid level, in which case the denser blood products are in the more dependent location (i.e., posteriorly in a supine patient).

D. There is no tumor within the subdural space, which is where the low attenuation is centered.

E. Aneurysms are not commonly seen in the subdural space.

■ References

1. Al-Nakshabandi NA. The swirl sign. Radiology 2001;218(2):433

2. Bricolo AP, Pasut LM. Extradural hematoma: toward zero mortality. A prospective study. Neurosurgery 1984;14(1):8–12

3. Cheung PS, Lam JM, Yeung JH, Graham CA, Rainer TH. Outcome of traumatic extradural haematoma in Hong Kong. Injury 2007;38(1):76–80

4. Maugeri R, Anderson DG, Graziano F, Meccio F, Visocchi M, Iacopino DG. Conservative vs. Surgical Management of Post-Traumatic Epidural Hematoma: A Case and Review of Literature. Am J Case Rep 2015;16:811–817

5. Bullock MR, Chesnut R, Ghajar J, et al. Surgical management of acute epidural hematomas. Neurosurgery 2006;58(3 Suppl):S7-15; discussion Si-iv

Top Tips

◆ The "swirl sign" refers to areas of low attenuation within predominately hyperdense extra-axial blood. The low attenuating areas are unclotted blood and suggest active bleeding.[1]

◆ Epidural hemorrhages have associated skull fracture in 74 to 95%.[2,3]

◆ Management of acute epidural hemorrhages are based on three factors: maximum thickness of the epidural hemorrhage (1.5–2.5 cm), volume of the epidural hemorrhage (30 cm^3), and amount of midline shift (0.5–1.2 cm).[4,5]

Details 1

■ Case

A 22-year-old woman with right-sided pelvic pain and a negative pregnancy test. Right ovary measures greater than 4 cm. Which ONE of the following is the MOST likely diagnosis?
   A. Ectopic pregnancy
   B. Ruptured hemorrhagic cyst
   C. Acute appendicitis
   D. Solid ovarian mass
   E. Ovarian torsion

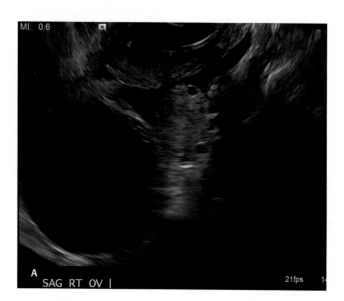

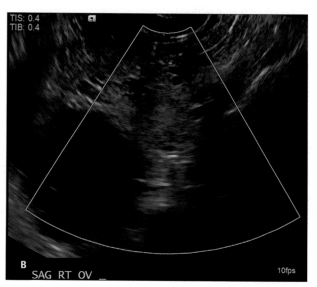

■ The following questions pertain to adnexal pathology.

1. Which of the following is the most consistent finding in ovarian torsion?
   A. Peripherally located follicles
   B. Enlargement of the ovary
   C. Heterogenous echotexture
2. Which of the following is the MOST common neoplasm associated with ovarian torsion?
   A. Large simple cyst
   B. Cystadenoma
   C. Cystadenocarcinoma
   D. Mature cystic teratoma
3. True or False. Blood flow within the ovary excludes ovarian torsion.
4. True or False. Pelvic inflammatory disease is a risk factor for ovarian torsion.
5. Which of the following is the modality of choice in evaluating ovarian torsion?
   A. Radiography
   B. Ultrasound
   C. Computed tomography
   D. Magnetic resonance imaging

6. True or False. Ovaries may move toward the midline in ovarian torsion.
7. What is the treatment of choice for ovarian torsion in a postmenopausal woman?
   A. Observation
   B. Untwisting of the vascular pedicle
   C. Oophorectomy
8. _____ is caused by ovarian stimulation treatment and consists of extravascular accumulation of fluid that results in ascites, pleural effusions, intravascular volume depletion, and oliguria.
9. _____ is a clinical syndrome characterized by amenorrhea, hirsutism, infertility, and obesity.

■ Answers and Explanations

E. Correct! Ovarian torsion is the most likely diagnosis. The images demonstrate free fluid, an enlarged right ovary (> 4 cm) with peripheral follicles, and lack of flow. These are all characteristics of ovarian torsion. With torsion, the ovarian stroma may be echogenic, hypoechoic, or heterogenous, depending on the amount of edema, hemorrhage, and/or necrosis.

Other choices and discussion

A. The patient's pregnancy test is reported as negative. Additionally, the round mass does not demonstrate internal flow or a "ring of fire" to suggest an ectopic pregnancy.

B. Free fluid is seen in the right adnexa, but a complex cyst is not demonstrated.

C. Free fluid is seen in the right adnexa, but a blind-ending tube is not demonstrated.

D. A solid mass would have flow on power Doppler imaging.

Question 1

B. Of the choices presented, the most consistent finding in ovarian torsion is enlargement of the ovary (> 4 cm).[1] Heterogenous echotexture may occur secondary to ischemia, edema, and/or hemorrhage. Peripherally located follicles are also common.

Question 2

D. Cyst, cystadenoma, and cystadenocarcinoma can all lead to ovarian torsion, but mature cystic teratoma (dermoid cyst) is the most common neoplasm that can lead to ovarian torsion.

Question 3

False. Although the lack of blood flow suggests ovarian torsion, the presence of blood flow does not exclude ovarian torsion. When ovarian torsion occurs, the venous system is compromised, causing ovarian congestion. This results in the accumulation of fluid within the ovarian stroma and into the follicles. This results in increased pressure and ultimately, arterial compromise and thrombosis. Torsion-detorsion phenomena can occur in the ovaries, sometimes causing hyperemia during the detorsion periods.

Question 4

False. Pelvic inflammatory disease leads to the formation of adhesions. This restricts the twisting of the adnexa and can actually be protective. This is also true for endometriosis.[2]

Question 5

Ultrasound is the modality of choice when evaluating ovarian torsion for many reasons, including wide availability, lack of ionizing radiation, inexpensive cost, and the ability to evaluate blood flow. Features of ovarian torsion on computed tomography or magnetic resonance imaging include enlargement of the ovary and twisting of the vascular pedicle.

Question 6

True. During ovarian torsion, the ovary sometimes migrates superiorly or toward the midline. This can cause difficulties in finding the ovary, since it is not in the normal location.

Question 7

C. Postmenopausal women with ovarian torsion should have a bilaterally oophorectomy performed at the time of the diagnosis.[2] Premenopausal women should have untwisting of the vascular pedicle, attempting to allow for the hemorrhage and edema to resolve. If the ovary is not salvageable, then oophorectomy can be pursued in a second operation.

Question 8

Ovarian hyperstimulation syndrome is a complication of ovarian stimulation treatment for in vitro fertilization. Imaging features include bilateral enlargement of the ovaries, multiple ovarian cysts, pleural effusions, and ascites. Conservative treatment with close monitoring is necessary. In severe cases, it is potentially life-threatening.

Question 9

Polycystic ovarian syndrome is depicted on imaging as an enlarged ovary containing multiple peripheral follicles. This can sometimes be misinterpreted as ovarian torsion. The clinical findings of irregular menses or amenorrhea, hirsutism, infertility, and obesity are helpful in making the diagnosis. In addition, unlike torsion, polycystic ovarian syndrome is bilateral. Major health consequences include infertility, type 2 diabetes mellitus, hypertension, dyslipidemias, cerebral vascular accidents, and coronary atherosclerosis.[3]

■ References

1. Chang HC, Bhatt S, Dogra VS. Pearls and pitfalls in diagnosis of ovarian torsion. Radiographics 2008;28(5):1355–1368

2. Oelsner G, Shashar D. Adnexal torsion. Clin Obstet Gynecol 2006;49(3):459–463

3. Lee TT, Rausch ME. Polycystic ovarian syndrome: role of imaging in diagnosis. Radiographics 2012;32(6):1643–1657

> ### Top Tips
>
> ◆ Predisposing conditions for ovarian torsion include large cysts, cystic neoplasms (benign or malignant), mature cystic teratomas (most common), and hemorrhagic cysts
>
> ◆ "Whirlpool" sign: twisted vascular pedicle seen with ovarian torsion
>
> ◆ "Spoke-wheel" sign: numerous large ovarian cysts in a spoke-wheel pattern seen with ovarian hyperstimulation syndrome

Details 2

■ Case

What is the MOST likely diagnosis for patient A?
- A. Acute cholecystitis
- B. Chronic cholecystitis
- C. Choledocholithiasis
- D. Acute hepatitis
- E. Hepatocellular carcinoma

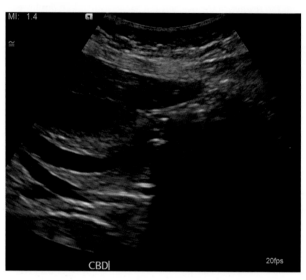

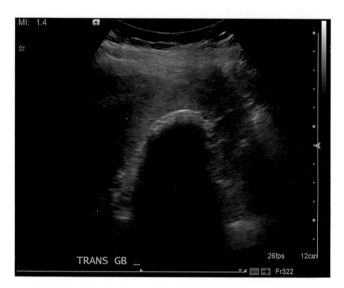

Patient A: A 30-year-old woman presenting with right upper quadrant pain.

Patient B: A 49-year-old woman presenting with right upper quadrant pain.

■ The following questions pertain to right upper quadrant pathology and relevant imaging.

1. What is the gold standard imaging modality for assessing choledocholithiasis?
2. True or False. As MRCP is the gold standard imaging modality for choledocholithiasis, it should be the first imaging study for right upper quadrant pain.
3. Which of the following is the MOST common serious complication of endoscopic retrograde cholangiopancreatography?
   - A. Hemorrhage
   - B. Pancreatitis
   - C. Perforation
   - D. Cholangitis
   - E. Cholecystitis
4. Which ultrasound sign is illustrated in the image for patient B?
5. True or False. WES complex is consistent with acute cholecystitis.

6. The most sensitive sonographic signs of acute cholecystitis include _____ and _____.
7. What is the most likely diagnosis of the following description? A round and echogenic structure along the gallbladder wall that is nonmobile, nonshadowing, and has Doppler flow.
   - A. Adherent sludge ball
   - B. Adherent gallstone
   - C. Gallbladder polyp
8. What is the most likely cause of a comet-tail artifact seen on a gallbladder ultrasound?
9. An impacted calculus within the cystic duct can lead to which of the following? (Select ALL that apply.)
   - A. Mirizzi syndrome
   - B. Acute cholecystitis
   - C. Gallbladder cancer

■ Answers and Explanations

C. Correct! This patient has choledocholithiasis. The test case image for patient A demonstrates an intraluminal echogenic focus within a tubular structure, with associated posterior acoustic shadowing. This is consistent with choledocholithiasis and dilatation of the common bile duct.

Other choices and discussion

A. The gallbladder is not fully imaged, but there is no demonstration of acute cholecystitis.

B. The gallbladder is not fully imaged, but there is no demonstration of chronic cholecystitis.

D. Acute hepatitis may have a "starry-sky" appearance on ultrasound, which is related to intralobular edematous swelling of the hepatocytes, decreased hepatic echogenicity, and accentuation of the venule wall.

E. Hepatocellular carcinoma is divided into solitary, multifocal, or diffuse types. Hepatocellular carcinoma might be associated with focal intrahepatic biliary ductal dilatation, but common bile duct involvement would be atypical.

Question 1

Magnetic resonance cholangiopancreatography (MRCP) is the gold standard and is highly accurate for the diagnosis of choledocholithiasis (97%). Note that MRCP sometimes underestimates the number of bile duct stones present. Although ultrasound is usually the first-line imaging modality, it has < 50% sensitivity for the diagnosis of choledocholithiasis. Computed tomography (CT) has moderate sensitivity. On CT, calculi within the biliary system can appear in the form of a "target sign," with radiodense calculi surrounded by low attenuating bile.

Question 2

False. A right upper quadrant ultrasound is the preferred study for acute right upper quadrant pain. Ultrasound is the most sensitive test for acute cholecystitis.

Question 3

B. The most common serious complication of endoscopic retrograde cholangiopancreatography is pancreatitis (3.5%). Intraluminal hemorrhage is a less common complication (~1%) and is usually mild. Infection can also occur.

Question 4

A wall-echo-shadow (WES) complex is illustrated in this right upper quadrant ultrasound. The WES complex is a sonographic sign representing a gallbladder filled with calculi. The "wall" corresponds to the wall of the gallbladder, the "echo" corresponds to the echogenic gallbladder calculi, and the "shadow" corresponds to the posterior acoustic shadowing from the calculi. There may be a small amount of bile that separates the "wall" from the "echo."

A porcelain gallbladder can sometimes be misinterpreted as a WES complex. With a porcelain gallbladder, however, a small amount of bile between the wall and the calculi is not seen.

Question 5

False. As described previously, WES complex is a sonographic finding that corresponds to a gallbladder filled with calculi. Not all cases are associated with acute cholecystitis. Note that the WES may actually cause difficulties in evaluating wall thickness.

Question 6

Sonographic Murphy sign and cholelithiasis are the most sensitive signs of acute cholecystitis. Other associated signs of acute cholecystitis include gallbladder wall thickening and pericholecystic fluid.

Question 7

That is the description of a gallbladder polyp. Sludge, gallstone, and polyp can all be round in shape and nonmobile. If small (< 3 mm), adherent gallstones may lack posterior acoustic shadowing. The key to this question is the Doppler flow, as only a polyp will have internal flow. Twinkle artifact can be seen with calculi and should not be confused with internal flow.

The vast majority of gallbladder polyps are benign and most are composed of cholesterol. Polyps that are > 1.5 cm are associated with an increased risk of malignancy. It is generally accepted that cholecystectomy should be considered in polyps > 1 cm. Polyps < 6 mm do not require additional follow up.

Question 8

Adenomyomatosis is the most likely cause of a comet-tail artifact in the gallbladder. Adenomyomatosis causes thickening of the gallbladder wall. It involves the mucosa and muscular wall with invaginations or diverticula called Rokitansky-Aschoff sinuses. These sinuses often accumulate cholesterol crystals that lead to the comet-tail artifact. Adenomyomatosis can sometimes mimic gallbladder cancer on imaging. These two can be differentiated on CT, if the gallbladder wall demonstrates small cystic-appearing spaces to confirm adenomyomatosis.

Question 9

All of the choices are correct. Mirizzi syndrome refers to gallstone impaction in the cystic duct causing extrinsic common bile duct compression and subsequent obstruction. An impacted calculus within the cystic duct can lead to acute cholecystitis, if it obstructs the duct. Gallbladder cancer risk factors include porcelain gallbladder, gallstones, and chronic cholecystitis.

Top Tips

- ◆ Most biliary calculi are composed of cholesterol and are not visible on plain film.
- ◆ Porcelain gallbladder is associated with an increased risk of gallbladder cancer and should be surgically removed.
- ◆ Gallbladder cancer and adenomyomatosis can mimic each other on imaging.

Details 3

■ Case

What is the MOST likely diagnosis of patient A (plain film image)?
   A. Small bowel obstruction
   B. Large bowel obstruction
   C. Ileus from pancreatitis
   D. Ileus from acute appendicitis

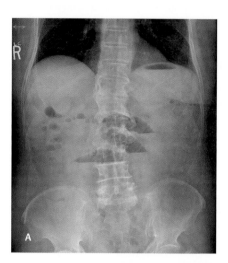

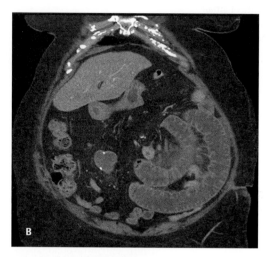

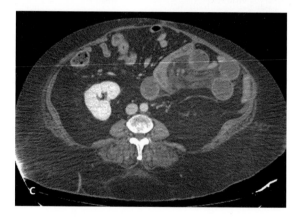

■ The following questions pertain to bowel obstruction.

1. What potential findings on plain film radiography could suggest the diagnosis of ileus from pancreatitis or acute appendicitis?
2. Two ominous findings of bowel ischemia on radiography include _____ and _____
3. In a suspected small bowel obstruction, what is the BEST initial study to obtain?
    A. Acute abdominal series
    B. Computed tomography (CT) of the abdomen and pelvis
4. What is the most likely diagnosis of patient B (CT images)?
    A. Partial small bowel obstruction
    B. Complete small bowel obstruction
    C. Closed-loop bowel obstruction
    D. Large bowel obstruction
5. What is the treatment for a closed-loop bowel obstruction?
6. True or False. In the United States, the most important risk factor for small bowel obstruction is abdominal or inguinal hernia.
7. True or False. A strangulated hernia is the same as an incarcerated hernia.
8. What is the most common cause of large bowel obstruction in adults?
9. True or False. In complete small bowel obstruction, the colon is always collapsed.

■ Answers and Explanations

A. Correct! This patient has a small bowel obstruction. Common findings in small bowel obstruction (seen in this case) include dilated segments of small bowel with air–fluid levels and relatively decompressed segments of colon. Ileus can have similar features, including distended segments of small bowel, but the multiple air–fluid levels in the test case should lead the radiologist to diagnose small bowel obstruction.

Question 1

Distended segments of small bowel in the mid abdomen (ileus) with calcifications in the expected region of the pancreas suggest chronic pancreatitis with superimposed acute pancreatitis.

An appendicolith on radiography with splinting (positional levoscoliosis) secondary to psoas muscle irritation and focal right lower quadrant ileus suggest acute appendicitis.

Question 2

Pneumatosis and portal venous gas are ominous findings that suggest bowel ischemia. Pneumoperitoneum may also be present, but this is nonspecific.

Question 3

B. The American College of Radiology appropriateness criteria state that for suspected high-grade, low-grade, or intermittent bowel obstruction, CT is the preferred initial study. This is due to the limited information that radiographs provide the radiologist and surgeon.

Question 4

C. Correct! The CT shows a closed-loop obstruction. Associated CT findings of closed-loop obstruction may include twisting of the mesenteric vessels ("whirl" sign), bowel ischemia depicted by feeble or absent bowel wall enhancement, pneumatosis, interloop fluid, and the presence of two transition points in close proximity.

Question 5

Closed-loop bowel obstruction should have surgical intervention due to the high propensity for bowel ischemia.

Question 6

False. In the United States, the most common cause of small bowel obstruction is adhesions from prior surgery. Other causes include abdominal and inguinal hernias, inflammation, and neoplasm. In underdeveloped countries, the most common cause of small bowel obstruction is abdominal or inguinal hernia.

Question 7

False. An incarcerated hernia is a hernia that is not reducible without surgery. A strangulated hernia is a hernia with vascular compromise. The majority of strangulated hernias are incarcerated, but the majority of incarcerated hernias are not strangulated. Strangulation of bowel demonstrates decreased bowel wall enhancement and sometimes bowel wall thickening. Typically, there are inflammatory changes, fluid, and stranding within the hernia sac. Incarcerated hernias have normal bowel wall enhancement, but may have mild free fluid within the sac.

Question 8

The most common cause of large bowel obstruction in adults is malignancy. Other potential causes include hernia and volvulus. Adhesions do not commonly cause large bowel obstruction.

Question 9

False. In complete small bowel obstruction, the colon is not always collapsed. An early complete obstruction may still have fecal material within the colon.

■ Reference

1. Butt MU, Velmahos GC, Zacharias N, Alam HB, de Moya M, King DR. Adhesional small bowel obstruction in the absence of previous operations: management and outcomes. World J Surg 2009;33(11):2368–2371

Top Tips

◆ Ileus can mimic small bowel obstruction on radiography.

◆ Acute appendicitis can cause ileus. Consider the diagnosis on plain film if there is an appendicolith, blurring of the psoas muscle reflection, and splinting of the patient with levoscoliosis.

◆ Adhesions are the most common cause of small bowel obstruction. These often develop from prior surgery, but can also occur in patients without surgery (i.e., Crohn's disease or prior adjacent diverticulitis[1]).

Details 4

■ Case

Which ONE of the following is the MOST likely diagnosis?
   A. Aortic pseudoaneurysm
   B. Aortic rupture
   C. Aortic dissection
   D. Intramural hematoma

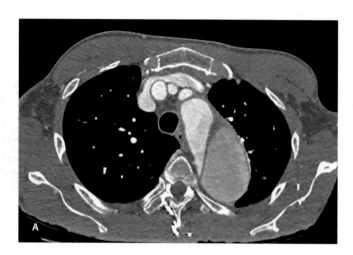

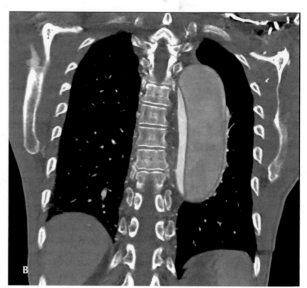

■ The following questions pertain to aortic pathology.

1. True or False. The most common cause of aortic dissection is trauma.
2. The type of aortic dissection depicted in the test case is classified as _____ and the treatment is _____
3. What is the recommended definitive test to evaluate for suspected thoracic aortic dissection?
4. What are three causes of acute aortic dissection related to acute elevated blood pressure?
5. True or False. In an aortic dissection, the true lumen is normally larger than the false lumen.
6. Five potential complications of ascending aortic dissection include _____.

7. Regarding the part of the aortic wall that makes up the false lumen in an aortic dissection, the false lumen is created _____
   A. between the intima and the media.
   B. within the media.
   C. between the media and the adventitia.
8. What are the three "acute aortic syndromes"?
9. True or False. The true lumen of an aortic dissection usually gives rise to the celiac axis and the superior mesenteric artery.

■ Answers and Explanations

C. Correct! This is an aortic dissection, which is depicted by an intimomedial flap. In the test case, the true lumen is densely opacified with contrast, and the false lumen has delayed filling and mixing of contrast. The dissection does not involve the branch vessels.

Other choices and discussion

A. Aortic pseudoaneurysm would have the same attenuation as the aorta on all phases of contrast enhancement.

B. Aortic rupture might have differences in attenuation. However, periaortic hemorrhage, which is not seen in this case, would be present.

D. Thoracic aortic intramural hematoma is classified and treated the same as a dissection. A discrete intimomedial flap is not seen with intramural hematoma, and the density is generally higher than nonopacified blood (60 to 70 HU). Intramural hematoma can be caused by hypertension, penetrating atherosclerotic ulcer, or sequela of trauma.

Question 1

False. The most common cause of aortic dissection is hypertension.

Question 2

Stanford type B, medical treatment. Since the dissection does not involve the ascending thoracic aorta or branch vessels, this a Stanford type B dissection. These types of dissections are often treated with blood pressure control. However, given the aneurysmal dilation of the aorta, surgical treatment may be considered.

Question 3

Computed tomography angiography chest and abdomen with contrast is the definitive test. Magnetic resonance angiography can be used if the patient is allergic to iodinated contrast.

Question 4

Cocaine use, pheochromocytoma, and weightlifting (heavy weights) have all been associated with aortic dissection.[1]

Question 5

False. The true lumen is normally smaller and has a higher velocity flow than the false lumen.

Question 6

1. Heart failure from acute aortic regurgitation. This is usually due to aortic leaflet prolapse or distortion of the leaflet alignment.

2. Cardiac tamponade. This may lead to hypotension.

3. Aortic rupture. This may lead to hypotension.

4. Vascular insufficiency from underperfusion of the branch vessels of the aortic arch. This may lead to pulse deficits.

5. Neurologic complications, which include stroke, spinal cord ischemia, ischemic neuropathy, and hypoxic encephalopathy.[1]

Question 7

B. The false lumen is created within the media. The inner wall is made up of the intima and media (intimomedial flap), and the outer wall is made up of the media and adventitia.

Question 8

The three acute aortic syndromes include aortic dissection, intramural hematoma, and penetrating ulcer. These are all classified into Type A and Type B, and have similar management. It is important to remember that all three of these pathologies are located within the media and can cause identical symptomatology.[2]

Question 9

True. The celiac axis and superior mesenteric artery usually arise from the true lumen.

■ References

1. Braverman AC. Acute aortic dissection: clinician update. Circulation 2010;122(2):184–188

2. Macura KJ, Corl FM, Fishman EK, Bluemke DA. Pathogenesis in acute aortic syndromes: aortic dissection, intramural hematoma, and penetrating atherosclerotic aortic ulcer. Am J Roentgenol 2003;181(2):309–316

Top Tips

◆ Aortic dissection: True lumen is usually smaller than the false lumen. True lumen usually gives rise to the celiac axis and superior mesenteric artery. Hypertension is the most common etiology.

◆ Intramural hematoma: Treated and classified the same as an aortic dissection. May be depicted by "hyperattenuating crescent" sign (on noncontrast computed tomography).

◆ Acute aortic syndromes occur within or extend into the media layer of the aortic wall.

Details 5

■ Case

In this non-contrast-enhanced computed tomography (CT), which ONE of the following is the MOST likely diagnosis?

A. Leptomeningeal carcinomatosis
B. Leptomeningitis
C. Subarachnoid hemorrhage
D. Hyperoxygenation therapy

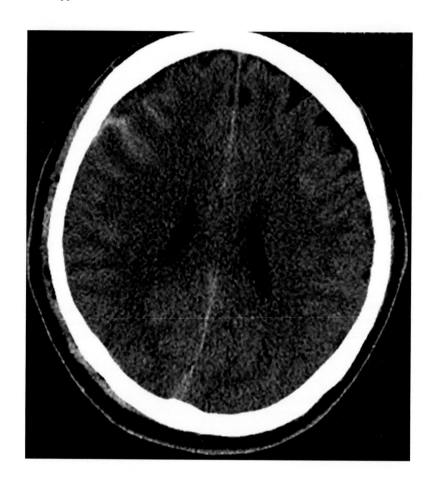

■ The following questions pertain to subarachnoid blood.

1. True or False. The most common cause of subarachnoid hemorrhage is trauma.
2. Ruptured saccular aneurysm is the second most common cause of subarachnoid hemorrhage. The third most common cause is _____.
3. What is the recommended FIRST diagnostic test to evaluate a clinically suspected nontraumatic subarachnoid hemorrhage?
4. What are the three patterns of subarachnoid hemorrhage, and which pattern is depicted in the test case?
5. True or False. Intracranial aneurysms most commonly develop near or at the branch points of the circle of Willis.
6. Three potential complications of subarachnoid hemorrhage include _____.
7. True or False. A lumbar puncture for subarachnoid blood is more likely to be diagnostic if it is performed within the first 2 hours of the onset of symptoms.
8. True or False. Pseudo-subarachnoid hemorrhage is an ominous sign.
9. Which classification system is used for grading subarachnoid hemorrhage on CT?

■ Answers and Explanations

C. Correct! On this non-contrast-enhanced CT, subarachnoid hemorrhage is the only choice that would result in hyperdensity within the sulci and subarachnoid space.

Other choices and discussion

A. Leptomeningeal carcinomatosis can occur in the same distribution as subarachnoid blood. This entity can be seen on contrast-enhanced CT and on magnetic resonance fluid-attenuated inversion recovery (FLAIR) sequences.

B. Leptomeningitis can look the same as leptomeningeal carcinomatosis on imaging.

D. Hyperoxygenation therapy can demonstrate hyperintense FLAIR signal along the subarachnoid space. This is due to the weakly paramagnetic effect of supplemental oxygen, which results in reduction of cerebrospinal fluid T1-weighted relaxation time.

Question 1

True. Trauma is the most common cause of subarachnoid hemorrhage.

Question 2

Nonaneurysmal perimesencephalic hemorrhage is the third most common cause of subarachnoid hemorrhage. As the name suggests, the blood is localized in the perimesencephalic cisterns. A specific cause is not found on angiography, and it is likely venous in origin. Complications are quite rare.

Question 3

When there is clinical suspicion for subarachnoid hemorrhage, the first diagnostic test is a non-contrast-enhanced CT of the head. If the CT demonstrates a subarachnoid hemorrhage, then further vascular imaging is needed. This could begin with either intra-arterial digital subtraction angiography or with CT angiography. If the source of the subarachnoid hemorrhage is not seen, then further workup is pursued by either lumbar puncture or CT angiography.

Question 4

The three patterns of subarachnoid hemorrhage include diffuse, perimesencephalic, and isolated cerebral convexity. The pattern depicted in the test case is the isolated cerebral convexity type. Recognition of the pattern is important to help predict causality and source of hemorrhage, as early in the time course, the hemorrhage localizes to the source of bleeding.

Question 5

True. The most common location of intracranial aneurysms is along the circle of Willis, and 90% of these arise in the anterior circulation.

Question 6

Three potential complications of subarachnoid hemorrhage include rebleeding, nonobstructive hydrocephalus, and vasospasm.

Within the first few days after hemorrhage, there is potential for rebleeding of a ruptured aneurysm. Larger aneurysms have a higher incidence of rebleeding. Additionally, subarachnoid hemorrhage can lead to nonobstructive hydrocephalus due to blockage of the cerebrospinal fluid resorption by the arachnoid villi. Lastly, vasospasm may develop in 4 to 10 days, which is treated with calcium channel blockers, most notably nimodipine.

Question 7

False. Xanthochromia usually requires at least 6 hours and sometimes up to 12 hours to develop following subarachnoid hemorrhage.

Question 8

True. Pseudo-subarachnoid hemorrhage refers to decreased parenchymal attenuation as a result of diffuse cerebral edema with increased intracranial pressure, causing dilatation of the superficial veins. This sign indicates severe brain injury and a poor prognosis.

Question 9

The modified Fisher scale is a method of grading subarachnoid hemorrhage from grade 0 to grade 4. The risk of vasospasm progressively increases with increasing grade. The grading system is based on subarachnoid hemorrhage thickness and presence or absence of intraventricular hemorrhage.

Grade 0	No subarachnoid hemorrhage
Grade 1	Thin subarachnoid hemorrhage
Grade 2	Thin subarachnoid hemorrhage with intraventricular hemorrhage
Grade 3	Thick subarachnoid hemorrhage
Grade 4	Thick subarachnoid hemorrhage with intraventricular hemorrhage

Thin = < 1 mm thickness. Thick = > 1 mm thickness.

Top Tips

◆ The most sensitive magnetic resonance imaging sequence for subarachnoid hemorrhage is FLAIR.

◆ Other pathologic and artifactual processes can cause increased FLAIR signal, including leptomeningitis, leptomeningeal carcinomatosis, hyperoxygenation therapy, and cerebrospinal fluid or vascular pulsation.

◆ Aneurysms usually occur at branch points, and the anterior circulation is most commonly involved. Anterior communicating artery aneurysms are twice as likely to rupture as other intracranial aneurysms.

Image Rich 1

■ Case

Match the ankle injury type with the Lauge-Hansen classification.
- A. Maisonneuve fracture pattern
- B. Supination adduction
- C. Supination external rotation (SER)
- D. Pronation external rotation (PER)

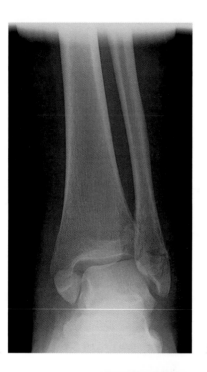

1.

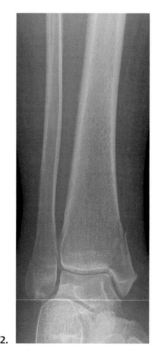

2.

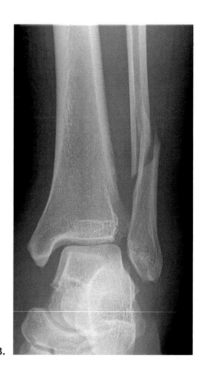

3.

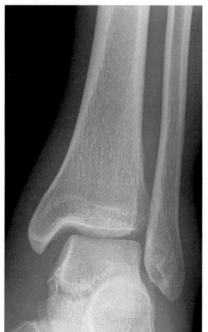

4a.

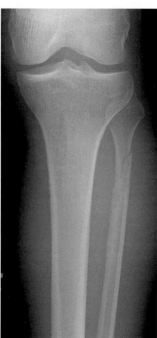

4b.

■ Answers and Explanations

1. C. The first image demonstrates a transverse fracture of the medial malleolus and a trans-syndesmotic fibular fracture (Weber B), which makes this a SER stage IV ankle injury. Ankle injuries follow a stepwise injury pattern. Stepwise progression for SER injury includes anterior inferior tibiofibular ligament rupture or avulsion of the anterior tibial tubercle, trans-syndesmotic fibular fracture, posterior tibiofibular ligament rupture or avulsion of the posterior malleolus, and lastly, transverse fracture of the medial malleolus or rupture of the deltoid ligaments.

2. B. The second image demonstrates an infrasyndesmotic fibular fracture (Weber A) with a vertical fracture of the medial malleolus, which is compatible with a supination adduction ankle injury. Stage I injury is either an intrasyndesmotic fibular fracture or a rupture of the talofibular ligament. Stage II is characterized as a vertical fracture of the medial malleolus. It is important to evaluate for marginal plafond impaction, as orthopedics will attempt to elevated the impacted articular component.[1]

3. D. The third image depicts a suprasyndesmotic fibular fracture (Weber C) with medial clear space widening and lateral talar shift. This is compatible with a PER ankle injury. The stepwise progression for PER injury includes transverse fracture of the medial malleolus or deltoid ligament injury, anterior inferior tibiofibular ligament rupture or anterior tibial tubercle avulsion fracture, suprasyndesmotic fibular fracture, and lastly, posterior malleolus fracture or rupture of the posterior inferior tibiofibular ligament.

4 a,b. A. The last two images demonstrate widening of the medial and lateral clear space with a fracture of the proximal fibular diaphysis. This is a Maisonneuve fracture pattern and should always be suspected when there is widening of the medial and lateral clear space without fracture on an ankle series. Tibia-fibular plain radiography should be obtained to evaluate for proximal fibular fracture.

It is important to learn both the Danis-Weber and Lauge-Hansen classifications, because both classifications describe the same ankle injury. The Danis-Weber classification is focused on anatomic location of the fibular fracture, whereas the Lauge-Hansen classification describes the mechanistic relationship of ankle injury.

Lauge-Hansen classification can predict injuries that are not conspicuous on plain radiography because it describes injuries occurring in a stepwise manner (i.e., stages).

Rules to remember:

1. Identify the location of the fibular fracture using the Danis-Weber classification (see Top Tips).

2. Classify the type of injury in the Lauge-Hansen classification (see Top Tips).

3. Look for the highest stage of injury.

■ Reference

1. McConnell T, Tornetta P, 3rd. Marginal plafond impaction in association with supination-adduction ankle fractures: a report of eight cases. J Orthop Trauma 2001;15(6):447–449

Top Tips

Location of fibular fracture	Danis-Weber classification	Lauge-Hansen classification
Infrasyndesmotic	Weber A	Supination adduction
Trans-syndesmotic	Weber B	SER
Suprasyndesmotic	Weber C	PER

A fourth type of injury, pronation abduction, is not discussed because it is an uncommon type of ankle injury.

If the medial clear space and lateral clear space are widened without fibular fracture on ankle series, image the leg to evaluate for proximal fibular fracture (i.e., Maisonneuve fracture pattern).

Image Rich 2

■ Case

The following patients all present to the emergency department with abdominal pain. Match the radiology images with the correct diagnoses.

    A. Epiploic appendagitis
    B. Acute appendicitis
    C. Diverticulitis
    D. Colon cancer

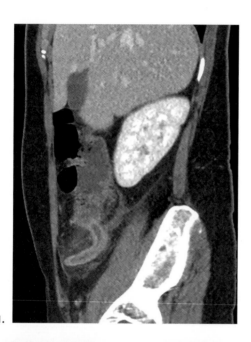

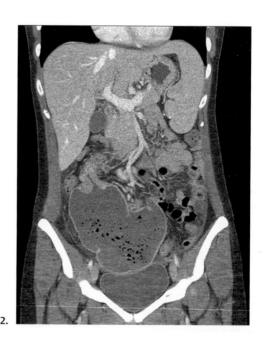

1.

2.

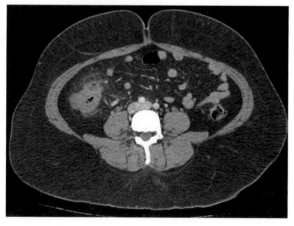

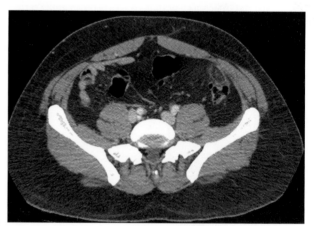

3.

4.

■ Answers and Explanations

1. B. Acute appendicitis. Acute appendicitis can be diagnosed with ultrasound, magnetic resonance imaging (MRI), computed tomography (CT), and even plain film radiography. In adults, CT is the imaging modality of choice for the evaluation of appendicitis. An enlarged appendix with periappendiceal fat stranding is the typical appearance for uncomplicated appendicitis. Appendicitis can be complicated by perforation and abscess formation that may alter management.

An appendiceal inflammatory mass, which refers to the inflammation that surrounds the appendix and other structures, may sometimes develop. This occurs in patients with an appendiceal perforation that typically has a gradual and less severe appendicitis presentation. As appendiceal inflammatory mass formation increases the complication rate for emergent appendectomy, interval appendectomy is usually performed following intravenous antibiotic therapy.[1]

In children, ultrasound is the imaging modality of choice. Ultrasound has several advantages over CT, including the lack of ionizing radiation, the lack of intravenous contrast, the ability to assess compression of the appendix, and the ability to assess the vascularity with Doppler ultrasound. Ultrasound findings of acute appendicitis include a noncompressible blind ending tubular structure measuring ≥ 7 mm with periappendiceal inflammation. An appendicolith can sometimes be seen as an echogenic focus with posterior acoustic shadowing. See the following example.

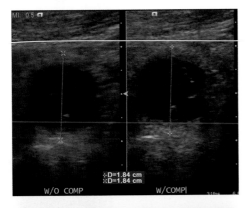

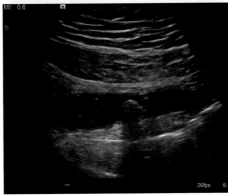

MRI is the second line modality of choice in a child when the appendix is not seen or the findings are equivocal on ultrasound. Findings of appendicitis on MRI include an enlarged appendix with periappendiceal inflammation. Diffusion restriction on MRI can be seen in early appendicitis.[2]

2. D. Colon cancer. Colorectal cancer is the fourth most common cancer in the United States (breast > lung > prostate > colorectal) and may present with different forms, including polyp (exophytic or sessile), focal colonic wall lesion, or circumferential invasion of the colonic wall with intraluminal narrowing. The test case image depicts the classic "apple-core" lesion, which was orginally described with barium studies. One can also appreciate the marked dilatation of the cecum, compatible with large bowel obstruction. Malignancy is the most common cause of large bowel obstruction. Perforated colon cancer can sometimes be difficult to differentiate from diverticulitis, both clinically and with imaging.

3. C. Diverticulitis. Diverticulitis is a common cause of abdominal pain in adults. Imaging findings for uncomplicated diverticulitis include colonic wall thickening and pericolonic inflammatory change. Complicated diverticulitis includes abscess formation and perforation. An inflamed diverticula is not always seen. Diverticulitis can result in bowel obstruction acutely, and it can also lead to bowel obstruction long after the inflammation has resolved, from subsequent adhesion formation. One potential sequela of diverticulitis is fistula formation (colovesicular, colovaginal, or coloenteric). As discussed previously, colon cancer can mimic diverticulitis. If malignancy is a consideration, a colonoscopy should be pursued after the inflammation resolves.

4. A. Epiploic appendagitis. Epiploic appendagitis refers to inflammation of one of the epiploic appendages of the colon. This process can cause symptoms that are similar to acute appendicitis or diverticulitis. This is a self-limiting process and does not need surgical treatment. This key to the diagnosis is that the inflammation surrounds a central ovoid clearing of fat attenuation without adjacent colonic wall thickening. A central round hyperdensity may be present, representing a thrombosed vessel within the appendage.

■ References

1. Deelder JD, Richir MC, Schoorl T, Schreurs WH. How to treat an appendiceal inflammatory mass: operatively or nonoperatively? J Gastrointest Surg 2014;18(4):641–645

2. Inci E, Kilickesmez O, Hocaoglu E, Aydin S, Bayramoglu S, Cimilli T. Utility of diffusion-weighted imaging in the diagnosis of acute appendicitis. Eur Radiol 2011;21(4):768–775

Top Tips

◆ Hyperemia is seen in early acute appendicitis. However, as the process progresses, decreased flow leading to necrosis is sometimes observed.

◆ Ultrasound should be the first-line study of choice for the evaluation of appendicitis in pediatric and pregnant patients.

◆ Epiploic appendagitis can mimic diverticulitis and appendicitis but is a nonsurgical lesion. Thus, accurate diagnosis is crucial.

Image Rich 3

■ Case

Match the image with appropriate recommended treatment.
   A. Retraction of a line/tube
   B. Advancement of a line/tube
   C. Removal of a line/tube
   D. Placement of a tube

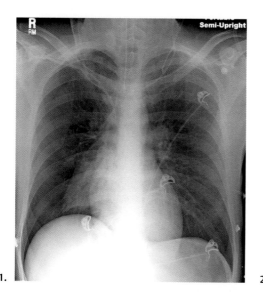

1.

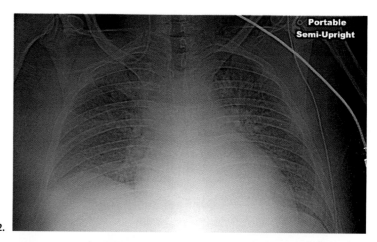

2.

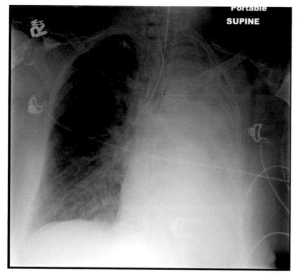

3.

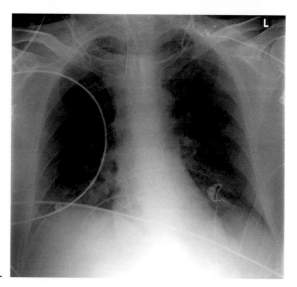

4.

■ Answers and Explanations

1. D. Placement of a tube. A right pneumothorax is present, which is a known complication for subclavian vein catheter placement. Other complications include failure to place the catheter, arterial access, hemithorax, and catheter malposition. It is also important to check for a contralateral pneumothorax, as line attempts may have occurred on both sides of the patient prior to imaging.

Radiographic findings of tension pneumothorax include visceral pleural line visualization, ipsilateral lung atelectasis, increased intercostal spaces, shift of the mediastinum away from the pneumothorax, and depression of the diaphragm.

2. C. Removal of a line. A malpositioned right subclavian catheter is present. The subclavian catheter courses cephalad into the right internal jugular vein. Malpositioned catheters can extend into various veins, including the internal mammary vein, azygous vein, superior intercostal vein, and the inferior thyroidal vein. Malpositioned lines should be repositioned or replaced. Once the sterile field is broken, a line may be pulled back but not advanced.

A lateral radiograph can evaluate the course of the central venous catheter in the anterior-posterior plane. If the catheter courses anteriorly along the sternum, it is likely within the internal mammary vein. If it courses posteriorly, it may be in the azygous vein. The normal position of a central venous catheter on a lateral radiograph is at the junction between the anterior third and middle third of the chest.

3. A. Retraction of a tube. There is a right main stem intubation with ipsilateral lung hyperinflation and collapse of the contralateral left lung. There is volume loss and deviation of the mediastinum to the left. Because the patient probably already has respiratory compromise (intubated), this tube placement will likely cause further hypoxemia. With the neck in a neutral position, the endotracheal tube should be 5 ± 2 cm from the carina. On portable radiography, the carina overlies T5–T7. If the carina is not visible, it can be assumed that a position at T3 or T4 is safe.[1]

4. B. Advancement of a tube. The Dobhoff tube tip overlies the proximal esophagus. It should be advanced and ideally placed past the pylorus. Dobhoff tubes are typically used for feeding and nutrition. The tube placement in the test case greatly increases the risk for aspiration. Enteric tubes can also coil in the hypopharynx. If this occurs, the tube should be removed completely and placement reattempted.

Bagging the patient before intubation can cause gaseous distention of the stomach and should not be confused with esophageal intubation. Look for the endotracheal tube overlying the tracheal air column and at the lung volumes.

■ References

1. Goodman LR, Conrardy PA, Laing F, Singer MM. Radiographic evaluation of endotracheal tube position. Am J Roentgenol 1976;127(3):433–434

Top Tips

◆ Lateral radiography can help determine whether a malpositioned central line is within the internal mammary vein (anterior location) or the azygous vein (posterior location).

◆ Complications for intubation include dental injury, pneumothorax, and malpositioned tube in the right mainstem bronchus or esophagus.

◆ Endotracheal tube positioning: 5 ± 2 cm above the carina. Carina is at the T5–T7 level on portable radiography.

Image Rich 4

■ **Case**

Match the computed tomography imaging with the morphology used in the thoracolumbar injury classification and severity score (TLICS).
- A. Compression
- B. Burst
- C. Translation
- D. Distraction

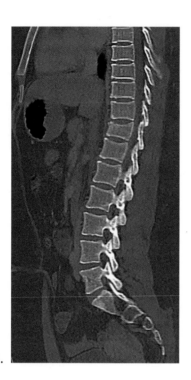

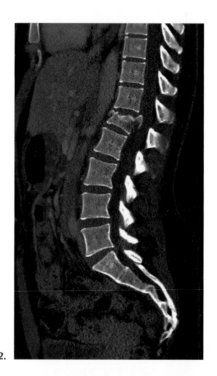

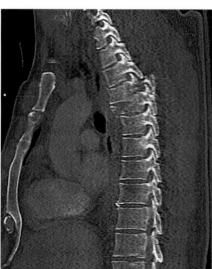

1.

2.

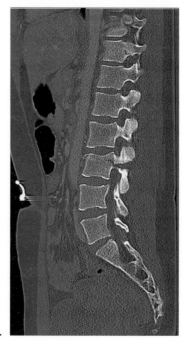

3.

4.

■ **Answers and Explanations**

Three major spinal injury classifications exist, including Denis classification, AO spine classification, and TLICS.

The Denis classification (three-column) evaluates which part of the spinal column is injured. The columns are divided into anterior, middle, and posterior. The anterior column includes the anterior longitudinal ligament and the anterior two-thirds of the disc and vertebral body. The middle column includes the posterior one-third of the vertebral body and the posterior longitudinal ligament. The posterior column includes the pedicles and structures posterior to the pedicles. Anterior column injuries are considered stable. Injury involving the anterior and middle columns may be unstable. If all three columns are involved, the spinal injury is considered unstable.

The AO spine classification and TLICS classification describe morphology of the injury. Both have neurologic modifiers. The AO spine classification categorizes injuries into Type A, Type B, or Type C.

TLICS describes the morphology of the injury (compression, burst, translation/rotation, or distraction), posterior ligamentous complex (PLC) integrity (intact, suspected injury, injury), and neurologic status. Based on the scoring criteria, this classification is used to predict the need for surgery. This classification gives points depending on the injury morphology (1–4), posterior ligamentous complex (0–3), and neurologic involvement (0–3). If the sum is > 4, then operative management is usually considered. If the sum is < 4, then nonoperative management is encouraged. If the sum is 4, then the injury may be treated either operatively or nonoperatively.

1. A. Compression fracture. Compression fractures are the most common type of osseous injury to the thoracic and lumbar spine. These types of injuries occur with axial loading and/or flexion forces. An important factor to consider is the extent of vertebral body loss of height. Multiple levels may be affected, and fractures may or may not be contiguous. One point is given for the compression fracture morphology in the TLICS classification.

Common findings include concavity of the superior endplate, buckling of the anterior cortex of the vertebral body, anterior-superior corner fracture, or slight height loss with a sclerotic band 1 to 2 mm below the superior endplate (trabecular impaction).

Compression fractures are typically considered a single (anterior) column injury in the Denis classification and a Type A1 injury in the AO spine classification.

2. B. Burst fracture. This has a similar mechanism of injury to that of compression fractures, but comminution occurs and fragments can extend anteriorly, laterally, and posteriorly. The test case image depicts both anterior and posterior fracture fragments. Retropulsion of the fracture fragment can cause compression of the thecal sac, cord, and nerve roots. Two points are given for the burst morphology in the TLICS classification.

The burst fracture morphology is considered a two-column injury in the Denis classification as it injures both the anterior and middle columns of the vertebrae.

The AO spine classification separates burst fractures into incomplete (only one endplate fractured) and complete (both endplates fractured) burst fractures. These are labeled as Type A3 and Type A4, respectively.

3. C. Translation injury. Translational injury refers to movement of a superior segment of the spine in relation to an inferior segment of the spine. Most commonly, there is anterior translation of the vertebrae, depicted by anterolisthesis with either subluxed/dislocated facets or fracture of the pars interarticularis. Lateral translation can also occur. Three points are given to the translation morphology in the TLICS classification. Rotational injury (e.g., unilateral facet dislocation) is also given three points.

Translational injury is considered a three-column injury in the Denis classification as this type of injury disrupts either bone or discoligamentous structures in each of the three columns.

The AO spine classification categorizes these injuries into Type C injuries.

4. D. Distraction injury. Distraction injury may be due to flexion or extension forces. Injury can be solely discoligamentous or may be transosseous in nature. The most commonly recognized distraction injury is the "Chance fracture," with a horizontal/axial fracture plane through the posterior elements/pedicles into the vertebral body, as depicted in the test case. This is a flexion-distraction type morphology. Extension-distraction can also occur, with disruption of the anterior longitudinal ligament and widening of the disc space, and it can continue into the posterior elements. Four points are given to this morphology in the TLICS classification. It is important to remember that flexion-distraction injuries can also have a compression/burst fracture component.

Distraction injury may be considered a three-column injury in the Denis classification, if the injury extends to the level of the anterior two-thirds of the vertebral body.

The AO spine classification categorizes these injuries into Type B injures. These are subdivided into B1 for transosseous tension band disruption (Chance fracture), B2 for posterior tension band disruption with concomitant compression/burst fracture, and B3 for hyperextension injuries.

Top Tips

◆ Chance fracture type injury is an unstable injury, classified as a distraction injury in TLICS and AO spine classification. It most commonly undergoes posterior fixation. There is a high association with intra-abdominal injuries.

◆ PLC described in TLICS anatomically includes supraspinous ligament, interspinous ligament, facet capsule/joint, and ligamentum flavum. The posterior longitudinal ligament is not part of the PLC.

◆ Incomplete cord injury has a higher point value than complete cord injury because surgery may prevent the progression to complete cord injury.

Image Rich 5

■ Case

Match the herniation imaging findings with the correct potential sequelae.
- A. Anterior cerebral artery territory infarction
- B. Fixed and dilated pupil
- C. Posterior inferior cerebellar artery (PICA) territory infarction and hydrocephalus
- D. Cardiorespiratory compromise

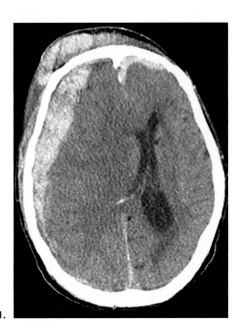

1.

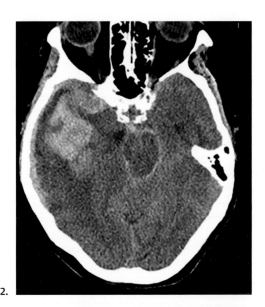

2.

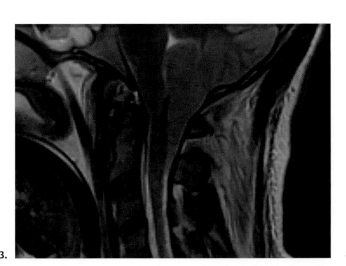

3.

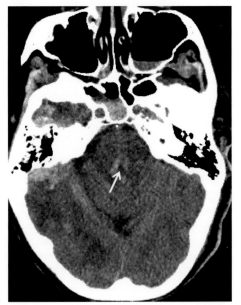

4.

Answers and Explanations

1. A. Anterior cerebral artery infarction. The first image demonstrates subfalcine herniation. Subfalcine herniation occurs when mass effect is exerted on the cerebral hemisphere with subsequent hemispheric displacement, particularly the cingulate gyrus, beneath the falx cerebri. One potential sequela of subfalcine herniation is compression of the anterior cerebral artery, which can lead to infarction. This can occur on the ipsilateral side or bilaterally.

2. B. Fixed and dilated pupil. The second image demonstrates uncal herniation. As the medial temporal lobe and uncus move medially and downward across the tentorial incisura, compression can result on the brainstem, posterior cerebral arteries, and cranial nerve III (oculomotor). Compression of the oculomotor nerve can lead to an ipsilateral fixed and dilated pupil. This type of herniation can also compress the posterior cerebral artery, with subsequent infarction of the occipital lobes and resultant homonymous hemianopsia.[1]

3. C. PICA infarct and hydrocephalus. Tonsillar herniation is shown in the third image. Tonsillar herniation can occur from a mass within the posterior fossa (neoplasm or hemorrhage), severe supratentorial mass effect, or a lumbar puncture in the setting of increased intracranial pressure. Tonsillar herniation can cause compression of the PICA, leading to cerebellar infarction. Compression of the fourth ventricle sometimes leads to obstructive hydrocephalus.

4. D. Cardiorespiratory compromise. Duret hemorrhages are noted on the fourth image, depicted by blood within the pons. Duret hemorrhages are commonly seen with central herniation (downward transtentorial herniation of the midbrain) that tears perforating vessels that extend into the pons. As the midbrain descends, there is compression of the medulla oblongata, which leads to cardiorespiratory compromise.[1]

References

1. Johnson PL, Eckard DA, Chason DP, Brecheisen MA, Batnitzky S. Imaging of acquired cerebral herniations. Neuroimaging Clin N Am 2002;12(2):217–228

2. Aboulezz AO, Sartor K, Geyer CA, Gado MH. Position of cerebellar tonsils in the normal population and in patients with Chiari malformation: a quantitative approach with MR imaging. J Comput Assist Tomogr 1985;9(6):1033–1036

3. Barkovich AJ, Wippold FJ, Sherman JL, Citrin CM. Significance of cerebellar tonsillar position on MR. Am J Neuroradiol 1986;7(5):795–799

SECTION III DIAGNOSTIC RADIOLOGY IMAGING

Top Tips

Cerebellar tonsil positioning can have a wide range in the normal population. If the cerebellar tonsils are below the basion-opisthion line by ≥ 5 mm, then pathologic tonsillar herniation is present. Normal variants can occur and the suggested measurements for normal are < 2 to 3 mm.[2,3]

Type of herniation	Territory of infarction
Subfalcine herniation	Anterior cerebral artery
Uncal herniation	Posterior cerebral artery
Tonsillar herniation	PICA

More Challenging 1

■ Case

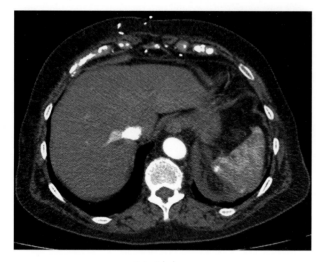
Arterial phase

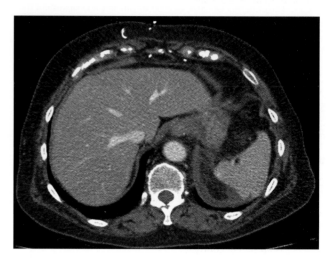
Portal-venous phase

■ Questions

1. What is the most likely diagnosis?
   A. Normal spleen enhancement pattern
   B. Splenic injury without vascular injury
   C. Splenic injury with pseudoaneurysm
   D. Splenic injury with active extravasation of contrast within the spleen
   E. Splenic injury with active extravasation of contrast into the peritoneum

2. What is the appropriate management of a stable patient with the above finding?
   A. No intervention needed
   B. Proximal embolization of the main splenic artery
   C. Distal embolization of the splenic pseudoaneurysm
   D. Laparotomy with partial resection of the spleen
   E. Laparotomy with splenectomy

3. What is the potential life-threatening consequence of an untreated splenic pseudoaneurysm?
   A. If < 2 cm in diameter, pseudoaneurysms are not life-threatening.
   B. Delayed splenic rupture
   C. Malignant hypertension
   D. Splenic pseudoaneurysm thrombosis

■ Answers and Explanations

Question 1

C. Correct! The test case images depict a splenic injury with a pseudoaneurysm. The pseudoaneurysm follows the aortic blood pool on both phases of contrast enhancement.

Other choices and discussion

A. The arterial phase of enhancement of the spleen often gives a "tiger-striped" appearance. This should not be seen on the portal-venous phase. In the test case, the low attenuating areas within the spleen on the portal-venous phase are lacerations. Splenic injuries can be graded with either the American Association for the Surgery of Trauma (AAST) grading system or with the computed tomography–based classification.

B. A vascular injury *is* present.

D. Active contrast extravasation can mimic a pseudoaneurysm on a single-phase study but should not follow the aortic blood pool on both phases. Also, contrast extravasation tends to grow in size on the portal venous phase.

E. There is no sign of contrast extravasation into the peritoneum. Intraperitoneal extravasation of contrast from the spleen can appear as a layer of contrast along the dependent portion of the perisplenic space or be surrounded by non-opacified hemorrhage.

Question 2

C. Correct! Splenic pseudoaneurysms should be embolized, and this should be performed as distally as possible. Selective embolization helps to maintain the majority of the splenic function.[1]

Other choices and discussion

A. Although splenic injuries can often be managed conservatively, a concomitant pseudoaneurysm should be embolized.

B. Proximal embolization (main splenic artery) is used to decrease the perfusion pressure to the spleen. Perfusion occurs through collateral pathways, including short gastric, pancreatic, gastroepiploic, and splenic capsular arteries.[2]

D. Partial resections of the spleen are usually reserved for benign splenic masses. Although partial splenic resection can be performed in the setting of trauma, if the patient is stable, endovascular embolization is preferred, and if the patient is unstable, total splenectomy is preferred.

E. Laparotomy with splenectomy is usually reserved for unstable patients or for high-grade injuries that are likely to fail conservative therapy.

Question 3

B. Correct! Delayed splenic rupture can be associated with splenic pseudoaneurysms. Rupture is potentially life-threatening.[3] Although the AAST grading system does not specifically address pseudoaneurysm, the radiology multidetector computed tomography grading system does.[4]

Other choices and discussion

A. Pseudoaneurysms of any size are life-threatening and need treatment.

C. Hypertension is the most common disease associated with *renal* artery aneurysms, not splenic pseudoaneurysms. It is unclear whether the renal artery aneurysm causes the hypertension or the hypertension causes the aneurysm.[5]

D. Thrombosis does occur in splenic pseudoaneurysms. It can actually be beneficial.

■ References

1. Madoff DC, Denys A, Wallace MJ, et al. Splenic arterial interventions: anatomy, indications, technical considerations, and potential complications. Radiographics 2005;25 Suppl 1:S191–211

2. Imbrogno BF, Ray CE. Splenic artery embolization in blunt trauma. Semin Intervent Radiol 2012;29(2):147–149

3. Freiwald S. Late-presenting complications after splenic trauma. Perm J 2010;14(2):41–44

4. Marmery H, Shanmuganathan K, Alexander MT, Mirvis SE. Optimization of selection for nonoperative management of blunt splenic injury: comparison of MDCT grading systems. Am J Roentgenol 2007;189(6):1421–1427

5. Henke PK, Cardneau JD, Welling TH 3rd, et al. Renal artery aneurysms: a 35-year clinical experience with 252 aneurysms in 168 patients. Ann Surg 2001;234(4):454–462; discussion 462–453

Top Tips

◆ The spleen is the most commonly injured organ in the adult population.

◆ The AAST grading system is a classification that helps direct management of splenic injuries.

◆ Splenic pseudoaneurysms are potentially life-threatening (delayed splenic rupture) and need treatment.

More Challenging 2

■ Case

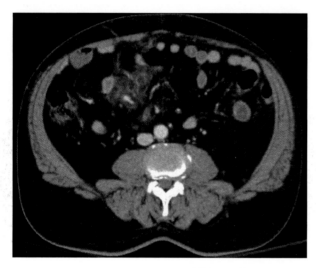

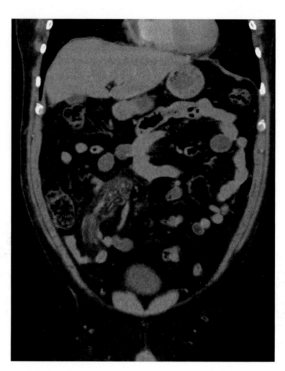

A 25-year-old man status post motor vehicle collision.

■ Questions

1. What is the MOST likely diagnosis?
   A. Mesenteric panniculitis
   B. Sclerosing mesenteritis
   C. Carcinoid tumor
   D. Lymphoma
   E. Mesenteric hematoma

2. Where do bucket-handle tears of the mesentery occur?
   A. Proximal portion of the superior mesenteric artery
   B. Proximal portion of the inferior mesenteric artery
   C. Superior mesenteric vein near the confluence of the superior mesenteric and splenic veins

   D. Inferior mesenteric vein near the drainage into the splenic vein
   E. Mesenteric vessels at the level of the bowel

3. What is the most SPECIFIC radiographic sign of bowel injury?
   A. Bowel wall thickening
   B. Discontinuity of the bowel wall
   C. Moderate density free fluid
   D. Interloop fluid
   E. Extraluminal gas

■ Answers and Explanations

Question 1

E. Correct! The test case images demonstrate stranding and hemorrhage along the mesenteric vasculature compatible with mesenteric hematoma. This type of injury can be seen in both blunt and penetrating trauma. The hemorrhage results from injury to the mesenteric vessels. Mesenteric injuries can be life-threatening because of hemorrhage and/or bowel ischemia. Several of the other provided choices could have a similar appearance on computed tomography, but the traumatic history here is the key to making the correct diagnosis.

Other choices and discussion

A. Mesenteric panniculitis is rare and characterized by chronic inflammation of the fat within the mesentery. This entity has been described as a mesenteric panniculitis fatty mass with associated well-defined, < 5 mm, soft tissue nodules.[1] Imaging findings are similar to the test case images. "Misty mesentery" is a term used to describe mesenteric panniculitis.

B. Sclerosing mesenteritis is considered a fibrotic stage of mesenteric panniculitis. Mesenteric panniculitis is the acute phase, depicted by fat necrosis and acute inflammation. Sclerosing mesenteritis is the later stage and is often associated with other chronic inflammatory diseases including retroperitoneal fibrosis, sclerosing cholangitis, Riedel thyroiditis, and orbital pseudotumor. Although the etiology of sclerosing mesenteritis is unknown, infection, trauma, ischemia, and coexistence with malignancy have all been suggested.[2]

C. Carcinoid tumor within the mesentery can have a similar appearance to sclerosing mesenteritis. With carcinoid, there are varying degrees of mesenteric fibrosis and calcification, including the classic "spoke-wheel" pattern of fibrosis.

D. Lymphoma can also have a similar appearance, with infiltration into the mesenteric fat and enlargement of mesenteric lymph nodes.

Question 2

E. Correct! Bucket-handle tears of the mesentery occur in the setting of blunt force trauma, where the more mobile bowel moves away from the mesentery, shearing off the mesenteric vessels at the level of the bowel. Depending on how much of the bowel is involved, ischemic bowel may ensue, requiring surgical resection. Other traumatic sequelae often found in association with mesenteric injury include bowel injury, spinal injury, and pelvic ring fractures.

The other choices are incorrect.

Question 3

B. Correct! Discontinuity of the bowel wall is the most specific sign for bowel injury; however, this is also the least common finding. The other choices are all nonspecific findings of bowel injury.

Other choices and discussion

A. Bowel wall thickening is seen in 75% of cases of transmural injury. However, this finding is not specific.

C. Moderate density free fluid has a high sensitivity for bowel injury. However, this finding is not specific.

D. Interloop fluid refers to fluid along the mesenteric side of small bowel segments and sometimes indicates the site of bowel injury. Interloop fluid is more likely to be associated with bowel or mesenteric injury than with solid organ injury.[3]

E. Pneumoperitoneum is seen in 44 to 55% cases of bowel injury. Other causes of pneumoperitoneum include barotrauma, mechanical ventilation, and Foley catheter–introduced air in patients with intraperitoneal bladder rupture.

■ References

1. Daskalogiannaki M, Voloudaki A, Prassopoulos P, et al. CT evaluation of mesenteric panniculitis: prevalence and associated diseases. Am J Roentgenol 2000;174(2):427–431

2. Horton KM, Lawler LP, Fishman EK. CT findings in sclerosing mesenteritis (panniculitis): spectrum of disease. Radiographics 2003;23(6):1561–1567

3. Brody JM, Leighton DB, Murphy BL, et al. CT of blunt trauma bowel and mesenteric injury: typical findings and pitfalls in diagnosis. Radiographics 2000;20(6):1525–1536; discussion 1536–1537

**SECTION III
DIAGNOSTIC RADIOLOGY
IMAGING**

Top Tips

◆ Mesenteric injury is a potentially life-threatening injury that can cause hemodynamic instability or bowel ischemia.

◆ Bucket-handle tears of the mesentery occur at the level of the bowel and may lead to bowel ischemia.

◆ When encountering mesenteric stranding on computed tomography, remember to consider trauma in the differential.

More Challenging 3

■ Case

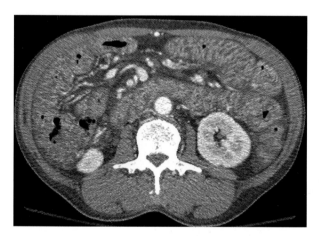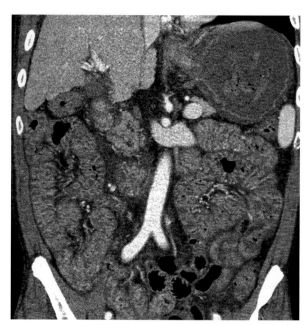

Contrast-enhanced computed tomography (CT) of the abdomen and pelvis.

■ Questions

1. What is the MOST likely diagnosis?
   A. Small bowel obstruction
   B. Small bowel contusion
   C. Mesenteric injury
   D. Shock bowel
   E. Celiac disease

2. Which ONE of the following is a component of the CT hypotension complex?
   A. Mucosal hypoenhancement of the bowel
   B. Slit-like/flattened inferior vena cava
   C. Increased diameter of the aorta
   D. Hypoenhancing adrenal glands
   E. Focal bowel wall thickening

3. How is shock bowel treated? Select the ONE correct answer.
   A. Fluid resuscitation and cessation of the bleeding source
   B. Resection of the small bowel segments that show the classic mucosal hyperenhancement
   C. Cross-clamping of the aorta
   D. Resuscitative endovascular balloon occlusion of the aorta catheter placement
   E. Antibiotic therapy

■ Answers and Explanations

Question 1

D. Correct! This is shock bowel. Shock bowel is thought to result from hypovolemia, with resultant sympathetic stimulation, splanchnic vasoconstriction, and reduced bowel perfusion.[1]

Other choices and discussion

A. Findings of small bowel obstruction would include dilated segments of fluid-filled small bowel and a transition from dilated to decompressed bowel.

B. Small bowel contusion can appear as focal wall thickening with a discrete hematoma or as circumferential wall thickening within a small bowel segment. Contusions are usually limited to a small segment of bowel. Mucosal hyperenhancement would be atypical with small bowel contusion.

C. Although mesenteric injury can lead to "bucket-handle" tears and concomitant bowel ischemia, focal findings are also usually present.

E. Celiac disease is a common but underdiagnosed disease of malabsorption, affecting 1 in 200 Americans. It is depicted on CT by ileojejunal fold pattern reversal and small bowel dilated with fluid. Other features include lymphadenopathy and transient small bowel intussusception.[2]

Question 2

B. Correct! The inferior vena cava becomes "slit-like" (anteroposterior dimension < 9 mm). The CT hypotension complex is most commonly seen in traumatic injury with hypovolemia leading to hypotension.

Other choices and discussion

A. Shock bowel has a characteristic appearance of diffuse bowel mucosal *hyper*enhancement and submucosal (wall) edema. This is thought to result from decreased bowel perfusion, which alters the permeability of the bowel and causes leakage of fluid and contrast.

C. The diameter of the aorta may *decrease* due to the hypovolemia.

D. Adrenal gland *hyper*enhancement may occur. However, this is more common in pediatric patients.

Question 3

A. Correct! Early fluid resuscitation and cessation of the bleeding source is generally sufficient for treating shock bowel. Soon after resuscitation, the bowel returns to normal.

Other choices and discussion

B. Although there is bowel hypoperfusion, the bowel is not infarcted when this appearance is seen on CT scan. Resection is not indicated.

C. Cross clamping the aorta is used to control bleeding distally, but could potentially cause visceral ischemia when the clamp is engaged and reperfusion injury after the cross clamp is released.

D. A resuscitative endovascular balloon occlusion of the aorta catheter is inserted into the femoral artery and is used to stop exsanguinating hemorrhage distal to the balloon. The balloon can be inflated above the celiac axis (for abdominal bleeding) or below the renal arteries (for pelvic bleeding). Although this maneuver may temporarily stop hemorrhage, resuscitation is the key component to reverse the hypotension complex.[3]

E. The use of antibiotic therapy is not a corrective action for shock bowel.

■ References

1. Ames JT, Federle MP. CT hypotension complex (shock bowel) is not always due to traumatic hypovolemic shock. Am J Roentgenol 2009;192(5):W230–235

2. Scholz FJ, Afnan J, Behr SC. CT findings in adult celiac disease. Radiographics 2011;31(4):977–992

3. Biffl WL, Fox CJ, Moore EE. The role of REBOA in the control of exsanguinating torso hemorrhage. J Trauma Acute Care Surg 2015;78(5):1054–1058

SECTION III
DIAGNOSTIC RADIOLOGY
IMAGING

Top Tips

- ◆ CT hypotension complex findings include shock bowel, slit-like/flattened inferior vena cava, small diameter aorta, and hyperenhancing adrenal glands.

- ◆ Shock bowel appears as diffuse hyperenhancing bowel mucosa and submucosal edema.

- ◆ Shock bowel is most often reversible by resuscitation and cessation of the source of bleeding.

More Challenging 4

■ Case

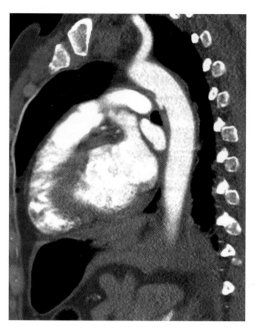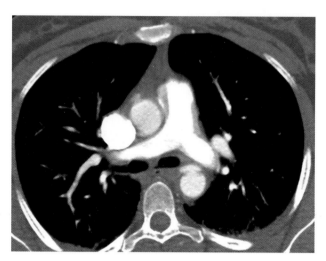

A 46-year-old woman status post motor vehicle collision.

■ Questions

1. What is the MOST likely diagnosis?
   A. Atypical ductus diverticulum
   B. Atypical infundibulum of the right third intercostal artery
   C. Aortic dissection
   D. Aortic pseudoaneurysm
   E. Intramural hematoma of the aorta

2. Which ONE of the following is the most common location for a thoracic aortic injury?
   A. Ascending aorta
   B. Aortic isthmus

   C. At the level of the diaphragm
   D. At a major branch vessel (i.e., carotid)

3. What is the definitive treatment for the traumatic pseudoaneurysm at the aortic isthmus depicted in the test case? (Select ALL that apply.)
   A. Blood pressure control
   B. Anticoagulation
   C. Endovascular stent-graft
   D. Open surgical repair

■ Answers and Explanations

Question 1

D. Correct! This is an aortic pseudoaneurysm. The computed tomography image demonstrates an external contour abnormality or "out-pouching" of contrast with acute angles at the site of injury. A pseudoaneurysm refers to a tear in one or more layers of the vessel and is sometimes termed a *contained rupture*. This is in contrast to a true aneurysm, which would dilate all three layers of the vessel and have a smooth contour. The aortic wall is made up of the intima, media, and adventitia.

Other choices and discussion

A. Although an atypical ductus diverticulum is a potential pitfall when diagnosing a pseudoaneurysm, atypical ductus diverticula maintain smooth shoulders and uninterrupted margins.[1]

B. Infundibula of the second and third right intercostal arteries are often found in this same region. However, infundibula extend perpendicular to the aorta, are usually conical in shape, and have smooth margins that lead to a vessel.[1]

C. Aortic dissection refers to an intimal-medial flap with true and false lumens in the vessel. A dissection does not lead to an external contour abnormality.

E. Although there is periaortic hemorrhage, the hemorrhage in this case is not within the wall of the aorta.

Question 2

B. Correct! The most common location for a traumatic thoracic aortic injury to occur is at the aortic isthmus (descending thoracic aorta), both at autopsy and at the time of imaging. The aortic isthmus is tethered by the ligamentum arteriosum, which is located just distal to the left subclavian artery.

Discussion

Other common locations of injury include the branch points of the vessels of the aortic arch, the ascending aorta, and the descending aorta near the diaphragm. (Note that these sites are all less common than at the aortic isthmus.)

At the time of imaging, ascending aortic injury makes up only 5% of aortic injuries. However, at the time of autopsy, ascending aortic injury makes up 20 to 25% of aortic injuries. A number of complications from ascending thoracic aortic injury can occur, including hemopericardium with subsequent tamponade, coronary artery injury, and aortic valve rupture.[2]

Question 3

C and D. Correct! Both open surgical repair and thoracic endovascular aortic repair (TEVAR) can be used for definitive treatment of traumatic pseudoaneurysms. Many centers are using TEVAR with promising results. TEVAR has a shorter procedure time and lower operative risk, but potential complications include endoleak, stent collapse, stroke, retrograde dissection, migration, and paralysis.[3,4] It is standard practice to treat life-threatening, nonaortic injuries first in patients with traumatic aortic pseudoaneurysm.

Other choices and discussion

A. Although blood pressure should be controlled in patients with traumatic pseudoaneurysm, this is not the definitive treatment. Blood pressure control is the first-line treatment for Stanford type B dissection or for intramural hematoma.

B. Anticoagulation is not the definitive treatment for traumatic pseudoaneurysm. Anticoagulation is used in conjunction with antihypertensive medication for minimal aortic injuries (i.e., intimal injury with or without adherent thrombus).

■ References

1. Fisher RG, Sanchez-Torres M, Whigham CJ, Thomas JW. "Lumps" and "bumps" that mimic acute aortic and brachiocephalic vessel injury. Radiographics 1997;17(4):825–834

2. Creasy JD, Chiles C, Routh WD, Dyer RB. Overview of traumatic injury of the thoracic aorta. Radiographics 1997;17(1):27–45

3. Nishimoto M, Fukumoto H, Nishimoto Y, Furubayashi K, Morita H, Sasaki S. Surgical treatment of traumatic thoracic aorta rupture: a 7-year experience. Jpn J Thorac Cardiovasc Surg 2003;51(4):138–143

4. Shan JG, Zhai XM, Liu JD, Yang WG, Xue S. Thoracic endovascular aortic repair for traumatic thoracic aortic injury: a single-center initial experience. Ann Vasc Surg 2016;32:104–110

5. Groskin SA. Selected topics in chest trauma. Semin Ultrasound CT MR 1996;17(2):119–141

SECTION III DIAGNOSTIC RADIOLOGY IMAGING

Top Tips

◆ A pseudoaneurysm is a contained aortic rupture in which at least one of the three layers is injured. All three layers of the aortic wall remain intact in true aneurysms.

◆ Intramural hematoma is treated the same as an aortic dissection. Stanford type A dissections (involving the ascending thoracic aorta, including the aortic arch) are managed surgically. Stanford type B dissections (located in the descending thoracic aorta, distal to the left subclavian artery) are usually managed medically.

◆ Up to 60% of patients with traumatic aortic rupture have no visible or palpable evidence of thoracic injury.[5] On chest radiography, look for the following signs of aortic injury: loss of the aortic arch contour, left apical cap, deviation of the trachea and nasogastric tube to the right, or depressed left main stem bronchus.

More Challenging 5

■ Case

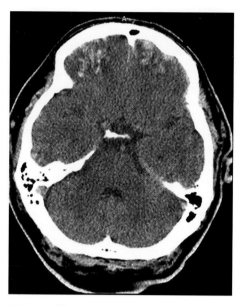

A 56-year-old man status post motor vehicle collision.

■ Questions

1. The findings in the test case are most likely the result of which ONE of the following?
   A. Epidural hemorrhage from adjacent skull fracture
   B. Injury to the bridging veins
   C. Amyloid angiopathy
   D. Coup-contrecoup injury
   E. Hemorrhagic tumor

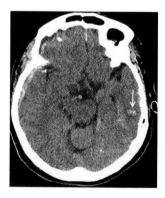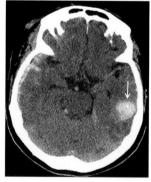

Another patient: noncontrast computed tomography (CT) status post motor vehicle collision.

Follow up noncontrast CT 4 hours later.

2. What is the MOST likely explanation for the hyperdense structure (*white arrows*) to enlarge on the follow-up study?
   A. Difference in the positioning of the patient; the lesion is likely the same size.
   B. Cerebral contusion has enlarged, which is not uncommon within the first 48 hours of injury.

   C. Subarachnoid hemorrhage has filled up the sulcus.
   D. Additional injury has occurred between studies; the patient may have fallen from the gurney.

3. What is the difference between *primary* and *secondary* cerebral contusion injury?
   A. Primary injury occurs at the site of impact and secondary injury occurs at the opposite site of impact.
   B. Primary injury is the site of intracranial injury and secondary injury is the consequence of this injury (i.e., hemiplegia if infarction occurs, pupillary dilation secondary to oculomotor nerve compression, etc.).
   C. Primary injury is the injury to the cells (neurons, astrocytes, and oligodendrocytes) within moments of the injury, whereas secondary injury is the continued insult secondary to ischemia, excitotoxic substances, and free radical damage.
   D. Primary injury is the injury to the patient and secondary injury is the effect on the family members (i.e., emotional, financial).
   E. Primary injury is the injury to the vehicle and secondary injury is the force that is transmitted to the patient.

■ Answers and Explanations

Question 1

D. Correct! The image demonstrates bifrontal cerebral contusions, which is a common location for coup-contrecoup injuries. Cerebral contusion is most commonly found in the cortical and subcortical regions near ridges of bone or along the calvarium.

Other choices and discussion

A. Epidural hemorrhage refers to extra-axial blood between the dura mater and the calvarium. The test case demonstrates (predominately) intra-axial blood.

B. Injury to the bridging veins normally results in a subdural hemorrhage, which is an extra-axial bleed between the potential space of the dura mater and the arachnoid mater.

C. Cerebral amyloid angiopathy is an age-dependent disease characterized by deposition of amyloid beta peptides. It is associated with intracerebral hemorrhage, but rarely causes symptoms in patients younger than 60 years of age. In addition, the test case reports a history of acute trauma, making parenchymal injury more likely.

E. Intra-axial hemorrhage is noted bilaterally, which could potentially occur with glioblastoma (grade IV astrocytoma), as these tumors can cross the midline and can have a hemorrhagic component; however, the appearance of the test case is classic for cerebral contusion.

Question 2

B. Correct! Cerebral contusion increases in size in approximately 50% of patients, and this usually occurs within the first 48 hours. This is sometimes referred to as "blooming." This can cause increasing mass effect and lead to worsening of the patient's symptoms and outcome.

Other choices and discussion

A. Although there are slight differences in positioning, there is a size increase of well over 25 to 30%, which is the recommended percentage to use when confirming an increase in size.

C. There is minimal subarachnoid blood in the left temporal convexity, but the enlarging hemorrhage is intra-axial and represents intraparenchymal blood products.

D. A second traumatic injury could absolutely occur, especially when transferring the patient, but this would be much less likely than "blooming" of the known intracerebral contusion.

Question 3

C. Correct! Cerebral contusions are comprised of both primary and secondary injury. *Primary* injury occurs at the time of the insult (direct injury to the cells), whereas *secondary* injury is the continued insult secondary to ischemia, excitotoxic substances, and free radical damage from the breakdown of blood products and tissue damage. Further injury occurring secondary to microvascular dysfunction includes vasoconstriction, vasospasm, and occlusion. This leads to tissue ischemia, edema, and the hemorrhagic progression of the contusion.[1]

It is important to understand that although imaging findings may be stable or even improving, damage continues to occur and patient status may decline.

Other choices and discussion

The other choices are incorrect. The mechanism in choice A describes the coup-contrecoup phenomenon.

Note that sometimes the evolution of an *intraparenchymal* hematoma can mimic a neoplastic process. Contrast-enhanced imaging of an intraparenchymal hematoma can show rim enhancement more than a year after development. An arterial spin labeling magnetic resonance imaging may be useful in distinguishing chronic intraparenchymal hematoma from hypervascular cystic neoplasm.[4]

■ References

1. Kurland D, Hong C, Aarabi B, Gerzanich V, Simard JM. Hemorrhagic progression of a contusion after traumatic brain injury: a review. J Neurotrauma 2012;29(1):19–31

2. Alahmadi H, Vachhrajani S, Cusimano MD. The natural history of brain contusion: an analysis of radiological and clinical progression. J Neurosurg 2010;112(5):1139–1145

3. Kim JJ, Gean AD. Imaging for the diagnosis and management of traumatic brain injury. Neurotherapeutics 2011;8(1): 39–53

4. Kamide T, Seki S, Suzuki KI, et al. A chronic encapsulated intracerebral hematoma mimicking a brain tumor: findings on arterial spin labeling of MRI. Neuroradiol J 2016;29:273–276

Top Tips

◆ Cerebral contusions increase in size in 50% of patients, and this usually occurs within the first 48 hours.[2] Follow-up studies in 6 to 8 hours are useful in evaluating progression.

◆ The most common locations for cerebral contusions are the frontal lobes and the temporal poles.

◆ CT may underestimate intracerebral injury, especially if imaged early (< 3 hours). More than 80% of traumatic axonal injuries are nonhemorrhagic and difficult to diagnose on CT.[3] Magnetic resonance imaging is more sensitive for diagnosing nonhemorrhagic contusions and traumatic axonal injuries.

Essentials 1

■ Case

This patient is status post a single gunshot wound to the abdomen, with an entrance and exit wound on physical examination.

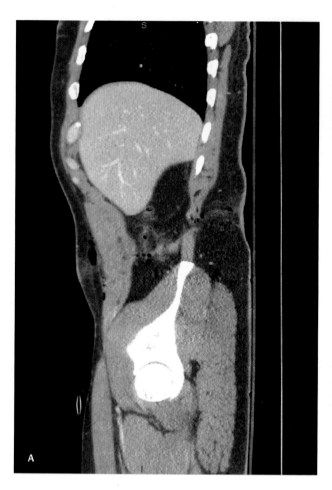

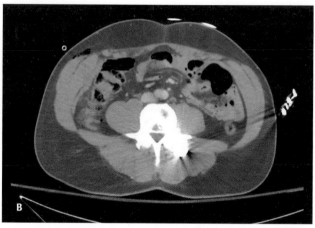

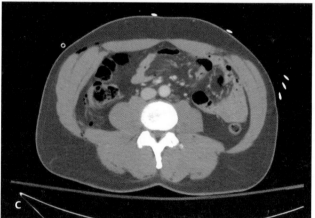

■ Questions

1. Which of the following best describes the computed tomography (CT) findings?
   A. Ectopic gas has been introduced by the bullet; there is no organ injury.
   B. Findings are concerning for colonic injury.
   C. Gunshot wounds are sterile, regardless of bullet path.
   D. No evidence of bowel injury, as there is no spillage of bowel contents.

2. What is the best next step?
   A. Supportive care
   B. Follow-up CT
   C. Surgical evaluation
   D. Barium enema

3. INDIRECT signs of penetrating bowel injury include which ONE of the following?
   A. Interloop fluid
   B. Bowel discontinuity
   C. Leakage of oral contrast
   D. Presence of an exit wound in the bowel wall

■ Answers and Explanations

Question 1

B. Correct! Findings are concerning for colonic injury. The path of the bullet is visible on the coronal and axial images. The proximity of the bullet path to the ascending colon must lead to a high index of suspicion for a bowel injury. The presence of pericolonic gas and fat stranding add further worry. In this patient, a through and through bowel injury was found at surgery.

Other choices and discussion

A. Ectopic gas is often introduced by bullet injuries. Indeed, the gas superficial to the anterior abdominal wall might be due to this mechanism. However, the deeper gas adjacent to the colon is not clearly due to the bullet alone, and colon injury should be suspected.

C. Gunshot injuries are not intrinsically sterile, especially when they traverse the gastrointestinal tract or the airways.

D. Spillage of bowel contents would be a direct sign of bowel injury, but the reverse is not true, and the absence of extraluminal bowel contents does not exclude injury.

Question 2

C. Correct! In the presence of penetrating trauma and bowel injury, surgical exploration is indicated.

Other choices and discussion

A. Supportive care is unlikely to result in resolution of the bowel injury without complications.

B. Follow up CT is not likely to provide any further diagnostic information at this point.

D. Barium enema is specifically contraindicated in this patient. Free barium from a leak can result in barium peritonitis, which can be difficult to treat or even life threatening. If a fluoroscopic examination is desired to confirm a bowel leak, this exam should be performed with water-soluble contrast.

Question 3

A. Correct! *Direct* signs of penetrating bowel injury are diagnostic of injury and include bowel wall discontinuity, wound tract extension to the bowel, leakage of oral or rectal contrast material, and active mesenteric vascular extravasation. Indirect signs may arise secondary to a bowel injury and should raise suspicion. *Indirect* signs of penetrating bowel injury include fat stranding, interloop fluid, and mesenteric hematoma.

Other choices and discussion

B. Bowel discontinuity is a direct sign of bowel injury.

C. Leakage of oral contrast is a direct sign of bowel injury.

D. The presence of an exit wound in the bowel wall is a direct sign of bowel injury.

■ Suggested Readings

Karanikas ID, Kakoulidis DD, Gouvas ZT, Hartley JE, Koundourakis SS. Barium peritonitis: a rare complication of upper gastrointestinal contrast investigation. Postgrad Med J 1997;73(859):297–298

Lozano JD, Munera F, Anderson SW, Soto JA, Menias CO, Caban KM. Penetrating wounds to the torso: evaluation with triple-contrast multidetector CT. Radiographics 2013;33(2):341–359

SECTION IV GASTROINTESTINAL IMAGING

Top Tips

- Direct CT signs of bowel injury: bowel wall discontinuity, wound tract extension to the bowel, leakage of oral or rectal contrast material, and active mesenteric vascular extravasation of contrast material. These are diagnostic of bowel injury.

- Indirect CT signs of bowel injury: fat stranding, mesenteric hematoma, and interloop fluid. These may arise secondary to an injury and should raise suspicion.

- Always look carefully for subtle signs of bowel injury, and never assume that ectopic gas is from bullet entry alone!

Essentials 2

■ Case

A 39-year-old woman presents with progressive abdominal pain. Computed tomography and fluorodeoxyglucose-positron emission tomography images are shown.

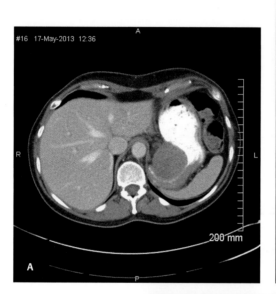

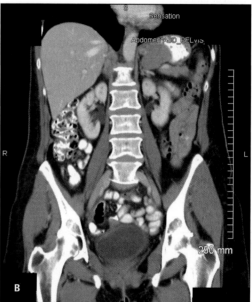

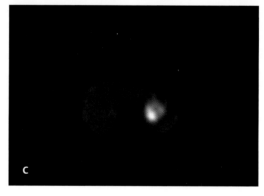

■ Questions

1. What is the MOST likely diagnosis?
   A. Adenocarcinoma
   B. Linitis plastica
   C. Breast cancer metastasis
   D. Gastrointestinal stromal tumor

2. What is the most common location for these tumors?
   A. Esophagus
   B. Stomach
   C. Small bowel
   D. Colon

3. What is the most likely site of metastasis for these tumors?
   A. Liver
   B. Lung
   C. Lymph nodes
   D. Adjacent organs/mesenteric

■ Answers and Explanations

Question 1

D. Correct! This smoothly marginated, partially exophytic, gastric mass is most consistent with a gastrointestinal stromal tumor (GIST). GIST is a mesenchymal tumor that arises from the gastric wall and is often indolent and asymptomatic. Occasionally, these tumors may be ulcerated and/or hemorrhagic. GIST is most often seen in adults over age 40.

Other choices and discussion

A. Although adenocarcinoma is a common primary gastric mass, it is mucosal in origin. Larger masses are typically ulcerated and heterogeneous, growing concentrically along the gastric wall, unlike the test case.

B. Linitis plastica is a term that refers to a diffuse infiltrative process of the gastric wall, usually involving the submucosa. This is a descriptive term rather than a pathologic diagnosis and may be due to either neoplastic or inflammatory causes.

C. Breast cancer metastases might occur in the stomach. However, an isolated large homogeneous gastric mass would be very unlikely for breast cancer.

Question 2

B. Correct! Although GIST can occur anywhere along the gastrointestinal tract, the majority are found in the stomach (60 to 70%).

Other choices and discussion

A. GIST may occur in the esophagus, but this is rare. Mural masses in the esophagus are far more likely to be muscular (e.g., leiomyoma).

C. The small bowel, especially the duodenum, is the second most common location for a GIST (30% of tumors).

D. The colon is the least common location for a GIST.

Question 3

A. Correct! A small percentage of GISTs are malignant. When metastatic, disease most commonly spreads to the liver.

Other choices and discussion

B. Pulmonary metastases are rare in GIST.

C. Lymph node metastases are rare in GIST.

D. Contiguous/mesenteric spread of GIST is uncommon in primary disease, but can be seen in recurrence after resection.

■ Suggested Readings

Sandrasegaran K, Rajesh A, Rydberg J, Rushing DA, Akisik FM, Henley JD. Gastrointestinal stromal tumors: clinical, radiologic, and pathologic features. Am J Roentgenol 2005;184:803–811

Top Tips

◆ The most common location for a GIST is the stomach.

◆ A GIST typically presents as a large, enhancing, solid mural mass.

◆ These are usually benign, but when malignant, metastases most commonly occur in the liver.

Essentials 3

■ Case

An elderly woman presents with bloating and abdominal pain.

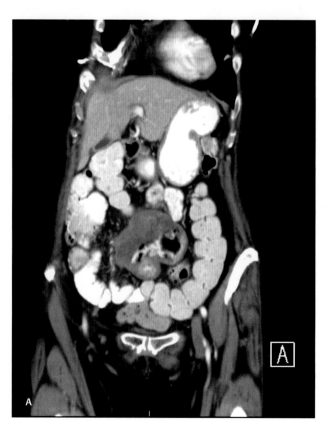

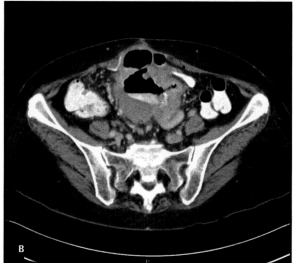

■ Questions

1. All of the following are in the differential diagnosis EXCEPT?
   A. Lymphoma
   B. Adenocarcinoma
   C. Carcinoid
   D. Metastasis

2. What is the most likely diagnosis?
   A. Metastatic breast cancer
   B. Adenocarcinoma
   C. Inflammatory bowel disease
   D. Small bowel lymphoma

3. Which ONE of the following is true regarding this disease process?
   A. Obstruction is common.
   B. Intussusception can occur.
   C. The most common cell type is a T-cell lymphoma.
   D. This most commonly occurs within the duodenum.

■ Answers and Explanations

Question 1

C. Correct! Small bowel carcinoid is unlikely to present as a large mass expanding the lumen of the small bowel.

Other choices and discussion

A. Small bowel lymphoma often has the appearance of the test case.

B. Adenocarcinoma is a common intrinsic small bowel mass and may rarely have the appearance of the test case.

D. Metastases may also have the appearance of the test case.

Question 2

D. Correct! This patient has one of the classic appearances of small bowel lymphoma. Lymphoma is the most common malignant tumor of the small bowel and may present with enlarged nodular folds, with diffuse mural thickening, or as an expansile and ulcerative, nonobstructing mass, as in this case. If disease is limited to the bowel and adjacent lymph nodes, it is termed primary small bowel lymphoma. Small bowel lymphoma may also be secondary.

Other choices and discussion

A. Breast cancer metastases may occur in the small bowel and might even have this appearance, but this is less common than lymphoma.

B. Adenocarcinoma of the small bowel is more likely to result in luminal obstruction than dilatation.

C. Inflammatory bowel disease would be very unlikely.

Question 3

B. Correct! Small bowel lymphoma can act as a lead point for intussusception.

Other choices and discussion

A. Obstruction is less common in small bowel lymphoma, as these tumors tend to be soft and pliable.

C. The most common cell type is B-cell lymphoma.

D. The most common location for small bowel lymphoma is the ileum.

■ Suggested Readings

Ghai S, Pattison J, Ghai S, O'Malley ME, Khalili K, Stephens M. Primary gastrointestinal lymphoma: spectrum of imaging findings with pathologic correlation. RadioGraphics 2007;27(5):1371–1388

SECTION IV
GASTROINTESTINAL
IMAGING

Top Tips

◆ Small bowel lymphoma most commonly occurs in the ileum.

◆ Obstruction from lymphoma is uncommon because these masses are soft and pliable tumors.

◆ Small bowel lymphoma may be primary or secondary.

Essentials 4

■ Case

A 56-year-old woman presents to the emergency room.

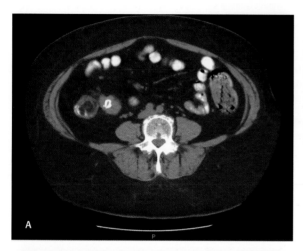
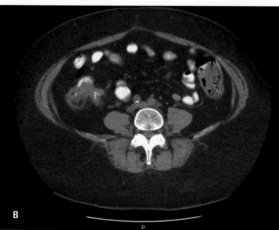
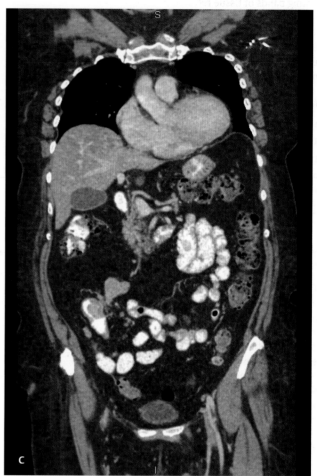

■ Questions

1. What is the MOST likely diagnosis?
   A. Carcinoid
   B. Lymphoma
   C. Desmoid tumor
   D. Epiploic appendagitis

2. What telltale symptom might this patient have?
   A. Intractable vomiting
   B. Dry mouth
   C. Flushing
   D. Constipation

3. Which of the following appearances might be expected for carcinoid metastases in the liver?
   A. Arterial hypoenhancement
   B. Uptake of hepatocyte-specific contrast agents
   C. Predominantly necrotic mass
   D. Portal venous phase isoattenuation

■ Answers and Explanations

Question 1

A. Correct! This is most likely a carcinoid tumor. Small bowel carcinoid occurs most commonly in the ileum. This patient has masslike mural thickening in the distal small bowel. There is an associated masslike process in the mesentery with radiating bands of tissue retraction (desmoplastic reaction). With carcinoid, sometimes only the mesenteric metastases are visible on imaging. A loose rule of thirds is sometimes used: one-third occur in the small bowel, one-third have metastases, one-third are multiple, one-third have a second malignancy, and one-third have carcinoid syndrome.

Other choices and discussion

B. Lymphoma can occur in the bowel wall and the mesentery, but this appearance is less typical.

C. Desmoid tumor could explain the partially calcified retractile process in the mesentery, but involvement of the bowel wall would be atypical.

D. Epiploic appendagitis presents as an inflammatory process centered around a fat lobule along the *serosal* margin of the colon. There may be a visible central thrombosed vessel.

Question 2

C. Correct! This patient might have flushing. Tumors releasing 5-hydroxytryptamine (serotonin) may cause a constellation of symptoms termed the "carcinoid syndrome." These symptoms may include flushing, diarrhea, abdominal pain, wheezing, and/or palpitations. There is high first-pass metabolism in the liver for serotonin released by bowel or mesenteric tumors, so carcinoid syndrome usually only occurs in the presence of liver metastases or in primary tumors outside of the gastrointestinal tract (especially the lung).

Other choices and discussion

A. Intractable vomiting might occur if the tumor has caused bowel obstruction. However, no bowel obstruction is present in the test case.

B. Dry mouth is classically seen with sympathetic overstimulation rather than with carcinoid syndrome.

D. Carcinoid tumor would be expected to cause diarrhea (not constipation).

Question 3

D. Correct! Portal venous phase isoattenuation. The classic enhancement pattern on computed tomography (CT) for carcinoid and other neuroendocrine metastases to the liver is arterial phase hyperenhancement, becoming somewhat isoattenuating to the liver on portal venous and delayed phases. Indeed, these tumors may be difficult to see on CT, if arterial phase imaging is not performed.

Other choices and discussion

A. Arterial hypoenhancement might be seen with treated metastases, but not in active metastatic disease.

B. Carcinoid metastases should be hypointense on the hepatobiliary phase during liver magnetic resonance imaging with hepatocyte-specific contrast. In fact, conspicuity on the hepatobiliary phase can be an excellent means of monitoring liver metastases.

C. Large amounts of necrosis would be atypical for carcinoid metastases in the liver.

■ Suggested Readings

Ganeshan D, Bhosale P, Yang T, Kundra V. Imaging features of carcinoid tumors of the gastrointestinal tract. Am J Roentgenol 2013;201:773–786

Top Tips

◆ The primary small bowel carcinoid may or may not be visible on CT.

◆ Metastatic carcinoid in the mesentery is classically a masslike process with desmoplastic reaction. The mass may or may not be calcified.

◆ Carcinoid liver metastases are typically hyperenhancing in the arterial phase.

Essentials 5

■ Case

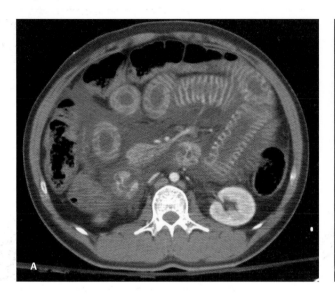 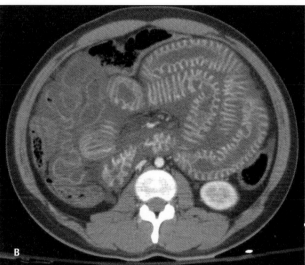

■ Questions

1. What is the best explanation for the small bowel abnormality?
   A. Inflammatory bowel disease
   B. Shock bowel
   C. Bowel ischemia
   D. Lymphoma

2. What is the most common underlying cause of the major finding in this case?
   A. Obstruction
   B. Volume overload
   C. Contrast reaction
   D. Acute severe blood loss

3. Which of the following structures may also be hyperattenuating with this entity?
   A. Spleen
   B. Liver
   C. Adrenal glands
   D. Inferior vena cava

■ Answers and Explanations

Question 1

B. Correct! This is shock bowel. Shock bowel is characterized by marked submucosal edema with mucosal hyperenhancement. Shock bowel occurs from massive sudden blood loss in trauma patients and is a poor prognostic indicator. The appearance may also be seen with other causes of severe volume loss or hypotension. The proposed mechanism is mesenteric vasoconstriction with altered perfusion dynamics. Of note, the changes are reversible with resuscitation and do not always lead to bowel infarction.

Other choices and discussion

A. Active inflammatory bowel disease may result in mural edema and enhancement, but is not the best choice in this case.

C. Bowel ischemia may result in some mural edema and/or mucosal hyperemia. However, the mesenteric arteries and veins appear patent on the provided images, and there is no evidence of aortic atherosclerosis. For vascular pathology to affect the number of small bowel loops seen in this patient, a large central arterial or venous abnormality would be expected.

D. Lymphoma would not be expected to have the provided appearance.

Question 2

D. Correct! Acute severe blood loss is the most common cause of shock bowel.

Other choices and discussion

A. Obstruction would not be expected to have this appearance.

B. The ascites in this patient is caused by altered bowel permeability, not by volume overload.

C. The demonstrated findings would not be the primary result of a contrast reaction. Systemic anaphylaxis in a contrast reaction might result in hypoperfusion, but would not be the most common cause of the shock bowel appearance.

Question 3

C. Correct! Adrenal glands. In addition to the bowel findings and the slit-like inferior vena cava (IVC) seen on these images, hypovolemic shock may result in adrenal hyperenhancement, small aorta, delayed nephrograms, variable pancreatic enhancement with peripancreatic edema, and hypoenhancement of the liver and spleen.

Other choices and discussion

A. The spleen would typically be hypoenhancing in the setting of hypovolemic shock.

B. The liver would typically be hypoenhancing in the setting of hypovolemic shock.

D. The IVC is typically slit-like in hypovolemic shock (as in our patient), but not hyperattenuating.

■ Suggested Readings

Ames JT, Federle MP. CT hypotension complex (shock bowel) is not always due to traumatic hypovolemic shock. Am J Roentgenol 2009;192(5):W230–W235

Top Tips

- Shock bowel is characterized by marked submucosal edema and mucosal enhancement.
- Associated findings can include hyperenhancement of the adrenal glands, flattening of the IVC and aorta, variable enhancement of the pancreas with peripancreatic edema, delayed nephrograms, and hypoenhancement of the spleen and liver.
- The changes are reversible with resuscitation and do not always lead to bowel infarction.

Essentials 6

■ Case

A patient presents to the emergency room with worsening crampy abdominal pain.

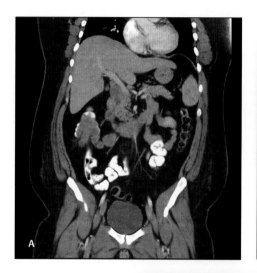

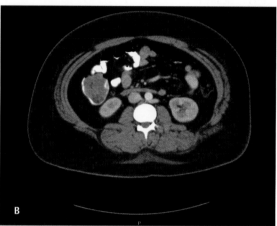

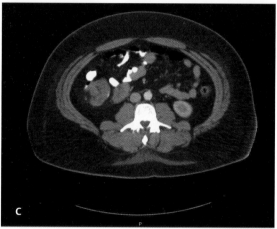

■ Questions

1. What is the best diagnosis?
   A. Colocolonic intussusception
   B. Infectious colitis
   C. Ischemia
   D. Meckel's diverticulum

2. Regarding this disease process, which ONE of the following statements is correct?
   A. Often self-limited
   B. Usually associated with adhesions
   C. Most often caused by a benign mass
   D. Most often caused by adenocarcinoma in adults

3. Which of the following describes the intussuscipiens?
   A. The donor loop of bowel
   B. The cause of the abnormality
   C. The recipient loop of bowel
   D. The layer of mesenteric fat within the associated mass on computed tomography

■ Answers and Explanations

Question 1

A. Correct! Both the axial and coronal images demonstrate a segment of bowel and accompanying mesentery entering a downstream loop consistent with a colocolonic intussusception.

Other choices and discussion

B. Infectious colitis typically manifests as long segment bowel inflammation with a gradual transition to normal upstream or downstream bowel.

C. Bowel ischemia may be focal but is not typically masslike and would not account for the mesenteric fat within the colon on these images.

D. A Meckel's diverticulum is a blind-ending diverticulum in the distal small bowel. A remnant of the Vitelline duct, a Meckel's diverticulum may contain gastric mucosa and may be a source of gastrointestinal bleeding. Various gastrointestinal masses may arise within a Meckel's diverticulum. A mass arising within a Meckel's diverticulum might have some of the imaging features shown, but this patient's abnormality is within the colon and appears characteristic of intussusception.

Question 2

D. Correct! Most often caused by adenocarcinoma in adults. In adults, colonic intussusception is most often caused by an underlying mass or other lead point. In children and adolescents, ileocolonic and colocolonic intussusception is most commonly spontaneous. In adults, small bowel–small bowel intussusception is also common, usually transient, and asymptomatic.

Other choices and discussion

A. Colonic intussusception is not usually self-limited in adults. Treatment of the underlying cause is usually indicated.

B. Colonic intussusception may be associated with a variety of causes, but adhesions are a less common cause than an underlying mass.

C. A benign mass such as a lipoma or leiomyoma may cause intussusception, but would be less common than adenocarcinoma.

Question 3

C. Correct! The recipient loop of bowel. It can help to remember that there are some similarities between the pronunciations of the words "intussuscipiens" and "recipient."

Other choices and discussion

A. The donor loop of bowel is referred to as the intussusceptum.

B. The underlying cause of the abnormality is referred to as the lead point.

D. The layer of mesenteric fat does not have a special name in the terminology of intussusception.

■ Suggested Readings

Gollub MJ. Colonic intussusception: clinical and radiographic features. Am J Roentgenol 2011;196(5):W580–W585

Warshauer DM, Lee JKT. Adult intussusception detected at CT or MR imaging: clinical-imaging correlation. Radiology 1999;212:853–860

Top Tips

- Large bowel intussusception in adults is often associated with a malignancy, such as adenocarcinoma.
- Small bowel intussusception in adults can be benign and transient.
- The intussusceptum is the donor loop and the intussuscipiens is the receiving loop.

Essentials 7

■ Case

A patient presents to the emergency room with recent development of progressive abdominal pain and nausea.

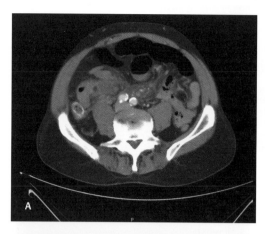

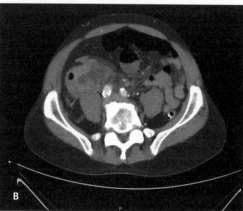

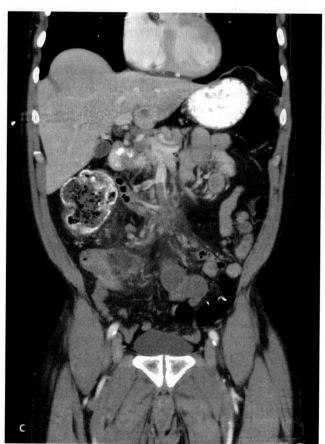

■ Questions

1. What is the correct diagnosis?
   A. Acute embolic superior mesenteric artery thrombosis
   B. Acute superior mesenteric vein thrombosis
   C. Portal hypertension
   D. Internal hernia

2. What secondary abnormality is also present?
   A. Mesenteric infarct
   B. Bowel obstruction
   C. Varices
   D. Pneumatosis

3. Which ONE of the following statements is true for this test case diagnosis?
   A. It has a low mortality.
   B. It is most commonly idiopathic.
   C. Resultant bowel involvement is usually segmental.
   D. The inferior mesenteric vein is more commonly involved than the SMV.

■ Answers and Explanations

Question 1

B. Correct! Acute SMV thrombosis. The images show a filling defect within the SMV and multiple mesenteric venous branches. Always be sure to look at the mesenteric vasculature, especially when there is bowel inflammation, segmental bowel edema, mesenteric edema, or otherwise unexplained abdominal pain.

Other choices and discussion

A. The abnormality is within the SMV, rather than the artery. If unsure on a single image, scroll up and down to convince yourself you are looking at the artery or the vein.

C. Portal venous thrombosis and portal hypertension can result from SMV thrombosis. However, there is no evidence of portal hypertension on this image.

D. There is no internal hernia on these images.

Question 2

A. Correct! There is geographic mesenteric fat necrosis in the right lower quadrant, consistent with mesenteric infarct. There is also generalized edema at the root of the mesentery.

Other choices and discussion

B. There is gaseous distention of small bowel loops in the anterior abdomen, but no primary evidence of bowel obstruction.

C. Chronic mesenteric venous thrombosis can lead to varices (i.e., collateral venous channels), but well-formed collaterals are not usually present in the acute setting.

D. Pneumatosis can result from bowel ischemia in the setting of mesenteric thrombosis. However, no pneumatosis is present on the provided images.

Question 3

C. Correct! Resultant bowel involvement is usually segmental. Bowel ischemia can result from mesenteric venous thrombosis and will be limited to the segments of bowel drained by the thrombosed vein.

Other choices and discussion

A. Severe SMV thrombosis has a high mortality.

B. SMV thrombosis is rarely idiopathic, after appropriate clinical investigation. Underlying causes include hypercoagulable states, malignancy, bowel inflammation/infection, portal hypertension, recent surgery, and medications. Primary SMV thrombosis is a diagnosis of exclusion.

D. The SMV is affected more commonly than the inferior mesenteric vein.

■ Suggested Reading

Duran R, Denys AL, Letovanec I, Meuli RA, Schmidt S. Multidetector CT features of mesenteric vein thrombosis. RadioGraphics 2012;32(5):1503–1522

Top Tips

◆ Remember to always look at the mesenteric vasculature, especially when there is bowel inflammation, segmental bowel edema, mesenteric edema, or otherwise unexplained abdominal pain.

◆ Scroll up and down until you are sure you know which mesenteric vessel you are looking at.

◆ The distribution of bowel involvement with mesenteric thrombosis is usually segmental.

Essentials 8

■ Case

An elderly patient presents with acute left lower quadrant pain.

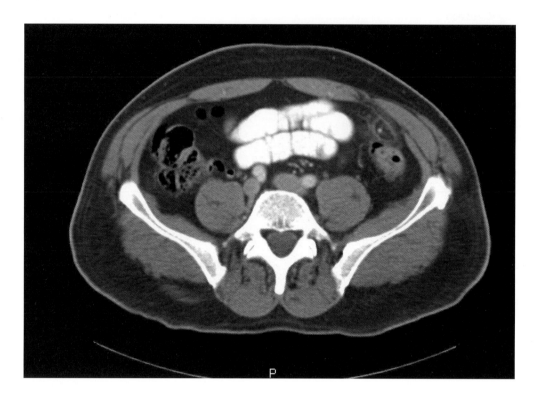

■ Questions

1. What is the most likely diagnosis?
   A. Diverticulitis
   B. Inflammatory bowel disease
   C. Bowel ischemia
   D. Epiploic appendagitis

2. What is the best next step?
   A. Surgical consultation
   B. Supportive therapy
   C. Additional imaging
   D. Colonoscopy

3. Which of the following is a potential etiology of this process?
   A. Torsion
   B. Luminal occlusion
   C. Autoimmune
   D. Infection

■ Answers and Explanations

Question 1

D. Correct! There is edema surrounding an oval fat lobule along the serosal margin of the descending colon, consistent with epiploic appendagitis.

Other choices and discussion

A. Acute diverticulitis is a common cause of left lower quadrant pain in adults. However, this image does not show any diverticula or peridiverticular inflammation.

B. This patient's inflammatory changes are not centered in the bowel wall, so inflammatory bowel disease is unlikely.

C. There is no computed tomography (CT) evidence of bowel ischemia in this patient.

Question 2

B. Correct! Supportive therapy. Complications of epiploic appendagitis are rare, and supportive care alone is sufficient for management in the acute setting.

Other choices and discussion

A. Surgical consultation may be avoided by making the correct diagnosis on imaging.

C. Additional imaging is not required when characteristic CT findings are present.

D. Colonoscopy is unnecessary in epiploic appendagitis.

Question 3

A. Correct! Commonly cited etiologies of epiploic appendagitis include torsion of the appendage or thrombosis of the venous drainage.

Other choices and discussion

B. Luminal occlusion is often a cause of acute diverticulitis.

C. Autoimmune factors do not play a role in epiploic appendagitis.

D. Signs of infection such as fever and elevated white blood cell count are not usually part of the presentation.

■ Suggested Readings

Singh AK, Gervais DA, Hahn PF, Sagar P, Mueller PR, Novelline RA. Acute epiploic appendagitis and its mimics. Radiographics 2005;25(6):1521–1534

Top Tips

◆ Epiploic appendagitis is a mimic of acute inflammatory conditions such as acute appendicitis or acute diverticulitis.

◆ On CT, there is edema surrounding an oval fat lobule along the serosal margin of the colon.

◆ Treatment is supportive. The correct diagnosis can avoid a surgical consultation.

SECTION IV
GASTROINTESTINAL
IMAGING

Essentials 9

■ Case

A 90-year-old man presents with acute abdominal pain. The image shows a scout X-ray prior to a fluoroscopy exam, but after a contrast computed tomography (CT).

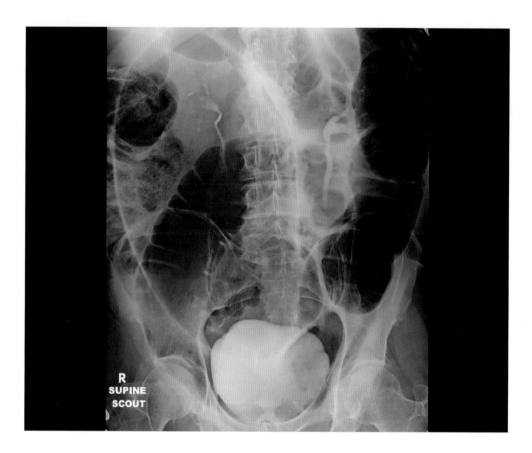

■ Questions

1. Based on this image, which ONE of the following is most likely?
   A. Cecal bascule
   B. Cecal volvulus
   C. Sigmoid volvulus
   D. Toxic megacolon

2. Regarding this abnormality, which ONE of the following statements is correct?
   A. The whirl sign has been described on radiographs.
   B. This abnormality is the second most common type of colonic volvulus.
   C. This abnormality is most commonly seen in young adulthood.
   D. Chronic constipation is a risk factor.

3. Which ONE of the following is true regarding management of this abnormality?
   A. There is no role for barium enema.
   B. Rectal tube decompression may be therapeutic.
   C. Surgical intervention is required for treatment.
   D. Nasogastric decompression is indicated.

■ Answers and Explanations

Question 1

C. Correct! Sigmoid volvulus. The image shows a massively dilated loop of bowel emanating from the left lower quadrant, which may be difficult to appreciate initially because it is almost too large to be seen on the image. There is mild gaseous distention of the upstream colon. Of the provided options, only sigmoid volvulus would result in this appearance.

Other choices and discussion

A. Cecal bascule is an upward folding of the cecum without volvulus. The cecum must have a mesentery and lie within the peritoneum for this to occur.

B. Cecal volvulus characteristically results in a dilated loop of bowel within the central abdomen or left upper quadrant, emanating from the right abdomen. There may be resultant small bowel obstruction.

D. Colonic dilatation is expected in toxic megacolon and, indeed, severe dilatation with mural ischemia is one potential cause of toxic megacolon. However, the pattern in this test case is most consistent with sigmoid volvulus.

Question 2

D. Correct! Chronic constipation may lead to redundancy of the sigmoid colon, which can result in hypermobility and volvulus. Long-term fiber use is also a risk factor.

Other choices and discussion

A. The whirl sign has been described on CT for volvulus, but is not visible on radiographs.

B. Sigmoid volvulus is the most common type of colonic volvulus, accounting for about 70% of cases.

C. Sigmoid volvulus is most commonly seen in older adults.

Question 3

B. Correct! Placement of a decompressing rectal tube may result in resolution of the volvulus. If unsuccessful, surgical management may be required.

Other choices and discussion

A. Radiographs and CT can successfully diagnose sigmoid volvulus in the majority of patients. In equivocal cases, barium enema may contribute to the diagnosis (by demonstrating beaking of the rectosigmoid junction with obstruction to upstream flow).

C. Surgical intervention may be avoided in cases of successful rectal tube decompression.

D. Nasogastric decompression is unlikely to resolve a sigmoid volvulus.

■ Suggested Readings

Peterson CM, Anderson JS, Hara AK, Carenza JW, Menias CO. Volvulus of the gastrointestinal tract: appearances at multimodality imaging. Radiographics 2009;29(5):1281–1293

**SECTION IV
GASTROINTESTINAL
IMAGING**

Top Tips

♦ Sigmoid volvulus usually occurs in the elderly population.

♦ Predisposing factors to sigmoid redundancy include chronic constipation and long-term fiber use.

♦ CT can demonstrate twisting of the mesentery and focal narrowing of the sigmoid colon.

Essentials 10

■ Case

An 81-year-old patient presents acute cramping abdominal pain.

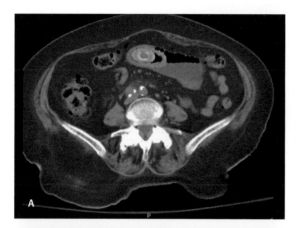

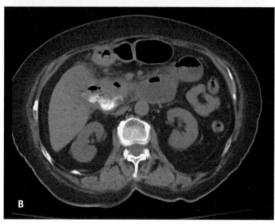

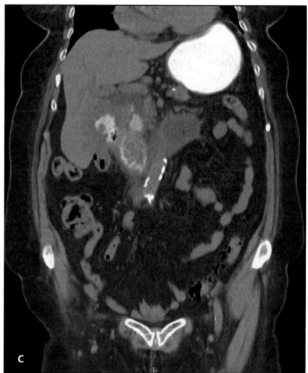

■ Questions

1. What is the most complete diagnosis?
   A. Gallstone ileus
   B. Small bowel obstruction
   C. Duodenal perforation
   D. Crohn's disease

2. All of the following are part of Rigler's triad on radiographs EXCEPT:
   A. Ectopic location of gallstone
   B. Pneumobilia
   C. Free intra-abdominal air
   D. Small bowel obstruction

3. Which ONE of the following statements about gallstone ileus is correct?
   A. Most patients present with Rigler's triad.
   B. There is a predilection for young women.
   C. Bowel obstruction is likely when stones are 15 mm or greater in diameter.
   D. The gallstone usually passes through a fistula between the gallbladder and the bowel.

■ Answers and Explanations

Question 1

A. Correct! Gallstone ileus. The first axial image demonstrates a concentrically calcified gallstone within the small bowel lumen. There is upstream small bowel dilatation due to obstruction at the level of the stone. The additional axial image and the coronal image demonstrate moderate edema in the gallbladder fossa and adjacent to the duodenum. There is extraluminal oral contrast extending from the second portion of the duodenum toward the gallbladder fossa, diagnostic of a cholecystic-enteric fistula.

Other choices and discussion

B. Small bowel obstruction is present. However, this is not the most complete diagnosis.

C. Duodenal perforation is present. However, this is not the most complete diagnosis.

D. Crohn's disease is not present in this patient.

Question 2

C. Correct! Rigler's triad describes three characteristic findings (ectopic location of gallstone, pneumobilia, and small bowel obstruction) that may be present on abdominal radiographs with gallstone ileus. Free intra-abdominal air is not part of Rigler's triad and would be unexpected with gallstone ileus.

Other choices and discussion

A. If calcified, the ectopic calcified gallstone may be seen on radiographs.

B. Pneumobilia results from the biliary fistula.

D. Small bowel obstruction is the third component of Rigler's triad.

Question 3

D. Correct! The gallstone usually passes through a fistula between the gallbladder and the bowel. The fistula forms between the gallbladder and an adjacent loop of bowel secondary to recurrent or chronic inflammation of the gallbladder, bowel, or both.

Other choices and discussion

A. Most patients do not present with Rigler's triad. Only 10% of patients present with all three findings. Obstruction is often visible on radiographs ("ileus" is a misnomer for this process). However, the gallstone may be relatively radiolucent, and pneumobilia may be subtle or absent.

B. Most patients with gallstone ileus are elderly, and there is a female predominance.

C. To result in bowel obstruction, the gallstone generally needs to be greater than 2.5 cm in diameter.

■ Suggested Readings

Lassandro F, Romano S, Ragozzino A, Rossi G, Valente T, Ferrara I, Romano L, Grassi R. Role of helical CT in diagnosis of gallstone ileus and related conditions. Am J Roentgenol 2005;185(5):1159–1165

Top Tips

- "Gallstone ileus" is not a true ileus. It is a mechanical obstruction due to a gallstone within the small bowel lumen.

- The gallstone usually passes through a cholecystic-enteric fistula with the duodenum or other portion of the bowel like the stomach.

- The impacting stones are usually greater than 2.5 cm in order to be large enough to cause obstruction.

Details 1

■ Case

A patient with known cirrhosis. Which ONE of the following is correct?
   A. Biopsy is not necessary to make this diagnosis.
   B. The differential diagnosis includes hemangioma.
   C. Serum alpha-fetoprotein (AFP) measurement is a sensitive screening test for this diagnosis.
   D. This would be a Liver Imaging Reporting and Data System (LI-RADS) 3 lesion.

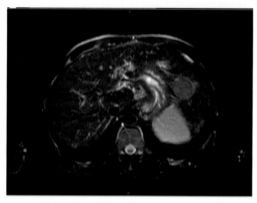

T2

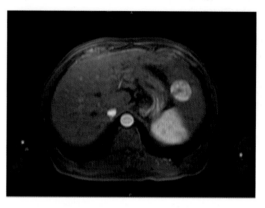

Arterial phase

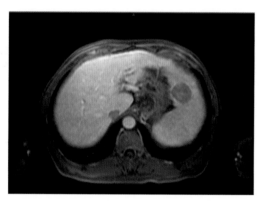

Portal venous phase

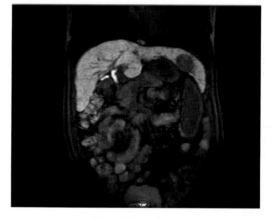

Hepatobiliary phase

■ The following pertain to cirrhosis, HCC, and relevant imaging.

1. What two classification systems have recently been introduced for liver lesions in the presence of chronic liver disease?
2. What phase in a dynamic contrast examination is the most critical for the detection of HCC?
3. What is the time delay usually needed to reach the hepatocyte phase following the administration of Eovist (Bayer Healthcare Pharmaceuticals, Whippany, NJ; gadoxetate disodium) intravenous (IV) contrast?
4. True or False. The presence of a capsule or pseudocapsule is a feature of HCC.

5. True or False. Regenerative nodules are typically bright on T2-weighted sequences.
6. True or False. Serum AFP levels are always elevated in the presence of HCC.
7. The most common distant organ of spread from HCC is _____.
8. True or False. HCCs can contain fat on in and out of phase images.
9. Is portal vein tumor invasion a characteristic of HCC?
10. What are the routes of elimination of Eovist (gadoxetate disodium) IV contrast?

■ Answers and Explanations

A. Correct! Biopsy is not necessary to make this diagnosis. This patient has hepatocellular carcinoma (HCC). In patients with chronic liver disease, well-established imaging criteria, provided by the American College of Radiology/LI-RADS and Organ Procurement and Transplantation Network, can establish the diagnosis of HCC without the need for biopsy. Biopsy is reserved for equivocal cases.

Other choices and discussion

B. A hemangioma would be expected to be much brighter than this lesion on the T2-weighted sequence. Arterial phase enhancement might be seen with an atypical/flash-filling hemangioma, but the portal venous phase washout in this case would not be expected.

C. AFP alone is insufficiently sensitive to be used for HCC screening. Typically, intermittent liver imaging is employed for patients with chronic liver disease.

D. A lesion with arterial enhancement, washout, and size over 2 cm would be categorized as LI-RADS 5, definitely HCC.

Question 1

Organ Procurement and Transplantation Network and LI-RADS are the two classification systems that have recently been introduced for liver lesions in the presence of chronic liver disease.

Question 2

The most critical phase of enhancement for the detection of HCC is the late arterial phase. This may be recognized by the presence of contrast in the hepatic arteries and portal vein, but not in the hepatic veins.

Question 3

Greater than 10 minutes are needed to reach the hepatocyte phase with Eovist magnetic resonance imaging. Many centers wait 15 or 20 minutes before image acquisition. Multihance (gadobenate dimeglumine) also has a hepatobiliary phase, although the delayed phase may not be reached for 1 to 2 hours, and the percentage of biliary excretion is much lower than is seen with Eovist.

Question 4

True. Although not always present, a capsule or pseudocapsule raises suspicion for HCC.

Question 5

False. Regenerative nodules are typically intermediate or dark on T2-weighted sequences.

Question 6

False. When elevated, AFP may serve as an effective tumor marker for HCC. The absence of elevated AFP does not exclude HCC.

Question 7

The lung is the most common site of distant HCC metastasis.

Question 8

True. Fat within a lesion is more common in hepatocellular adenoma than in HCC, but the presence of fat does not exclude HCC.

Question 9

Yes. Portal vein invasion is a characteristic of HCC.

Question 10

In patients with normal renal and hepatic function, approximately 50% of the IV Eovist (gadoxetate sodium) bolus is excreted by kidneys in urine, and 50% of the bolus is excreted by the liver in bile.

■ Suggested Readings

American College of Radiology. Liver imaging reporting and data system. http://www.acr.org/lirads

Wald C, Russo MW, Heimbach JK, Hussain HK, Pomfret EA, Bruix J. New OPTN/UNOS policy for liver transplant allocation: standardization of liver imaging, diagnosis, classification, and reporting of hepatocellular carcinoma. Radiology 2013;266(2):376–382

SECTION IV
GASTROINTESTINAL
IMAGING

Top Tips

◆ In patients with chronic liver disease, imaging criteria can establish the diagnosis of HCC without biopsy.

◆ The most critical phase of enhancement for HCC is the late arterial phase, highlighted by contrast in the hepatic arteries and portal veins, but not the hepatic veins.

◆ In patients with normal renal and hepatic function, approximately half of Eovist (gadoxetate disodium) is excreted by the liver and half by the kidneys.

Details 2

■ Case

A 59-year-old man presents with recent deep venous thrombosis and weight loss. There is no history of acute pancreatitis. Two axial computed tomography images are shown. What is the most likely diagnosis?

A. Mucinous cystadenoma
B. Serous cystadenoma
C. Adenocarcinoma
D. Walled off necrosis

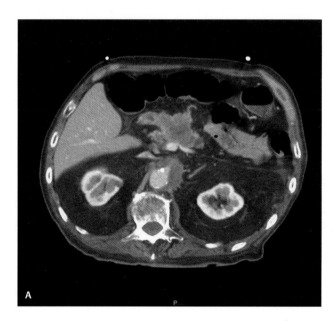 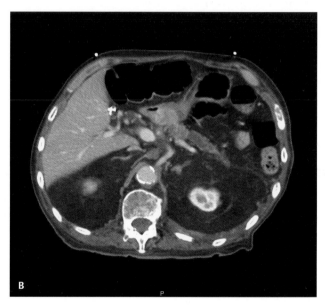

■ The following questions pertain to pancreatic ductal adenocarcinoma.

1. What approximate level of encasement of the superior mesenteric artery (SMA) would make this patient's tumor unresectable?
2. What organ is the most common site of distant spread?
3. True or False. Atrophy of the tail of the pancreas is an indirect sign of pancreatic adenocarcinoma.
4. At what diameter is the pancreatic duct considered dilated?
5. Name two ways that imaging during the pancreatic phase is helpful.
6. True or False. Typically, these tumors are hypervascular.
7. What percentage of these tumors is resectable at presentation?
8. According to the TNM staging, up to what T stage would a patient be considered resectable?
9. True or False. Portal venous occlusion related to tumor extension can still be managed with surgery.
10. True or False. Tumors centered in the head present earlier than those centered in the tail of the pancreas.

■ Answers and Explanations

C. Correct! This is adenocarcinoma. The images demonstrate an irregular hypoenhancing mass in the pancreatic neck with upstream ductal dilatation and atrophy. There is abutment of mesenteric vessels and infiltrative retroperitoneal tissue abutting the aorta.

Other choices and discussion

A. Mucinous cystadenoma is a common cause of cystic pancreatic lesions but would not have the features shown.

B. Serous cystadenoma is a common cause of cystic pancreatic lesions but would not have the features shown.

D. Walled off necrosis may present as an irregular hypoattenuating area within the pancreas, and there may even be vascular abutment or involvement of additional retroperitoneal spaces. However, there will also be a history of necrotizing pancreatitis, which is absent in this case.

Question 1

Encasement of the SMA by > 180 degrees is typically considered unresectable.

Question 2

The liver is the most common site of distant metastases in pancreatic adenocarcinoma.

Question 3

True. Except for small tumors in the uncinate, or tumors in the distal tail, pancreatic adenocarcinoma can result in upstream ductal dilatation and glandular atrophy. This is an indirect sign of pancreatic adenocarcinoma.

Question 4

The pancreatic duct is usually considered enlarged when the diameter is > 3 mm.

Question 5

The pancreatic phase, which occurs after a delay of approximately 40 seconds, provides optimal contrast between normal and abnormal pancreatic parenchyma. This phase is also helpful because the peripancreatic arteries are usually well visualized.

Question 6

False. Adenocarcinoma of the pancreas is typically hypoenhancing to the adjacent normal pancreas.

Question 7

Unfortunately, only 15 to 20% of patients have resectable disease at presentation.

Question 8

T3 tumors (tumor extends beyond the pancreas but does not involve the celiac axis or SMA) are generally resectable, as long as there are no distant metastases.

Question 9

False. In general, if direct tumor extension has resulted in occlusion of a major regional blood vessel, the tumor is unresectable.

Question 10

True. The tumor itself is usually asymptomatic in early stages, but masses in the pancreatic head may occlude the common bile duct and lead to the presenting system of jaundice. Head masses present earlier than tail masses.

■ Suggested Readings

Brennan DDD, Zamboni GA, Raptopoulos VD, Kruskal JB. Comprehensive preoperative assessment of pancreatic adenocarcinoma with 64-section volumetric CT. RadioGraphics 2007;27(6):1653–1666

Wong JC, Raman S. Surgical resectability of pancreatic adenocarcinoma: CTA. Abdom Imaging 2010;35(4):471–480

SECTION IV
GASTROINTESTINAL
IMAGING

Top Tips

- ◆ Pancreatic adenocarcinoma is usually hypoenhancing to normal pancreatic tissue and is best identified in the pancreatic phase of enhancement (approximately 40-second delay).

- ◆ Always carefully examine the celiac axis, SMA, superior mesenteric vein, and portal vein for involvement.

- ◆ Careful examination of the liver is also critical. Liver metastases may be subtle but will usually preclude resection.

Details 3

■ **Case**

A patient presents for magnetic resonance imaging (MRI) following colonoscopy. What is the most likely diagnosis?
- A. Adenocarcinoma of the rectum
- B. Focal colitis
- C. Perirectal fistula
- D. Squamous cell carcinoma of the anus

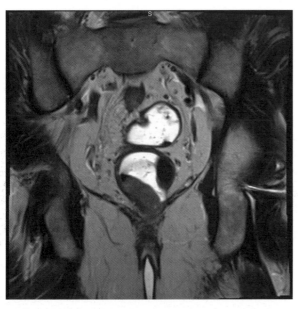

Coronal T2

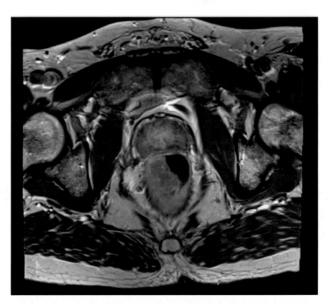

Axial T1 postcontrast

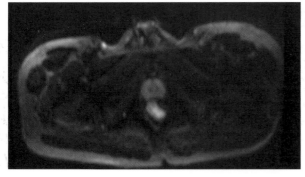

Axial diffusion-weighted imaging

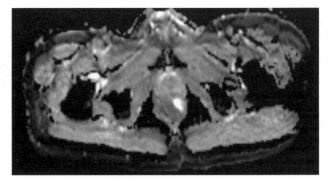

Axial apparent diffusion coefficient

■ **The following questions pertain to rectal carcinoma.**

1. In this case, what is the patient's T staging?
2. T3 lesions involve up to what layer of the bowel wall?
3: What size of perirectal lymph node is considered malignant?
4. Malignant lymph nodes demonstrate _____ signal on apparent diffusion coefficient map.
5. What location is the most common for spread of disease to lymph nodes?

6. T2 lesions involve how deep into the bowel wall?
7. The mesorectal fascia contains which structures?
8. How far above the anal verge is a lesion considered low versus high in the rectum?
9. What are the advantages of MRI over ultrasound for staging of rectal carcinoma?
10. What are the advantages of MRI over computed tomography for staging of rectal carcinomas?

■ Answers and Explanations

A. Correct! There is an enhancing T2-hypointense mass within the rectum centered above the dentate line, with restricted diffusion. This is most likely rectal adenocarcinoma.

Other choices and discussion

B. Focal colitis may result in wall thickening, but the features of this mass are more suggestive of enhancing neoplasm.

C. Perirectal fistula would manifest as a low signal tract extending from the rectum with adjacent enhancement, possibly containing T2-hyperintense fluid.

D. Squamous cell carcinoma of the anus would arise from squamous mucosa below the dentate line.

Question 1

This is a T2 mass that involves at least the mucosa and muscularis. There is some possible irregularity of the perirectal fascia which might signify transmural tumor extension, but this is not definitive. The provided images would probably not support a T3 categorization.

Question 2

T3 lesions extend beyond the muscularis propria into the perirectal tissues but do not involve adjacent organs or the visceral peritoneum.

Question 3

There is no consensus for size alone. A size cutoff of 5 mm in short axis dimension provides reasonable sensitivity and specificity. Adding suspicious characteristics such as round morphology, irregular or spiculated margins, or heterogeneous signal can increase diagnostic accuracy.

Question 4

The primary tumor and metastatic lymph nodes typically demonstrate restricted diffusion. The apparent diffusion coefficient signal should therefore be decreased.

Question 5

Perirectal lymph nodes near the primary tumor are a common initial site of disease spread.

Question 6

T2 lesions extend to the level of the muscularis propria.

Question 7

The mesorectal fascia contains fat, lymphatics, lymph nodes, and the rectum itself.

Question 8

Surgical approach may depend on the position of a rectal tumor relative to the anus. A cutoff of 5 cm above the anal verge has been used to define high versus low rectal tumors.

Question 9

Like MRI, transrectal ultrasound may demonstrate the primary tumor and depth of mural involvement. However, MRI provides better visualization of the surrounding structures and regional lymph nodes.

Question 10

MRI is superior to computed tomography for the delineation of rectal wall invasion and defining involvement of adjacent organs.

■ Suggested Readings

Jhaveri KS, Hosseini-Nik H. MRI of rectal cancer: an overview and update on recent advances. Am J Roentgenol 2015;205(1):W42–W55

Kaur H, Choi H, You YN, Rauch GM, Jensen CT, Hou P, Chang GJ, Skibber JM, Ernst RD. MR imaging for preoperative evaluation of primary rectal cancer: practical considerations. Radiographics 2012;32(2):389–409

Taylor FGM, Swift RI, Blomqvist L, Brown G. A systematic approach to the interpretation of preoperative staging MRI for rectal cancer. Am J Roentgenol 2008;191(6):1827–1835

Top Tips

◆ Rectal cancer staging is best performed with MRI.

◆ Tumor staging depends on the depth of invasion relative to the bowel wall and adjacent structures and the presence of any abnormal lymph nodes.

◆ It is useful to comment in the radiology report how far the tumor is above the anal verge.

Details 4

■ Case

A 21-year-old woman presents with slowly progressive right midabdominal pain and leukocytosis. Coronal and axial T2-weighted images are shown. What is the diagnosis?

A. Pregnancy-related pain
B. Ovarian torsion
C. Appendicitis
D. Ureteral stone

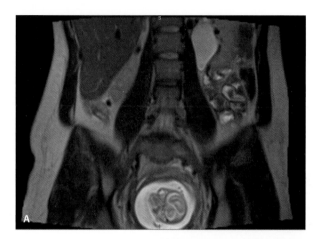
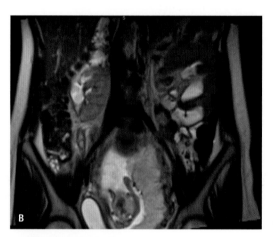
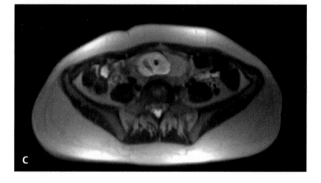

■ The following questions pertain to appendicitis.

1. Is the presence of a stone in the appendix (appendicolith) on computed tomography (CT) diagnostic of appendicitis?
2. What is the maximum maternal radiation dose that is considered safe for a fetus?
3. What is the estimated radiation dose to the fetus in the first trimester from a standard abdomen and pelvis CT exam?
4. True or False. When maternal appendicitis is suspected, the need for accurate diagnosis should take precedence when deciding whether to use gadolinium-based contrast material.
5. True or false. Iodinated intravenous contrast is considered safe in the setting of pregnancy.

6. Classic findings of acute appendicitis on CT include _____.
7. The location of pain in the setting of acute appendicitis is classically known as _____.
8. Why are retained appendicoliths problematic after surgery?
9. True or False. In the third trimester, evaluation for appendicitis should be limited to the deep right lower quadrant.
10. The accuracy of CT for acute appendicitis has been reported to be in the range of _____.

■ Answers and Explanations

D. Correct! Appendicitis. This patient has a thick-walled and distended appendix in the right lower quadrant, with edema in the periappendiceal fat. The patient is also pregnant.

Other choices and discussion

A. This patient's pain is not related to the pregnancy. Magnetic resonance imaging (MRI) is, however, an excellent modality for evaluating suspected acute appendicitis in pregnancy, due to the absence of ionizing radiation.
B. Ovarian torsion can cause right lower quadrant pain but is not demonstrated in this case.
C. Ureteral stone can cause right lower quadrant pain but is not demonstrated in this case.

Question 1

No. The presence of an appendicolith alone does not indicate appendicitis on CT.

Question 2

There is some uncertainty in discussing radiation dose and the developing fetus. However, a dose of 50 mGy has been considered a safe limit, below which there will be no harm from deterministic effects and a < 1% risk of stochastic effects.

Question 3

Phantom studies have suggested a dose of approximately 20 to 30 mGy in the first trimester and approximately 30 to 44 mGy in the second trimester.

Question 4

False! Although maternal health takes precedence over fetal health in many circumstances, gadolinium use would be contraindicated. Furthermore, intravenous contrast is unnecessary for the MRI diagnosis of acute appendicitis.

Question 5

True. Intravenous iodinated contrast may be administered in the setting of pregnancy, if indicated for the mother's care.

Question 6

The classic CT findings of appendicitis include mural thickening, mural enhancement, dilatation of the appendix, and adjacent inflammatory changes. Variable size thresholds have been employed, typically ranging from diameters of 7 to 8 mm.

Question 7

McBurney's point is the term used to describe the location of pain in the setting of acute appendicitis.

Question 8

Retained appendicoliths may be a source of infection and can lead to abscess formation.

Question 9

False. The enlarging uterus in the third trimester may displace the cecum and appendix into the upper abdomen. Evaluation for appendicitis in the third trimester may need to cover a larger area.

Question 10

CT accuracy for acute appendicitis has been reported to be 92 to 98%.

■ Suggested Readings

Abbasi N, Patenaude V, Abenhaim HA. Management and outcomes of acute appendicitis in pregnancy-population-based study of over 7000 cases. BJOG 2014;121:1509–1514

Andersen B, Nielsen TF. Appendicitis in pregnancy: diagnosis, management and complications. Acta Obstet Gynecol Scand 1999;78:758–762

Long SS, Long C, Lai H, Macura KJ. Imaging strategies for right lower quadrant pain in pregnancy. Am J Roentgenol 2011;196(1):4–12

Mazze RI, Källén B. Appendectomy during pregnancy: a Swedish registry study of 778 cases. Obstet Gynecol 1991;77:835–840

Mourad J, Elliott JP, Erickson L, Lisboa L. Appendicitis in pregnancy: new information that contradicts long-held clinical beliefs. Am J Obstet Gynecol 2000;182:1027–1029

Spalluto LB, Woodfield CA, DeBenedectis CM, Lazarus E. MR imaging evaluation of abdominal pain during pregnancy: appendicitis and other nonobstetric causes. Radiographics 2012;32(2):317–334

Woodfield CA, Lazarus E, Chen KC, Mayo-Smith WW. Abdominal pain in pregnancy: diagnoses and imaging unique to pregnancy—review. Am J Roentgenol 2010:194(6):WS14–WS30

SECTION IV
GASTROINTESTINAL
IMAGING

Top Tips

◆ The clinical findings of appendicitis in pregnant patients may differ from nonpregnant patients.

◆ If the appendix is not identified by ultrasound, MRI is the imaging modality of choice for suspected appendicitis in pregnancy.

◆ Gadolinium-based contrast administration is contraindicated in pregnancy.

Details 5

■ **Case**

A middle-aged patient presents 5 weeks after the onset of gallstone pancreatitis. What is the best term to describe the current finding in the pancreatic bed?
  A. Complex pseudocyst
  B. Walled-off necrosis
  C. Necrotizing pancreatitis
  D. Acute necrotic collection

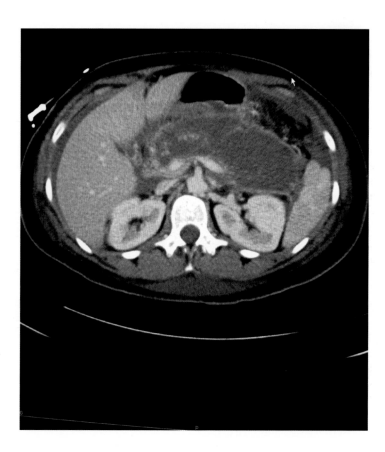

■ **The following questions pertain to pancreatitis.**

1. What is the name of the most recent classification system for the staging of pancreatitis?
2. What terms are used to describe fluid collections in IEP, and what distinguishes one from the other?
3. What terms are used to describe collections in necrotizing pancreatitis, and what distinguishes one from the other?
4. What vascular complication may classically occur from acute pancreatitis?
5. What are the two most common causes of pancreatitis in the United States?

6. What imaging is necessary for the diagnosis of acute pancreatitis?
7. How long after symptom onset should a patient with acute pancreatitis be imaged?
8. Imaging findings of simple (IEP) pancreatitis include

   _____.
9. What is the most critical imaging feature for identifying pancreatic necrosis?
10. What imaging feature is the hallmark of chronic pancreatitis?

■ Answers and Explanations

B. Correct! This is walled-off necrosis. This mixed-attenuation, thick-walled collection occupies the expected location of the pancreas, indicating previous necrotizing pancreatitis.

Other choices and discussion

A. The term "pseudocyst" has often been used to describe any postpancreatitis fluid collection. In the current terminology, however, a pseudocyst specifically refers to a peripancreatic fluid collection persisting more than 4 weeks after an episode of interstitial edematous pancreatitis.

C. Necrotizing pancreatitis refers to pancreatic inflammation leading to glandular necrosis and is not used to describe a fluid collection.

D. An acute necrotic collection is a pancreatitis-associated fluid collection occurring within the first 4 weeks of an episode of necrotizing pancreatitis.

Question 1

The Revised Atlanta classification outlines the standardized terminology for describing acute pancreatitis and associated fluid collections. Acute pancreatitis is classified as either necrotizing pancreatitis or interstitial edematous pancreatitis (IEP), depending on the presence or absence of glandular necrosis.

Question 2

Fluid collections in IEP are classified as acute peripancreatic fluid collections if they are present for fewer than 4 weeks after symptom onset, and as pseudocysts if they are present for more than 4 weeks after symptom onset.

Question 3

Collections in necrotizing pancreatitis are classified as acute necrotic collections if they develop fewer than 4 weeks after symptom onset, and as walled-off necrosis if they develop more than 4 weeks after symptom onset and develop a discrete wall.

Question 4

Splenic artery aneurysm classically occurs secondary to acute pancreatitis. Other vascular complications might include aneurysm of the gastroduodenal artery and splenic vein thrombosis. Always look carefully at the vessels on contrast-enhanced studies of the pancreas.

Question 5

Alcohol and choledocholithiasis are the two most common causes of acute pancreatitis in the United States.

Question 6

None! Despite ever-increasing imaging use, remember that the diagnosis of acute pancreatitis can be made based on clinical and laboratory findings. Contrast-enhanced computed tomography (CT) is used to establish the diagnosis in equivocal cases. CT may be used to identify and follow complications. Almost all patients will also have an ultrasound to assess for the presence of gallstones, and many will have a magnetic resonance cholangiopancreatography to assess for choledocholithiasis.

Question 7

CT is indicated in cases that do not resolve within 48 to 72 hours, in order to confirm the diagnosis and identify any complications. Earlier imaging may be indicated in severe cases.

Question 8

IEP will exhibit enlargement of the pancreas with peripancreatic edema and accumulation of simple fluid.

Question 9

Lack of glandular enhancement is the defining feature of pancreatic necrosis on CT.

Question 10

Coarse pancreatic calcifications are the hallmark of chronic pancreatitis.

■ Suggested Readings

O'Connor OJ, Buckley JM, Maher MM. Imaging of the complications of acute pancreatitis. Am J Roentgenol 2011;197(3):W375–W381

O'Connor OJ, McWilliams S, Maher MM. Imaging of acute pancreatitis. Am J Roentgenol 2011;197(2):W221–W225

Shyu JY, Sainani NI, Sahni VA, Chick JF, Chauhan NR, Conwell DL, Clancy TE, Banks PA, Silverman SG. Necrotizing pancreatitis: diagnosis, imaging, and intervention. Radiographics 2014;34(5):1218–1239

Thoeni RF. Revised Atlanta classification of acute pancreatitis: its importance for the radiologist and its effect on treatment. Radiology 2012;262(3):751–764

Top Tips

♦ Alcohol and choledocholithiasis are the two most common causes of pancreatitis in the United States.

♦ The Revised Atlanta classification provides clear terminology for discussing acute pancreatitis and pancreatitis-associated fluid collections.

♦ In current terminology, a pseudocyst is a peripancreatic fluid collection that is present more than 4 weeks after an episode of interstitial edematous pancreatitis.

Image Rich 1

■ Case

Four liver magnetic resonance imaging examinations in patients with indeterminate liver lesions on computed tomography are presented. Which set(s) of images depict probably malignant lesions?

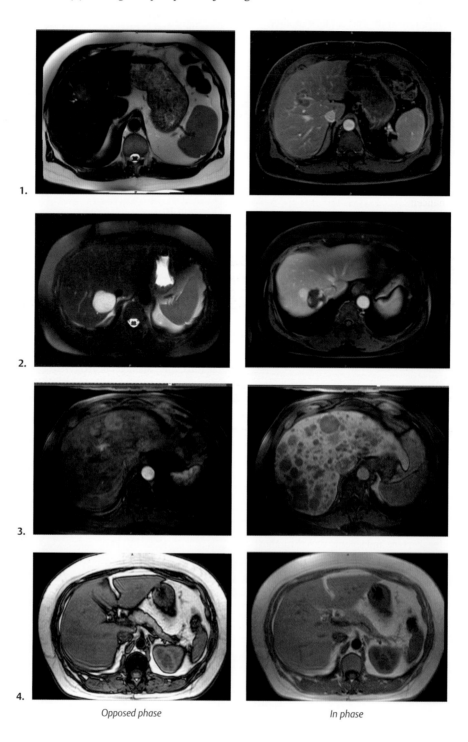

1.

2.

3.

4.

Opposed phase   *In phase*

■ Answers and Explanations

Option 1 is likely malignant. The images show a mildly T2 hyperintense mass, with continuous peripheral enhancement on the portal venous phase. This is likely malignant, possibly representing an adenocarcinoma metastasis. The enhancement is somewhat reminiscent of a hemangioma. However, the T2 signal is less than expected for a hemangioma, and the enhancement is not nodular or discontinuous.

Option 2 is likely benign. The images show a markedly T2 hyperintense mass with discontinuous peripheral nodular enhancement after contrast administration. This is a classic-appearing hepatic hemangioma. This pattern of enhancement is known as type 2 enhancement. Type 1 enhancement is characterized by immediate uniform enhancement (small capillary or "flash filling" hemangioma) and is typically found in smaller hemangiomas. Type 3 enhancement is characterized by peripheral nodular enhancement with centripetal progression but persistent central hypointensity (e.g., giant hemangioma).

Option 3 is likely malignant. The images show multiple masses with arterial phase enhancement and no uptake on the hepatobiliary phase. These are likely metastatic, as there are no obvious findings of chronic liver disease. Hypervascular metastases typically arise from neuroendocrine tumors (e.g., pancreatic islet cell tumor, carcinoid tumor, or pheochromocytoma), renal cell carcinoma, thyroid carcinoma, choriocarcinoma, melanoma, and sarcomas. This was a case of carcinoid metastases.

Option 4 is likely benign. The images show a focal lesion along the free edge of hepatic segment 4 adjacent to the falciform ligament. The lesion is occult on the in-phase image and hypointense to liver on the opposed phase image. This is consistent with focal fatty deposition. Classic locations include the liver edge adjacent to the falciform ligament, adjacent to the gallbladder fossa, and adjacent to the portal vein in the central liver.

■ Suggested Readings

Danet I-M, Semelka RC, Leonardou P, Braga L, Vaidean G, Woosley JT, Kanematsu M. Spectrum of MRI appearances of untreated metastases of the liver. Am J Roentgenol 2003;181(3):809–817

Silva AC, Evans JM, McCullough AE, Jatoi MA, Vargas HE, Hara AK. MR imaging of hypervascular liver masses: a review of current techniques. Radiographics 2009;29(2):385–402

Top Tips

◆ Signal loss of the opposed-phase images relative to the in-phase images is diagnostic of fatty deposition within the liver.

◆ Sources of hypervascular liver metastases include neuroendocrine tumors (e.g., pancreatic islet cell tumor, carcinoid tumor, or pheochromocytoma), renal cell carcinoma, thyroid carcinoma, choriocarcinoma, melanoma, and sarcomas.

◆ The classic appearance of adenocarcinoma metastases to the liver includes T1 hypointensity, mild T2 hyperintensity, and heterogeneous nonprogressive enhancement (sometimes target-like).

Image Rich 2

■ Case

All of these patients were referred for magnetic resonance imaging (MRI) for indeterminate liver lesions on computed tomography (CT). Match the appropriate diagnosis to the provided images.

A. Hepatocellular carcinoma
B. Focal nodular hyperplasia (FNH)
C. Cyst
D. Hepatic adenoma

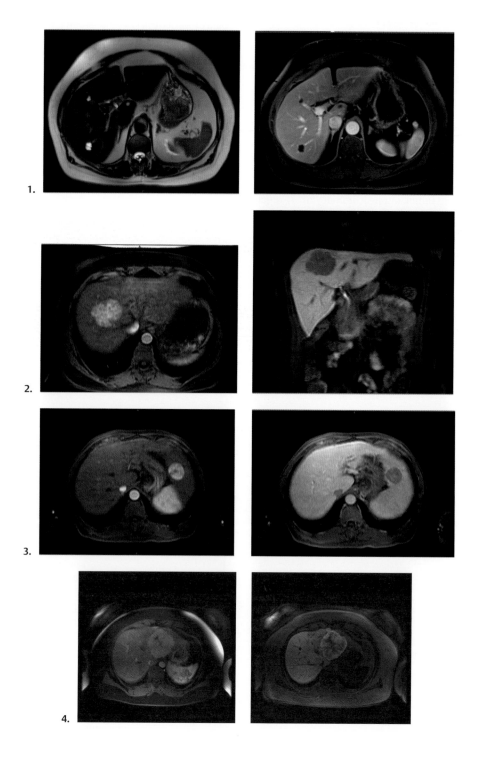

1.

2.

3.

4.

■ Answers and Explanations

1. C. Cyst. Option 1 shows three small circumscribed lesions (anterior right lobe, posterior right lobe, and caudate lobe) that are markedly T2 hyperintense and nonenhancing after contrast administration. These lesions are most consistent with simple hepatic cysts. In situations when ultrasound or CT is inconclusive in determining a benign etiology of small hepatic lesions, MRI can often be used for confirmation.

2. D. Hepatic adenoma. Option 2 demonstrates a mass that is moderately hyperenhancing on the arterial phase and is without uptake on the hepatobiliary phase. The hyperenhancement might raise concern for hepatocellular carcinoma. However, the lesion is lacking a capsule, and there are no signs of chronic liver disease. Additionally, the alpha-fetoprotein was negative. Not shown here, there was no evidence of washout on the portal venous or equilibrium phases. This lesion is a hepatic adenoma.

3. A. Hepatocellular carcinoma. Option 3 does have classic findings of hepatocellular carcinoma. The mass in the left hepatic lobe demonstrates hyperenhancement on the arterial phase and washout on the portal venous phase. This patient had chronic liver disease.

4. B. FNH. Option 4 is an example of FNH. The lesion is hyperenhancing to adjacent liver in the arterial phase, has a hypointense central scar, and demonstrates uptake on the hepatobiliary phase. This is classic for FNH. FNH is also typically minimally hyperintense on T2, isointense on T1, and may exhibit delayed enhancement of the central scar.

■ Suggested Readings

Danet I-M, Semelka RC, Leonardou P, Braga L, Vaidean G, Woosley JT, Kanematsu M. Spectrum of MRI appearances of untreated metastases of the liver. Am J Roentgenol 2003;181(3):809–817

Silva AC, Evans JM, McCullough AE, Jatoi MA, Vargas HE, Hara AK. MR imaging of hypervascular liver masses: a review of current techniques. Radiographics 2009;29(2):385–402

Top Tips

◆ On MRI with gadoxetate disodium (Eovist; Bayer Healthcare Pharmaceuticals Inc., Whippany, NJ), FNH and adenoma both demonstrate hyperenhancement on the arterial phase images, but only FNH will retain contrast in the hepatobiliary phase.

◆ FNH classically has a T2 hyperintense central scar, is isointense to adjacent liver parenchyma on precontrast images, enhances homogeneously on arterial phase images, and is similar to adjacent liver on portal venous phases.

◆ MRI can often confirm benign etiology of even small hepatic cysts.

SECTION IV GASTROINTESTINAL IMAGING

Image Rich 3

■ Case

The following four patients have pancreatic abnormalities. Match the appropriate diagnosis to the provided images.
(Case courtesy of Dr. Desiree Morgan.)

A. Pancreatic adenocarcinoma
B. Acute necrotic collection
C. Mucinous cystadenoma
D. Serous cystadenoma

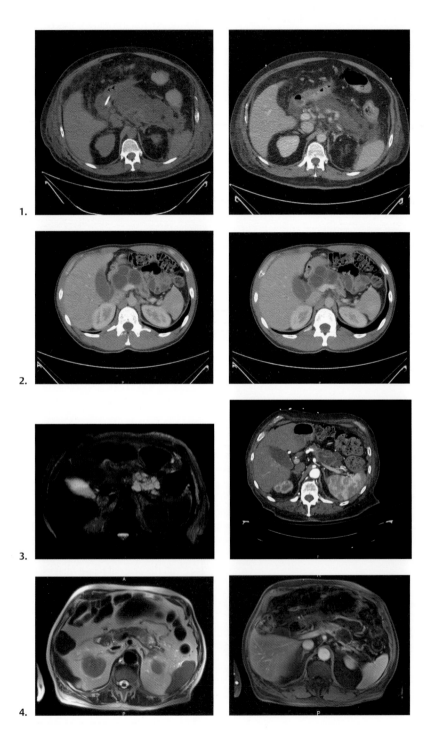

■ Answers and Explanations

1. B. Acute necrotic collection. Option 1 shows an ill-defined, large, heterogeneous fluid attenuation area with peripancreatic stranding. The overall appearance suggests an inflammatory process (e.g., pancreatitis). This is an example of an acute necrotic collection.

2. C. Mucinous cystadenoma. Option 2 shows a complex cystic lesion with septa and upstream pancreatic duct dilatation. The cystic portions of the lesion are approximately 2 cm in size. Of the presented lesions, this is the most likely to represent a mucinous cystadenoma. The visible septations appear thin. Many mucinous cystadenomas have larger cysts than shown here. These lesions are more likely to be malignant than are serous lesions, so intervention is sometimes necessary. The appearance of a mucinous cystadenoma and an oligocystic serous adenoma can overlap.

3. D. Serous cystadenoma. Option 3 shows a mass with smaller and more numerous cystic spaces. Of the four lesions shown, this one is most consistent with a serous cystadenoma. Typical serous cystadenomas will have many cystic spaces, each smaller than 2 cm in size. There is often a central scar, which may be calcified, although there is none in this case. Serous cystadenomas are typically benign lesions. If the patient is asymptomatic and there are no other complications on imaging, the lesion may be followed, rather than biopsied or removed.

4. A. Pancreatic adenocarcinoma. Option 4 shows a solid, heterogeneous, hypoenhancing lesion without obvious signs of current or prior pancreatitis. There is upstream pancreatic atrophy. This was found to be an adenocarcinoma of the pancreas.

■ Suggested Readings

Sahani DV, Kadavigere R, Saokar A, Fernandez-del Castillo C, Brugge WR, Hahn PF. Cystic pancreatic lesions: a simple imaging-based classification system for guiding management. Radiographics 2005;25(6):1471–1484

Shyu JY, Sainani NI, Sahni VA, Chick JF, Chauhan NR, Conwell DL, Clancy TE, Banks PA, Silverman SG. Necrotizing pancreatitis: diagnosis, imaging, and intervention. Radiographics 2014;34(5):1218–1239

SECTION IV GASTROINTESTINAL IMAGING

Top Tips

◆ Classic serous cystadenomas of the pancreas have cystic spaces < 2 cm in size, a central scar, septations, and calcifications.

◆ Typical-appearing serous cystadenomas are benign and do not necessarily need to be resected.

◆ Mucinous pancreatic lesions should be more closely monitored or resected, due to a small malignant potential.

Image Rich 4

■ Case

Biliary abnormalities. Which image(s) depict probably malignant lesions?

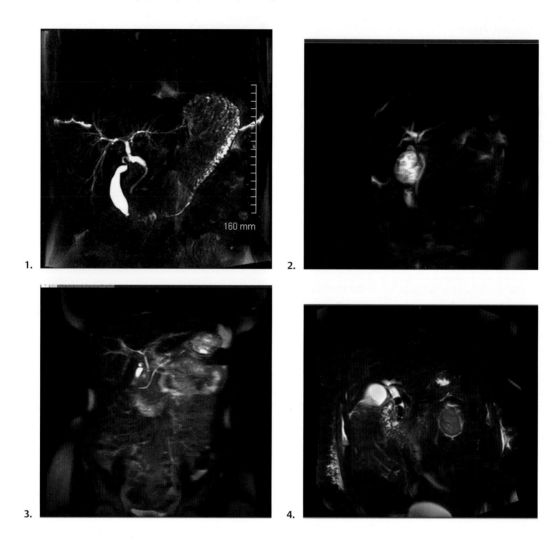

1.

2.

3.

4.

■ Answers and Explanations

Option 1 is most likely benign and represents an example of primary sclerosis cholangitis (PSC). PSC is an inflammatory condition of the bile ducts, which can lead to cirrhosis and also predispose to cholangiocarcinoma. The principal imaging finding is the presence of intermittent areas of narrowing and dilatation throughout the intrahepatic biliary tree. The common bile duct is sometimes involved. About 70% of patients with PSC have inflammatory bowel disease, most commonly ulcerative colitis. The overall incidence of PSC among patients with inflammatory bowel disease is about 1 to 4%.

Option 2 is most likely malignant. The image demonstrates intrahepatic biliary ductal dilatation, with focal severe narrowing of the bile ducts at the liver hilum. This appearance is suspicious for a centrally located cholangiocarcinoma, or Klatskin tumor.

Option 3 is most likely benign. The image demonstrates a separation between the common bile duct and the main pancreatic duct. This is a benign congenital variant termed pancreatic divisum. Pancreatic divisum, with an incidence of 3 to 7%, results from the failure of fusion of the dorsal and ventral pancreatic ducts. There can be an increased incidence in idiopathic recurrent pancreatitis in these patients, suggesting an association between these entities. In pancreas divisum, the larger dorsal pancreatic duct (duct of Santorini), which drains the pancreatic tail, body, and superior head, courses anterior to the common bile duct and drains into the minor papilla. The smaller ventral duct (duct of Wirsung), which drains the inferior pancreatic head and uncinate process, accompanies the common bile duct into the major papilla. Complete divisum occurs with complete separation of the draining ducts of the dorsal and ventral pancreas. Incomplete divisum occurs when there is a small branch communication between these ducts.

Option 4 is most likely benign. The image demonstrates multiple oval, T2 hypointense filling defects within a mildly dilated common bile duct. This is most consistent with choledocholithiasis. The differential diagnosis of common bile duct filling defects also includes tumor, blood products, sludge, air, parasites, and ingested food products. The patient's clinical condition and history as well as the appearance on other sequences can help confirm the diagnosis.

■ Suggested Readings

Chung YE, Kim M-J, Park YN, Choi J-Y, Pyo JY, Kim YC, Cho HJ, Kim KA, Choi SY. Varying appearances of cholangiocarcinoma: radiologic-pathologic correlation. Radiographics 2009;29(3):683–700

Vitellas KM, Keogan MT, Spritzer CE, Nelson RC. MR cholangiopancreatography of bile and pancreatic duct abnormalities with emphasis on the single-shot fast spin-echo technique. Radiographics 2000;20(4):939–957

Top Tips

◆ About 70% of patients with PSC have inflammatory bowel disease, especially ulcerative colitis. The incidence of PSC among patients with inflammatory bowel disease is about 1 to 4%.

◆ Filling defects in the common bile duct on magnetic resonance cholangiopancreatography may be due to stones, blood, tumor, sludge, parasites, or air.

◆ A Klatskin tumor is a hilar cholangiocarcinoma occurring at the junction of the left and right hepatic ducts.

Image Rich 5

■ **Case**

Four patients with esophageal abnormalities are presented. Match the appropriate diagnosis to the provided images. (Case courtesy of Dr. Christine Menias.)

A. Malignant intraluminal mass
B. Eosinophilic esophagitis
C. Extrinsic mass
D. Benign stricture

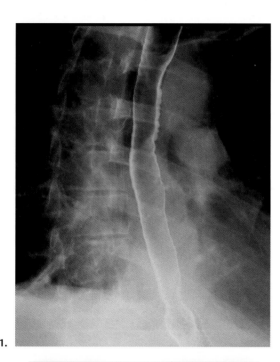

1.

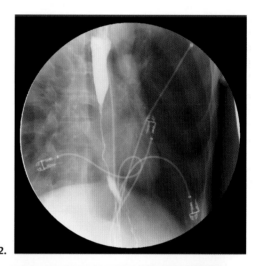

2.

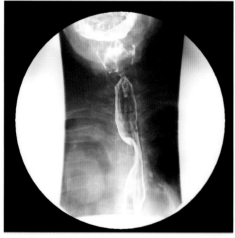

3.

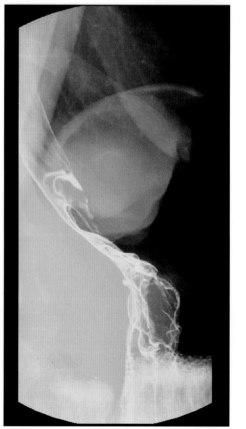

4.

■ Answers and Explanations

1. B. Eosinophilic esophagitis. Option 1 is an example of eosinophilic esophagitis. On fluoroscopic examination, the esophagus has ringed indentations along an area of narrowing. These rings appear as multiple, fixed, closely spaced, concentric rings that traverse the stricture. The length of the stricture is moderate in extent and the location can occur in any section of the thoracic esophagus. The clinical presentation in adults is typically young men with longstanding dysphagia and recurrent food impactions.

2. D. Benign stricture. Option 2 demonstrates a long smooth stricture. With the length and smooth appearance, a benign cause is favored. The typical differential of a lower esophageal structure would include entities such as reflux disease, scleroderma, prolonged nasogastric tube intubation, and alkaline reflux esophagitis. In this case, the patient had undergone radiation to the lower mediastinum.

3. C. Extrinsic mass. Option 3 also has a focal area of narrowing, this time along the upper thoracic esophagus. The contour of the narrowing has obtuse angles, suggesting an intramural or extrinsic process. Upon careful inspection, there is a density along the right side of the mediastinum and a mass in the lung from an invasive non–small cell lung cancer. The esophageal contour abnormality is due to extrinsic compression.

4. A. Malignant intraluminal mass. Option 4 demonstrates an ulcerated intraluminal mass with resultant luminal narrowing. In this case, the follow-up endoscopy confirmed an esophageal mass, which was felt to be a metastasis from the patient's known melanoma.

■ Suggested Readings

Luedtke P, Levine MS, Rubesin SE, Weinstein DS, Laufer I. Radiologic diagnosis of benign esophageal strictures: a pattern approach. Radiographics 2003;23(4):897–909

Zimmerman SL, Levine MS, Rubesin SE, Mitre MC, Furth EE, Laufer I, Katzka DA. Idiopathic eosinophilic esophagitis in adults: the ringed esophagus. Radiology 2005;236(1):159–165

Top Tips

- Eosinophilic esophagitis is typically seen in young men with longstanding dysphagia and with complaints of recurrent food impactions.
- Findings of eosinophilic esophagitis at fluoroscopy include ringed indentations, which are multiple, fixed, and closely spaced along an area of narrowing.
- Long smooth strictures of the esophagus are often benign.

More Challenging 1

■ Case

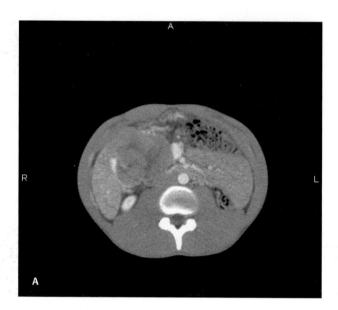

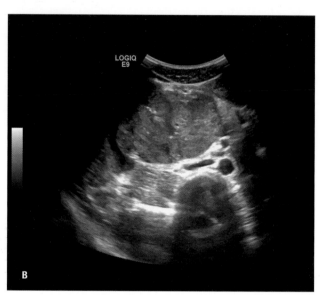

■ Questions

1. A 22-year-old African-American patient presents with low-grade upper abdominal pain for the past week. No significant past medical history. In addition to these findings, other images (not shown) demonstrate multiple liver lesions. What is the most likely etiology of this pancreatic mass?
   A. Pancreatic adenocarcinoma
   B. Nonfunctioning islet cell tumor
   C. Complicated pseudocyst
   D. Solid pseudopapillary tumor of the pancreas

2. Which of the following populations is most likely to have this tumor?
   A. Elderly
   B. Male
   C. African-American
   D. Pediatric

3. Which ONE of the following is true regarding solid pseudopapillary tumors of the pancreas?
   A. The most common site of spread is the lung.
   B. These lesions are typically benign.
   C. The most common location for the primary lesion is the pancreatic body.
   D. The average size of the primary tumor at diagnosis is under 3 cm.

■ Answers and Explanations

Question 1

D. Correct! This is a young male patient with a large mixed-attenuation pancreatic mass. Solid pseudopapillary tumor is the most likely diagnosis. These masses are heterogeneously cystic and solid and tend to present in the second or third decade of life. If present, internal hemorrhage on computed tomography or magnetic resonance imaging can be a distinguishing feature.

Other choices and discussion

A. Pancreatic adenocarcinoma would be unusual in a patient of this age. Additionally, this mass is larger and less infiltrative than expected for a pancreatic adenocarcinoma in this location.

B. Nonfunctioning islet cell tumor is in the differential diagnosis for this case. Islet cell tumors are typically hyperenhancing in the pancreatic phase, which could help differentiate this mass.

C. A complicated pseudocyst may be heterogeneous, but is still predominantly cystic. This mass is predominantly solid on both computed tomography and ultrasound.

Question 2

C. Correct! Solid pseudopapillary tumors have a predisposition for African-American and Asian populations. In addition, they are most commonly found in young, non-Caucasian, female patients.

Other choices and discussion

A. Solid masses in elderly patients are more likely to be malignant.

B. Although this patient is male, men are much less likely than women to have a solid pseudopapillary tumor.

D. This tumor is rare in children.

Question 3

B. Correct! The large majority of solid pseudopapillary tumors of the pancreas are benign.

Other choices and discussion

A. When aggressive, the most common site of metastasis is the liver. This patient, in fact, has liver metastases (not shown). Regional lymph nodes may also be involved.

C. These masses have a predilection for the pancreatic head and the tail.

D. The average tumor size at diagnosis is over 6 cm.

■ Suggested Readings

Coleman KM, Doherty MC, Bigler SA. Solid-pseudopapillary tumor of the pancreas. Radiographics 2003;23(6):1644–1648

Top Tips

◆ Solid pseudopapillary tumors of the pancreas have a predilection for young females of African-American or eastern Asian descent.

◆ These are typically benign tumors. If metastatic, spread is usually to the liver and lymph nodes.

◆ The masses tend to be large and heterogeneous at presentation. The presence of internal hemorrhage can be a distinguishing feature.

More Challenging 2

■ Case

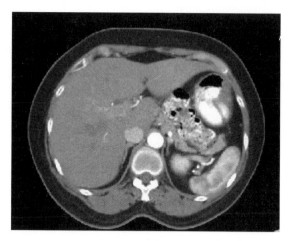

Arterial phase

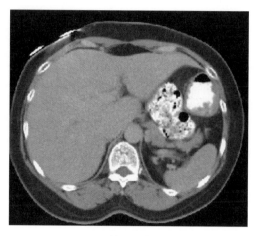

Equilibrium phase

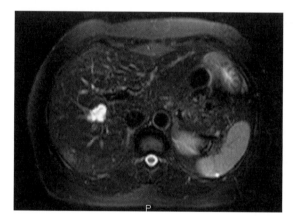

Postcontrast T1 portal venous phase

■ Questions

1. A 55-year-old woman presents with a 3-month history of nonspecific abdominal pain. An incidental liver lesion was found. There is no history of malignancy and liver serologies are negative. Selected computed tomography images and magnetic resonance imaging (MRI) are presented. What is the most likely diagnosis?
   A. Sclerosed hemangioma
   B. Focal nodular hyperplasia
   C. Hepatocellular carcinoma
   D. Colon carcinoma metastasis

2. Which ONE of the following may assist in differentiating a hepatic adenoma from an HCC?
   A. Arterial phase hyperenhancement
   B. Portal venous phase hypoenhancement

C. Absence of enhancement on hepatobiliary phase imaging
D. Elevated serum AFP

3. Hepatocyte-specific contrast is superior to other intracellular contrast agents for the diagnosis of which ONE of the following lesions?
   A. Hepatocellular carcinoma
   B. Focal nodular hyperplasia
   C. Focal fatty deposition
   D. Hemangioma

■ Answers and Explanations

Question 1

A. Correct! Of the choices provided, a sclerosed hemangioma is the most likely. The computed tomography shows no arterial phase enhancement. The lesion is isoattenuating to the liver on the equilibrium phase image, suggesting delayed enhancement. On MRI, the marked T2 hyperintensity is most suggestive of a liver cyst or a hemangioma. There are some enhancing components on the portal venous phase, which should not be seen with a simple liver cyst. However, the appearance is also atypical for a hemangioma. This is a difficult diagnosis to make and, indeed, follow up imaging was performed in this patient to ensure a benign etiology. The lesion decreased in size on follow-up imaging, consistent with a sclerosed hemangioma.

Other choices and discussion

B. FNH would exhibit hyperenhancement on the arterial phase relative to the liver. Uptake of the hepatocyte-specific contrast agent on the delayed phase MRI would also be expected (not shown).

C. HCC would also typically exhibit hyperenhancement on the arterial phase, classically with washout and a capsule or pseudocapsule. There may or may not be uptake on the hepatobiliary phase. With HCC, the serum alpha-fetoprotein (AFP) may be elevated and chronic liver disease is often seen, neither of which are present in this case.

D. A liver metastasis might have a similar appearance to this lesion, especially if it were a treated metastasis. Colon cancer metastases would be expected to have more definitive enhancement, some degree of washout, and somewhat less T2 hyperintensity than is seen in the test case.

Question 2

D. Correct! Elevated serum AFP. In patients without chronic liver disease, there is considerable overlap in the appearance of hepatic adenoma and HCC. For these patients, an elevated AFP raises suspicion for HCC. The inverse is not true; a normal AFP does not exclude HCC.

Other choices and discussion

A. Arterial phase enhancement is present in both hepatic adenoma and HCC.

B. Portal venous phase hypoenhancement ("washout") is present in both hepatic adenoma and HCC.

C. Absence of enhancement on hepatobiliary phase imaging is expected for both hepatic adenoma and most HCCs.

Question 3

B. Correct! An FNH will accumulate hepatocyte-specific contrast, demonstrating signal on the hepatobiliary phase images. This can facilitate the differentiation of FNH from other hyperenhancing masses (such as hepatic adenoma and atypical hemangioma) and is one of the main indications for using Eovist (Bayer Healthcare Pharmaceuticals, Inc., Whippany, NJ; gadoxetate disodium). Another area of superiority with hepatocyte-specific contrast is the identification and monitoring of hepatic metastases, which are conspicuous on the delayed phase. The delayed phase can also be useful for the assessment of the biliary tree.

Other choices and discussion

A. HCC does not typically concentrate hepatocyte-specific contrast, although well-differentiated forms may demonstrate uptake on the hepatobiliary phase. For this reason, the hepatobiliary phase does not contribute to the diagnosis of HCC.

C. Focal fatty deposition is successfully identified on MRI by comparing the in-phase and opposed-phase images. Aside from the differences in fat concentration, areas of focal fat behave like the surrounding liver. Do not let enhancement within an area of suspected focal fat confuse you; enhancement is normal and expected.

D. The diagnosis of hemangioma is not facilitated by hepatocyte-specific contrast. Indeed, the diagnosis can be more challenging because the progressive enhancement of the adjacent liver parenchyma can obscure the presence of enhancement within the hemangioma.

■ Suggested Readings

Doyle DJ, Khalili K, Guindi M, Atri M. Imaging features of sclerosed hemangioma. Am J Roentgenol 2007;189(1):67–72

Gupta RT, Iseman CM, Leyendecker JR, Shyknevsky I, Merkle EM, Taouli B. Diagnosis of focal nodular hyperplasia with MRI: multicenter retrospective study comparing gadobenate dimeglumine to gadoxetate disodium. Am J Roentgenol 2012;199(1):35–43

Top Tips

◆ Sclerosed hemangiomas can be difficult to diagnosis and often require follow up to ensure stability or decrease in size as the lesion becomes more fibrotic.

◆ In patients without chronic liver disease, an elevated AFP may help distinguish hepatic adenoma from HCC.

◆ Hepatocyte-specific contrast facilitates the diagnosis of certain lesions such as FNH and liver metastases, but is not superior to other intracellular contrast agents for many other liver lesions.

More Challenging 3

■ Case

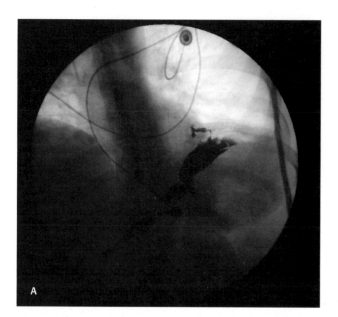

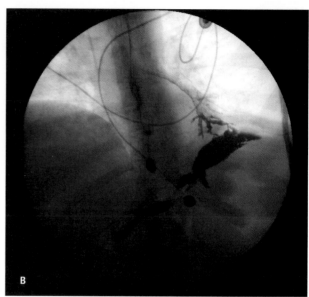

■ Questions

1. A patient presents with left-sided chest and abdominal pain. She describes coughing episodes after meals. Images from an upper gastrointestinal (GI) examination are presented. Which ONE of the following may have predisposed the patient to her current diagnosis?
   A. Hiatal hernia
   B. Previous gastric sleeve procedure
   C. Previous median sternotomy
   D. Gastric volvulus

2. What is the best diagnosis?
   A. Bronchopleural fistula
   B. Diaphragmatic rupture

   C. Gastric outlet obstruction
   D. Gastrobronchial fistula

3. What is the most common complication after gastric band surgery?
   A. Band slippage
   B. Malpositioned band
   C. Pouch dilatation
   D. Perforation

■ Answers and Explanations

Question 1

B. Correct! This patient had a previous gastric sleeve procedure. The images show progressive filling of the left lower lobe airways through a fistula from the stomach. Of the choices, previous abdominal surgery is the most likely etiology.

Other choices and discussion

A. Chronic inflammation within a hiatal hernia might lead to fistulization. However, this patient does not have a hernia, and the fistula is transdiaphragmatic.

C. Previous median sternotomy should not involve the stomach and should not predispose to this complication.

D. Gastric volvulus is not present in this patient, and would not be expected to lead to a fistula in isolation.

Question 2

D. Correct! There is a gastrobronchial fistula. There is passage of contrast from the stomach to the tracheobronchial tree through the left hemidiaphragm. This patient had a postoperative abscess, which eventually led to fistulization.

Other choices and discussion

A. Bronchopleural fistula can be a cause of pneumothorax. This should not be visualized on an upper GI examination and would not explain the contrast communicating with the tracheobronchial tree.

B. This patient does have a fistula passing through the diaphragm, but there is no evidence of diaphragmatic rupture.

C. Gastric outlet obstruction will result in delayed or absent emptying of the stomach on upper GI, but should not result in fistulization.

Question 3

A. Correct! Band slippage is the most common complication. With gastric band slippage, there is herniation of stomach superiorly through the band or slippage of the band farther distal along the stomach than intended. If untreated, this can lead to chronic stomal stenosis. This may manifest as malalignment of the band on radiographs, with an enlarged gastric pouch on

fluoroscopy. The normal phi angle for a laparoscopic adjustable band is between 4 and 58 degrees. The stomal diameter is typically 3 to 4 mm in transverse measurement, and the proximal pouch is typically < 4 cm at its greatest dimension.

Other choices and discussion

B. Band malpositioning (i.e., misplaced at the time of surgery) is rare, especially for experienced surgeons.

C. Pouch dilatation can occur without band slippage if the band is too tight, if there are constricting adhesions, or if oral intake is too great.

D. Perforation and fistulization are uncommon after gastric band placement, occurring in < 1 to 3% of patients. The likelihood increases to 8% after a second operation.

■ Suggested Readings

Alharbi SR. Gastrobronchial fistula a rare complication post laparoscopic sleeve gastrectomy. Ann Thorac Med 2013;8(3):179–180

Graif A, Conde K, DeMauro CA. Imaging of a gastrobronchial fistula after gastric bypass surgery and the contrast dilemma. Del Med J 2015;87(4):113–116

Levine MS, Carucci LR. Imaging of bariatric surgery: normal anatomy and postoperative complications. Radiology 2014;270(2):327–341

Sakran N, Assalia A, Keidar A, Goitein D. Gastrobronchial fistula as a complication of bariatric surgery: a series of 6 cases. Obes Facts 2012;5:538–545

Sonavane SK, Menias CO, Kantawala KP, Shanbhogue AK, Prasad SR, Eagon JC, Sandrasegaran K. Laparoscopic adjustable gastric banding: what radiologists need to know. Radiographics 2012;32(4):1161–1178

Top Tips

- The development of a gastrobronchial fistula may occur secondary to a subphrenic abscess with secondary spread across the diaphragm.

- Band slippage is the most common complication after gastric band surgery. This can be seen as malalignment on radiographs with an enlarged pouch on fluoroscopy.

- An enlarged pouch without band malalignment may indicate pouch dilatation from overtightening of the band, constricting adhesions, or hyperalimentation.

More Challenging 4

■ **Case**

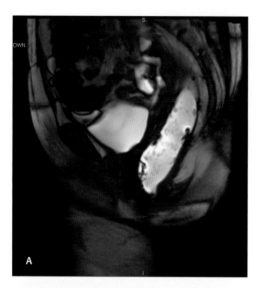

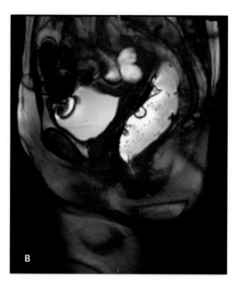

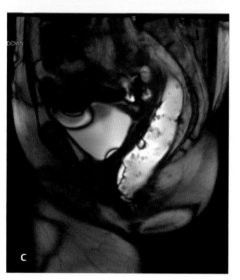

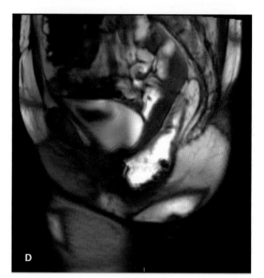

■ **Questions**

1. A 48-year-old woman with a long-term history of chronic constipation and pelvic pain presents for a pelvic floor magnetic resonance imaging (MRI). Selected images from different phases of the exam are presented. Which dynamic maneuver is used to evaluate for puborectalis muscle contraction?
   A. Squeeze/clench
   B. Valsalva
   C. Rest
   D. Defecation

2. Which of the following is used as the anatomic reference point of the pelvic floor on MRI?
   A. H line
   B. M line
   C. Pubococcygeal line
   D. Puborectalis muscle

3. What is the key finding on these images?
   A. Middle compartment prolapse
   B. Paradoxical motion of the puborectalis muscle
   C. Rectal prolapse
   D. Enterocele

■ Answers and Explanations

Question 1

A. Correct! Squeeze/clench. Dynamic pelvic floor MRI can help in the diagnosis and management of problematic pelvic floor disorders, which occur in as many as 24% of women. There are usually four dynamic maneuvers during pelvic floor MRI. During the squeeze/clench sequence, the patient is asked to tighten the pelvic floor musculature. The radiologist assesses for appropriate elevation of the pelvic floor. The second image shows this maneuver.

Other choices and discussion

B. Valsalva maneuver is performed to assess for weakness in the pelvic floor, as well as any associated organ prolapse. The third image was performed with Valsalva maneuver.

C. Rest imaging is performed to evaluate the baseline alignment of the pelvic floor and pelvic organs. The first image was performed at rest.

D. A defecation phase is vital to assess the functional changes that occur in the pelvic floor during defecation. The fourth image was performed during defecation.

Question 2

C. Correct! The pubococcygeal line demarcates the pelvic floor on sagittal MRI. This line is drawn from the inferior border of the symphysis pubis to the last coccygeal joint (i.e., between the last two coccygeal vertebrae).

Other choices and discussion

A. The "H line" is drawn from the inferior border of the symphysis pubis to the posterior border of the anorectal junction. This measures the anteroposterior width of the pelvic hiatus.

B. The "M line" is drawn from the anorectal junction to the pubococcygeal line. An M line longer than 2 cm at rest is indicative of rectal prolapse. Greater than 2 cm but less than 3 cm can be graded as mild, 3 to 6 cm can be graded as moderate, and greater than 6 cm can be graded as severe.

D. The puborectalis muscle is a pelvic floor structure and plays an important role in defecation, but is not the anatomic reference on MRI.

Question 3

C. Correct! The images demonstrate rectal prolapse at rest, which worsens with Valsalva. An M line < 2 cm is diagnostic of rectal prolapse.

Other choices and discussion

A. The middle compartment contains the uterus and vagina, which remain orthotopic on the provided images.

B. There is no paradoxical motion of the puborectalis muscle.

D. Enterocele refers to prolapse of small bowel through a defect between the rectum and vagina. This is different from a rectocele, which refers to the anterior wall of the rectum protruding into the posterior vagina.

■ Suggested Readings

Bitti GT, Argiolas GM, Ballicu N, et al. Pelvic floor failure: MR imaging evaluation of anatomic and functional abnormalities. Radiographics 2014;34:429–448

Colaiacomo MC, Masselli G, Polettini E, Lanciotti S, Casciani E, Bertini L, Gualdi G. Dynamic MR imaging of the pelvic floor: a pictorial review. Radiographics 2009;29(3):e35

Top Tips

◆ Pelvic floor prolapse is common, affecting up to 24% of women in their lifetime.

◆ On sagittal images, the pubococcygeal line is drawn from the inferior border of the pubic symphysis to the last coccygeal joint.

◆ The M line is drawn from the anorectal junction to the pubococcygeal line. Pelvic floor prolapse is diagnosed with an M line longer than 2 cm, and may be graded as mild (< 3 cm), moderate (3 to 6 cm), or severe (> 6 cm).

More Challenging 5

■ Case

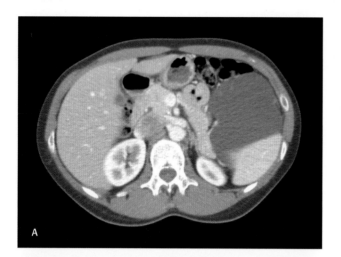

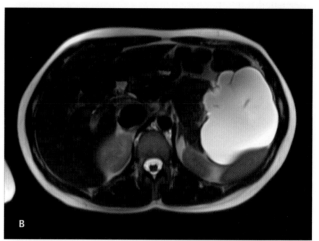

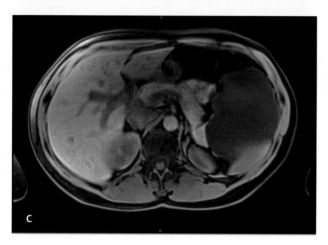

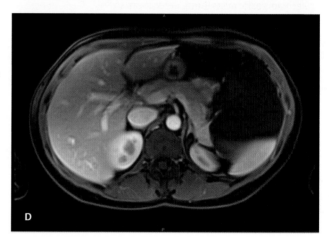

■ Questions

1. A middle-aged woman presents for workup of micro-scopic hematuria. No previous pertinent medical or surgical history. Based on the images shown, which ONE of the following is the most likely diagnosis?
   A. Mucinous cystadenoma
   B. Pancreatic lymphoepithelial cyst
   C. Lymphangioma
   D. Pancreatic pseudocyst

2. Which ONE of the following statements is true for serous cystadenomas?
   A. They should always be resected.
   B. Associated pancreatic ductal dilatation is common.
   C. Cysts within the lesion are typically > 2 cm in size.
   D. A fibrous central scar with or without calcification can be seen.

3. Which ONE of the following statements is true for lymphangiomas?
   A. They usually present as a large unilocular cystic mass.
   B. In the abdomen, they most commonly occur in the peritoneal space.
   C. They sometimes cross more than one retroperito-neal compartment.
   D. They rarely contain calcifications.

■ Answers and Explanations

Question 1

Answer: B. **Correct!** This is a pancreatic lymphoepithelial cyst. The computed tomography image demonstrates a smoothly marginated, fluid-attenuation mass in the left upper quadrant. The magnetic resonance images demonstrate homogeneous T2 hyperintensity and no evidence of internal enhancement. There is a "claw" sign with the pancreatic tail, suggestive of a pancreatic origin of the cyst. Although rare, a lymphoepithelial cyst is the most likely option provided. This lesion was symptomatic and surgically resected.

Other choices and discussion

A. Mucinous cystadenomas are macrocystic and might have the demonstrated appearance, although they typically have more septations, heterogeneous components, and/or nodular components than does the test case.

C. Lymphangioma might have a similar appearance, but should not arise from the pancreas itself.

D. Pancreatic pseudocyst is in the differential for pancreatic or peripancreatic cysts, but a history of pancreatitis would be expected.

Question 2

D. Correct! A fibrous central scar with or without calcification can be seen. Serous cystadenomas are sometimes referred to as microcystic adenomas due to the presence of multiple small cysts. There is often an enhancing central scar, which may be calcified.

Other choices and discussion

A. Serous cystadenoma is a benign lesion and is typically not resected.

B. Pancreatic ductal dilatation is uncommon with serous cystadenoma.

C. The individual cysts of a serous cystadenoma are typically smaller than 2 cm in size.

Question 3

C. Correct! They sometimes cross more than one retroperitoneal compartment. A lymphangioma is a lymphatic malformation, which may be quite large and can characteristically cross multiple anatomic borders.

Other choices and discussion

A. Lymphangiomas are typically lobulated and multilocular.

B. In the abdomen, lymphangiomas are typically retroperitoneal.

D. Lymphangiomas often contain calcifications.

■ Suggested Readings

Adsay NV, Hasteh F, Cheng JD, et al. Lymphoepithelial cysts of the pancreas: a report of 12 cases and a review of the literature. Mod Pathol 2002;15:492–501

Nam SJ, Hwang HK, Kim H, Yu J-S, Yoon D-S, Chung J-J, Kim JH, Kim KW. Lymphoepithelial cysts in the pancreas: MRI of two cases with emphasis of diffusion-weighted imaging characteristics. J Magn Reson Imaging 2010;32:692–696

Sahani DV, Kambadakone A, Macari M, Takahashi N, Chari S, Fernandez-del Castillo C. Diagnosis and management of cystic pancreatic lesions. Am J Roentgenol 2013;200(2):343–354

Yang DM, Jung DH, Kim H, Kang JH, Kim SH, Kim JH, Hwang HY. Retroperitoneal cystic masses: CT, clinical, and pathologic findings and literature review. Radiographics 2004;24(5):1353–1365

Top Tips

◆ Large unilocular cysts of the pancreas have a differential diagnosis including pseudocyst, mucinous cystadenoma, unilocular serous cystadenoma, and lymphoepithelial cyst.

◆ Mucinous cystadenomas usually have cysts larger than 2 cm, whereas serous cystadenomas usually have cysts smaller than 2 cm.

◆ A lymphangioma typically presents as a cystic retroperitoneal mass, which sometimes crosses anatomic borders.

Essentials 1

■ Case

A 34-year-old woman presents with left flank pain.

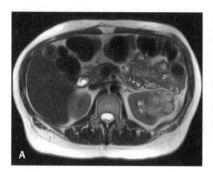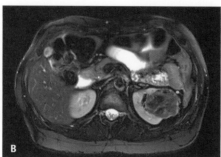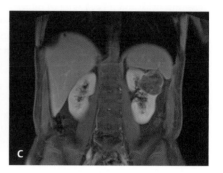

■ Questions

1. Which ONE of the following is the correct diagnosis?
   A. Myelolipoma
   B. Angiomyolipoma
   C. Liposarcoma
   D. Renal cell carcinoma

2. The left renal mass measures 5.3 cm maximally. What is the MOST appropriate treatment?
   A. Conservative management with 6-month follow up imaging
   B. None, as this lesion is benign
   C. Embolization/ablation
   D. Surgical excision

3. With which syndrome are AMLs associated?
   A. Tuberous sclerosis (TS)
   B. Von Hippel-Lindau
   C. Neurofibromatosis 2
   D. Birt-Hogg-Dube

■ Answers and Explanations

Question 1

B. Correct! This is an angiomyolipoma (AML). Images demonstrate a lesion containing macroscopic fat arising from the lateral aspect of the left kidney. *Macroscopic* fat typically demonstrates loss of signal on fat-suppressed images. *Microscopic* fat does not demonstrate loss of signal on fat-suppressed images; rather, it exhibits a loss of signal between in- and out-of-phase chemical shift imaging. The components of an AML include blood vessels (angio), smooth muscle (myo), and fat (lipoma).

Other choices and discussion

A. A myelolipoma is typically a macroscopic fat-containing lesion of the adrenal gland. In this case, the lesion clearly arises from the kidney. Note the "claw" sign. The "claw" represents normal renal parenchyma around the lesion, suggesting the organ of origin.

C. In this anatomic region, liposarcomas generally arise from the retroperitoneum and exert mass effect on the kidney. They rarely arise de novo from the kidney. Liposarcomas are usually hypovascular. The key to making the diagnosis of liposarcoma is determining that the site of origin is the retroperitoneum rather than the kidney.

D. Although 5% of RCCs contain fat, that fat is usually microscopic. Sonographically, however, AML and RCC may be indistinguishable. In some challenging cases, a lipid-poor AML may be indistinguishable from RCC with any type of imaging, and surgery may be indicated to exclude RCC.

Question 2

C. Correct! Embolization/ablation is recommended. The greatest risk for an AML is hemorrhage. The risk increases when the lesion reaches 4 cm in size or when the patient is pregnant.

Other choices and discussion

A. Conservative management with imaging is acceptable if the lesion is small (< 4 cm) and the patent is asymptomatic.

B. This lesion is benign but its size warrants treatment.

D. This lesion is usually successfully treated with embolization and ablation, which have lower risks than surgery.

Question 3

A. Correct! Renal AMLs are associated with TS. TS, also known as Bourneville disease, is a neurocutaneous disorder. A total of 20% of all AMLs are associated with TS, and up to 75% of individuals with TS have AMLs. When associated with TS, AMLs tend to be bilateral and multiple. Classically, TS is associated with the triad of mental retardation, seizures, and adenoma sebaceum. However, that classic triad is often absent. Other manifestations of TS include facial angiofibromas, cortical/subcortical tubers, subependymal giant cell astrocytomas, lymphangiomyomatosis of the lungs, and cardiac rhabdomyomas. This disorder is inherited in an autosomal dominant fashion but can be sporadic.

Other choices and discussion

B. Von Hippel-Lindau is associated with multiple renal/liver/pancreatic cysts as well as clear cell–type RCC. There is an increased risk of pheochromocytoma, papillary cystadenoma of the epididymis, and pancreatic neoplasms (serious cystadenoma and islet cell tumors). There is an association with central nervous system hemangioblastomas and retinal angiomas. This disorder can be inherited (autosomal dominant) or sporadic.

C. Neurofibromatosis 2 is an autosomal dominant condition classically associated with multiple schwannomas, meningiomas, and ependymomas.

D. Birt-Hogg-Dube syndrome is an autosomal dominant multisystem disease involving the kidneys, skin, and lung. It is characterized by multiple bilateral renal tumors (chromophobe/clear cell RCC and oncocytoma), multiple lung cysts (with an increased risk of spontaneous pneumothorax), and cutaneous lesions (papules and angiofibromas).

■ Suggested Readings

Bharwani N, Christmas TJ, Jameson C, et al. Epithelioid angiomyolipoma: imaging appearances. Br J Radiol 2009;82: e249–252

Hidalgo J, Chéchile G. Familial syndromes coupling with small renal masses. Adv Urol 2008.

Israel GM, Hindman N, Hecht E, et al. The use of opposed-phase chemical shift MRI in the diagnosis of renal angiomyolipomas. Am J Roentgenol 2005;184:1868–1872

Jinzaki M, Tanimoto A, Narimatsu Y, et al. Angiomyolipoma: imaging findings in lesions with minimal fat. Radiology 1997;205:497–502

Maclean DF, Sultana R, Radwan R, et al. Is the follow-up of small renal angiomyolipomas a necessary precaution? Clin Radiol 2014;69:822–826

Sherman JL, Hartman DS, Friedman AC, et al. Angiomyolipoma: computed tomographic-pathologic correlation of 17 cases. Am J Roentgenol 1981;137:1221–1226

Top Tips

◆ A macroscopic fat-containing lesion of the kidney is essentially diagnostic of an AML.

◆ AML > 4 cm should be treated (by embolization/ablation, or less often, partial nephrectomy) because of the risk of hemorrhage.

◆ Make sure to confirm that the macroscopic fat-containing lesion arises from either the kidney or the adrenal. If not, retroperitoneal liposarcoma must be considered.

Essentials 2

■ Case

A 19-year-old woman presents with chronic dull pelvic pain. The low density portion of the adnexal mass has a hounsfield unit of −53.

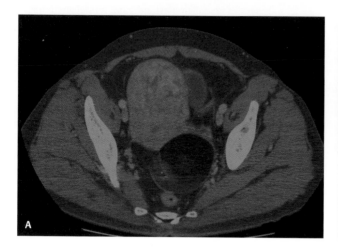

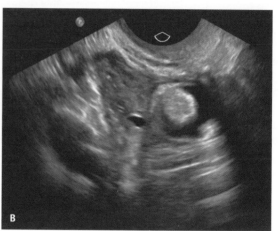

■ Questions

1. Which ONE of the following is the MOST likely diagnosis?
   A. Hemorrhagic cyst
   B. Endometrioma
   C. Mature ovarian teratoma
   D. Ovarian serous cytadenoma

2. What is the MOST likely complication associated with this test case?
   A. Malignant transformation
   B. Hemorrhage
   C. Ovarian torsion
   D. Rupture

3. What entity is the rounded hyperechoic structure within the mass on the ultrasound image?
   A. Rokitansky nodule
   B. Calcification
   C. Retracted clot
   D. Fat

■ Answers and Explanations

Question 1

C. Correct! This is a teratoma. A mature teratoma is a slowly growing ovarian tumor having at least two of the three germ cell layers. In this case, the computed tomography (CT) demonstrates fat density (matching the density of the surrounding pelvic fat) and soft tissue density. Although CT and magnetic resonance imaging are excellent at diagnosing a teratoma, ultrasound is the modality of choice because of its convenience, lack of ionizing radiation, and high accuracy. Ultrasound typically demonstrates a cystic adnexal mass with mural components, often including an echogenic mass with posterior shadowing.

Other choices and discussion

A. A hemorrhagic cyst would not demonstrate fat on CT. On ultrasound, a hemorrhagic cyst appears as a complex cyst with internal blood products. Acute blood is hyperechoic and becomes increasingly hypoechoic over time.

B. An endometrioma would not demonstrate fat on CT. Its appearance on ultrasound can mimic that of a hemorrhagic cyst.

D. Ovarian serous cystadenomas do not contain fat. They tend to be cystic, large, and often bilateral. In addition, they are more common in older women.

Question 2

C. Correct! Torsion is the most common complication of a teratoma, occuring in 5 to 15% of cases. For this reason, these masses are often resected when they are large. The risk of torsion increases once the ovary reaches 5 cm in size.

Other choices and discussion

A. The rate of malignant transformation is < 2%. It can occur in any of the three germ cell layers (ectoderm, mesoderm, and endoderm). Squamous cell carcinoma arising from the lining of the cyst is the most common type. Factors associated with malignant transformation of a dermoid include patient age > 45 years, tumors > 10 cm, elevated serum tumor markers, and a predominantly enhancing soft tissue component.

B. Hemorrhage is a rare complication.

D. Rupture is a rare complication (1 to 4% of patients). Infection is also a rare complication.

Question 3

A. Correct! This is a Rokitansky nodule, which is also referred to as a dermoid plug. It is typically composed of hair, dermal elements, teeth, and/or sebacious material. A Rokitansky nodule has an echogenic and nodular appearance on ultrasound.

Other choices and discussion

B. Calcification can contribute to (but is not the only component of) the Rokitansky nodule.

C. If the lesion were simply a cyst with blood products, a retracted clot would be the correct choice. However, the additional elements shown on CT confirm a teratoma.

D. Fat can contribute to (but is not the only component of) the Rokitansky nodule.

■ Suggested Readings

Friedman AC, Pyatt RS, Hartman DS, et al. CT of benign cystic teratomas. Am J Roentgenol 1982;138:659–665

Outwater EK, Siegelman ES, Hunt JL. Ovarian teratomas: tumor types and imaging characteristics. Radiographics 2001;21:475–490

Patel MD, Feldstein VA, Lipson SD, et al. Cystic teratomas of the ovary: diagnostic value of sonography. Am J Roentgenol 1998;171:1061–1065

SECTION V
GENITOURINARY IMAGING

Top Tips

- Mature teratomas are common, slowly growing ovarian neoplasms that contain at least two of the three germ cell layers.

- Ultrasound is the modality of choice for teratoma and can usually make the definitive diagnosis. Typically, there is an echogenic component, shadowing, and a fluid-fluid level.

- Several useful ultrasound signs for teratoma: The "tip of the iceberg" sign refers to the echogenic structures within the lesion obscuring deeper portions because of poor sound penetration. The "dot-dash" sign refers to multiple thin echogenic bands due to hair within the cystic lesion.

Essentials 3

■ Case

A 51-year-old woman status post motor vehicle accident.

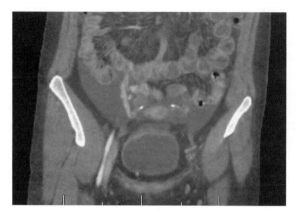

Portal venous phase

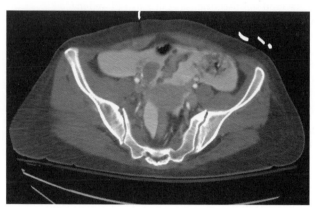

Twenty-five minutes post contrast injection delay

■ Questions

1. What is the correct diagnosis?
   A. Bowel perforation
   B. Intraperitoneal bladder rupture
   C. Extraperitoneal bladder rupture
   D. Rupture of a hemorrhagic cyst

2. What is the MOST appropriate management?
   A. Close observation with serial imaging
   B. Surgery with bladder repair
   C. Radical cystectomy
   D. Foley catheter placement

3. What is the MOST appropriate way to instill contrast solution for a voiding cysturethrogram on a trauma patient?
   A. Manually inject 100 mL by hand into the Foley catheter.
   B. Power inject 300 mL into the Foley catheter.
   C. By gravity, use a bag raised above the patient with a volume of 300 mL (or until the patient can tolerate).
   D. Inject contrast intravenously and wait for its excretion into the urinary bladder.

■ Answers and Explanations

Question 1

B. Correct! This is an intraperitoneal bladder rupture. The initial images demonstrate thickening of the superior bladder wall with adjacent fluid, and the delayed images demonstrate contrast surrounding loops of bowel with tracking into the paracolic gutters. Intraperitoneal bladder rupture represents 10 to 20% of all bladder injuries. It occurs with individuals that sustain a direct blow to a distended urinary bladder. On imaging, extravasated contrast insinuates between bowel loops. This is known as a type 2 injury by cystography.

Other choices and discussion

A. There is no evidence of bowel injury. The density of the contrast within the abdomen on the delayed images matches that in the ureter, confirming its origin from the urinary system/bladder. Additionally, there is no oral contrast on these images. The standard computed tomography protocol for blunt abdominal trauma is computed tomography of the abdomen and pelvis with intravenous contrast but no oral contrast.

C. Extraperitoneal bladder rupture is the most common type of bladder injury (80 to 90%). It is most often associated with pelvic fractures or penetrating trauma. Extravasated contrast tends to accumulate within the prevesicle space (also known as the retropubic space or space of Retzius). This is known as a type 4 injury by cystography.

D. A ruptured hemorrhagic cyst would not produce such extensive and dense fluid throughout the abdomen. Furthurmore, this would not account for the irregular morphology of the bladder on the coronal image.

Question 2

B. Correct! Intraperitoneal bladder rupture requires surgery. Given the risk of chemical peritonitis, there is significant potential morbidity if the defect is not surgically corrected.

Other choices and discussion

A. Conservative management is only appropriate for *extraperitoneal* bladder rupture.

C. Radical cystectomy is a drastic measure and represents major surgery. In most cases, the urinary bladder is salvagable following trauma.

D. An indwelling Foley catheter is the treatment for extraperitoneal bladder rupture.

Question 3

C. Correct! The gravity method allows the least traumatic direct entry for contrast. Contrast administration should stop when the patient feels full or can no longer tolerate the instillation.

Other choices and discussion

A. Manually injecting contrast is too intrusive and may cause additional injury/discomfort.

B. Power injecting contrast is too intrusive and may cause additional injury/discomfort.

D. The indirect method of intravenous contrast administration would not ensure optimal urinary bladder filling, and a significant finding might potentially be missed.

■ Suggested Readings

Ramchandani P, Buckler PM. Imaging of genitourinary trauma. Am J Roentgenol 2009;192:1514–1523

Vaccaro JP, Brody JM. CT cystography in the evaluation of major bladder trauma. Radiographics 2000;20:1373–1381

Top Tips

◆ Computed tomography cystography or voiding cysturethrogram are the studies of choice to diagnose a bladder rupture. Plain film may demonstrate a "pear-shaped bladder."

◆ Intraperitoneal bladder rupture: caused by blunt force or penetrating trauma to a full bladder; requires surgical repair.

◆ Extraperitoneal bladder rupture: caused by adjacent pelvic fracture; can be treated conservatively.

◆ Driving with a full bladder places one at an increased risk for a bladder injury. Void first!

Essentials 4

■ Case

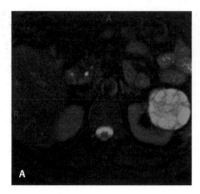 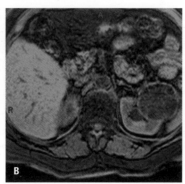 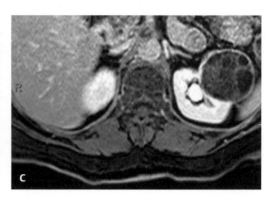

■ Questions

1. Imaging features of this lesion are classic for which entity?
    A. Multilocular cystic nephroma
    B. Hemorrhagic cyst
    C. Renal cell carcinoma
    D. Oncocytoma

2. What Bosniak category does this lesion fall into?
    A. Bosniak 1
    B. Bosniak 2
    C. Bosniak 3
    D. Bosniak 4

3. What is the standard management for this test case?
    A. Observation
    B. Resection
    C. Embolization
    D. Further imaging

■ Answers and Explanations

Question 1

A. Correct! This is the classic appearance for a multilocular cystic nephroma. Multilocular cystic nephroma (MLCN) is typically encapsulated, T2 hyperintense, herniates into the renal pelvis, and has variable septal enhancement. This lesion has a bimodal age distribution which includes young men and middle-aged women.

Other choices and discussion

B. Hemorrhagic cysts are typically homogenously T1 hyperintense and nonenhancing.

C. This could represent a cystic RCC. Although it does have the the classic appearance of a MLCN, RCC is much more common than MLCN. These two lesions are often difficult to differentiate by imaging, and both lesions are often resected.

D. Oncocytomas are large, well-demarcated lesions that are less cystic than the test case. They classically have a nonenhancing central stellate scar (which is T2 hypointense), a finding seen in 30% of cases. Relatively homogeneous enhancement is common. Oncocytomas can be multiple and bilateral. There is also an association of oncocytomas with tuberous sclerosis and Birt-Hogg-Dube.

Question 2

C. Correct! This is Bosniak 3. Bosniak 3 lesions are indeterminate for malignancy and usually require resection or ablation. Key findings of Bosniak 3 lesions include thick/nodular septa and a wall with measurable enhancement (both are seen here). Malignant potential is 55%.

Other choices and discussion

A. Boniak 1 lesions are simple cysts with imperceptible walls. There is no malignant potential, and follow up is not necessary.

B. Bosniak 2 lesions are minimally complex cysts. These include hemorrhagic cysts < 3 cm, cysts with few thin septations (< 1 mm), and cysts with thin calcifications. There is no malignant potential, and follow up is not necessary.

Bosniak 2F lesions are slightly more complex cysts. These include hemorrhagic cysts > 3 cm in size, an increased number of (or minimal thickening of) septa, and nodular or thickened calcifications, but still no measurable contrast enhancement. The malignant potential is 5%. These require follow up at 6 months.

D. Bosniak 4 lesions are clearly malignant. These includes cysts with a solid-enhancing nodule or mass.

Question 3

B. Correct! Resection is the treatment of choice.

Other choices and discussion

A. While this entity is benign, it is not readily distinguished from RCC by imaging, and observation could be a mistake.

C. Embolization is not the standard of care. If performed, embolization is generally reserved for small tumors. One drawback of embolization is that it would probably require multiple treatments, thus prolonging the time period for therapy. In addition, because malignancy is not definitively excluded by imaging, resection is indicated.

D. Further imaging would not result in a more definitive diagnosis.

■ Suggested Readings

Israel GM, Bosniak MA. How I do it: evaluating renal masses. Radiology 2005;236:441–450

Madewell JE, Goldman SM, Davis CJ, et al. Multilocular cystic nephroma: a radiographic-pathologic correlation of 58 patients. Radiology 1983;146:309–321

Palmer WE, Chew FS. Renal oncocytoma. Am J Roentgenol 1991;156:1144

Silver IM, Boag AH, Soboleski DA. Best cases from the AFIP: Multilocular cystic renal tumor: cystic nephroma. Radiographics 2008;28:1221–1225

Top Tips

- Multilocular cystic nephroma is a benign lesion that is often difficult to distinguish from RCC in adults and from Wilms tumor in children.

- Bimodal distribution of MLCN: young men (< 5 years old) and women in the fifth and sixth decades of life.

- MLCN imaging: multiloculated cystic lesion, well encapsulated, septations with variable enhancement, often herniating into the renal pelvis.

Essentials 5

■ Case

A 72-year-old woman presents with dysparunia and a history of dribbling.

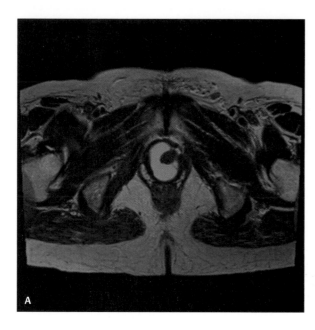

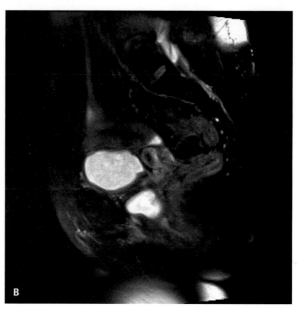

■ Questions

1. What is the correct diagnosis?
   A. Bartholin gland cyst
   B. Skene gland cyst
   C. Urethral diverticulum
   D. Gartner duct cyst

2. What is the MOST important magnetic resonance imaging (MRI) sequence for making this diagnosis?
   A. T2-weighted sequence
   B. T1-weighted sequence
   C. Contrast-enhanced T1-weighted sequence
   D. Diffusion-weighted imaging

3. What type of cancer MOST commonly arises within a urethral diverticulum?
   A. Transitional cell carcinoma
   B. Adenocarcinoma
   C. Squamous cell carcinoma
   D. Small cell carcinoma

■ Answers and Explanations

Question 1

C. Correct! The patient has a urethral diverticulum. These occur posterolateral to the urethra and above the level of the pubic symphysis. They can grow and surround the ureter posteriorly ("Saddlebag" morphology), as in this case. Symptoms include dysuria, dribbling, and dysparunia (the 3 Ds) as well as urinary frequency and urgency. A connection to the urethral lumen is demonstrated in most cases.

Other choices and discussion

A. Bartholin gland cysts typically occur posterior to the lower vagina and below the level of the pubic symphysis. They are associated with the labia majora and result from chronic inflammation leading to ductal obstruction. These cysts are usually asymptomatic but may require drainage due to superimposed infection.

B. Skene gland cysts are rentention cysts that form secondary to inflammation/obstruction of the paraurethral ducts. These are typically located lateral to the external urethral meatus and below the level of the pubic symphysis. Skene gland cysts are usually asymptomatic but may require drainage or excision due to superimposed infection.

D. Gartner duct cysts typically occur anterior to the superior vagina and above the level of the inferiormost aspect of the pubic symphysis. They result from the incomplete regression of the wolffian ducts. When Gartner duct cysts are located at the level of the urethra, they can cause mass effect on the urethra, giving rise to urinary tract symptoms.

Question 2

A. Correct! T2 is the MRI sequence of choice and should be obtained in all three planes. T2 is the most sensitive for the detection of small cystic lesions. MRI is the current test of choice for the diagnosis of urethral diverticulum. Historically, either contrast-enhanced radiography (voiding cystourethrography or double-balloon urethrography) or fiberoptic urethroscopy were used to make the diagnosis. However, these methods are invasive, difficult to perform, and uncomfortable for the patient. Additionally, if the urethral diverticulum contains hemorrhage, pus, or stones, the diverticulum may be missed.

Other choices and discussion

B. T1-weighted sequence is less sensitive than T2 for the detection of small cystic lesions. However, T1 is useful in detecting the sometimes-found internal hemorrhage.

C. Postcontrast images are less sensitive than T2 for making this diagnosis. However, contrast is useful in detecting underlying inflammation, infection, or malignancy.

D. Diffusion-weighted imaging is not the sequence of choice. However, diffusion-weighted imaging is to supplement the detection of underlying infection/malignancy.

Question 3

B. Correct! Adenocarcinoma is the most common cancer type to arise within a urethral diverticulum. Note that the overall incidence of malignancy within a diverticulum is low. Adenocarcinoma also occurs within urachal remnants and diverticula.

Other choices and discussion

A. Transitional cell carcinoma is the most common cell type in the genitourinary tract and is found most commonly within the bladder, urethra, and ureters.

C. Sqamous cell carcinoma is not common within the genitourinary tract. About 5% of bladder cancers are of squamous cell origin.

D. Small cell carcinoma is not common within the genitourinary tract.

■ Suggested Readings

Chou CP, Levenson RB, Elsayes KM, et al. Imaging of female urethral diverticulum: an update. Radiographics 2008;28: 1917–1930

Hahn WY, Israel GM, Lee VS. MRI of female urethral and periurethral disorders. Am J Roentgenol 2004;182:677–682

Patel AK, Chapple CR. Female urethral diverticula. Curr Opin Urol 2006;16:248–254

Siegelman ES, Outwater EK, Banner MP, et al. High-resolution MR imaging of the vagina. Radiographics 1997;17:1183–1203

Top Tips

◆ A urethral diverticulum should be distinguished from other cystic lesions of the lower female pelvis by its location, which is superior to the bottom of the pubic symphysis and posterior to the urethra.

◆ T2 is the most sensitive MRI sequence for detection of a urethral diverticulum (or other cystic lesions of the female pelvis).

◆ Adenocarcinoma is the most common malignancy in both urethral diverticula and urachal remnants. Transitional cell carcinoma is the most common malignancy in the remainder of the urinary tract.

Essentials 6

■ Case

A retrograde pyelogram was performed for hematuria.

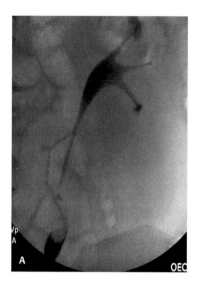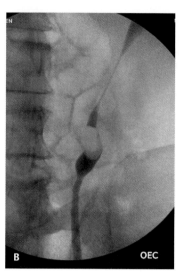

■ Questions

1. What is the MOST likely cause for this patient's hematuria?
   A. Renal calculus
   B. Blood clot
   C. Transitional cell carcinoma
   D. Renal cell carcinoma

2. Which ONE of the following is a risk factor for the development of the diagnosis in the test case?
   A. Smoking
   B. Alcohol
   C. Infection
   D. Intravenous iodinated contrast

3. Metachronous tumors of the urinary tract are most common with:
   A. Bladder transitional cell carcinoma
   B. Upper urinary tract transitional cell carcinoma
   C. Urethral transitional cell carcinoma
   D. Renal cell carcinoma

Answers and Explanations

Question 1

C. Correct! This is a case of transitional cell carcinoma (TCC). This is the classic appearance of a ureteral tumor by plain film urography, with the formation of a meniscus or a "goblet" sign. The lack of upstream ureteral dilatation suggests that this process developed slowly. TCC is most commonly found in an older population (average age of 65) with a 4:1 predilection for males. A total of 96% of cases are found in the urinary bladder, 3% in the renal pelvis, and 1% in the ureter. These tumors are usually characterized as either papillary or nonpapillary.

Other choices and discussion

A. Renal calculus is unlikely given lack of upstream dilation, which would be expected with a stone of this size. In addition, this stone would have to be radiolucent, and a stone would not produce the meniscus effect seen here.

B. A blood clot of this size would be expected to cause upstream dilatation of the collecting system.

D. RCC is extremely rare in the ureter.

Question 2

A. Correct! Risk factors and industrial exposures linked to TCC cancer development include smoking, certain amine and phenyl dyes, cyclophosphamide, phenacetin, and aristolochic acid (Balkan nephropathy).

The other choices are all incorrect.

Question 3

B. Correct! Metachronous tumors of the urinary tract are more common with upper urinary tract TCC. Metachronous tumors are those that occur at different times. Approximately 40% of patients with upper urinary tract TCC will develop additional sites of tumor distally (usually in the bladder). The surgical treatment of choice for an upper tract TCC (involving the kidney or ureter) is a nephroureterectomy (where the ipsilateral kidney and ureter are removed).

Other choices and discussion

A. Only 2 to 4% of patients with bladder TCC develop tumor elsewhere within the urinary tract. Surgical treatment for bladder TCC typically consists of radical cystectomy with ileal conduit formation. (The bladder is first removed. Then a portion of the ileum is removed and connected to the ureters to serve as the urinary bladder.) The conduit drains through an ostomy.

C. Urethral TCC is extremely rare. Most carcinomas of the urethra are squamous cell.

D. There is an increased risk of metachronous RCC in patients von Hippel-Lindau disease, patients diagnosed with RCC before the age of 40, and patients with familial RCC.

Suggested Readings

Browne RF, Meehan CP, Colville J, et al. Transitional cell carcinoma of the upper urinary tract: spectrum of imaging findings. RadioGraphics 2005;25:1609–1627

Kawashima A, Goldman SM. Neoplasms of the renal collecting system, pelvis and ureters. In: Pollack HM, McClennan BL, Dyer RB, Kenney PJ, eds. Clinical Urography. New York, NY: Saunders; 2000:1560–1641

Vikram R, Sandler CM, Ng CS. Imaging and staging of transitional cell carcinoma. Lower urinary tract. Am J Roentgenol 2009;192:1481–1487

Top Tips

- TCC is the most common tumor of the urinary tract and occurs most frequently in the bladder.

- Upper TCC is more prone to metachronous lesions than bladder TCC. The surgical treatment differs depending on the site of disease.

- In the ureter, look for the "goblet" sign when differentiating from a calculus. TCC may variably result in obstruction.

Essentials 7

■ Case

Follow-up imaging for a condition diagnosed in early childhood.

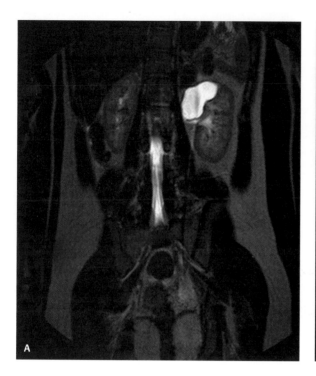 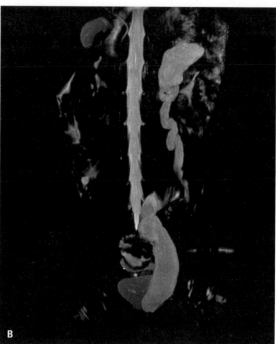

■ Questions

1. Which ONE of the following is the MOST likely cause for these imaging findings?
   A. Ureterovesical stone
   B. Duplex kidney
   C. Congenital megaureter
   D. Renal sinus cyst

2. In a duplicated collecting system, which system typically refluxes and which system obstructs?
   A. Upper pole both obstructs and refluxes
   B. Lower pole obstructs and upper pole refluxes
   C. Upper pole obstructs and lower pole refluxes
   D. Lower pole both obstructs and refluxes

3. What is the MOST accurate way to diagnose this condition?
   A. Ultrasound
   B. Multiphase CT
   C. Portal venous phase CT
   D. Intravenous pyelogram

■ Answers and Explanations

Question 1

B. Correct! This is a duplex kidney. The first image demonstrates a cystic structure in the left upper pole, which is contiguous with the dilated ureter seen on the magnetic resonance urogram (second image). There is also focal atrophy at the upper pole of the left kidney. This atrophy is the result of chronic obstruction. The remaining lower portion of the kidney is normal and has a nondilated collecting system. These are all typical findings of a duplicated collecting system with two ureters. The visible ureter is dilated and extends from the upper pole moiety. The ureter of the lower pole moiety is not visible. A duplicated system is one of the most common congenital renal anomalies. The extent of duplication is on a spectrum. It may be a simple as duplication of only the renal pelvis, draining with a single ureter, or two distinct collecting systems that drain into the bladder. When the latter occurs, the anatomy usually follows the Weigert-Meyer rule (see below). Duplication is seen in 0.7% of the population, and mild forms are often overlooked with imaging. Most cases are asymptomatic, but complications of infection, obstruction, and reflux sometimes occur.

Other choices and discussion

A. If a left ureterovesical junction stone were to cause this degree of ureteral dilatation, atrophy of the *entire* kidney would be expected. Additionally, given lack of perinephric edema, this process appears to be chronic.

C. A congenital megaureter could be the answer, if a normal collecting system wasn't visualized in the lower portion of the left kidney. A true primary congenital megaureter is related to a distal adynamic segment with proximal dilatation. This is analogous to primary achalasia in the esophagus. This entity is often diagnosed in children. This can rarely be associated with congenital megacalyces. Vesicoureteric reflux can also result in ureteral dilatation.

D. The cystic structure in the first image is a part of the dilated collecting system. A renal sinus cyst does not connect to the renal pelvis and collecting system.

Question 2

C. Correct! The upper pole obstructs and lower pole refluxes. According to the Weigert-Meyer law, the lower pole ureter inserts orthotopically (in its normal location), and the upper pole ureter inserts ectopically, inferiorly, and medially relative to the lower pole ureter. The ectopic insertion is often associated with a ureterocele, which can cause obstruction of the upper pole moiety. There is often distortion of the ectopic ureter insertion, resulting in reflux. On pyelogram, sometimes only the lower pole opacifies (due to upper pole obstruction). Mass affect from the dilated upper pole forms the classic "drooping lily" sign.

The other choices are incorrect.

Question 3

B. Correct! Use of contrast to confirm or exclude communication of the "cyst" with the collecting system is the best way to differentiate a renal sinus cyst from hydronephrosis. (A cystic structure filling with contrast that subsequently passes into the collecting system does not represent a renal sinus cyst.) In terms of which contrast study to select, the important point is to be able to compare precontrast to postcontrast, possibly including delayed imaging. Of the answer choices, multiphase CT is the best option.

A multiphase magnetic resonance imaging study is equally as effective as a contrast-enhanced CT for this purpose.

Note that a cystic structure in this region that opacifies could represent either hydronephrosis or a calyceal diverticulum, which also communicates with the collecting system. The morphology should be able to differentiate these choices.

Other choices and discussion

A. Renal ultrasound can often (but not always) differentiate parapelvic cysts from hydronephrosis.

C. A single phase of a contrast study can have limitations in making this diagnosis.

D. An intravenous pyelogram can demonstrate hydronephrosis and can often demonstrate deformities of the collecting system by adjacent renal sinus cysts, but the anatomic assessment is limited and intravenous pyelogram cannot demonstrate the cysts themselves.

■ Suggested Readings

Callahan MJ. The drooping lily sign. Radiology 2001;219: 226–228

Fernbach SK, Feinstein KA, Spencer K, et al. Ureteral duplication and its complications. Radiographics 1997;17:109–127

Lebowitz RL, Avni FE. Misleading appearances in pediatric uroradiology. Pediatr Radiol 1980;10:15–31

Top Tips

◆ Duplex kidney is a common congenital renal tract anomaly. The site and extent of duplication may vary.

◆ With complete duplication of the collecting system, the two ureters insert separately (according to the Weigert-Meyer rule). The upper pole moiety ureter inserts ectopically, inferomedially to the orthotopic lower pole moiety ureter.

◆ With a complete duplex system, the upper pole moiety obstructs, while the lower pole moiety refluxes.

Essentials 8

■ Case

The left kidney was not visualized on ultrasound.

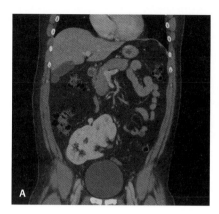
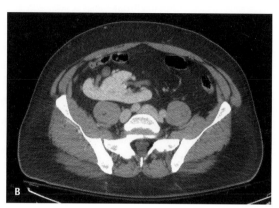

■ Questions

1. Which ONE of the following is the correct diagnosis?
   A. Crossed fused renal ectopia
   B. Duplicated right renal collecting system
   C. Horseshoe kidney
   D. Low-lying right kidney

2. In this test case, where is the left ureter likely inserting into the urinary bladder?
   A. Inferiorly from the right ureteral insertion
   B. Together with the right ureter at its insertion
   C. Orthotopically
   D. Superior to the right ureteral insertion

3. Unilateral renal agenesis is commonly associated with which of the following? Choose ALL that are correct.
   A. Caroli disease
   B. Chromosomal anomalies
   C. Müllerian duct anomalies
   D. Budd-Chiari syndrome

■ Answers and Explanations

Question 1

A. Correct! The kidneys are not in their expected location on these images, and a fused kidney is seen in the right lower quadrant. This is the characteristic appearance of crossed-fused renal ectopia. Computed tomography depicts the parenchymal band connecting the kidneys. Potential complications of this anomaly include nephrolithiasis, infection, and hydronephrosis. Crossed fused renal ectopia results from abnormal renal ascent in embryogenesis. Normally by the eighth week of life, the kidneys reach their appropriate position at the L2 level.

Other choices and discussion

B. A duplicated collecting system would not explain both the absence of a contralateral kidney and the pelvic kidney location.

C. A horseshoe kidney refers to fusion of both kidneys (either with a parenchymal or a fibrous band) with the respective kidneys remaining on their own side. With a horseshoe kidney, the inferior pole of each kidney is medially positioned while the superior pole is laterally positioned. This is the reverse of normotopic kidneys.

D. While the right kidney is low lying, a pelvic kidney is an incomplete diagnosis. Additionally, this would not account for the fusion of the kidneys.

Question 2

C. Correct! The abnormally fused kidney's ureter inserts into its normal location (orthotopically); in this case, on the left side of the bladder.

Other choices and discussion

A. An inferior insertion of the ureter may be seen with a duplicated renal collecting system.

B. A fused insertion with the right ureter might occur along the spectrum of a duplicated collecting system.

D is incorrect.

Question 3

B. Correct! Renal agenesis can be association with a number of chromosomal anomalies, including Down syndrome and Turner syndrome.

C. Correct! Unilateral renal agenesis is commonly associated with müllerian duct anomalies.

Renal agenesis results from absence of induction of the metanephros by the ureteral bud at 6 to 7 weeks gestation. The metanephros becomes the adult kidney, and absence of its formation results in the complete absence of the structure. The metanephros is also important for normal internal genital formation, explaining the association of renal anomalies with wolffian and müllerian duct anomalies. In the absence of a kidney, always check the pelvic structures, as uterine anomalies in females and ipsilateral seminal vesicle agenesis in males are commonly associated. Adrenal agenesis is extremely rare and can be associated with renal agenesis.

Other choices and discussion

A. Caroli disease is a congenital disorder with multifocal cystic dilatation of the segmental intrahepatic bile ducts. It is associated with autosomal recessive and autosomal dominant polycystic kidney disease as well as medullary sponge kidney.

D. Budd-Chiari is hepatic venous obstruction and is not associated with renal agenesis.

■ Suggested Readings

Bauer BS. Anomalies of form and fusion, crossed renal ectopia with and without fusion. In: Alan J, ed. Wein: Campbell-Walsh Urology Book. 9th ed. Philadelphia: WB Saunders; 2007:3269–3304

Dyer RB, Chen MY, Zagoria RJ. Classic signs in uroradiology. Radiographics 2004;24(suppl 1):S247–280

Gay SB, Armistead JP, Weber ME, et al. Left infrarenal region: anatomic variants, pathologic conditions, and diagnostic pitfalls. Radiographics 1991;11:549–570

Kaufman MH, Findlater GS. An unusual case of complete renal fusion giving rise to a "cake" or "lump" kidney. J Anat 2001;198:501–504

Top Tips

- After horseshoe kidney, cross-fused renal ectopia is the next most common congenital renal anomaly.

- Differentiating between renal agenesis, a pelvic kidney, and an atrophic kidney has significant clinical relevance. A nuclear medicine renal scan can sometimes detect occult renal function.

- Because of their embryologic origins, renal anomalies sometimes occur in association with pelvic genitalia anomalies. When you see one, make sure to check the other as well.

Essentials 9

■ Case

A 34-year-old woman presents with infertility.

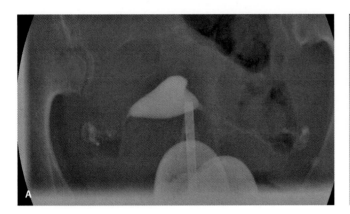
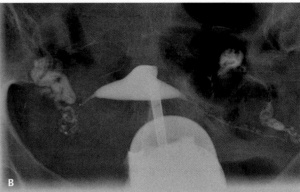

■ Questions

1. What diagnosis is visible on the hysterosalpingogram (HSG) to explain the infertility?
   A. Salpingitis isthmica nodosa
   B. Asherman syndrome
   C. Fibroids
   D. Occluded fallopian tubes

2. What else is this patient at risk for?
   A. Pelvic inflammatory disease
   B. Ectopic pregnancy
   C. Endometriosis
   D. Tuberculosis

3. Which ONE of the following is a contraindication to performing an HSG?
   A. Pelvic infection
   B. Menstruation
   C. Prior uterine surgery
   D. Pelvic pain

■ Answers and Explanations

Question 1

A. Correct! SIN is demonstrated in this case. SIN refers to nodular scarring of the fallopian tubes. Characteristic findings include multiple nodular diverticular spaces involving the tubes (usually the proximal two-thirds). In this case, tiny outpouchings instilled with contrast are seen along the course of the fallopian isthmus.

Other choices and discussion

B. Asherman syndrome (uterine synechiae) refers to the presence of intrauterine adhesions, usually from injury to the endometrium. There is an association with infertility. However, the endometrial cavity distends normally on the test case images, and no irregular linear filling defects are seen within the uterus.

C. Fibroids (if submucosal) will form filling defects of the endometrial cavity. Sometimes this is best seen during early filling, rather than with peak filling. However, no filling defects are visualized in this case. Intramural or subserosal fibroids may be missed with HSG.

D. There is appropriate spillage of contrast beyond the fallopian tubes, indicating that they are patent. The cornual portion of the fallopian tube is encased by uterine smooth muscle. If there is spasm of the muscle during an HSG, one or both tubes may not completely fill, mimicking a fixed tubal occlusion. Some institutions use the spasmolytic agent glucagon to combat spasm. Administration of glucagon can minimize uterine muscle contraction and optimize tubal opacification. This aids in differentiating cornual spasm from true tubal occlusion.

Question 2

B. Correct! There is an increased risk of tubal ectopic pregnancy in patients who have SIN. The scarred fallopian tube sometimes prevents appropriate travel of the ovary.

Other choices and discussion

A. Pelvic inflammatory disease is a proposed *etiology* for tubal scarring and the development of SIN.

C. Endometriosis can potentially mimic the appearance of SIN.

D. Tuberculosis can potentially mimic the appearance of SIN.

Question 3

A. Correct! If contrast is instilled into a potential nidus of infection, the infection could spread from the fallopian tubes into the peritoneum. If there is intravasation of contrast into the uterine veins, the patient could become septic. Some referring clinicians give prophylactic antibiotics prior to the procedure, especially if there is a history of pelvic inflammatory disease. However, antibiotics are not routinely required, and this decision is up to the discretion of the referrer.

Other choices and discussion

B. Although it is not ideal to perform an HSG during menstruation (since the blood could obscure the findings), menstruation is not an absolute contraindication. Pregnancy is a contraindication.

C. Prior uterine surgery is not a contraindication. In fact, HSGs are often performed to evaluate postoperative patients for possible adhesions.

D. Pain is not a contraindication.

■ Suggested Readings

Bolaji II, Octaba M, Mohee K, et al. An odyssey through salpingitis isthmica nodosa. Eur J Obstet Gynaecol Reprod Biol 2015;184:73–79

Creasy JL, Clark RL, Cuttino JT, et al. Salpingitis isthmica nodosa: radiologic and clinical correlates. Radiology 1985;154:597–600

Sathyamoorthy P. Salpingitis isthmica nodosa: review of four cases from the general hospital, Kota Bharu. Singapore Med J 1994;35:65–66

Simpson W, Beitia LG, Mester J. Hysterosalpingography: a reemerging study. Radiographics 2006;26:419–431

Top Tips

◆ HSG is usually performed to identify a cause for infertility, to evaluate for patency of the fallopian tubes, or to assess efficacy of surgical sterilization techniques such as Essure devices.

◆ SIN results from fallopian tube scarring, and HSG shows multiple (often subtle) diverticula arising from the proximal fallopian tube. There is an associated increased risk for ectopic pregnancy and infertility.

◆ Three portions of the fallopian tube are the cornual portion (at the junction with the uterus), the isthmic portion, and the ampullary portion (near the ovary). Remember the mnemonic CIA.

Essentials 10

■ Case

The patient presents with left scrotal pain. Selected images from a left scrotal ultrasound and a computed tomography are shown.

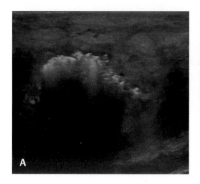 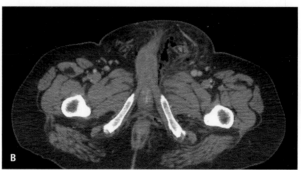 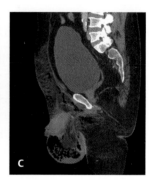

■ Questions

1. What is the next BEST step in management of this patient?
   A. Intravenous antibiotics
   B. Surgical debridement
   C. Steroids
   D. Careful observation, as this often resolves spontaneously

2. This patient most likely has which underlying condition?
   A. Hydrocele
   B. Orchitis
   C. Diabetes
   D. Undescended testicle

3. What would you expect to see on scrotal ultrasound with this diagnosis?
   A. Echogenic foci with dirty shadowing
   B. Echogenic foci with clean shawdowing
   C. Comet tail artifact
   D. Multiple cystic foci

■ Answers and Explanations

Question 1

B. Correct! Surgery is indicated. Ultrasound and computed tomography demonstrate subcutaneous gas of the left perineum and scrotum with overlying skin thickening. This is diagnostic of Fournier gangrene, which is a life-threatening, rapidly progressive, necrotizing fascitis of the perineum. Presenting symptoms typically include fever, leukocytosis, perineal/scrotal pain, and crepitus from soft tissue gas.

Other choices and discussion

A. This is a urologic emergency. Given the associated mortality risk, intravenous antibiotics alone will not suffice. Broad spectrum antibiotics are administered in association with surgery, as Fournier gangrene is typically a polymicrobial infection.

B. Steroids do not play a role in the treatment of this condition.

D. This is a urologic emergency, and this process does not resolve spontaneously.

Question 2

C. Correct! Diabetes is a risk factor for Fournier gangrene. Other risk factors include immunosuppressed status, human immunodeficiency virus, male gender, and alcoholism.

Other choices and discussion

A. Hydrocele is not a risk factor.

B. Spread of infection from the testicle is usually not the etiology. Commonly, the infection originates from anorectal fistulas or perineal abscesses.

D. Cryptorchidism is not a risk factor.

Question 3

A. Correct! Air within the scrotal wall and perineal tissues will manifest as small echogenic foci with dirty shadowing and ring down artifact (no narrowing of the ring down beam).

Other choices and discussion

B. Echogenic foci with clean shadowing typically indicates calcification/stones.

C. Comet tail artifact, which eminates from calcific or crystalline structures (highly reflective), is a form of reverberation artifact that shows narrowing. Comet tail may be seen with small stones, colloid nodules, and adenomyomatosis of the gallbladder.

D. Multiple cystic foci would not be expected.

■ Suggested Readings

Rajan DK, Scharer KA. Radiology of Fournier's gangrene. Am J Roentgenol 1998;170:16

Uppot RN, Levy HM, Patel PH. Case 54: Fournier gangrene. Radiology 2003;226:115–117

You JS, Chung YE, Cho KS, et al. The emergency computed tomography as important modality for early diagnosis of Fournier gangrene. Am J Emerg Med 2010;29(959):e1–2

Top Tips

- Fournier gangrene is a fulminant necrotizing fasciitis of the scrotum/perineum. It is usually polymicrobial.
- Fournier is usually found in diabetics, the elderly, or the immunocompromised. There is a male predominance, and there may be a history of infection in the skin or adjacent pelvis.
- This is a surgical emergency!

SECTION V
GENITOURINARY IMAGING

Details 1

■ Case

A 31-year-old woman presents with pelvic pain. Which ONE of the following is the correct diagnosis for the adnexal mass on the patient's RIGHT?
- A. Endometrioma
- B. Ovarian dermoid
- C. Serous cystadenoma
- D. Simple cyst

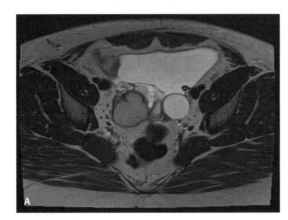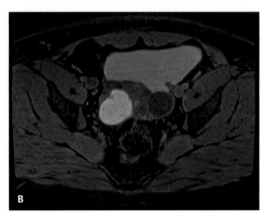

■ The following questions pertain to endometriosis and ovarian masses.

1. What symptoms might this patient present with?
2. What demonstrated magnetic resonance characteristic on these images is classic for the diagnosis?
3. True or False. A T1-weighted fat-saturated magnetic resonance sequence would help differentiate this diagnosis from a teratoma.
4. How can an endometrioma be differentiated from a hemorrhagic cyst?
5. An ovarian lesion that demonstrates uptake on an iodine-123 whole-body nuclear medicine scan is called _____.

6. The second most common ovarian tumor (after an ovarian dermoid) is _____.
7. Are serous cystadenomas or mucinous tumors of the ovary more likely to be bilateral?
8. Which ovarian tumor causes endometrial hyperplasia?
9. What is Meigs syndrome, and which ovarian tumor causes it?
10. True or False. Once diagnosed, paraovarian cysts should be followed with annual imaging.

■ Answers and Explanations

A. Correct! The lesion on the patient's right is an endometrioma. An endometrioma refers to endometrial tissue that has implanted on the ovary. It is also known as a "chocolate cyst" and can be bilateral. The signal intensity is the result of blood products of variable age (owing to repeated hemorrhage). Deep endometriosis is a manifestation of the process beyond the ovaries, with implantation on the uterine or bowel serosal tissue. Adhesions form with deep endometriosis, and tethering of the ovaries to surrounding structures is often found. Classically, the normal physiologic fluid does not gather in the normal cul-de-sac, but rather is displaced. There is an inceased risk of clear cell and endometroid epithelial ovarian malignancies in patients with endometriosis. Intralesional enhancing nodules raise the possibility of malignancy.

Other choices and discussion

B. There is no evidence of fat signal intensity within the lesion to confirm the diagnosis of ovarian dermoid.

C. Serous cystadenomas may be blood tinged but are not typically fully comprised of blood products, as in the test case.

D. The test case mass on the patient's right does not follow simple fluid signal on both of the images; however, the mass on the left does and is a simple cyst.

Question 1

This patient might present with cyclical pain, as this is endometrial tissue that has implanted on the ovary.

Question 2

These magnetic resonance images demonstrate "T2 shading," which is characterized by T2-hypointensity due to the presence of deoxyhemoglobin and methaemoglobin. The T1-weighted image is typically light bulb bright from repeated hemorrhage and subacute blood products.

Question 3

True. A T1-weighted fat-saturated image helps to differentiate blood products from fat, as both are hyperintesne on T1 without fat saturation. Fat saturation is necessary in the evaluation of a potential endometrioma.

Question 4

Like an endometrioma, a hemorrhagic cyst is bright on T1-weighted images. However, a hemorrhagic cyst is usually also bright on T2-weighted images (i.e., no "shading"). This is because a hemorrhagic cyst typically has acute or subacute blood products, whereas an endometrioma has the repeated or chronic blood products that causes T2 shading. Sometimes, T2 shading is not obvious, and it may be difficult to differentiate the two entities based only on signal intensity. Hemorrhagic cysts sometimes exhibit crescentic layering and tend to resolve or retract during the subsequent menstrual cycle. Additional findings of deep endometriosis include pelvis adhesions and implants on other pelvic structures including the uterine serosa.

Question 5

Struma ovari. This rare condition refers to thyroid tissue arising from the ovary, and this may be seen with iodine scintigraphy.

Question 6

Serous cystadenoma. After ovarian dermoid, serous cystadenoma is the next most common ovarian tumor.

Question 7

Serous cystadenomas have an increased propensity for bilaterality (15%). Mucinous ovarian tumors are usually unilateral.

Question 8

Brenner tumor of the ovary can cause endometrial hyperplasia. This rare epithelial tumor is bilateral in 30% of the cases.

Question 9

Meigs syndrome refers to the combination of pleural effusion, ascites, and an ovarian lesion. The implicated ovarian lesion is generally a fibroma (90%), thecoma, or fibrothecoma.

Question 10

False. Once diagnosed, no follow up imaging is necessary for paraovarian cysts (assuming no suspicious features). Paraovarian cysts are congenital, separate from the ovary, and do not resolve.

■ Suggested Readings

Glastonbury CM. The shading sign. Radiology 2002;224:199–201

Lee SI. Radiological reasoning: imaging characterization of bilateral adnexal masses. Am J Roentgenol 2006;187:S460–466

SECTION V GENITOURINARY IMAGING

Top Tips

- ◆ An endometrioma is endometrial tissue that implants on the ovary and causes cyclic pain. Its imaging features reflect repeated hemorrhage within a cyst. T1-hyperintense with "T2 shading" is classic.

- ◆ Differential diagnoses of T1-hyperintense adnexal lesions: fat (dermoid), blood (endometrioma or hemorrhagic cyst), and proteinaceous material. Use fat saturation to narrow the differential.

- ◆ Endometriomas should be followed at least annually to exclude neoplasm. Malignant transformation is more common in patients older than 45 and for endometriomas > 6 cm.

Details 2

■ Case

The left adrenal nodule seen on these noncontrast and contrast-enhanced computed tomography (CT) images has the following measurements: unenhanced 18 HU, portal venous phase 66 HU, and delayed phase 25 HU. What is the correct diagnosis for this left adrenal nodule?
- A. Lipid poor adenoma
- B. Adrenal carcinoma
- C. Indeterminate nodule
- D. Lipid rich adenoma

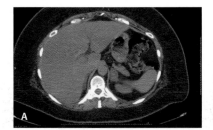 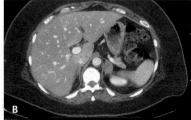 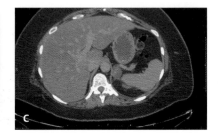

■ The following questions pertain to adrenal lesions.

1. What is the appropriate postcontrast administration time delay for a CT adrenal mass protocol?
2. The minimum relative percentage washout used to diagnose an adrenal adenoma when unenhanced CT is not available is _____.
3. A 2-cm left adrenal nodule measures 6 HU. What is the BEST next step?
4. Name the elements that make up a myelolipoma.
5. True or False. Loss of signal on dual-gradient chemical shift imaging is expected with a myelolipoma.

6. What adrenal lesion is often characterized as "light bulb bright" on T2-weighted images?
7. Which nuclear medicine studies can be used to assess for pheochromocytoma?
8. Which features of an adrenal mass raise concern for adrenocortical carcinoma?
9. What is a collision tumor of the adrenal gland?
10. What does calcification of the adrenal gland imply?

■ Answers and Explanations

A. Correct! This is a lipid poor adenoma. Unenhanced CT demonstrates a density measurement > 10 HU. Therefore, this is not a lipid rich adenoma. Absolute washout > 60% is diagnostic of an adrenal adenoma. In this case, the absolute washout is 85%. If washout is < 60%, the study is indeterminate, and other etiologies including carcinoma or metastasis must be considered.

Question 1

To adequately assess potential washout, a 10- to 15-minute delay is considered appropriate.

Question 2

At least 40% *relative* washout is diagnostic of an adrenal adenoma. At least 60% *absolute* washout (that is, when compared to a noncontrast study) is diagnostic of an adrenal adenoma.

Relative washout = (delayed HU − enhanced HU)/enhanced HU × 100.

Absolute washout = (delayed HU − enhanced HU) (enhanced HU − unenhanced HU) × 100.

Question 3

No further workup is necessary. This is consistent with a lipid-rich adrenal adenoma. Clinically, this could be functioning, and biochemical and laboratory workup may be appropriate.

Question 4

A myelolipoma is comprised of mature adipocytes and hematopoietic cells (*myelo* = bone marrow elements). A myelolipoma is a benign entity and usually incidentally discovered on imaging. One-third of these masses contain calcification. The magnetic resonance imaging example provided demonstrates loss of signal on the T2 fat-saturated images in the right adrenal gland. This indicates the presence of macroscopic fat and is diagnostic of a myelolipoma.

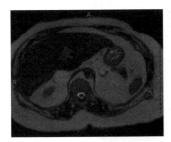
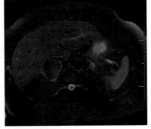
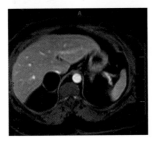

Question 5

False. On dual-gradient chemical shift imaging, a myelolipoma shows the same signal on both in-phase and out-of-phase sequences. Myelolipomas contain macroscopic fat, not microscopic fat. A drop-in signal on out-of-phase images indicates microscopic (or intracellular) fat, as is seen with an adrenal adenoma.

Question 6

Pheochromocytoma is the classic "T2 light bulb bright" adrenal lesion. However, light bulb bright is not specific for pheochromocytoma. For example, cystic necrosis of an adrenal cortical carcinoma can have a similar appearance on T2. In addition, this finding is sometimes not even present with pheochromocytoma.

Question 7

Both In-111-pentetreotide (Octreoscan) and I-123 metaiodobenzylguanidine scans are useful in the diagnosis and localization of pheochromocytoma.

Question 8

Adrenocortical carcinoma should be considered in an adrenal mass with the following features: large size (> 4 cm, 70% malignant), calcification, hemorrhage, and necrosis. Pheochromocytomas can have similar features but are differentiated by biochemical markers.

Question 9

A collision tumor refers to the situation when two histologically distinct tumors are in very close proximity to (or actually abut) each other in the same adrenal gland. This is uncommon, but when it occurs, one of the two lesions is typically an adrenal adenoma and the other a metastatic lesion.

Question 10

Calcification of the adrenal gland implies prior hemorrhage (sepsis, trauma, or Waterhouse-Friderichsen syndrome), infection (tuberculosis or histoplasmosis), or underlying neoplasm (adrenal cortical carcinoma, myelolipoma, pheochromocytoma).

SECTION V GENITOURINARY IMAGING

Top Tips

- *Lipid-rich* adenomas are accurately diagnosed with a density measurement of 10 HU or less on unenhanced CT or with a loss of signal between in-phase and out-of-phase imaging on magnetic resonance imaging.

- If the above criteria are not met, *lipid-poor* adenomas can be diagnosed with the calculation of absolute or relative washout, which should be > 60% and > 40%, respectively.

- Myelolipoma is a benign (usually adrenal) mass that is composed of macroscopic fat and hematopoietic cells. Look for drop of signal on fat-saturated magnetic resonance imaging (denotes macroscopic fat).

Details 3

■ Case

A 45-year-old woman presents. What is the MOST likely diagnosis?
  A. Staghorn calculus
  B. Renal sinus hemorrhagic cyst
  C. Retained contrast
  D. Xanthogranulomatous pyelonephritis

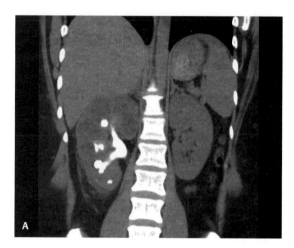 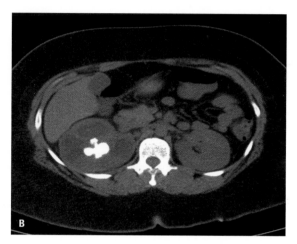

■ The following questions pertain to renal infection.

1. The pathologic hallmark of XGP is _____.
2. What is the management of XGP?
3. What is the classic appearance of pyelonephritis on contrast-enhanced computed tomography?
4. True or False. Renal abscesses 2 cm or greater should be drained percutaneously.
5. What is ureteritis cystica?
6. What is leukoplakia, and is there malignant potential?

7. What is malakoplakia, and is there malignant potential?
8. What is the next best step if is pus suspected in a febrile patient with a dilated renal collecting system?
9. True or False. Intravenous antibiotics alone can typically treat emphysematous pyelonephritis.
10. Homogenous calcification of the kidney associated with tuberculosis is referred to as _____.

■ Answers and Explanations

D. Correct! This is a case of xanthogranulomatous pyelonephritis (XGP). The kidney is enlarged, contains dilated calyces with a multiloculated appearance ("bear paw" sign), and there is a staghorn calculus. There is also slight thickening of the surrounding renal fascia. These findings are characteristic of diffuse type XGP. Variant forms involve less than the entire kidney. XGP is a granulomatous infection with a female predilection and is usually found in middle-aged to elderly patients. The most commonly implicated bacteria are *Escherichia coli* and *Proteus mirabilis*.

Other choices and discussion

A. A staghorn calculus is present, but this is an incomplete diagnosis.

B. Renal sinus hemorrhagic cyst would be somewhat hyperdense (although not as dense as in the test case). Further, this would not satisfactorily explain the dilated calyces.

C. Retained contrast is unlikely, as there is no evidence of any contrast elsewhere, and this would not explain the dilated yet not opacified calyces.

Question 1

The pathologic hallmark of XGP is lipid-laden macrophages. In this noncontrast test case, the low attenuation deposits in the region of the calyces are the lipid-laden macrophages.

Question 2

Management for XGP is typically nephrectomy (or sometimes partial nephrectomy). These patients often progress to significant complications, most commonly pyelocutaneous and ureterocutaneous fistulae. With appropriate treatment, prognosis is generally good with low mortality.

Question 3

With pyelonephritis, there is classically a striated nephrogram (owing to areas of edema within the infected kidney) and perinephric fascial standing. Remember to search for contralateral disease, because the process is sometimes bilateral, and to exclude a drainable abscess.

Question 4

False. Percutaneous catheter drainage placement is generally chosen over intravenous antibiotics alone when the renal abscess reaches 3 cm, not 2 cm.

Question 5

Ureteritis cystica is a benign condition of the ureters that demonstrates multiple small submucosal cysts. It is typically found in diabetics with chronic infections or stones, and it may be associated with *E. coli* or tuberculosis. On the excretory phase of a computed tomography urogram (or by conventional intravenous excretory urography), ureteritis cystica appears as multiple small (2 to 5 mm), smooth-walled, rounded, lucent filling defects projecting into the lumen of the ureter.

Question 6

Leukoplakia of the urinary tract refers to squamous metaplasia of the urothelium and is associated with infection (majority) or stones. It occurs more commonly in the bladder than in the renal pelvis or ureter. Radiographically, leukoplakia presents as mucosal thickening/filling defects. Leukoplakia does have malignant potential.

Question 7

Malakoplakia is an uncommon chronic granulomatous inflammatory disease that affects the bladder wall. It predominantly affects women and is associated with *E. coli*. Radiographically, malakoplakia presents as bladder masses or wall thickening. There is no malignant potential, but malakoplakia may be locally aggressive.

Question 8

Emergent decompression of the dilated collecting system is indicated if pus is present, as there may be impending sepsis. Generally, this is accomplished by placement of a percutaneous nephrostomy tube or stent.

Question 9

False. Emphysematous pyelonephritis is not easily treated with intravenous antibiotics. This entity is a life-threatening necrotizing infection in which gas is found within the renal collecting system. Antibiotics and nephrectomy are the standard of care. The prognosis is worse when there is also air in the perinephric space.

Question 10

Homogenous calcification of the kidney associated with tuberculosis is referred to as a "putty" kidney.

■ Suggested Readings

Clapton WK, Boucaut HA, Dewan PA, et al. Clinicopathological features of xanthogranulomatous pyelonephritis in infancy. Pathology 1993;25:110–113

Hayes WS, Hartman DS, Sesterbenn IA. Xanthogranulomatous pyelonephritis. Radiographics 1991;11:485–498

Merchant S, Bharati A, Merchant N. Tuberculosis of the genitourinary system-urinary tract tuberculosis: renal tuberculosis-part I. Indian J Radiol Imaging 2013;23:46–63

Rajesh A, Jakanani G, Mayer N, et al. Computed tomography findings in xanthogranulomatous pyelonephritis. J Clin Imaging Sci 2011;1:45

Top Tips

- XGP is a granulomatous infection with the imaging findings of renal enlargement, staghorn calculus, and dilated calyces with low attenuation deposits. The pathologic hallmark is lipid-laden macrophages, and the treatment is nephrectomy.

- Leukoplakia has malignant potential, whereas malakoplakia does not.

- Pyonephrosis requires urgent decompression. Emphysematous pyelonephritis requires urgent antibiotics followed by nephrectomy.

Details 4

■ Case

This patient had an essentially normal contrast-enhanced computed tomography abdomen 1 day prior to the film shown on the left. Comparison study from 1 week earlier is shown on the right. What is the correct diagnosis?

A. Normal study
B. Nephrocalcinosis
C. Bilateral staghorn calculus
D. Acute tubular necrosis
E. Mechanical obstuction

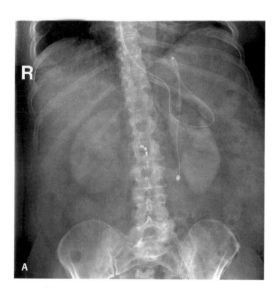
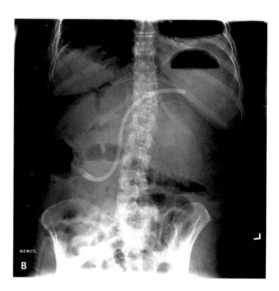

■ The following questions pertain to renal injury.

1. What numeric rise in creatinine is considered diagnostic of CIN following contrast administration?
2. What is the greatest risk factor for developing nephrogenic systemic fibrosis (NSF) following gadolinium administration?
3. What is an appropriate time delay after contrast injection to assess for trauma to the ureter and/or collecting system?
4. What is a Page kidney, and what are the clinical consequences?
5. According to the American Association for the Surgery of Trauma, a renal laceration on computed tomography that measures 2 cm is classified as a grade _____ injury.

6. A subcapsular hematoma without renal compression is classified as what grade injury?
7. Urinary extravasation on delayed imaging is considered what grade injury?
8. Name a common cause of bladder flap hematoma.
9. The most common cause of ureteral injury is _____.
10. The most common mechanism for urethral injury in a male is _____ .

■ Answers and Explanations

D. Correct! This patient has acute tubular necrosis. The film on the left demonstrates opacified kidneys. There is no hydronephrosis to suggest mechanical obstruction, and the normal study performed 1 week earlier (on the right) excludes calcifications. Thus, the kidneys are demonstrating prolonged contrast retention. As intravenous contrast was given 24 hours earlier, this is most likely acute tubular necrosis caused by contrast-induced nephropathy (CIN). Risk factors include a low glomerular filtration rate (GFR), a high dose of contrast, and an intra-arterial (as opposed to intravenous) injection.

Question 1

According to the most recent American College of Radiology manual on contrast media, there is no absolute definition for CIN. However, one of the most frequently used criteria is an absolute increase of 0.5 mg/dL over a baseline serum creatinine.

Question 2

The greatest risk factor for developing NSF is impaired renal function. If the kidneys are unable to eliminate the gadolinium from the system (which typically occurs when the eGFR < 30), then the chelates dissociate, leaving free gadolinium ions to deposit into the soft tissues. NSF can develop weeks or even months after gadolinium administration. Physical manifestations include skin thickening, edema, fibrous plaques, involvement of internal organs, and sometimes death. There is no effective therapy. NSF has been demonstrated on bone scan as diffuse soft tissue radiotracer uptake and on fluorodeoxyglucose-positron emission tomography as skin and muscle activity.

Question 3

A total of 6 to 10 minutes after contrast injection is an appropriate delay to assess for trauma to the ureter and/or collecting system. At this point, the contrast should opacify the renal collecting system, the ureters, and the early bladder lumen, whereas contrast in most of the other abdominal structures should have largely washed out.

Question 4

Page kidney refers to hypertension that develops after long-term external compression of the renal parenchyma, typically from a subcapsular fluid collection. The compression of the renal vessels leads to a decrease in blood flow and subsequent activation of the renin-angiotensin system, which causes a rise in blood pressure. With a Page kidney, the renal parenchyma is usually noticably distorted.

Question 5

Grade 3. Grade 3 injuries are > 1 cm in size, without renal pelvis or collecting system extension. Grade 2 injuries are superficial lacerations < 1 cm in size without extention to the collecting system, or a nonexpanding perirenal hematoma.

Question 6

Grade 1 injury. This is defined as a contusion or a nonenlarging subcapsular perirenal hematoma.

Question 7

Grade 4 injury. This is a laceration which extends to the renal pelvis or demonstrates urinary extravasation. Grade 4 also involves injury to the main renal vessels with contained hemorrhage, or an expanding subcapsular hematoma compressing the kidney.

Question 8

Bladder flap hematoma is an uncommon complication of Cesarean section. It is a hematoma located between the posterior urinary bladder wall and the anterior uterus, and usually results from dehisence of the incision in the lower uterine segment. Bladder flap hematomas are generally small (< 5 cm).

Question 9

Gynecologic surgery is the most common cause of ureteral injury.

Question 10

Traumatic straddle injury is the most common mechanism for urethral injury in a male. The depicted picture is a retrograde urethrogram (which is always indicated as the initial study when urethral injury is suspected), which shows leakage of contrast from the anterior urethra into the surrounding soft tissues of the penis. Injury should be suspected clinically when there is blood at the urethral meatus, hematuria, and/or an inability to void.

Top Tips

- The definition of CIN is debated. One reasonable definition is an absolute increase of 0.5 mg/dL over a baseline serum creatinine.

- Gadolinium carries the risk of NSF. The risk is much less when the eGFR is > 30.

- American Association for the Surgery of Trauma grading system for renal injury:

  - Grade I: Subcapsular hematoma

  - Grade 2: Superficial renal laceration < 1 cm

  - Grade 3: Superficial renal laceration > 1 cm

  - Grade 4: Injury to the collecting system or main renal vessels with contained hemorrhage

Details 5

■ Case

A 42-year-old woman presents with a history of myomectomy. She tested negative for beta-human chorionic gonadotropin. What is the MOST likely diagnosis?

A. Uterine arteriovenous malformation
B. Gestational trophoblastic disease
C. Retained products of conception
D. Endometrial carcinoma

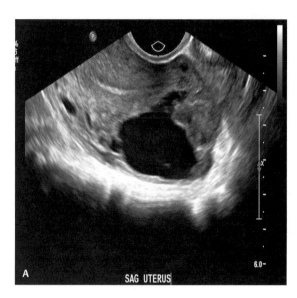
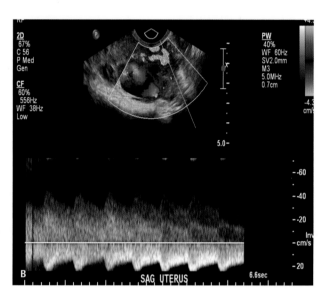

■ The following questions pertain to conditions related to uterine masses or the gravid uterus.

1. Embolization of the uterine artery was performed to treat the AVM. From where does the uterine artery arise?
2. "Snowstorm" or "bunch of grapes" signs are seen with which uterine entity?
3. Name the condition where the placenta covers the internal cervical os, as seen in this image.
4. What are common risk factors for placenta previa?
5. True or False. Placenta accreta is associated with intraplacental bands.

6. What are some common risk factors associated with placenta accreta?
7. An endometrial mass with a single feeding vessel is most likely a _____.
8. Endometrial polyps and nondegenerating fibroids are of which signal intensity on T2-weighted images?
9. The most common type of fibroid degeneration is _____.
10. Which type of fibroid degeneration is common in pregnant women?

■ Answers and Explanations

A. Correct! This is a uterine AVM. This relatively rare entity can be life-threatening. It is usually the result of prior surgical intervention (i.e., Cesarean section, myomectomy), but is sometimes congenital. As demonstrated in the test case, color Doppler ultrasound is a noninvasive method for diagnosis, demonstrating a highly vascular structure in the wall of the uterus with both arterial and venous flow. Typically, serpiginous/tubular anechoic structures are seen in the myometrium and demonstrate a low resistance (0.2 to 0.5) and a high velocity flow pattern.

Other choices and discussion

B. Gestational trophoblastic disease could have a somewhat similar appearance, but the beta- human chorionic gonadotropin would be markedly elevated.

C. Retained products of conception would present with abnormal and often hypervascular material centered in the endometrium, not within the myometrial wall.

D. The anechoic appearance of the test case is not typical of uterine carcinoma.

Question 1

The uterine artery arises from the anterior division of the internal iliac artery. Additional branches of the anterior division of the internal iliac artery are the umbilical (only patent in the fetus), superior vesicle (branch of the umbilical artery), obturator, vaginal, inferior vesicle, middle rectal, internal pudendal, and inferior gluteal arteries.

Question 2

"Snowstorm" or "bunch of grapes" signs describe a complete molar pregnancy. The characteristic appearance is diffuse, solid-appearing echoes with small, interspersed anechoic spaces.

Question 3

Placenta previa. This condition describes an abnormally low position of the placenta that lies close to or covers the internal cervical os. A low-lying placenta is present when the lower placental edge lies 0.5 to 3.0 cm from internal os.

Question 4

Risk factors for placenta previa include prior history of placenta previa, prior Caesarean section, high maternal age, and smoking.

Question 5

True. The general term placenta accreta describes abnormal placental adherence with the villi, extending beyond the confines of the endometrium, to attach to the myometrium. This attachment is known as intraplacental bands, which can sometimes be seen on magnetic resonance imaging. Placenta accreta is attachment to the superficial aspect of the myometrium without deep invasion. Placenta increta is invasion into the myometrium. Placenta percreta is invasion beyond the myometrium with serosal breach.

Question 6

Risk factors associated with placenta accreta include placenta previa, prior Caesarean section, prior uterine surgery/procedure, and advanced maternal age.

Question 7

An endometrial mass with a single feeding vessel is most likely an endometrial polyp. This feature usually helps to differentiate a polyp from a submucosal fibroid.

Question 8

Endometrial polyps are T2-hyperintense. Fibroids (nondegenerating) are generally T2-hypointense.

Question 9

The most common type of fibroid degeneration is hyaline (or calcific) degeneration. This shows areas of absent enhancement on magnetic resonance imaging.

Question 10

Red (or carneous) fibroid degeneration due to hemorrhagic infarction is associated with pregnancy. Myxoid and cystic fibroid degeneration demonstrate increased T2 signal.

Top Tips

♦ A uterine AVM represents multiple arteriovenous fistulous communications, with no intervening capillary network, within the uterus. It is usually caused by instrumentation or trauma but may be congenital.

♦ Ultrasound with Doppler is usually able to make the diagnosis of uterine AVM. Magnetic resonance imaging is useful for problem cases and sometimes for therapeutic planning purposes. Catheter angiography, the traditional gold standard for diagnosis, is less commonly performed because it is invasive.

♦ Placenta previa occurs when the placenta lies close to or on top of the internal cervical os. Placenta accreta describes a spectrum of abnormal villous projections into the myometrium. Both conditions place pregnant patients at an increased risk of hemorrhage.

Image Rich 1

■ Case

Match the appropriate diagnosis to the provided images.
- A. Retroperitoneal fibrosis
- B. Lymphoma
- C. Erdheim-Chester
- D. Metastatic testicular cancer

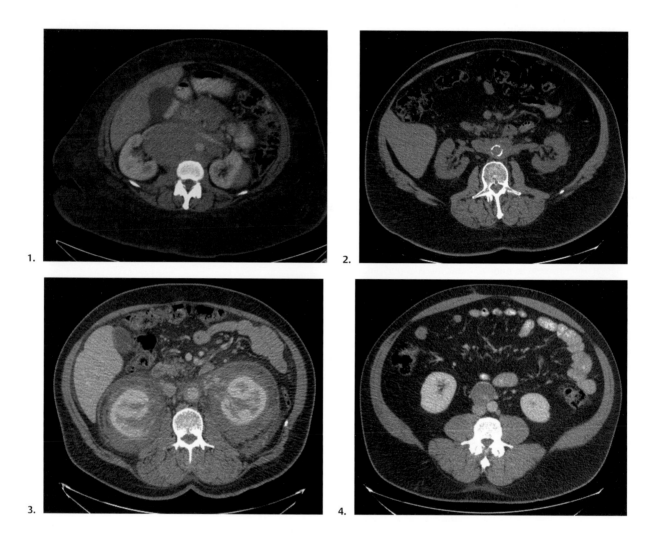

1.

2.

3.

4.

■ Answers and Explanations

1. B. Lymphoma. This is usually thought of as a "soft" lesion. It tends to encase and displace structures with causing obstruction. Lymphoma sometimes lifts the aorta off the spine (in contrast to RPF). Additional features more common in lymphoma than in RPF include predominantly suprarenal location, heterogeneity, perirenal extension, additional adenopathy, and a larger size (> 1.5 cm).

2. A. RPF. This entity tends to present with ureteral obstruction. Medial deviation of both ureters with pelvic extension is more common with RPF than with lymphoma. There is a male predominance with RPF. Most cases of RPF are idiopathic, but other causes that have been implicated include radiation, inflammation, retroperitoneal bleeding, and a variety of medications (e.g., methylsergide [an outdated migraine medication], hydralazine, methyldopa, and ergotamyl). RPF tissue enhances with contrast administration.

3. C. Erdheim-Chester. This rare multisystem granulomatosis has variable manifestations and severity. Pathologically, there is infiltration by lipid-laden histiocytes. Bone pain and fibrosis in the retroperitoneum are often present. Renal involvement (shown here) can result in renal failure. There is fibrosis surrounding the kidneys but sparing of the inferior vena cava and pelvic ureters (in contrast to typical retroperitoneal fibrosis). Cardiac failure and pulmonary fibrosis are common causes of death.

4. D. Metastatic testicular cancer. It is important to understand the drainage pattern for testicular cancer. Testicular cancer tends to spread to the paraaortic and paracaval regions. It does NOT drain to the pelvic iliac lymph node chains.

One other uncommon consideration for nodular retroperitoneal tissue is extramedullary hematopoiesis. This rare entity should only be considered when the patient has a known hemoglobinopathy and when characteristic skeletal changes are present.

■ Suggested Reading

Cronin CG, Lohan DG, Blake MA, et al. Retroperitoneal fibrosis: a review of clinical features and imaging findings. Am J Roentgenol 2008;191:423–431

Frampas E. Lymphomas: Basic points that radiologists should know. Diagn Interv Imaging 2013;94:131–144

Fortman BJ, Beall DP. Erdheim-Chester disease of the retroperitoneum: a rare cause of ureteral obstruction. Am J Roentgenol 2001;176:1330–1331

Top Tips

◆ Fluorodeoxyglucose-positron emission tomography cannot be used to differentiate lymphoma from retroperitoneal fibrosis, as both entities are typically fluorodeoxyglucose-avid.

◆ In comparison to lymphoma, RPF more commonly obstructs the ureters, remains smaller in anteroposterior and transverse diameter, and tends NOT to lift the aorta.

◆ Testicular cancers drain to the para-aortic and paracaval regions at the level of the kidneys, not to the pelvic nodes. If you see isolated retroperitoneal lymphadenopathy in a male patient, recommend a testicular ultrasound.

Image Rich 2

■ **Case**

Match the appropriate diagnosis to the provided images.

A. Obstructive uropathy
B. Renal vein thrombosis (RVT)
C. Renal artery stenosis (RAS)
D. Diabetic nephropathy

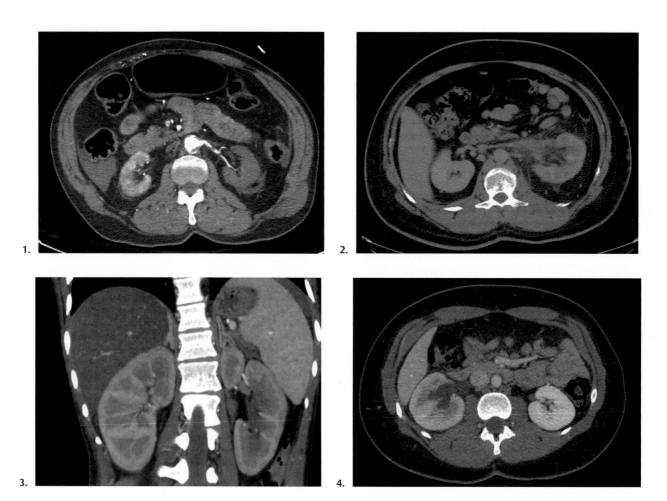

1.

2.

3.

4.

■ Answers and Explanations

1. C. RAS. There is markedly decreased perfusion of the left kidney, no hydronephrosis, and no renal enlargement. There is atherosclerosis and a high-grade clot in the left main renal artery. RAS can be diagnosed with computed tomography angiography, magnetic resonance angiography, ultrasound, or captopril renography.

Some findings that have been used to diagnose RAS on ultrasound include renal arterial resistive index difference > 5% between kidneys, peak systolic velocity renal artery to aorta ratio > 3.5, and an increased peak systolic velocity > 180 cm/sec.

2. B. RVT. There is enlargement of the left kidney (but no significant hydronephrosis), fascial stranding in the left renal pelvis region, and an expanded (visibly thrombosed) left renal vein. Acute renal vein thrombosis initially causes unilateral renal enlargement. Later, it can result in atrophy. Thrombus is either bland or tumor thrombus. The most common causes of renal vein thrombosis include nephrotic syndrome, lupus, glomerulonephritis, diabetes, dehydration, hypercoagulable state, underlying malignancy, sepsis, and trauma.

Common causes of RVT in children include dehydration, sickle cell, indwelling umbilical venous catheters, and maternal diabetes. Renal vein thrombosis can be diagnosed by computed tomography venogram, magnetic resonance venogram, or ultrasound. Ultrasound is sometimes technically challenging.

3. D. Diabetic nephropathy. There is bilateral nephromegaly (sometimes defined as kidneys > 13 cm in length) without focal masses. This is usually either the result of a systemic process or a central venous obstruction distal to the level of the individual renal veins. Specific causes of nephromegaly include diabetic nephropathy (~50% of cases), acute glomerulonephritis, systemic lupus erythematosus, other vasculitis/autoimmune disease (i.e., Wegner, Goodpasture, Henoch-Schönlein), human immunodeficiency virus nephropathy, lymphoma/leukemia, and acute interstitial nephritis.

During infancy/in utero, autosomal recessive polycystic kidney disease classically demonstrates bilaterally enlarged and sonographically echogenic kidneys.

4. A. Obstructive uropathy. There is enlargement of the right kidney, unilateral hydronephrosis, and a unilateral delayed nephrogram. In this case, the right kidney is still in the corticomedullary phase, whereas the left kidney has progressed to the nephrographic phase. A distal obstructive process is present (but not shown). The most common cause of an acute ureteral obstruction is a calculus, but other intrinsic or extrinsic processes (i.e., pelvic mass, retroperitoneal fibrosis, or ureteral blood clot) are also possible.

Some causes of unilateral renal enlargement include obstructive uropathy, acute pyelonephritis, acute arterial obstruction, and acute venous obstruction.

■ Suggested Readings

Chen MY, Zagoria RJ, Dyer RB. Radiologic findings in acute urinary tract obstruction. J Emerg Med 1997;15:339–343

Kawashima A, Sandler CM, Ernst RD, et al. CT evaluation of renovascular disease. Radiographics 2000;20:1321–1340

Zagoria RJ, Tung GA. The kidney: the diffuse parenchymal abnormality. In Genitourinary Radiology: The Requisites. Maryland Heights, MO: Mosby; 2004:139–140

Top Tips

- Differential diagnoses for a delayed nephrogram with hydronephrosis: obstructive uropathy from a ureteral stone, ureteral mass, blood clot, fungus ball, or extrinsic mass.

- Differential diagnoses for a delayed nephrogram without hydronephrosis: renal artery stenosis or renal vein thrombosis. Both can result in initial enlargement and eventual atrophy.

- Differential diagnoses for bilateral enlarged kidneys without mass: acute inferior vena cava thrombosis, other causes of central venous obstruction, human immunodeficiency virus or diabetic nephropathy, acute glomerulonephritis, systemic lupus erythematosus, and lymphoma.

SECTION V
GENITOURINARY IMAGING

Image Rich 3

■ **Case**

Match the appropriate diagnosis to the provided images.
   A. Ovarian dermoid
   B. Endometrioma
   C. Hemorrhagic cyst
   D. Cystic epithelial neoplasm

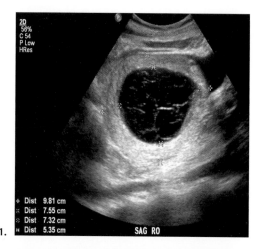

1.

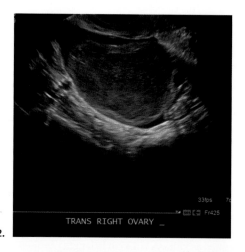

2.

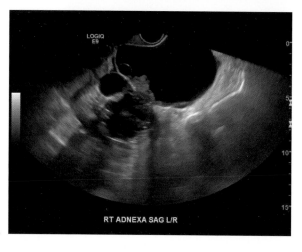

3.

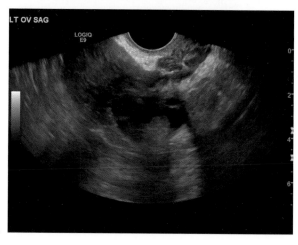

4.

■ Answers and Explanations

1. C. Hemorrhagic cyst. This case demonstrates a complex cystic lesion with internal echos in a lacy or reticular pattern. This is the classic ultrasound appearance of a hemorrhagic cyst. This cyst markedly expands the ovary, and it is important to exclude torsion with color Doppler imaging. According to the Society of Radiologic Ultrasound guidelines, cysts > 5 cm require a 6-week follow up ultrasound to ensure resolution. A short-term follow up ultrasound should show at least partial resolution for a simple hemorrhagic cyst, whereas an endometrioma will be unchanged.

2. B. Endometrioma. This case demonstrates a complex cystic lesion (evidenced by posterior accoustic enhancement) with homogenous internal echoes. This is the characteristic ultrasound appearance of an endometrioma. Echogenic mural foci are sometimes present, and these lesions can be multiloculated. Endometriomas are usually extremely hyperintense on T1-weighted magnetic resonance imaging with a degree of "shading" on T2-weighted images.

3. D. Cystic epithelial neoplasm. This case demonstrates a complex cystic lesion in the right adnexa. There are solid papillary projections within the larger cystic component. This sonographic appearance is very suspicious for neoplasm and, indeed, this lesion was surgically proven to represent a benign papillary serous cystadenoma. Cystic epithelial neoplasms are the second most common tumor of the ovary (after dermoids). They are the most common type of ovarian malignancy.

4. A. Ovarian dermoid. This case demonstrates an echogenic lesion with posterior acoustic shadowing. This is the classic appearance for a Rokitansky nodule in an ovarian dermoid. When this hyperechoic tissue with posterior shadowing is present, the diagnosis can be made on ultrasound with a high degree of certainty. Dermoids are bilateral in 10% of cases. They are sometimes responsible for ovarian torsion (the most common complication), and a small percentage will undergo malignant transformation. In equivocal cases, computed tomography or magnetic resonance imaging are usually diagnostic.

■ Suggested Readings

Alcázar JL, Laparte C, Jurado M, et al. The role of transvaginal ultrasonography combined with color velocity imaging and pulsed doppler in the diagnosis of endometrioma. Fertil Steril 1997;67:487–491

Kawamoto S, Urban BA, Fishman EK. CT of epithelial ovarian tumors. Radiographics 1999;19:S85–S102

Kurjak A, Zalud I, Alfirevic Z. Evaluation of adnexal masses with transvaginal color doppler ultrasound. J Ultrasound Med 1991;10:295–297

Levine D, Brown DL, Andreotti RG, et al. Management of asymptomatic ovarian and other adnexal cysts imaged at US: Society of Radiologists in Ultrasound consensus conference statement. Radiology 2010;256:943–954

Top Tips

- The 2010 Society of Radiologists in Ultrasound guidelines are the most widely accepted recommendations for cystic ovarian lesion followup.

- If premenopausal:

  - Benign cystic lesion (simple cyst, hemorrhagic cyst) ≤ 5 cm: No imaging follow up needed.

  - Benign simple cyst 5 to 7 cm: yearly ultrasound follow up.

  - Hemorrhagic cyst > 5 cm: Imaging follow up in 6 to 12 weeks to ensure resolution.

  - Anything suspicious (with vascular solid components/septations): Requires magnetic resonance imaging and/or surgical consultation.

- If postmenopausal:

  - Simple cyst up to 1 cm: No imaging follow up needed.

  - Simple cyst between 1 and 7 cm: Requires yearly imaging surveillance ultrasound.

  - Any size cyst with complexity (including hemorragic cysts) or suspicious lesion: Requires surgical consultation (if in early menopause, can image to resolution)

- At any age:

  - Endometrioma of any size: Initial follow up of 6 to 12 weeks, then yearly if not sugically removed.

  - Dermoid: Yearly ultrasound follow up to to ensure stability.

  - Hydrosalpinx/peritoneal inclusion cyst: As clinically indicated.

Image Rich 4

■ Case

Match the appropriate diagnosis to the provided images.
   A. Medullary sponge kidney
   B. Chronic lithium use
   C. Renal papillary necrosis
   D. Medullary nephrocalcinosis

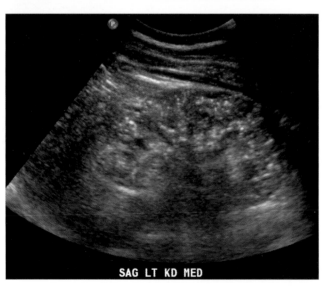

1.

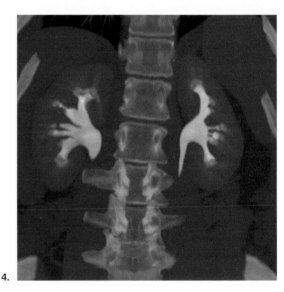

2.

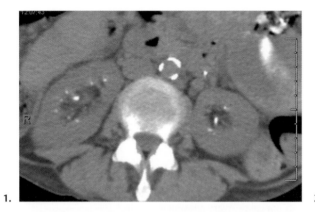

3.

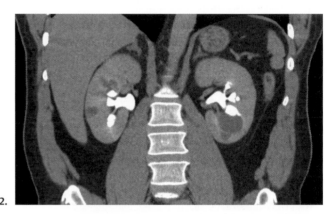

4.

■ Answers and Explanations

1. D. Medullary nephrocalcinosis. This case demonstrates calcification within the bilateral medullary pyramids. Medullary nephrocalcinosis is much more common than cortical nephrocalcinosis. The conditions that cause this entity can also lead to stone formation (urolithiasis). The most common causes of medullary calcinosis include hyperparathyroidism, medullary sponge kidney, and type 1 renal tubular acidosis. Less common causes include milk-alkali syndrome, sarcoidosis, and hypervitaminosis D. (Cortical nephrocalcinosis can be caused by **c**ortical necrosis, **o**xalosis, **A**lport syndrome, and [chronic] **g**lomerulonephritis. The mnemonic is COAG.)

2. C. Renal papillary necrosis. This case demonstrates contrast pooling within the renal papilla, creating a "ball on tee" appearance. Renal papillary necrosis refers to ischemic necrosis of the renal papillae. Classic features include forniceal excavation, a lobster claw appearance, the signet ring sign, and sloughed papillae with clubbed calyces. There is eventual sloughing of the tissue, and this can pass into the urinary tract. The most common causes of papillary necrosis are **n**onsteroidal anti-inflammatory use, **s**ickle cell disease, **a**nalgesic abuse, **i**nfection, **d**iabetes, and **d**ehydration (mnemonic is NSAID). Additional causes include cirrhosis, renal vein thrombosis, tuberculosis, and obstructive uropathy.

3. B. Chronic lithium nephropathy. This case demonstrates multiple small echogenic foci. These foci are not the result of calcification, however. They are actually due to multiple tiny cysts in which the sound reverberates within the walls. Multiple tiny cysts can be associated with chronic lithium nephropathy and are present in about 50% of patients undergoing this treatment. The magnetic resonance imaging appearance is very characteristic and can be helpful in making the diagnosis. Knowledge of the clinical history is paramount.

4. A. Medullary sponge kidney. This case demonstrate a "paintbrush" appearance of the collecting tubules. The calcyces are broad, shallow, and distorted, with striated saccular collections of contrast in the renal papilla. This is a case of medullary sponge kidney (benign renal tubular ectasia). There is cystic dilatation of the collecting tubules, and urine stasis in the tubules eventually leads to stone formation. The exact etiology is unknown, and this condition is usually incidental and asymptomatic. It occurs more commonly in males than in females, and is usually bilateral. The kidneys remain normal in size. Plain film can demonstrate nephrocalcinosis. There is an association with Caroli disease (congential cystic dilatation of intrahepatic ducts).

■ Suggested Readings

Di Salvo DN, Park J, Laing FC. Lithium nephropathy: unique sonographic findings. J Ultrasound Med 2012;31:637–644

Dyer RB, Chen MY, Zagoria RJ. Abnormal calcifications in the urinary tract. Radiographics 1998;18:1405–1424

Joffe SA, Servaes S, Okon S, et al. Multi-detector row CT urography in the evaluation of hematuria. Radiographics 2003;23:1441–1455

Roque A, Herédia V, Ramalho M, et al. MR findings of lithium-related kidney disease: preliminary observations in four patients. Abdom Imaging 2012;37:140–146

SECTION V GENITOURINARY IMAGING

Top Tips

◆ It is important to differentiate urolithiasis from other calcifications in the kidney, which include medullary nephrocalcinosis, cortical nephrocalcinosis, and vascular calcifications.

◆ Papillary necrosis differential diagnoses: The mnemonic is NSAID (**n**onsteroidal anti-inflammatory drugs [most common], **s**ickle cell disease, **a**nalgesic abuse, **i**nfection, **d**iabetes, and **d**ehydration).

◆ Medullary nephrocalcinosis differential diagnoses: Most commonly caused by hyperparathyroidism, medullary sponge kidney (ectatic tubules, "paintbrush" appearance), and type 1 renal tubular acidosis.

Image Rich 5

■ Case

Match the appropriate diagnosis to the provided images.
A. Seminoma
B. Burned out germ cell tumor
C. Microlithiasis
D. Fourier gangrene

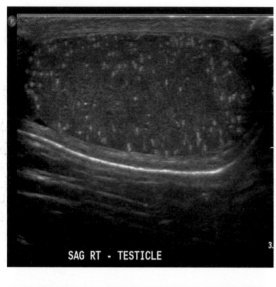

1.

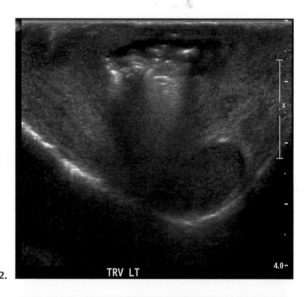

2.

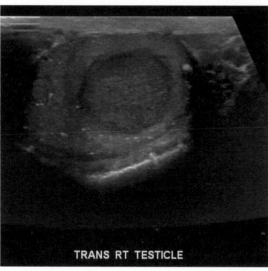

3.

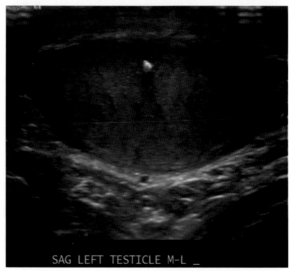

4.

■ Answers and Explanations

1. C. Testicular microlithiasis (TM). This case demonstrates multiple tiny calcifications throughout the testes. TM is a benign and common idiopathic condition that is defined by at least five calcific foci seen on one testicular ultrasound image. If fewer than five foci are present, some refer to this as "limited microlithiasis." There is a somewhat controversial association with germ cell tumors. Management of patients with TM is also controversial. Most experts recommend that asymptomatic patients should at least perform self-physical examinations, and those with symptoms or other risk factors should be followed with an annual ultrasound. Risk factors for germ cell testicular neoplasm include personal or family history of germ cell tumor, testicular maldescent, orchiopexy, and testicular atrophy.

2. D. Fournier gangrene. This case demonstrates echogenic foci with dirty shadowing. This is consistent with air, rather than calcification, in the scrotal tissues. When this finding of probable air is found, Fournier gangrene must be excluded. Fournier is a urologic emergency requiring surgical debridement, and that was the diagnosis here.

3. A. Testicular seminoma. This case demonstrates a homogenous hypoechoic mass in the right testicle (with a background of testicular microlithiasis). Testicular seminoma is the most common testicular tumor. In young men, 95% of testicular cancers are germ cell tumors, and 5% are sex cord-stromal tumors. Approximately half of germ cell tumors are seminoma, and half are nonseminomatous germ cell tumors. Seminoma tends to be hypoechoic and more homogeneous than nonseminomatous testicular tumors. This was seminoma.

4. B. Burned-out germ cell tumor. This case demonstrates a single calcification in the left testicle. The differential diagnosis for this calcification includes a burnt-out germ cell tumor, sequelae of prior infection, and sequelae of prior trauma. This is too large and coarse (and solitary) to represent microlithiasis. Regarding germ cell tumor, a testicular calcification may be the only finding on ultrasound, and a soft tissue component need not be present. This can be a difficult sonographic diagnosis, and a high level of suspicion is needed when evaluating testicular calcifications. This turned out to be a clinically occult, intratesticular, primary germ cell malignancy that was discovered in a man with abdominal lymphadenopathy. Because primary extragonadal germ cell tumors are rare, identification of a germ cell neoplasm in a retroperitoneal, visceral, or mediastinal mass should prompt sonographic evaluation of the testes.

■ Suggested Readings

Cast JE, Nelson WM, Early AS, et al. Testicular microlithiasis: prevalence and tumor risk in a population referred for scrotal sonography. Am J Roentgenol 2000;175:1703–1706

Top Tips

♦ TM is defined by at least five tiny echogenic foci seen on a single testicular ultrasound image. If several (but fewer than five) foci are seen, then the term "limited microlithiasis" is used.

♦ An increased risk of malignancy in TM is controversial. Current urologic guidelines advocate periodic routine physical self-examination to exclude a testicular mass. Some clinicians opt for annual surveillance ultrasound, particularly if there are additional risk factors.

♦ A solitary coarse calcification, with or without an associated soft tissue mass, should raise concern for a possible occult burned out germ cell tumor.

More Challenging 1

■ Case

A 52-year-old man presents with elevated PSA.

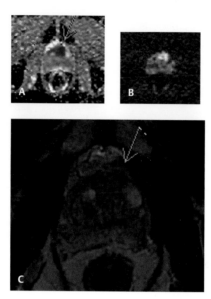

■ Questions

1. Regarding prostate cancer, based on the provided magnetic resonance imaging (MRI), which ONE of the following is the patient's diagnosis?
   A. Normal study. No evidence of prostate cancer or suspicious nodule.
   B. Suspicious nodule in the transition zone. No evidence for extracapsular disease.
   C. Suspicious nodule in the transition zone. Positive for extracapsular disease.
   D. Suspicious nodule in the transition zone. Positive for extracapsular disease. Positive for distant metastatic disease.
   E. Prostatitis. No evidence of prostate cancer or suspicious nodule.

2. Which of the following multiparametric MRI sequences are very useful for the diagnosis of prostate cancer? Select ALL that apply.
   A. T2
   B. Dynamic contrast-enhanced (DCE) T1
   C. DWI
   D. Gradient echo
   E. Fluid-attenuated inversion recovery (FLAIR)

3. Regarding prostate cancer, which of the following are correct? Select ALL that apply.
   A. Clinically significant disease is recognized as Gleason score 3 + 3 = 6 or greater.
   B. Detectable prostate-specific antigen following radical prostatectomy suggests recurrent disease.
   C. Problems with TRUS biopsy include high false-negative rates and understaging of disease.
   D. The most common complications with prostatectomy include impotence and incontinence.
   E. About 50% of patients aged 50 will have at least microscopic prostate cancer.

■ Answers and Explanations

Question 1

C. Correct! There is a suspicious nodule in the anterior transition zone and there is direct extension beyond the capsule. Extracapsular extension upstages the cancer from T2 to T3, which is a pivotal finding when staging prostate cancer, as this may alter management from prostatectomy to radiation and hormonal therapy. Even with state-of-the-art multiparametric prostate MRI, accuracy at extracapsular detection is sometimes marginal. Some readers believe that if extracapsular extension is a soft call, leaning toward nonextension is recommended, giving the patient "a chance at surgical cure." Conversely, more recent literature suggests that extracapsular extension is under-called on MRI.

Other choices and discussion

A. The study is not normal. Multiparametric prostate MRI can exclude clinically significant cancer with > 90% accuracy. The negative predictive value for Gleason 4 + 3 = 7 is 97%, and the negative predictive value for Gleason 3 + 4 = 7 is 90%. For comparison, the negative predictive value for the current standard of care transrectal ultrasound (TRUS) biopsy is 65 to 70%.

B. Extracapsular disease is present. For uniformity and clarity in communication, prostate nodules are reported with Prostate Imaging Reporting and Data System (PI-RADS). PI-RADS nodules range from 1 to 5, with 1 benign and 5 malignant. A total of 70% of prostate cancer occurs in the peripheral zone, where MRI accuracy is the greatest.

D. There is a suspicious nodule and extracapsular disease, but no evidence for distant metastatic disease demonstrated. Most of the prostate MRI protocol is performed with high resolution and small field of view imaging to assess the gland, seminal vesicles, and immediately surrounding soft tissues. However, at least one large field of view sequence is recommended to assess the whole pelvis for osseous metastases and pelvic lymphadenopathy.

E. Prostatitis may result in interpretation error and confusion with prostate cancer if the inflammation is focal. More commonly, however, prostatitis presents as patchy or diffuse T2 signal abnormality and in these cases, is easy to distinguish from cancer. Hyperintense signal within the prostate gland on precontrast T1 imaging is usually the result of prior biopsy.

Question 2

A. Correct! T2 is the traditional sequence for prostate MRI and utilizes anatomic variation to identify masses. Prostate cancer demonstrates T2 hypointense signal relative to the normal gland. T2 is the most important sequence in the central gland, where it is the primary determinant of the PI-RADS classification.

B. Correct! Cancers enhance. DCE utilizes contrast injection and software with kinetic models to optimally graph the enhancement. Cancer tends to demonstrate rapid dynamic contrast enhancement. DCE has become less important, based on the latest research, and plays a reduced role in PI-RADS V2.

C. Correct! Cancers demonstrate restricted diffusion. DWI is the most important sequence in the peripheral zone. PI-RADS V2 is almost entirely based on DWI/apparent diffusion coefficient in the peripheral zone.

Other choices and discussion

D. Gradient echo is not a standard parameter for prostate cancer assessment. Gradient echo, in general, is quite useful in detecting blood products.

E. FLAIR is not a standard parameter for prostate cancer assessment. FLAIR, in general, is an inversion recovery technique that nullifies fluid.

Question 3

B. Correct! Detectable PSA following radical prostatectomy suggests recurrent disease. The most widely accepted definition of biochemical recurrence is a PSA > 0.2 ng/mL that has risen on two consecutive samples taken at least 2 weeks apart by the same laboratory.

C. Correct! TRUS biopsy has a false-negative rate of 35% and understages Gleason scores by 35%.

D. Correct! The most common complications with prostatectomy include impotence and incontinence. These complications have led some urologists to instead perform focal therapy in low-risk prostate cancer.

E. Correct! About 50% of patients aged 50 will have at least microscopic prostate cancer. Pathology results describe the incidence of prostate cancer to be similar to the age of the patient. For example, a 40-year-old has a 40% chance of at least microscopic cancer. However, most of these cancers are clinically insignificant (similar to some well-differentiated thyroid and ductal carcinoma in situ breast cancers).

Other choices and discussion

A. Although there is some debate, clinically significant disease is recognized as Gleason 3 + 4 = 7 or greater. Gleason 6 or less is usually considered "clinically insignificant." The index lesion is typically the largest and most aggressive lesion and has the highest Gleason score. It is the index lesion that is the most important in determining prognosis, and multiparametric MRI can greatly assist in detecting this index lesion.

Top Tips

- ◆ Multiparametric prostate MRI can exclude clinically significant cancer with > 90% accuracy.

- ◆ DWI is the most important sequence in the peripheral zone. T2 is the most important sequence in the central gland. DCE is important in posttreatment patients.

- ◆ A total of 70% of prostate cancer occurs in the peripheral zone, where MRI accuracy is the greatest.

More Challenging 2

■ Case

A 68-year-old woman presents with vaginal bleeding. Ultrasound and magnetic resonance imaging (MRI) of uterus are provided.

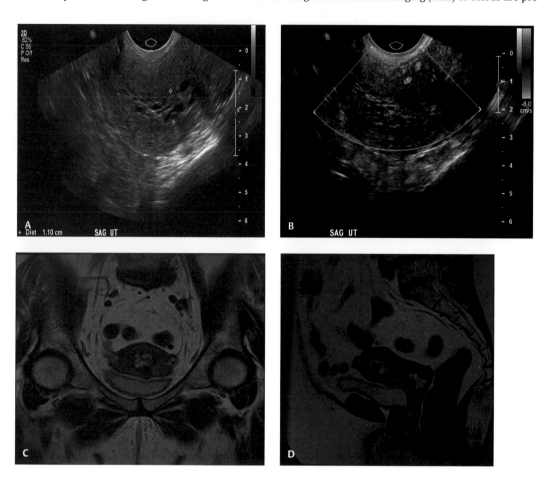

■ Questions

1. What is the diagnosis? Think about what pertinent history would be helpful.
   A. Cystic endometrial hyperplasia
   B. Endometrial cancer
   C. Adenomyosis
   D. Trophoblastic disease

2. What is the next best step?
   A. Continued surveillance imaging
   B. Endometrial sampling
   C. Hysterectomy
   D. Discontinuation of tamoxifen

3. What is normal endometrial thickness in the pre- and postmenopausal patient?
   A. Up to 15 mm for both pre- and postmenopausal patients
   B. Up to 20 mm for premenopausal patients and up to 10 to 13 mm for postmenopausal patients
   C. Up to 15 mm for premenopausal patients and up to 5 to 8 mm for postmenopausal patients
   D. Up to 20 mm for premenopausal patients and up to 5 mm for postmenopausal patients

■ Answers and Explanations

Question 1

A. Correct! This patient has CEH. The endometrium is thickened (measuring 11 mm) and is associated with mutliple cysts. CEH is associated with tamoxifen use, which is pertinent to know when interpreting this study. CEH is the most common and relatively benign form of endometrial hyperplasia. However, vigilance for endometrial malignancy should be high.

Other choices and discussion

B. Endometrial cancer could look similar, which is why direct sampling is usually performed in cases of CEH. On ultrasound, endometrial cancer typically appears as thickening of the endometrial stripe, but may appear as a polypoid mass or as cystic areas in the stripe. The majority of cases develop in the setting of unopposed hyperestrogen stimulation and endometrial hyperplasia. Less commonly, cancer develops in the setting of endometrial atrophy.

C. Adenomyosis represents cystic change within the myometrium (not the endometrium) from submucosal deposition of endometrial tissue. Detection and characterization of adenomyosis is variable and limited by ultrasound unless cystic foci are seen in the myometrium. MRI is much more sensitive and accurate in detection of adenomyosis.

D. Trophoblastic disease could also look similar and mimic CEH. Supporting clinical information of an elevated beta- Human chorionic gonadotropin would be needed.

Question 2

B. Correct! Endometrial sampling with cytology is generally indicated as any atypia puts the patient at increased risk for endometrial cancer.

The other choices are incorrect.

Question 3

C. Correct! Normal endometrial thickness is up to 15 mm for premenopausal patients and up to 5 to 8 mm for postmenopausal patients. In a postmenopausal patient without bleeding, 5 mm is the limit without hormone replacement therapy (HRT) and 8 mm if on HRT (such as tamoxifen). In a postmenopausal patient with bleeding, the endometrium should measure < 5 mm (whether on HRT or not).

The other choices are incorrect.

■ Suggested Readings

Fleischer AC. Sonographic assessment of endometrial disorders. Semin Ultrasound CT MR 1999;20:259–266

Jorizzo JR, Chen MY, Martin D, et al. Spectrum of endometrial hyperplasia and its mimics on saline hysterosonography. Am J Roentgenol 2002;179:385–389

Top Tips

◆ Endometrial stripe thickness:

If premenopausal, the endometrial stripe can be up to 15 mm.

If postmenopausal and no bleeding, the stripe should be < 5 mm or < 8 mm if on HRT/tamoxifen.

If postmenopausal with bleeding, the stripe should be < 5 mm regardless of HRT status.

◆ The most common cause of postmenopausal bleeding is atrophy of the uterine/vaginal lining.

◆ Tamoxifen causes endometrial hyperplasia, usually in a benign cystic fasion.

More Challenging 3

■ Case

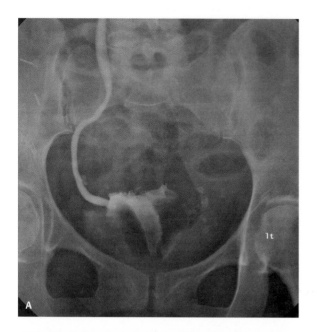

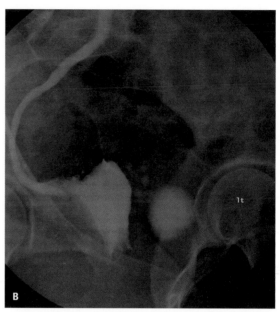

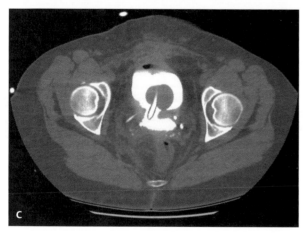

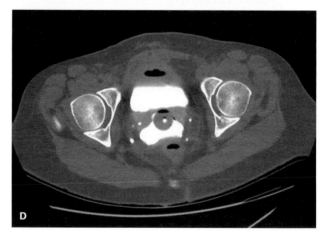

■ Questions

1. Status post right ureteroscopy with right nephrostomy tube placement. Images shown are after injection of the right nephrostomy tube. Computed tomography (CT) was subsequently performed. No history provided. What is the diagnosis?
   A. Colovesicular fistula
   B. Vesicovaginal fistula
   C. Bladder rupture
   D. Colovaginal fistula

2. What is the MOST common cause of this entity in the Western world?
   A. Infection
   B. Prolonged birth
   C. Gynecologic surgery
   D. Diverticulitis

3. If the abnormality cannot be seen by CT cystogram, what imaging modality is recommended?
   A. Transrectal ultrasound
   B. Pelvic magnetic resonance imaging (MRI)
   C. Renal scintigraphy
   D. Hysterosalpinography

■ Answers and Explanations

Question 1

B. Correct! This is a vesicovaginal fistula. There is opacification of the vagina on this CT cystogram. Because contrast was instilled into the urinary bladder, there must be a connection between the lower urinary tract and the anterior vagina. Clinically, this presents with draining of urine through the vagina. Fluoroscopic cystogram is the most common method used for this evaluation. CT cystography is also a good diagnostic choice.

The other choices are incorrect.

Question 2

C. Correct! Gynecologic surgery (usually hysterectomy) is the most common cause of a vesicovaginal fistula in the developed world. Prolonged obstructed labor is the most common cause in undeveloped countries. Pelvic malignancy, radiotherapy, trauma, and uterine rupture are other causes of vesicovaginal fistula. If discovered within a few days of surgery, a suprapubic catheter should be placed for up to 30 days and small fistulae may heal on their own. Sometimes surgery and graft placement is necessary for larger communications or for patients who fail conservative therapy. Surgery is usually performed fairly early unless the tissue has been irradiated or is infected. Radiated tissue is usually left up to 1 year before surgical repair to ensure optimal tissue healing.

The other choices are incorrect.

Question 3

B. Correct! Sometimes subtle fistulas of the lower genitourinary system can be picked by MRI (especially high-resolution T2 sequences), even though there is no abnormality detected by cystogram. A fluid-filled track can be readily apparent on T2-weighted images. The tract also tends to enhance.

Other choices and discussion

A. Sonography will not demonstrate a fistula unless it is fairly large.

C. Renal scintigraphy is less sensitive than CT cystogram for this purpose.

D. Hysterosalpinography is less sensitive than CT cystogram for this purpose.

■ Suggested Readings

Jafri SZ, Roberts JL, Berger BD. Fistulas of the genitourinary tract. In: Pollack HM, McClennan BL, eds. Clinical Urography. Philadelphia, PA: Saunders; 2000:2992–3011

Yu NC, Raman SS, Patel M, et al. Fistulas of the genitourinary tract: a radiologic review. Radiographics 2004;24:1331–1352

Top Tips

◆ Vesicovaginal fistulas are most commonly caused by gynecologic surgery and prolonged labor.

◆ Colovesicular fistulas are most commonly caused by diverticulitis and colon cancer.

◆ Fluoroscopic exams help evaluate for genitourinary fistulas. If a vesicovaginal or colovesicular fistula is suspected, a cystogram should be performed. If a rectovaginal fistula is suspected, a barium enema should be performed. The CT equivalents of these are also suitable. Subtle fistulas and their sinus tracts can be picked up by MRI.

More Challenging 4

■ Case

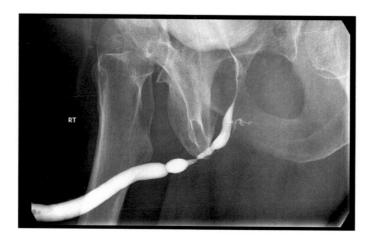

■ Questions

1. Where is the abnormality located?
    A. Prostatic urethra
    B. Membranous urethra
    C. Bulbar urethra
    D. Penile urethra

2. What is the MOST likely cause of this finding?
    A. Radiation
    B. Pelvic fracture
    C. Infection
    D. Congenital anomaly

3. What examination is performed in this case, and what is a typical indication for this study?
    A. Antegrade urethrogram, to assess ureteral integrity following trauma
    B. RUG, to assess ureteral integrity following trauma
    C. RUG, to assess the periurethral glands
    D. Antegrade urethrogram, to assess the periurethral glands

■ Answers and Explanations

Question 1

C. Correct! The image demonstrates narrowing/stricture of the bulbar urethra.

Other choices and discussion

The other choices are incorrect.

The male urethra is made of the anterior urethra and the posterior urethra. The anterior urethra is divided into the penile and bulbar portions. The posterior urethra is divided into the membranous and prostatic urethra. The penile urethra is the longest portion. The glands of Littré and bulbourethral glands (Cowper glands) enter the urethra at the bulbous portion. The membranous urethra is the shortest portion and passes through the urogenital diaphragm. The prostatic urethra is surrounded by the prostate. The smooth muscle verumontanum lies on its posterior wall. The ejaculatory ducts enter the urethra at this site.

Incidentally, the Cowper glands are opacified in this case, and these are not usually seen. These normal structures tend to opacify in the setting of stricture or infection. Opacification of the prostatic ducts, Cowper ducts, and periurethral Littré glands are often associated with urethral inflammatory and stricture disease.

Question 2

C. Correct! Infection is the most common cuase of urethral stricture. The most common infectious etiology in a young male is gonococcal urethritis, followed second in frequency by *Chlamydia*. Other common causes include trauma and instrumentation. Less common causes of urethra stricture include radiation, inflammatory balanitis xerotica obliterans, and congenital anomalies.

Other choices and discussion

A. Radiation is a less common cause of stricture than infection.

B. Pelvic fracture is a less common cause of stricture than infection. An anterior urethral injury is usually caused by straddle-type trauma, whereas a posterior urethral injury is caused by crushing forces with associated pelvic fractures. If there is blood at the urethral meatus following trauma, a retrograde urethrogram (RUG) should be performed PRIOR to a cysturethrogram. Catheterization is contraindicated prior to evaluation of the urethra.

D. Congenital anomaly is a less common cause of stricture than infection.

Question 3

B. Correct! RUG is the primary method used to image the urethra and is performed in the setting of trauma, or to assess urethral strictures and fistulas. Technique: The balloon of a 16 or 18-F Foley catheter is inserted in the fossa navicularis of the penile urethra and inflated with 1 to 1.5 mL saline. A total of 20 to 30 mL of 60% iodinated contrast material is then hand injected with a syringe under fluoroscopic guidance until the anterior urethra is opacified. Spasm of the external urethral sphincter is common and may prevent filling of the deep bulbar, membranous, and prostatic urethra. Application of slow, gentle pressure is helpful in minimizing this spasm. Visual confirmation of flow into the urinary bladder is desired. This procedure is not used to assess the periurethral glands, which are sometimes incidentally seen.

Voiding cystorethrogram, an antegrade study, is commonly used to evaluate the posterior urethra. Sometimes, both RUG and voiding cystorethrogram are performed for thorough assessment.

■ Suggested Readings

Amis ES, Jr, Newhouse JH, Cronan JJ. Radiology of male periurethral structures. Am J Roentgenol 1988;151:321–324

Sandler CM, Corriere JN Jr. Urethrography in the diagnosis of acute urethral injuries. Urol Clin North Am 1989;16:283–289

McCallum RW. The adult male urethra: normal anatomy, pathology, and method of urethrography. Radiol Clin North Am 1979;17:227–244

Kawashima A, Sandler CM, Wasserman NF. Imaging of urethral disease: a pictorial review. Radiographics 2004;24(suppl 1):S195–S216

Top Tips

- RUG is indicated in the setting of trauma with blood at the meatus to exclude injury to the urethra. RUG must be performed PRIOR to placement of a Foley catheter. RUG is also used to assess strictures and fistulae.

- It is important to know the anatomy of the urethra. From proximal to distal, the prostatic and membranous portions make up the posterior urethra, and the bulbar and penile portions make up the anterior urethra. Tip: "PM-BP": At night (in the PM), you take your blood pressure (BP) medication.

- Injury or strcture of the anterior urethra is due to straddle injury/infection. Injury to the posterior urethra is due to pelvic fractures.

More Challenging 5

■ Case

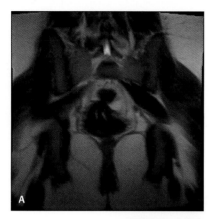
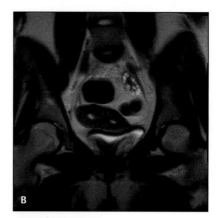

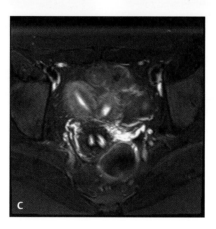

■ Questions

1. A patient presents with pelvic pain. What type müllerian duct anomaly (MDA) is this?
   A. Arcuate uterus
   B. Unicornuate uterus
   C. Bicornuate uterus
   D. Septate uterus

2. What type of MDA is MOST associated with miscarriage?
   A. Arcuate uterus
   B. Unicornuate uterus
   C. Bicornuate uterus
   D. Septate uterus

3. What causes a "T-shaped" uterus?
   A. In utero exposure to diethylstilbestrol (DES)
   B. Exposure to herpes simplex virus-1
   C. Not related to any exposure
   D. Genetically inherited

■ Answers and Explanations

Question 1

C. Correct! This is a bicornuate bicollis MDA. There are two uterine horns and two cervices separated by a septum. MDAs are associated with renal anomalies, such as agenesis and cross fused renal ectopia, in 29% of cases. They are not associated with ovarian anomalies. Hysterosalpingogram is limited in its ability to diagnose these anomalies, as assessing the external uterine contour is necessary for diagnosis. Ultrasound is often able to accurately assess, and magnetic resonance imaging is the gold standard in diagnosis and characterization.

Other choices and discussion

A. An arcuate uterus is characterized by a mild indentation of the external fundal contour. Two separate uterine horns and cervices would not be present.

B. Uterine didelphys could have a similar appearance. However, the cervices are more divergent with didelphys.

D. A sepate uterus would not have two separate cervices. Although not optimally demonstrated here, differentiation of a bicornuate uterus from a septate uterus can be accomplished by assessing the external uterine fundal contour. Lack of a cleft in the external uterine fundal contour is consistent with a septate uterus. A prominent cleft is seen with a bicornuate uterus.

Question 2

D. Correct! Septate uterus is the most common MDA associated with miscarriage (90% miscarriage rate), and it is also the most common MDA among women who experience difficulty with conception. Miscarriage in a septate uterus is due to the variable blood supply of the septum, which can be muscular and fibrous. Resection of the septum improves the rate of successful pregnancy.

Other choices and discussion

A. An arcuate uterus is the most common of the MDA in the general population, affecting 3.9% of all women. Arcuate and septate are resorption anomalies, whereas didelphys and bicornuate are fusion anomalies.

B. A unicornuate uterus is one with absence of a second uterine horn, or only a rudimentary uterine horn. If endometrium is seen within a rudimentary horn, it should be reported, as endometrial tissue at this site may cause symptoms of endometriosis and pregancy issues including uterine rupture.

C. A bicornuate uterus is usually asymptomatic.

Question 3

A. Correct! A "T-shaped" uterus is caused by in utero exposure to DES, a synthetic estrogen used to decrease the rate of spontaneous abortion. This anomaly is present in 31% of exposed women. DES exposure is also associated with clear cell carcinoma of the vagina/cervix.

The other choices are incorrect.

■ Suggested Readings

Behr SC, Courtier JL, Qayyum A. Imaging of müllerian duct anomalies. Radiographics 2012;32:E233–E250

Troiano RN, McCarthy SM. Mullerian duct anomalies: imaging and clinical issues. Radiology 2004;233:19–34

Zagoria RJ. Genitourinary Radiology: The Requisites. Maryland Heights, MO: Mosby Inc.; 2004

Top Tips

◆ Hysterosalpingogram is limited in the assessment of MDA.

◆ It is particularly important to differentiate a bicornuate from a septate uterus, as this has treatment and prognostic implications. Look for an external uterine fundal cleft. If present and > 1 cm, bicornuate is favored over sepate.

◆ With a unicornuate uterus, if a rudimentary horn is found, assess for endometrium.

Essentials 1

■ Case

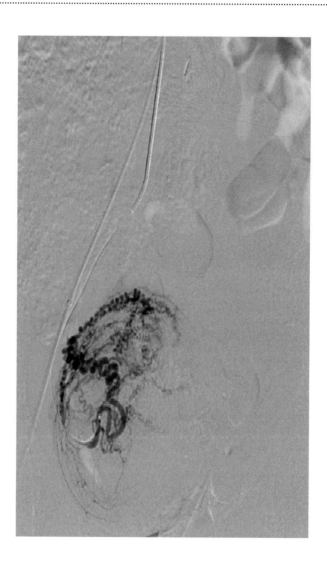

■ Questions

1. The uterine artery anatomically arises from which major pelvic arterial branch?
   A. The posterior division of the internal iliac artery
   B. The anterior division of the internal iliac artery
   C. The inferior mesenteric artery
   D. The anterior division of the inferior gluteal artery

2. Uterine fibroid embolization (UFE) is typically performed using which type of embolic material?
   A. Coils
   B. Glue
   C. Ethanol
   D. Particles

3. What is the best preprocedural planning study for uterine fibroid embolization?
   A. Magnetic resonance imaging
   B. Ultrasound
   C. Computed tomography
   D. Hysterosalpingogram

■ Answers and Explanations

Question 1

B. Correct! The uterine artery traditionally arises from the anterior division of the internal iliac artery on each side of the pelvis.

Other choices and discussion

A. The uterine artery traditionally arises from the *anterior*, not the posterior, division of the internal iliac artery.

C. The inferior mesenteric artery supplies the left colon and rectum.

D. The inferior gluteal artery (like the uterine artery) is a branch of the anterior division of the internal iliac artery, but it does not supply the uterus.

Question 2

D. Correct! Particles, in various forms, are used to provide optimal distal embolization of fibroids during UFE. Either spherical embolic beads or irregular polyvinyl alcohol particles are employed. A total of 500 to 700 micron and 700 to 900 micron particles are the most common sizes used. Studies have shown that smaller particles do not provide a benefit over these larger particles, except in cases of adenomyosis.

Following treatment, intracavitary fibroids may slough and pass as fragments. Retained fragments have the potential to become infected. Uterine necrosis is a rare post z embolization phenomenon.

Other choices and discussion

A. Coils are good at achieving vessel occlusion, but do not provide enough distal occlusion for an optimal UFE result.

B. Glue is a liquid embolic and can achieve deeper penetration than coils. However, it is not traditionally used for fibroid embolization. It is expensive and, at times, challenging to work with.

C. Ethanol is a liquid embolic that is a powerful sclerosing agent. Potential limitations include risk of tissue necrosis and difficulty in achieving predictable results.

Question 3

A. Correct! MRI is the preferred study in the United States to evaluate a patient prior to fibroid embolization. MRI provides information on fibroid vascularity (based on enhancement), fibroid location, potential presence of adnexal or additional uterine masses, potential presence of adenomyosis, and helps to define other vessels that may supply the fibroids. MRI may also be used to evaluate posttreatment efficacy.

Fibroid embolization should not be performed if there is a suspicion for leiomyosarcoma. Differentiating leiomyosarcoma from uterine fibroids can be quite challenging with imaging. Patients that have tremendous bulk symptoms, or patients that demand guaranteed eradication of their fibroids, may benefit from hysterectomy or myomectomy over UFE. If uterine artery embolization does not successfully treat all of the fibroids, an ovarian supply to the residual fibroids should be considered.

Other choices and discussion

B. Ultrasound is also a very good way to evaluate the uterus and ovaries. MRI has advantages over ultrasound, as listed above. However, ultrasound is a reasonable preprocedural approach for UFE when MRI is not available.

C. Computed tomography does not provide the detail needed for UFE that MRI and ultrasound offer.

D. HSG is typically used to evaluate female patients for an anatomic source of infertility or to assess the efficacy of implantable contraception devices in the fallopian tube. HSG does not provide robust information about fibroids. Theoretically, HSG could be helpful in evaluating intracavitary fibroids.

■ Suggested Readings

Deshumkh SP, Gonsalves CF, Guglielmo FF, Mitchell DG. Role of MRI imaging of uterine leiomyomas before and after embolization. Radiographics 2012;32(6):E251–E281

Top Tips

- A total of 500 to 700 micron or 700 to 900 micron particles are typically used for uterine artery embolization.

- Cervical fibroids do not respond as well to UFE because they often have alternate blood supply.

- The symptom that drives most women to seek treatment for fibroids is menorrhagia.

Essentials 2

■ Case

This patient is status post cardiac catheterization.

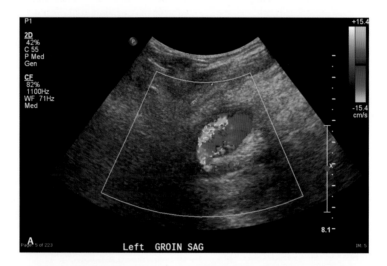

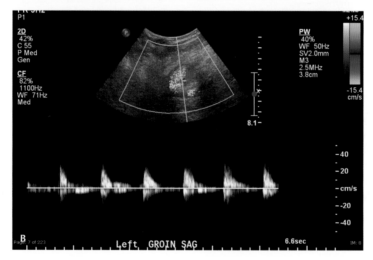

■ Questions

1. The test image depicts what abnormality?
   A. Arteriovenous fistula
   B. Pseudoaneurysm
   C. Arterial thrombus
   D. Arterial dissection

2. Which of the following methods of treatment for a pseudoaneurysm in this location is LEAST desirable?
   A. Ultrasound-guided compression
   B. Thrombin injection
   C. Surgical repair
   D. Covered stent placement

3. Which pseudoaneurysm characteristics are most amenable to safe treatment with thrombin injection?
   A. Short, wide neck
   B. Long, wide neck
   C. Long, narrow neck
   D. All of the above

■ Answers and Explanations

Question 1

B. Correct! This represents a pseudoaneurysm. To-and-fro flow is depicted as red and blue color Doppler flow (yin-yang sign). This is seen within a hypoechoic sac adjacent to an artery. This is the typical sonographic appearance of a pseudoaneurysm. These usually occur after catheterization or other trauma. Pseudoaneurysms that are symptomatic and/or are > 2 cm are frequently treated. Small pseudoaneurysms often thrombose without treatment.

Other choices and discussion

A. An AV fistula would present with arterial flow in the adjacent vein, not the to-and-fro color Doppler appearance shown here.

C. Pseudoaneurysms may contain thrombus, but no thrombus is present here.

D. Iatrogenic dissection is a potential complication of catheterization, but no dissection flap is identified here.

Question 2

D. Correct! Covered stent placement across a joint, such as the hip, is undesirable because of the risk of stent fracture from the motion of the joint.

Other choices and discussion

A. Ultrasound-guided compression is a traditional treatment used for common femoral artery pseudoaneurysm. Ultrasound is less invasive than surgery and yields good results. Ultrasound-guided compression is less successful in patients on anticoagulation.

B. Thrombin injection into the pseudoaneurysm sac has now become the standard treatment for common femoral artery pseudoaneurysm.

C. Historically, surgery was the first-line treatment for pseudoaneurysm that failed manual compression.

Question 3

C. Correct! A long, narrow neck to a pseudoaneurysm is the most favorable configuration to allow for safe thrombin injection. A long distance to the parent artery and a narrow channel of flow between the pseudoaneurysm and artery make the likelihood of inadvertent introduction of thrombin into the native artery less likely.

Thrombin is usually reconstituted to 1000 U per mL. However, some practitioners dilute it further to 100 U per mL. Another consideration in choosing a therapy is that some patients may be allergic to thrombin.

The other choices have increased risk of complications.

■ Suggested Readings

Webber GW, Jang J, Gustavson S, Olin JW. Contemporary management of postcatheterization pseudoaneurysms. Circulation 2007;115:2666–2674

Top Tips

♦ Thrombin injection should be performed in a part of the pseudoaneurysm sac away from the neck. This reduces the chance of embolization of thrombin down the extremity.

♦ The success rate for thrombin injection is > 90%.

♦ Thrombin injection should not be attempted on pseudoaneurysms that arise from arterial anastomoses or from mycotic pseudoaneurysms.

Essentials 3

■ Case

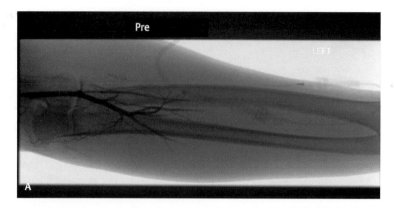

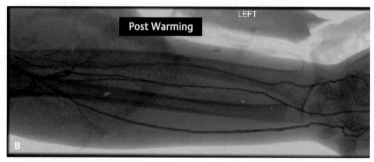

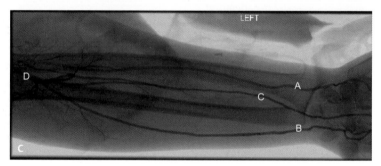

■ Questions

1. What is the most likely clinical history for this 25-year-old patient?
   A. Atrial fibrillation
   B. Renal failure on dialysis
   C. Cold hands
   D. Post trauma with pain
   E. Unilateral arm swelling

2. Match the letter to the correct vessel on the test image.
   _ Brachial artery
   _ Interosseous artery
   _ Radial artery
   _ Ulnar artery

3. The deep palmar arch is typically supplied by which artery?
   A. Radial artery
   B. Ulnar artery
   C. Princeps pollicis artery
   D. Radialis indicis artery

4. How does a Barbeau test differ from an Allen test?
   A. A blood pressure cuff is used in an Allen test.
   B. A pulse oximeter is used in a Barbeau test.
   C. There are four classifications for the result of an Allen test.
   D. The Barbeau test determines the patency of the radial artery.

■ Answers and Explanations

Question 1

C. Correct! The patient presented with bilateral cold hands. This patient has vasoconstriction that is reversible when the extremity is warmed. This finding is consistent with a thermally related vasoconstrictive process (Raynaud syndrome). Raynaud syndrome is not typically diagnosed with angiography or any given endovascular treatment.

Other choices and discussion

A. Atrial fibrillation resulting in emboli to all of the forearm arteries is unlikely in this 25-year-old. Additionally, reversal of impaired circulation with warming of the arm would not be expected.

B. Although it is unknown if the patient has renal failure, there does not appear to be calcification of the arteries, and no fistula is identified. If a fistula was present, steal could be considered.

D. There is no evidence of active extravasation/bleeding, aneurysm, or pseudoaneurysm to support a history of trauma. It is unlikely for changes from trauma to reverse after warming the extremity.

E. Ischemia can present with swelling, but in this case the impeded arterial flow is reversible when the extremity is warmed. This patient is more likely to complain of cold hands than of swelling. In addition, the patient's arms are rather slender on the unsubtracted angiogram images (rather than swollen).

Question 2

A. Brachial artery

B. Interosseous artery

C. Radial artery

D. Ulnar artery

Question 3

A. Correct! The radial artery typically provides the dominant supply to the deep palmar arch.

Other choices and discussion

B. The ulnar artery usually supplies the superficial arch.

C. There is no thenar artery in the hand. The thumb is supplied by the princeps pollicis artery.

D. The radialis indicis does not supply the deep arch but arises close to the princeps pollicis artery.

Question 4

B. Correct! A pulse oximeter is used in a Barbeau test. A pulse oximeter is typically placed on the thumb, whereas the radial artery is occluded during a Barbeau test.

Other choices and discussion

A. A blood pressure cuff is typically not used in either test. Both the Allen and the Barbeau involve manually occluding one or both of the major arteries to the hand (ulnar and radial).

C. There are four classifications of the results of a Barbeau test. An Allen test is usually positive or negative.

D. The Barbeau test typically tests the sufficiency of the ulnar artery to supply the hand as the radial artery is occluded during the test. It is not a test of radial artery patency.

■ Suggested Readings

Kim YH, Ng SW, Seo HS, Chang AH. Classification of Raynaud's disease based on angiographic features. J Plast Reconstr Aesthest Surg 2011;64(11):1503–1511

Kotowycz MA, Dzavik V. Radial artery patency after transradial catheterization. Circ Cardiovasc Interv 2012;5:127–133

Top Tips

◆ Raynaud syndrome can be a primary or secondary disorder, with secondary Raynaud syndrome related to an underlying disease (usually connective tissue disease).

◆ A Barbeau test is typically performed prior to radial artery catheterization to determine the patient's ability to tolerate radial artery occlusion. If there is no change in pulse oximetry or plethysmographic waveform, then the radial artery is likely to be safe to use for catheterization.

◆ The radial artery typically supplies the deep palmar arch, and the ulnar artery supplies the superficial palmar arch.

Essentials 4

■ Case

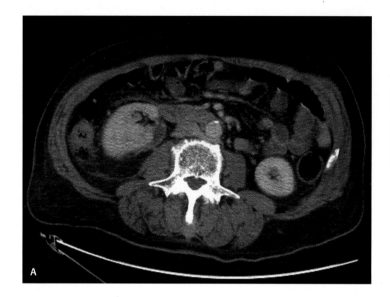
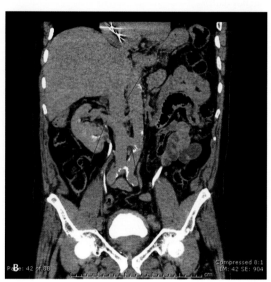

■ Questions

1. This patient, who is in need of an inferior vena cava (IVC) filter, has which of the following anatomic variants?
   A. Duplicated IVC
   B. Retroaortic left renal vein
   C. Circumaortic left renal vein
   D. Standard caval anatomy
   E. Caval agenesis

2. In patients with more than one left renal vein, the preferred position for placement of an IVC filter is? (Select the ONE best answer.)
   A. In between the renal veins
   B. Below the lowest renal vein
   C. Over the ostium of the superior renal vein
   D. In the left iliac vein
   E. In the superior vena cava

3. The incidence of new DVT in patients after placement of an IVC filter is:
   A. Increased compared to those patients without IVC filters
   B. The same as those patients without IVC filters
   C. Decreased compared to those patients without IVC filters
   D. Unknown
   E. Dependent on the anticoagulation status of the patient

■ Answers and Explanations

Question 1

C. Correct! This patient has a circumaortic left renal vein. Circumaortic left renal veins can be seen in up to 17% of the population.

The other choices are all incorrect.

Question 2

B. Correct! Below the lowest renal vein is an acceptable placement for an IVC filter. A filter below the lowest renal vein does not permit clot to potentially circumvent the filter. IVC filters can either be placed from an internal jugular or a femoral approach. The choice of approach is determined by the operator and by clinical factors. For example, if a patient has a right common femoral deep venous thrombosis, a left common femoral or internal jugular approach is preferable. Some filters are low profile enough to permit placement from a brachial or large basilic vein of the arm.

Other choices and discussion

A. Placement between the renal veins is suboptimal because of the theoretical risk of clot entering a lower renal vein, which is below the filter, and subsequently emerging from a higher renal vein, which is above the filter, permitting a pulmonary embolism to occur.

C. Placement over the ostium of a renal vein is suboptimal because this impedes venous drainage from that kidney, which could lead to renal vein thrombosis. Most filters are intended to be positioned 1 cm below the ostium of the renal vein. In this case, placement of the filter either below the lowest renal vein or above the highest renal vein (which is off-label use) is optimal, in terms of reducing the chance of thrombus circumventing the filter.

D. A filter in the left iliac vein is sometimes placed in the setting of a duplicated IVC (not present in this case). In that instance, a second filter would need to be placed in the IVC or in the right iliac vein to protect against a right lower extremity DVT.

E. A superior vena cava filter would not protect against lower extremity DVT.

Question 3

A. Correct! The chance of developing DVT is increased in patients with an IVC filter in place. This is counterintuitive, but has been borne out in the literature. This is one of the reasons there is a push to remove retrievable filters when caval filtration is no longer needed.

Radiologists looking at imaging on patients with IVC filters should note: penetration of the legs beyond the confines of the IVC, filter tilt, migration of position from the prior study, and filter fracture. All of these may indicate an IVC filter complication.

The other choices are all incorrect.

■ Suggested Readings

Fedullo PF, Roberts A. Placement of vena cava filters and their complications. UpToDate. September 2015. http://www .uptodate.com/contents/placement-of-vena-cava-filters-and-their-complications

Karazincir S, Balci A, Gorur S, Sumbas H, Kiper AN. Incidence of the retroaortic left renal vein in patients with varicocele. J Ultrasound Med 2007;26(5):601–604

Top Tips

◆ IVC filters come in permanent and retrievable varieties. Nevertheless, all US Food and Drug Administration–approved filters are approved for permanent use.

◆ The US Food and Drug Administration recommends removal of retrievable filters if there is no longer a clinical necessity. It is believed that there is an increased risk of adverse events (filter fracture, penetration of legs, etc.) with longer indwelling times.

◆ In general, the longer a filter has been in, the harder it will be to remove. Each manufacturer of retrievable filters has a suggested retrieval window for each of their products.

Essentials 5

■ **Case**

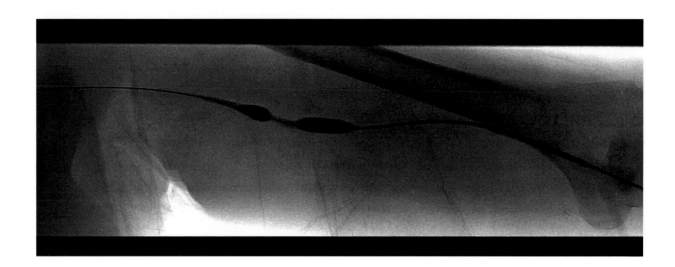

■ **Questions**

1. What finding on physical exam is expected based on this image taken from an elderly patient on dialysis with an antecubital fossa fistula?
   A. Weak thrill
   B. Mottled hand
   C. Swollen arm
   D. Pulsatility
   E. Strong thrill

2. In the event of contrast extravasation after angioplasty of a fistula, which ONE of the following is an appropriate initial maneuver?
   A. Placing a tourniquet in the axillary region
   B. Putting up a balloon at the site of rupture
   C. Placing coils at the site of rupture
   D. Injecting thrombin at the site of rupture
   E. Using a suture to ligate the fistula

3. In an arteriovenous dialysis graft, where is the most common site of stenosis?
   A. Arterial anastomosis
   B. Venous anastomosis
   C. Intragraft
   D. Subclavian
   E. Superior vena cava

■ Answers and Explanations

Question 1

D. Correct! Pulsatility would be expected. When a patient has outflow stenosis of the fistula back to the heart, there is back-pressure. This backpressure presents on physical exam with absence of a thrill and increased pulsatility, as the arterial pressure pushes against a fixed obstruction.

Other choices and discussion

A. Arterial stenosis would cause a weak or absent thrill.

B. The patient's arterial flow to the hand is not likely compromised by the fistula outflow stenosis. There is an entity known as a steal phenomenon whereby there is relatively increased flow through the fistula compared to the hand, resulting in symptoms. In this case, the outflow stenosis may function to force more blood to the hand than through the fistula, so the hand is less likely to be ischemic than when the fistula is fully patent.

C. The patient's arm is unlikely to be swollen, as swelling in these patients is often due to outflow stenosis at the level of the axillary, subclavian, or brachiocephalic veins. This stenosis is in the upper arm but not at the level of the subclavian, which would inhibit all venous drainage of that extremity and more likely result in swelling.

E. A thrill is created by turbulent flow through a fistula. A strong thrill is a reassuring physical exam finding. In the case of a stenosis in the fistula circuit, the normal thrill may be diminished or absent. In this patient with outflow stenosis, increased pulsatility would be expected rather than a strong thrill. This is due to the preservation of arterial pulsations as the arterial pressure is transmitted against a fixed obstruction.

Question 2

B. Correct! A balloon at the site of rupture will often arrest further bleeding. The efficacy of this treatment may be confirmed by excluding further bleeding after taking down the balloon. A balloon is also useful in temporizing the situation, until the operator is prepared to place a covered stent across the area of rupture. After angioplasty, technical success is defined as having < 30% residual stenosis.

Other choices and discussion

A. A tourniquet in the axillary region to stop arterial inflow into the arm may be used as a final effort after other measures have failed. A tourniquet is not a good initial treatment for extravasation, as it causes increased backpressure by obstructing venous outflow, and this may lead to further bleeding from the site of rupture.

C. While coils can cause thrombus that will stop the bleeding, they create an irreversible occlusion and are therefore not typically used to treat contained fistula ruptures.

D. Thrombin is not typically used to treat bleeding after angioplasty because of the potential risk of creating fistula thrombosis or generate a clot that may enter the central circulation.

E. Ligation of the fistula with a suture would make the dialysis access permanently unusable. This would only be considered as an emergent surgical procedure for life-threatening bleeding.

Question 3

B. Correct! The venous anastomosis is the most common site for stenosis in dialysis grafts.

The other choices are all incorrect. Although intragraft, subclavian, and central stenosis may occur, they are all less common sites than at the venous anastomosis.

■ Suggested Readings

Beathard GA. Physical examination of the dialysis vascular access. Semin Dial 1998;11:231–236

Kornfield ZN, Kwak A, Soulen MC, Patel AA, Kobrin SM, Cohen RM, Mantell MD, Chittams JL, Tereotola SO. Incidence and management of percutaneous transluminal angioplasty–induced venous rupture in the "fistula first" era. J Vasc Interv Radiol 2009;20:744–751

Top Tips

- Fistulas (native veins) have longer patency than grafts (synthetic material), so fistulas are often placed first.

- Grafts have both a venous and an arterial anastomosis, and fistulas only have an arterial anastomosis.

- Fistulas with outflow stenosis may have prolonged bleeding after removal of dialysis needles, in addition to increased fistula pulsatility on physical exam.

Essentials 6

■ Case

A 65-year-old asymptomatic man presents for follow up of a renal mass (not shown).

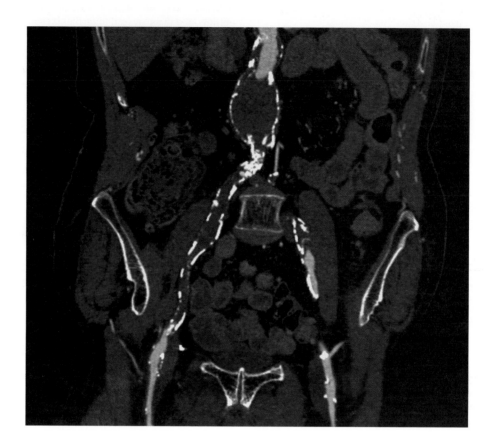

■ Questions

1. What is the most common etiology for this finding?
   A. Infectious
   B. Atherosclerotic
   C. Hypoplastic
   D. Iatrogenic
   E. Congenital

2. Patients with these imaging findings may present with a classic triad of symptoms, which includes which ONE of the following?
   A. Abdominal pain
   B. Renal failure
   C. Back pain
   D. Impotence
   E. Thigh claudication

3. Why are many patients asymptomatic?
   A. Longevity of the findings
   B. Coexisting diabetes
   C. Collateral pathways preserving distal blood flow
   D. Nerve injury from ischemia
   E. Muscular atrophy

■ Answers and Explanations

Question 1

B. Correct! This patient has distal aortic occlusion. Atherosclerotic disease is the most common etiology.

The other options are all incorrect—that is, although all of the other options (infectious, hypoplastic, iatrogenic, and congenital pathologies) can lead to aortic occlusion, none are more common than atherosclerosis.

Question 2

D. Correct! These patients, if symptomatic, classically present with a triad of buttock claudication, absent or decreased femoral pulses, and impotence. This patient has flow in his common femoral arteries, so he likely has palpable femoral pulses.

Other choices and discussion

A. These patients do not usually present with abdominal pain.

B. The occlusion does not extend to the renal arteries, so these patients do not typically present with renal failure.

C. These patients do not usually present with back pain.

E. These patients classically present with buttock claudication, although thigh claudication is possible.

Question 3

C. Correct! These patients are sometimes asymptomatic because collateral pathways maintain blood flow to the pelvis and lower extremities. These collateral pathways include systemic-systemic pathways (e.g., internal mammary artery to inferior epigastric artery), visceral-visceral pathways, and visceral-systemic pathways.

Aortoiliac disease can be described by the TransAtlantic Inter-Society Consensus criteria, with lesion complexity increasing from type A to type D. Type A is a short (usually under 3 cm) common iliac or external iliac lesion that can be treated from an endovascular approach, whereas Type D is a > 10 cm iliac stenosis or occlusion that may need surgical treatment.

The other choices are all incorrect. Many of these patients do have diabetes, but there is a better answer for why these patients are often asymptomatic.

■ Suggested Readings

Jaffan AAA, Murphy TP. Aortoiliac revascularization. In Mauro MA, Murphy KPJ, Thomson KR, et al (eds). Image-Guided Interventions. Philadelphia, PA: Saunders; 2013: 189–209

Top Tips

◆ Leriche syndrome describes the triad of buttock claudication, impotence, and absent or decreased femoral pulses that occurs in the setting of chronic aortoiliac occlusive disease. Risk factors include smoking, diabetes, hypertension, and hyperlipidemia.

◆ Many such patients are asymptomatic, due to rich collateral pathways that allow for lower extremity blood flow.

◆ Treatment may be purely endovascular or surgical. Higher TransAtlantic Inter-Society Consensus lesions are at an increased risk for loss of patency.

Essentials 7

■ Case

A 60-year-old man presents with bright red blood per rectum. Image is from a gastrointestinal (GI) bleed protocol computed tomography angiogram (CTA).

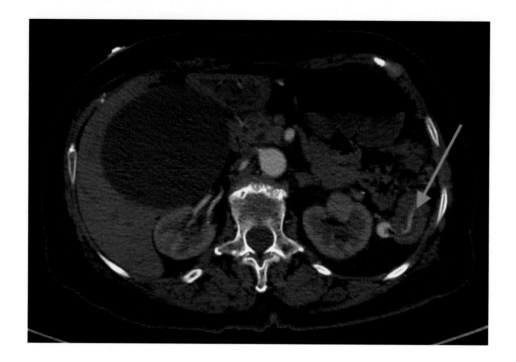

■ Questions

1. The vessel that normally supplies the splenic flexure also supplies which other organ?
   A. Small bowel
   B. Rectum
   C. Spleen
   D. Pancreas
   E. Cecum

2. Which ONE of the following is a potential advantage of a tagged red blood cell scan over a CTA for a GI bleed?
   A. Detection of slower bleeding rates
   B. Precise anatomic bleed localization
   C. Detailed depiction of arterial anatomy
   D. Shorter acquisition time
   E. More readily available

3. Assuming normal anatomy, from which location should catheter-based therapy for this GI bleed take place?
   A. Proximal SMA
   B. Proximal IMA
   C. Proximal middle colic artery
   D. Proximal left colic artery
   E. Distal to the marginal artery

■ Answers and Explanations

Question 1

B. Correct! The rectum is supplied by the inferior mesenteric artery (IMA), which also supplies the splenic flexure.

Other choices and discussion

A. The small bowel is supplied by the superior mesenteric artery (SMA).

C. The spleen is supplied by the splenic artery, which arises from the celiac artery.

D. The pancreas is supplied by multiple arteries originating from the celiac artery and the SMA.

E. The cecum is supplied by the SMA.

Question 2

A. Correct! Detection of slower bleeding rates is an advantage of the nuclear medicine study. A tagged red blood cell scan can detect bleeding rates as low as 0.1 mL/min, compared to CTA, which can detect bleeding rates as low as 0.3 to 0.7 mL/min. Catheter angiography can detect bleeding rates as low as 0.5 to 1 mL/min.

A GI bleed CTA protocol usually includes a noncontrast CT, an arterial phase intravenous contrast CT, and a venous phase delayed CT. No oral contrast is given. With this technique, any new high-density material in the bowel on the arterial phase that becomes more prominent on the venous phase is likely active bleeding. At most centers, angiography with embolization is attempted prior to surgery given its decreased morbidity.

The other choices are all incorrect.

Precise anatomic localization of the bleed, detailed depiction of arterial anatomy, shorter acquisition time, and more readily available modality are all advantages of CTA over nuclear scintigraphy.

Question 3

E. Correct! Distal to the marginal artery. The treatment of lower GI bleeds should occur as distally as possible, to minimize the risk of infarction of a large segment of bowel and prevent collateral flow to the source of bleeding. Treatment should originate beyond the mesenteric border of the colon (marginal or terminal artery in the IMA distribution, or vasa rectae in the SMA distribution). If initial angiography does not reveal active extravasation, then provocative angiography may be considered. Although the yield is low, it may be a worthwhile effort in patients with occult and recurrent lower GI bleeding.

Other choices and discussion

A. The SMA does not normally supply the splenic flexure.

B. A branch of the IMA should be treated, but treatment should be *distal*, not proximal.

C. The middle colic artery is usually a branch off the SMA, not the IMA.

D. A *distal* left colic artery branch should be treated, not the proximal left colic artery.

■ Suggested Readings

Darcy M. Management of lower gastrointestinal bleeding. In Mauro MA, Murphy KPJ, Thomson KR, et al (eds). Image-Guided Interventions. Philadelphia, PA: Saunders; 2013: 374–379

Funaki B. On-call treatment of acute gastrointestinal hemorrhage. Semin Intervent Radiol 2006;23(3):215–222

Top Tips

◆ Both CTA and tagged red blood cell scans are appropriate noninvasive exams to investigate lower GI bleeding. Colonoscopy may also be considered. Common etiologies for lower GI bleeding are diverticular hemorrhage and angiodysplasia.

◆ Patients with a positive CTA or tagged red blood cell scan are usually then investigated with angiography. In rare cases where angiography is not available or the patient is too unstable, surgery is considered.

◆ When treating lower GI bleeding with interventional techniques, the use of superselective catheterization and embolization is imperative to minimize the risk of bowel infarction or re-bleeding. The microcatheter should be placed as close as possible to the bleeding source prior to embolization.

Essentials 8

■ Case

A 25-year-old man has these findings on magnetic resonance angiography.

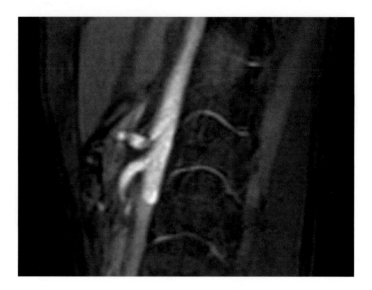

■ Questions

1. These findings are more likely to be significant:
   A. If present during expiration
   B. If the narrowing is > 50%
   C. If the patient has clinical symptoms
   D. If the lactate level is elevated
   E. Regardless of the patient presentation

2. The first-line treatment for this patient if he is symptomatic is:
   A. Surgery
   B. Endovascular stent placement
   C. Celiac ganglion block
   D. Medical management
   E. No treatment

3. The usual location of the median arcuate ligament is:
   A. Anterior to the celiac artery
   B. Posterior to the celiac artery but anterior to the aorta
   C. Inferior to the celiac artery
   D. Superior to the celiac artery
   E. Posterior to the aorta

■ Answers and Explanations

Question 1

C. Correct! These findings are more likely to be significant if the patient has clinical symptoms. The diagnosis of median arcuate ligament syndrome is based on clinical and radiologic findings. This patient suffered from abdominal pain and weight loss. The characteristic finding on imaging is focal narrowing of the proximal celiac axis with a hooked shape. This appearance can be transient on expiration, but is more concerning if seen during inspiration. Poststenotic dilatation or collateral vessels are adjunct findings concerning for pathologic narrowing.

Median arcuate ligament syndrome commonly occurs in young females 20 to 40 years old with symptoms of epigastric pain, which may or may not be postprandial, and weight loss. On physical exam, an abdominal bruit that varies with respiration may be audible in the epigastric region. The symptoms are believed to be due to stenosis of the celiac artery, although some believe that celiac ganglion irritation also contributes. Complications of median arcuate ligament syndrome include aneurysm formation of the pancreaticoduodenal arcades, gastroepiploic, or celiac arteries.

Other choices and discussion

A. This appearance is concerning if present during *inspiration*, as in this case. Conversely, this narrowing may be transient on expiration and is often clinically insignificant in those instances. On inspiration, the diaphragm lowers and the compression by the median arcuate ligament should be the least severe.

B. The degree of narrowing itself does not often directly correlate with the severity of patient symptoms.

D. An elevated lactate level does not contribute to the diagnosis.

E. This appearance is not concerning if the patient is asymptomatic.

Question 2

A. Correct! Surgical release of the median arcuate ligament is the best first treatment for this patient. The patient in this case did, in fact, have surgical release of the median arcuate ligament with subsequent improvement in his symptoms.

Other choices and discussion

B. Endovascular stent placement before surgery has a high failure rate. If symptoms persist after surgery, stent placement may be considered.

C. Although the symptoms of median arcuate ligament syndrome may be due in part to celiac ganglion irritation, a celiac ganglion block alone is not standard treatment for median arcuate ligament syndrome.

D. Medical management is not appropriate.

E. Given the presence of symptoms with this radiologic appearance, treatment is warranted.

Question 3

D. Correct! Normally the median arcuate ligament is superior to the celiac artery.

The other choices are incorrect. The median arcuate ligament is anterior to the celiac axis in a minority of cases, where it may cause compression of the celiac artery.

■ Suggested Readings

Horton K, Talamini M, Fishman E. Median arcuate ligament syndrome: evaluation with CT angiography. Radiographics 2005;25:1117–1182

Tracci M. Median arcuate ligament compression of the mesenteric vasculature. Tech Vasc Interv Radiol 2015;18(1):43–50

Top Tips

◆ The median arcuate ligament is a fibrous ligament connecting the diaphragmatic crura. It is normally situated superior to the celiac artery, but may be found anterior to the celiac artery in 10 to 24% of patients.

◆ While this diagnosis is traditionally made on conventional angiography, computed tomography angiography and magnetic resonance angiography are now increasingly used for this purpose. The imaging findings are exacerbated/exaggerated on expiration.

◆ Treatment initially consists of surgical decompression. Endovascular revascularization of the celiac artery may be performed at the same time or afterward. Endovascular treatment alone (without surgical treatment) has a high failure rate.

Essentials 9

■ Case

A young female patient presents with left lower extremity swelling, deep venous thrombosis, and this finding on magnetic resonance angiography and angiography.

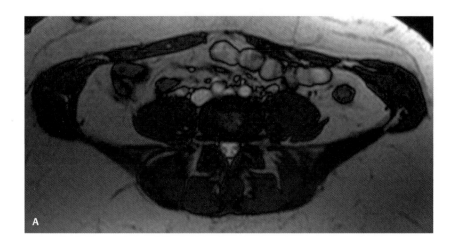

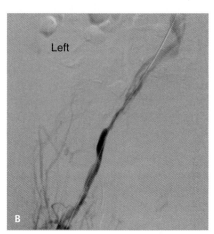

■ Questions

1. What is the most likely etiology for this finding?
   A. Iatrogenic
   B. Mechanical
   C. Traumatic
   D. Inflammatory
   E. Degenerative

2. The affected vessel is the:
   A. Left common iliac artery
   B. Left common iliac vein
   C. Left external iliac vein
   D. Right common iliac artery
   E. Right common iliac vein

3. What is the best treatment strategy for this patient?
   A. Endovascular techniques, including angioplasty with possible stent placement
   B. Surgical management
   C. Conservative management
   D. Systemic anticoagulation alone
   E. More workup is needed before a treatment plan can be made

■ Answers and Explanations

Question 1

B. Correct! This patient has May-Thurner syndrome. The most likely etiology is mechanical. The compression defect in the left common iliac vein is the result of compression by the passing right common iliac artery anteriorly and the lumbar vertebral body posteriorly. The presentation may be acute, with left lower extremity pain or swelling, or chronic, with chronic venous insufficiency. A rare presentation is that of pulmonary emboli.

Anatomic compression of the left common iliac vein is seen in up to 25% of asymptomatic patients. Degree of luminal stenosis > 50% and the presence of collateral veins are imaging clues that suggest May-Thurner syndrome. This syndrome likely contributes to the slightly higher incidence of left-sided deep venous thrombosis (DVT). High clinical suspicion is necessary to recognize the syndrome.

Other choices and discussion

A. Although oral contraceptives can contribute to this syndrome, they cannot by themselves explain the specific imaging findings.

C. There is no given history of trauma or findings to support this diagnosis on the provided image.

D. Inflammation alone cannot account for the imaging finding.

E. Degenerative changes do not result in DVT.

Question 2

B. Correct! The compression defect is in the left common iliac vein, which is compressed by the right common iliac artery that passes anterior to the left common iliac vein. Although ultrasound is often used as the initial imaging study, this modality can be quite limited in visualization of the pelvic veins. Both computed tomography and magnetic resonance venography are very useful in delineating the anatomy and estimating the degree of stenosis. Intravascular ultrasound can also demonstrate the degree of stenosis and spur.

The other choices are all incorrect.

Question 3

A. Correct! Endovascular techniques, including angioplasty with possible stent placement, is the best treatment strategy and has been shown to result in the best long-term venous patency rates.

Other choices and discussion

B. Surgical management is associated with higher rates of morbidity than is endovascular treatment.

C. Given the compressive nature of this syndrome, conservative management alone is not sufficient for treatment in symptomatic individuals.

D. Systemic anticoagulation alone results in high rates of rethrombosis.

E. The diagnosis of May-Thurner syndrome can, indeed, be made based on the imaging findings in the appropriate clinical setting.

■ Suggested Readings

Brinegar K, Sheth R, Khademhosseini A, et al. Iliac vein compression syndrome: clinical, imaging, and pathologic findings. World J Radiol 2015;7(11):375–381

Mousa A, AbuRahma A. May-Thurner syndrome: update and review. Ann of Vasc Surg 2013;27(7):984–995

Top Tips

◆ May-Thurner syndrome refers to the extrinsic compression of the left common iliac vein by the right common iliac artery anteriorly and the lumbosacral spine posteriorly. This syndrome results in left lower extremity pain, swelling, and DVT.

◆ May-Thurner syndrome is estimated to occur in 2 to 5% of patients who present with a lower extremity venous disorder. It is more common in women and tends to present in the second or third decade.

◆ Endovascular techniques have been shown to result in lower rates of rethrombosis when compared to systemic anticoagulation alone. Although many interventional radiologists will begin with angioplasty, stent placement is often necessary. Surgery has variable success and carries higher morbidity than does endovascular treatment.

Essentials 10

■ Case

A 34-year-old woman presents with mild left flank pain and asymptomatic hematuria.

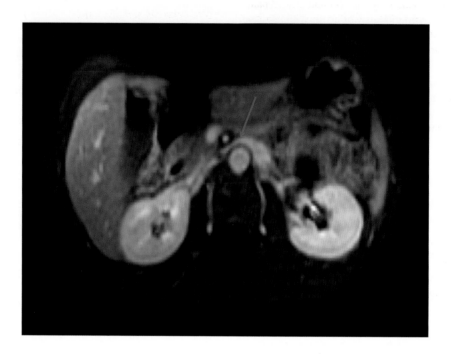

■ Questions

1. What is the pathophysiology of these clinical symptoms?
   A. Narrowing of the left renal vein between the aorta and superior mesenteric artery
   B. Narrowing of the left renal vein between the aorta and vertebral body
   C. Narrowing of the left renal vein by a mass
   D. Incompetent valve
   E. Narrowing of the left renal vein due to an iatrogenic stricture

2. What is a common sequela of this syndrome?
   A. Thrombosis
   B. Renal failure
   C. Left varicocele
   D. Premature menopause
   E. Malignancy

3. What is the most common treatment strategy?
   A. Surgical resection of the mass
   B. Left renal vein transposition
   C. Venous stent
   D. Weight loss
   E. Symptom management

■ Answers and Explanations

Question 1

A. Correct! The nutcracker syndrome is compression of the left renal vein between the aorta and superior mesenteric artery, with resultant varicosities in the renal pelvis, ureter, and gonadal vein. Symptoms include left flank (or abdominal) pain with asymptomatic hematuria. Men may develop a left varicocele from reflux of the left renal vein into the left gonadal vein. Women may develop pelvic congestion syndrome from reflux into the ovarian and parametrial venous plexus.

A retrograde venogram with a pressure gradient > 3 mm Hg is considered diagnostic of nutcracker syndrome. Ultrasound is helpful in measuring velocities of the left renal vein. A velocity of > 100 cm/sec taken where the superior mesenteric artery crosses the left renal vein is very sensitive and specific for the diagnosis of nutcracker syndrome. Computed tomography and magnetic resonance angiography can demonstrate compression of the left renal vein and associated collateral veins. Both imaging findings and clinical symptomatology are necessary to make the diagnosis.

Other choices and discussion

B. Narrowing of the left renal vein between the aorta and vertebral body may cause symptoms if the left renal vein took a retroaortic path (so-called posterior nutcracker syndrome).

C. A mass is much less likely to cause this problem.

D. An incompetent valve would not result in narrowing.

E. An iatrogenic stricture is much less likely to cause this problem.

Question 2

C. Correct! Left varicocele, as well as its female correlate, pelvic congestion syndrome, have both been described with this syndrome.

The other choices are incorrect. A thrombosis is a possible sequela, but a varicocele is more common.

Question 3

E. Correct! Symptom management (conservative treatment) is most common, especially for younger patients with mild cases, as there is a high spontaneous remission rate.

Other choices and discussion

A. There is no mass that would necessitate surgical resection.

B. Venous stenting may be pursued in severe cases, but this is not the most common treatment strategy.

C. Surgical techniques, including gonadocaval bypass and left renal vein transposition, may be pursued in severe cases, but this is not the most common treatment strategy.

D. Weight *gain* may be helpful in mild cases, if the patient is very thin.

■ Suggested Readings

Butros SR, Liu R, Oliveira GR, et al. Venous compression syndromes: clinical features, imaging findings and management. Br J Radiol 2013;86(1030):20130284

Eliahou R, Sosna J, Bloom A. Between a rock and a hard place: clinical and imaging features of vascular compression syndromes. Radiographics 2012;32:E33–E49

Top Tips

- Nutcracker syndrome often occurs in young, healthy women in their third to fourth decades. A narrow angle between the aorta and superior mesenteric artery is believed to contribute to the pathophysiology.

- The diagnostic gold standard is retrograde venography with renocaval pressure gradient measurements.

- Treatment is usually conservative, as this syndrome often resolves without intervention. Conservative treatments may include pain medication and hydration. Various surgical and endovascular treatments are only pursued in severe cases.

Essentials 11

■ Case

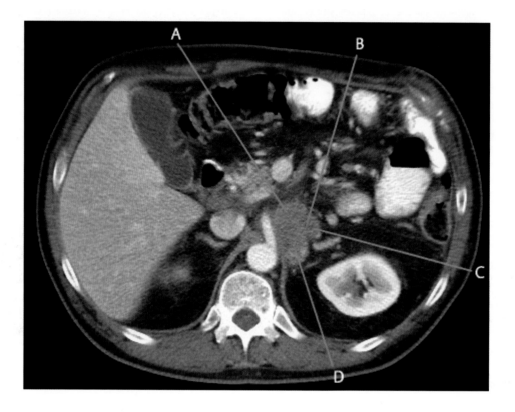

■ Questions

1. Which letter marks the best percutaneous route for biopsy of this mass?
   A. A
   B. B
   C. C
   D. D
   E. None of these routes is safe.

2. Which ONE of the following is the generally preferred route for an infected deep pelvic collection drainage in a female patient (assuming the collection is accessible without traversal of vital structures)?
   A. Transgluteal
   B. Transabdominal
   C. Transrectal
   D. Transvaginal
   E. Due to location, percutaneous drainage should be avoided.

3. According to the SIR guidelines, what is the recommendation regarding antibiotic prophylaxis in a septic patient prior to percutaneous abscess drainage?
   A. No antibiotics needed
   B. Gram-negative coverage only
   C. Gram-positive coverage only
   D. Broad-spectrum coverage
   E. Antibiotics should be withheld to prevent altering culture results

■ Answers and Explanations

Question 1

D. Correct! This route is the shortest and avoids traversing vital structures. Once the coaxial needle (if utilized) is in the retroperitoneum, a blunt stylet can be placed to avoid injury to the small vessels posterior to the mass. Intra-abdominal, intrathoracic, chest wall, and retroperitoneal abscess drainages/biopsies are considered to have a moderate risk of bleeding, according to Society of Interventional Radiology (SIR) guidelines.

Ultrasound and computed tomography are the most common modalities used for image guidance. In general, ultrasound is preferred when the collection is well visualized. Computed tomography may be used for small or deep collections, or for collections containing air. Often, fluoroscopy is helpful after initial access to guide wire and catheter manipulations.

Either the trocar or Seldinger technique can be used to access a collection. The trocar technique involves direct access of the collection with a coaxial combination of a catheter, stiffening cannula, and sharp stylet. This method is faster than the Seldinger technique, but requires real-time visualization of the catheter during placement to avoid nontarget catheter placement.

When planning a route to the collection, one should use the safest, most direct, and shortest route, while ideally avoiding intervening organs or vital anatomic structures. Sterile areas should not be contaminated. In cases of catheter drainage, the catheter should be placed in the most dependent portion of the collection.

Other choices and discussion

A. This route is not preferred because it traverses bowel, pancreas, and the splenic vein.

B. This route is not preferred because it passes adjacent to or through multiple larger vessels.

C. This route is safer than A or B but longer than D.

E. There is a safe route to this mass, so this answer is incorrect.

Question 2

D. Correct! A transvaginal approach is preferred when possible, except in very young female patients. In general, for any access route, relatively common complications include pain at the catheter entry site, bleeding, and sepsis. Other complications are more site-specific. The size and shape of the catheter are important factors in technical and clinical success. Smaller catheters can often be used to drain simple fluid collections, whereas larger catheters are required for more complex collections. Locking pigtail catheters are preferred over straight catheters.

Other choices and discussion

A. A transgluteal approach is preferred when there is no safe transvaginal, transrectal, or transabdominal approach.

B. A transabdominal route is preferred when there is no safe transvaginal or transrectal route.

C. A transrectal route is generally preferred when a transvaginal route is not possible. A transrectal route is considered by some to be less painful than a transvaginal route.

E. Despite the location in the deep pelvis with intervening bowel, vessels, and urinary bladder, a percutaneous route is often possible. Placing the patient prone or in a lateral decubitus position often presents new routes not possible in the supine position. Placement of a Foley catheter for urinary bladder decompression and administration of oral contrast for bowel opacification are ancillary steps that can also help with preprocedure planning.

Question 3

D. Correct! Because abscesses are often polymicrobial, broad-spectrum coverage is needed. There is no consensus for the first-choice antibiotic regimen, but most commonly, a second- or third-generation cephalosporin or ampicillin/sulbactam can be used for gram-positive coverage, and an aminoglycoside can be used for gram-negative coverage.

Other choices and discussion

A. The SIR guidelines consider percutaneous drainage of abscesses a dirty procedure, and therefore preprocedural antibiotic coverage is recommended.

B. Abscesses are often polymicrobial with gram-positive and gram-negative organisms, so gram-negative coverage alone is often not sufficient.

C. Abscesses are often polymicrobial with gram-positive and gram-negative organisms, so gram-positive coverage alone is often not sufficient.

E. While some may argue for withholding of broad-spectrum antibiotics in an asymptomatic patient prior to drainage, in a septic patient, antibiotics are indicated and should be initiated prior to drainage.

■ Suggested Readings

Charles HW. Abscess drainage. Semin Intervent Radiol 2012;29(4):325–336

Venkatesan AM, Kundu S, Sacks D. Practice guideline for adult antibiotic prophylaxis during vascular and interventional radiology procedures. J Vasc Interv Radiol 2010;21:1611–1630

Top Tips

♦ Percutaneous image-guided abscess drainage has largely replaced surgery as the first-line therapy for most intra-abdominal and intrathoracic fluid collections.

♦ Percutaneous abscess drainage is considered a dirty procedure, and preprocedural prophylactic antibiotics are recommended.

♦ The catheter should be removed when the patient has improved clinically, drainage is < 20 mL per day for at least 2 days, and there is no evidence of an associated fistula. Repeat imaging to demonstrate resolution of the abscess may be obtained but is not always necessary.

SECTION VI
INTERVENTIONAL IMAGING

Essentials 12

■ Case

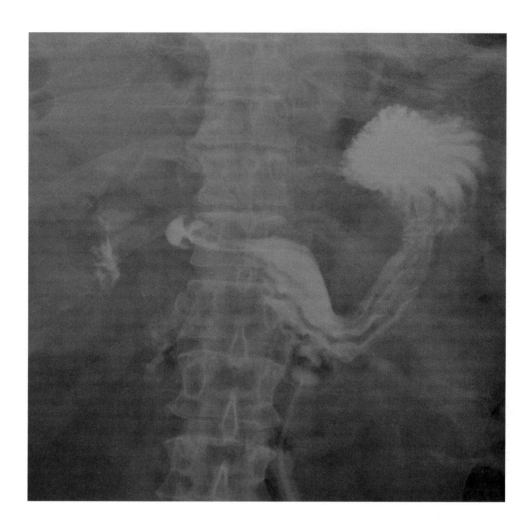

■ Questions

1. What is the optimal gastric puncture site for percutaneous gastrostomy tube placement?
   A. Antrum
   B. Pylorus
   C. Fundus
   D. Proximal body
   E. Gastroesophageal junction

2. What is the purpose of administering glucagon during gastrostomy tube placement?
   A. To reduce the risk of infection
   B. To reduce the risk of bleeding
   C. To maintain gastric distention
   D. To minimize peristalsis of adjacent bowel
   E. To prevent hypoglycemia during the procedure

3. Which artery is most likely to be injured during percutaneous gastrostomy tube placement?
   A. Aorta
   B. Celiac artery
   C. Splenic artery
   D. Left gastric artery
   E. Inferior epigastric artery

■ Answers and Explanations

Question 1

A. Correct! The antrum, or distal body, is the ideal position for puncture. One should aim to be equidistant from the greater and lesser curvatures to avoid vessel injury. An appropriate position for gastric puncture is determined under fluoroscopy after the stomach has been adequately insufflated with air. Glucagon or hyoscine-*N*-butylbromide is given to maintain adequate insufflation. Evaluation to exclude overlying colon should be performed. In cases of insufficient gaseous distention, the colon may be opacified by oral barium 12 hours prior to the procedure. The liver edge can be demarcated by palpation or ultrasound.

There is some controversy regarding the routine use of gastropexy. If gastropexy is utilized, several T-fasteners are initially deployed to allow for apposition of the stomach to the anterior abdominal wall. Then an incision is made between the gastropexy sites, and a needle is passed into the stomach through which a wire is introduced. The tract is subsequently dilated prior to catheter placement.

Various types of gastrostomy catheters are available, which differ by their length, diameter, and retention mechanism. Pigtail-retained and balloon-retained catheters are two common types. Button gastrostomies are low-profile catheters with a short hub and a valve at the skin with a feeding extension that may be removed after feeding.

The other choices are all incorrect.

Question 2

C. Correct! The purpose of administering glucagon is to maintain adequate gastric distention.

Other choices and discussion

A. Glucagon does not reduce the risk of infection.

B. Glucagon does not reduce the risk of bleeding.

D. Although glucagon decreases adjacent bowel peristalsis, this is not the main purpose of administering glucagon.

E. Although glucagon may raise blood glucose, this is not the main purpose of administering glucagon.

Question 3

E. Correct! The inferior epigastric artery is the most likely artery to be injured during percutaneous gastrostomy tube placement. Care should be taken to choose an approach lateral to the rectus muscle to avoid this complication.

The other choices are all incorrect. Although the aorta, celiac artery, splenic artery, and left gastric artery can all be injured during percutaneous gastrostomy tube placement, none of them is more likely to be injured than the inferior epigastric artery.

■ Suggested Readings

Lyon SM, Pascoe DM. Percutaneous gastrostomy and gastrojejunostomy. Semin Intervent Radiol 2004;21(3):181–189

Power S, Lee MJ. Gastrostomy and gastrojejunostomy. In Mauro MA, Murphy KPJ, Thomson KR, et al (eds). Image-Guided Interventions. Philadelphia, PA: Saunders; 2013: 969–975

Top Tips

◆ Percutaneous gastrostomy tubes are placed in a wide variety of patients who cannot maintain their nutrition orally. These often include patients with neurologic impairment or head and neck malignancies.

◆ After placement, the patient should remain fasting for at least 12 to 24 hours; however, it varies by type of tube and practitioner.

◆ Major complications from percutaneous gastrostomy tube placement include peritonitis, gastrointestinal perforation, and hemorrhage requiring transfusion. Minor complications include peristomal leakage, tube dislodgement, and superficial wound infections. Tube-related complications vary with the type of tube placed.

SECTION VI INTERVENTIONAL IMAGING

Essentials 13

■ Case

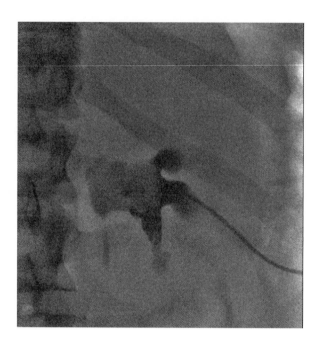

■ Questions

1. The ideal placement of a percutaneous nephrostomy (PCN) is through the
   A. Upper pole, anterior calyx
   B. Upper pole, posterior calyx
   C. Lower pole, anterior calyx
   D. Lower pole, posterior calyx
   E. Renal pelvis

2. Which patient factor is particularly important to consider prior to percutaneous nephrostomy placement?
   A. Airway assessment
   B. White blood cell count
   C. Heart rate
   D. Blood pressure
   E. Allergies

3. Which ONE of the following is the Society of Interventional Radiology guideline for antibiotic prophylaxis before PCN placement?
   A. This is considered a clean procedure, so prophylactic antibiotics are not recommended.
   B. This is considered a clean procedure, so prophylactic antibiotics are recommended.
   C. This is considered at least a clean-contaminated procedure, so prophylactic antibiotics are not recommended.
   D. This is considered at least a clean-contaminated procedure, so prophylactic antibiotics are recommended.
   E. The use of prophylactic antibiotics depends upon the patient status.

■ Answers and Explanations

Question 1

D. Correct! The ideal placement of a PCN is through the lower pole, posterior calyx. The long axis of the lower pole, posterior calyx is usually aligned with a relatively avascular zone called Brodel's line, and targeting this area provides the least risk of significant arterial injury.

Several techniques exist for PCN placement. In the one-stick technique, the same needle is used both for opacification of the collecting system and placement of the nephrostomy tube. Ultrasound is most commonly used for guidance, although fluoroscopy can alternatively be used, especially if a radiopaque stone is available as a target.

With the two-stick method, the first needle is used to opacify the collecting system, which allows for placement of a second needle into an appropriate posterior calyx under fluoroscopy. This can be helpful if visualization of the needle or calyces is poor under ultrasound. The first needle can be directed toward the renal pelvis, as it will not be converted into a nephrostomy.

There are no absolute contraindications to PCN. If possible, severe hyperkalemia, especially with changes on electrocardiogram, should be treated with emergent dialysis prior to nephrostomy placement. Coagulopathy should ideally be corrected prior to the procedure.

The other choices are all incorrect. Accessing the renal pelvis for catheter placement carries a higher risk of larger vessel injury.

Question 2

A. Correct! Given that the patient is typically lying prone during the PCN procedure, airway assessment is particularly important. Proper airway monitoring and airway access in case of an emergency is more difficult with the patient in the prone position, and there should be a lower threshold for anesthesia support in these cases.

The other choices are all incorrect. White blood cell count, heart rate, blood pressure, and allergies are all important to consider, but the prone positioning should make one think first of the airway.

Question 3

D. Correct! PCN is considered at least a clean-contaminated procedure but may be contaminated or dirty. Prophylactic antibiotics are recommended. There is no consensus for a first-choice antibiotic, but common choices include cefazolin, ceftriaxone, and ampicillin/sulbactam.

The other choices are all incorrect. A clean procedure is one where the gastrointestinal, genitourinary, or respiratory tract is not entered. Therefore, PCN is not considered a clean procedure. Society of Interventional Radiology guidelines recommend prophylactic use of antibiotics regardless of patient status.

■ Suggested Readings

Dagli M, Ramchandani P. Percutaneous nephrostomy: technical aspects and indications. Semin Intervent Radiol 2011;28(4):424–437

Stokes LS, Meranze SG. Percutaneous nephrostomy, cystostomy, and nephroureteral stenting. In Mauro MA, Murphy KPJ, Thomson KR, et al (eds). Image-Guided Interventions. Philadelphia, PA: Saunders; 2013: 1076–1088

Top Tips

- The most common indication for PCN is urinary obstruction. Other indications include urinary diversion in case of urinary fistula, urinary leak, or hemorrhagic cystitis. PCN may also be used for diagnostic testing, when the diagnosis of obstruction is uncertain based on clinical and noninvasive tests.

- The pleura and diaphragm are the most commonly injured structures during PCN. Nephrostomy placement should be below the 12th rib when possible to minimize pleural and diaphragmatic injury. Evaluation of prior cross-sectional imaging or evaluation under fluoroscopy for a retrorenal colon should also be performed.

- Transient minor bleeding and transient low-grade fever are very common after PCN placement. Severe bleeding requiring transfusion or other intervention occurs in 1 to 4% of cases. Minimizing the volume used to opacify the renal collecting system during access is recommended to reduce the risk of postprocedural sepsis.

Essentials 14

■ Case

Abduction and adduction right subclavian venography.

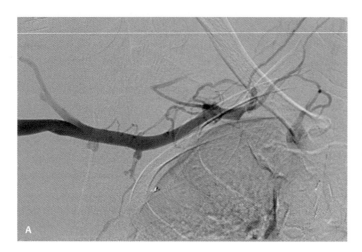

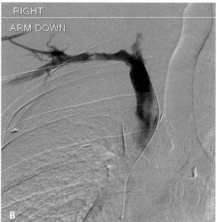

■ Questions

1. Which ONE of the following is the most likely clinical presentation?
   A. Elderly patient with longstanding midline catheter and new arm swelling
   B. Young male baseball pitcher with sudden onset arm swelling and redness
   C. Middle-aged female with hypertension and shoulder pain
   D. Elderly male smoker with facial swelling
   E. Young female patient with shortness of breath

2. Which arm motion characteristically produces symptoms?
   A. Abduction
   B. Adduction
   C. Flexion
   D. Extension
   E. Rotation

3. What is the best management for this patient?
   A. Stenting alone
   B. Thrombolysis alone
   C. Thrombolysis with balloon angioplasty
   D. Thrombolysis with systemic anticoagulation followed by surgery
   E. Systemic anticoagulation with intermittent arm elevation

■ Answers and Explanations

Question 1

B. Correct! This patient has subclavian venous effort thrombosis (also known as Paget Schroetter syndrome). A young male baseball pitcher with sudden onset arm swelling and redness is the most common clinical presentation of this condition. It typically occurs acutely in a young, healthy, active individual, with swelling of an entire arm. Over time, scar formation (both within and outside of the subclavian vein at the level of the first rib) occurs, which eventually leads to thrombotic occlusion.

Other choices and discussion

A. Although an elderly patient with catheter-induced thrombosis is possible, the position of the arm on the image suggests an alternative diagnosis.

C. Subclavian vein occlusion would not classically result in hypertension and shoulder pain.

D. Subclavian vein occlusion would not classically result in facial swelling.

E. Pulmonary embolism is possible, but the incidence of clot at this site in a young patient resulting in pulmonary embolism is low.

Question 2

A. Correct! Abduction characteristically produces the symptoms and accentuates the imaging findings, as in this case.

The other choices are all incorrect.

Question 3

D. Correct! Thrombolysis with systemic anticoagulation followed by surgery is the best management. Initial thrombolysis is used to provide relief of upper extremity symptoms, to prevent pulmonary embolism, to reduce the risk of post thrombotic syndrome, and to reduce the likelihood of recurrent thrombosis. Surgery is then performed to decompress the subclavian vein through the thoracic outlet. The first rib and scalene and subclavius muscles are removed and direct venous reconstruction is performed. Anticoagulation should be initiated when the diagnosis is first suspected and may be discontinued 12 weeks after surgical decompression.

Other choices and discussion

A. Stent placement, especially before surgical intervention, has a high rate of failure in this condition.

B. Thrombolysis alone has a high technical success rate but does not correct the underlying pathophysiology.

C. Thrombolysis with balloon angioplasty may be utilized in conjunction with thrombolysis, but neither corrects the underlying pathophysiology.

E. Systemic anticoagulation without catheter-directed thrombolysis and subsequent surgical management results in high rates of recurrent thrombosis (ranging from 50 to 70%), as well as high rates of chronic venous congestion.

■ Suggested Readings

Kurli V, Pryluck DS, Singh CK, et al. Acute upper extremity deep venous thrombosis. In Mauro MA, Murphy KPJ, Thomson KR, et al (eds). Image-Guided Interventions. Philadelphia, PA: Saunders; 2013: 766–771

Thompson R. Comprehensive management of subclavian vein thrombosis. Semin Intervent Radiol 2012;29:44–51

Top Tips

- ◆ Subclavian vein effort thrombosis is a mechanical condition caused by extrinsic compression of the subclavian vein between the clavicle and the first rib, the anterior scalene muscle, the subclavius muscle, and the costoclavicular ligament.

- ◆ Arm elevation or exertion particularly causes venous compression.

- ◆ Computed tomography or magnetic resonance imaging with the arm in abducted and adducted positioning should be performed to elicit positional compression of the subclavian vein.

Essentials 15

■ Case

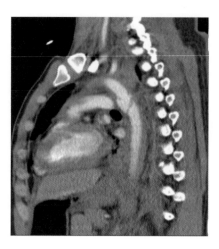

■ Questions

1. The most likely clinical history is:
   A. Fall from standing
   B. Motor vehicle accident
   C. Recent endovascular treatment of middle cerebral artery aneurysm
   D. Recent hospitalization for sepsis
   E. Shortness of breath

2. The most common location for this finding is:
   A. Aortic root
   B. Ascending aorta
   C. Descending aorta
   D. Aortic diaphragmatic hiatus
   E. Aortic isthmus

3. Which of the following is the diagnostic test of choice for suspected aortic injury due to blunt chest trauma?
   A. Conventional aortography
   B. Chest radiograph
   C. Ultrasound
   D. Chest computed tomography angiography
   E. Chest magnetic resonance angiography

■ Answers and Explanations

Question 1

B. Correct! This patient has an aortic traumatic pseudoaneurysm. Motor vehicle accidents with significant deceleration can result in this type of injury. There are several potential mechanisms of injury, including rapid deceleration, shearing forces, compression of the aorta between osseous structures, and injury due to sudden increases in intrathoracic pressure. Associated injuries include sternal and multiple rib fractures, especially the first rib. If untreated, traumatic aortic injuries can evolve into chronic pseudoaneurysms, which may develop peripheral calcification and thrombus.

The presence of mediastinal hematoma should prompt a careful search for aortic or great vessel injury. If none is seen, then the hematoma is likely of venous origin and may be related to a vertebral body fracture. The presence of a fat plane between the aorta and the mediastinal hematoma is a reassuring finding and argues against aortic injury.

Other choices and discussion

A. There is insufficient deceleration from a fall from standing to account for this type of injury.

C. While endovascular intervention can result in vessel injury, there is a more likely answer given the typical location of the finding in the test case.

D. While infected aortic aneurysm is a possibility, the lack of adjacent fat stranding and wall thickening in the test case makes this option less likely.

E. While this patient may have shortness of breath, there is likely additional clinical history to account for this finding.

Question 2

E. Correct! A total of 90% of traumatic injuries to the aorta occur at the aortic isthmus. The isthmus is the portion of the descending thoracic aorta between the left subclavian artery and the ligamentum arteriosum. The ascending aorta and the diaphragmatic hiatus each account for 5% of aortic injuries. These locations are more fixed compared to other parts of the thoracic aorta and are thus more prone to injury. Surgical and imaging series report relatively higher rates of injury at the aortic isthmus compared to autopsy reports. This is because of the lower fatality rate of aortic injuries at the isthmus compared to other locations.

Treatment options for aortic injuries include open surgical repair, endovascular repair, or medical management. Traditionally, open surgical repair is preferred for traumatic aortic injuries, but some centers are now using endovascular repair as a first-line treatment. One important tip to note is that technical factors such as motion artifact can mimic the appearance of an aortic injury.

Other choices and discussion

A. The aortic root is more prone to traumatic pseudoaneurysm formation as it is relatively fixed, but it is injured less commonly than the aortic isthmus.

B. The ascending thoracic aortic is more mobile and less prone to injury.

C. The descending thoracic aortic is more mobile and less prone to injury.

D. The diaphragmatic hiatus is more prone to traumatic pseudoaneurysm formation as it is relatively fixed, but it is injured less commonly than the aortic isthmus.

Question 3

D. Correct! Chest computed tomography angiography has 100% sensitivity and specificity for diagnosing aortic injury.

Other choices and discussion

A. Conventional aortography is the gold standard and was the preferred exam in the past, but is no longer preferred because of its invasive nature and limited assessment for luminal thrombus.

B. Chest radiograph is insensitive for this potentially life-threatening diagnosis.

C. Ultrasound is insensitive for this potentially life-threatening diagnosis.

E. Magnetic resonance angiography may be appropriate in certain problem-solving situations, but computed tomography is preferred because of its excellent sensitivity and specificity, easy accessibility, and short time needed to complete the study.

■ Suggested Readings

Beslic S, Beslic N, Beslic S, et al. Diagnostic imaging of traumatic pseudoaneurysm of the thoracic aorta. Radiol Oncol 2010;44(3):158–163

Cullen EL, Lantz EJ, Johnson M, et al. Traumatic aortic injury: CT findings, mimics, and therapeutic options. Cardiovasc Diag Ther 2014;4(3):238–244

Top Tips

◆ Traumatic aortic injuries are rare but lethal in > 80% of cases.

◆ Direct findings of aortic injury include intramural hematoma, intimal flap, and pseudoaneurysm. Indirect findings include irregular aortic contour, change in aortic caliber, and periaortic hematoma.

◆ A ductus bump or infundibulum, a remnant of the ductus arteriosus, is a mimic of acute injury. This is typically smooth walled and forms an obtuse margin with the aorta.

Essentials 16

■ Case

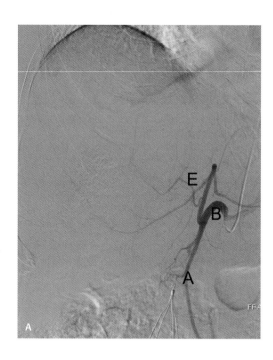
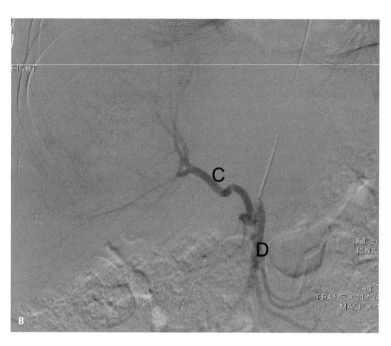

■ Questions

1. Match the letter with the appropriate vessel from this transradial celiac and superior mesenteric artery angiogram:
   __ Replaced right hepatic artery
   __ Superior mesenteric artery
   __ Common hepatic artery
   __ Gastroduodenal artery
   __ Left hepatic artery

2. Which chemotherapeutic agent is used in conventional chemoembolization for hepatocellular carcinoma?
   A. Sorafenib
   B. Doxorubicin
   C. Irinotecan
   D. Fluorouracil
   E. Bevacizumab

3. Which ONE of the following is a common symptom of postembolization syndrome?
   A. Fever
   B. Hematuria
   C. Rigors
   D. Rash
   E. Hypertension

■ Answers and Explanations

Question 1

C. Replaced right hepatic artery

D. Superior mesenteric artery

B. Common hepatic artery

A. Gastroduodenal artery

E. Left hepatic artery

Question 2

B. Correct! Doxorubicin, often mixed with Ethiodol (poppy seed oil), is administered intra-arterially to treat hepatocellular carcinoma. The classic mixture had previously involved triple drug therapy, with doxorubicin, cisplatin and mitomycin C. Due to availability, most centers now only use doxorubicin.

Other choices and discussion

A. Sorafenib is an oral tyrosine kinase inhibitor used to treat advanced hepatocellular carcinoma. It is not administered during the chemoembolization procedure.

C. Irinotecan is a chemotherapeutic agent used to treat colon cancer liver metastases and is not traditionally used to treat hepatocellular carcinoma.

D. Fluorouracil is a chemotherapeutic agent used to treat some gastrointestinal malignancies, but is not given during chemoembolization for hepatocellular carcinoma.

E. Bevacizumab (aka Avastin) is used to treat a variety of types of cancer. However, it is not traditionally administered during the chemoembolization procedure.

Question 3

A. Correct! Fever is a common symptom (as are pain and nausea) of the postembolization syndrome. This is a self-limited process that lasts 7 to 10 days. This should not be confused with sepsis or other pathologic processes that last longer and do not resolve on their own. After 10 days, symptoms should be worked up for more aggressive complications. Postembolization syndrome is treated conservatively with symptom management.

The other choices are all incorrect.

■ Suggested Readings

Brown DB, Nikolic B, Covey AM, Nutting CW, Saad WEA, Salem R, Sofocieous CT, Sze DY. Quality improvement guidelines for transhepatic arterial chemoembolization, embolization and chemotherapeutic infusion for hepatic malignancy. J Vasc Intervent Radiol 2012;23:287–294

Clark TWI. Complications of hepatic chemoembolization. Semin Intervent Radiol 2006;23(2):119–125

Top Tips

- An *accessory* hepatic artery occurs when a variant artery is found in addition to the normal arterial supply. A *replaced* hepatic artery occurs when a variant artery is found in place of the normal arterial supply. A replaced right hepatic artery is said to have a 10% prevalence in the population.

- Doxorubicin is the drug most commonly used in chemoembolization. It can be mixed with a poppy seed oil derivative and administered in a liquid form, or it can be loaded onto beads and administered intra-arterially, in which case the drug will elute over time.

- Postembolization syndrome is the constellation of fever, nausea, emesis, malaise, and fatigue. It is self-limited, and can last 7–10 days.

Essentials 17

■ Case

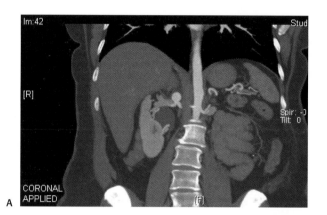

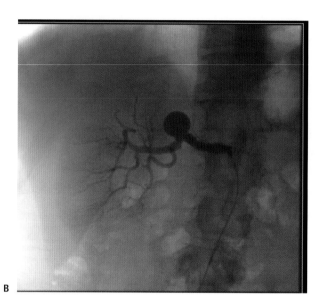

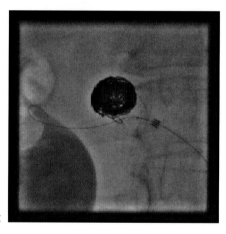

■ Questions

1. The renal computed tomography angiogram and angiogram depict what abnormality?
   A. Renal artery dissection
   B. Renal artery transection
   C. Renal artery aneurysm
   D. Renal artery stenosis
   E. Renal artery arteriovenous malformation

2. What is an accepted threshold size for intervention of visceral artery aneurysms?
   A. 0.5 cm
   B. 1 cm
   C. 1.5 cm
   D. 2 cm
   E. 5 cm

3. What treatment technique is depicted with this image?
   A. Glue embolization
   B. Stent graft placement
   C. Coiling
   D. Thrombin injection
   E. "Front door–back door" embolization

■ Answers and Explanations

Question 1

C. Correct! There is a main renal artery aneurysm.

The other answers are all incorrect.

Question 2

D. Correct! Visceral/renal aneurysms > 2 cm are often considered for treatment. This is especially true for high-risk or symptomatic patients. Note that this size indication is largely by consensus and not by randomized studies.

Other choices and discussion

A. Considered a very small aneurysm, those that are 0.5 cm are usually not treated because of small size. However, some radiologists will treat an aneurysm of any size, if the patient is symptomatic, has multiple aneurysms, is pregnant, or is a female of childbearing age.

B. Aneurysms that are 1 cm are often observed if they are discovered incidentally and if the patient is not a female of childbearing age. While each visceral aneurysm may behave differently, the risk for a devastating complication (like rupture) is low for an aneurysm of this size in a low-risk patient.

C. The range of 1 to 2 cm is a gray zone. Here, some practitioners consider treatment, but the majority consensus is that asymptomatic aneurysms < 2 cm can be safely observed.

E. Aneurysms > 5 cm are considered very large for a visceral aneurysm and should clearly be treated. Ideally, however, these aneurysms should be treated much sooner, when they reach 2 cm.

Question 3

C. Correct! This image depicts coil embolization of the renal artery aneurysm, which is one of the techniques used for treating an aneurysm. The technical difficulty with coiling is keeping the coils in the aneurysm sac without letting them spill into the parent vessel. This can be best achieved with meticulous technique and with tight packing of the coils.

Often, balloon-assisted or stent-assisted coiling can help. With balloon-assisted coiling, a balloon is inflated in the parent artery across the neck of the aneurysm, and a separate catheter (which is trapped by the balloon in the aneurysm) is used to introduce coils into the closed space. At the end of the procedure, the balloon is removed and the coils are left behind.

A similar technique is used with stent-assisted coiling. Here, an uncovered stent is placed in the parent vessel across the neck of the aneurysm, and a second catheter is trapped or placed through the stent interstices into the aneurysm. The general structure of the stent keeps the coils from prolapsing out of the aneurysm.

Other choices and discussion

A. Glue can be used to treat a variety of endovascular conditions, but that is not what is shown in the test case.

B. A stent graft (also known as a covered stent) can be used to exclude an aneurysm while maintaining arterial flow in the parent vessel. This graft is a good choice for end arteries that do not have collateral supply, in which sacrificing the parent vessel would result in distal ischemia.

D. Thrombin injection can be performed percutaneously for pseudoaneurysms, but it is not being used to treat this true aneurysm.

E. The "front door–back door" technique allows the interventionalist to embolize both beyond the aneurysm and the vessel leading into the aneurysm (or pseudoaneurysm). This prevents backfilling of the aneurysm. This is best done in vascular territories where there is collateral supply, not in end arteries where front door embolization alone will lead to infarction of that vascular territory.

■ Suggested Readings

Nosher JL, Chung J, Brevetti LS, Graham AM, Siegel RL. Visceral and renal artery aneurysms: a pictoral essay on endovascular therapy. Radiographics 2006;26(6):1687–1704

Top Tips

◆ An accepted size indication for treating incidental renal artery aneurysms is 2 cm. There is also generalized agreement that pregnant women or women of childbearing age are at an increased risk for rupture, and even smaller aneurysms in these patients should be treated.

◆ Aneurysms can be treated by exclusion via a covered stent, embolization of the native artery beyond and before the aneurysm (front door, back door embolization), or filling the aneurysm itself with embolic material (coils, glue, Onyx [Medtronic, Minneapolis, MN]).

◆ Renal artery aneurysms may be associated with hypertension.

Essentials 18

■ Case

A 23-year-old with cystic fibrosis presents with massive hemoptysis. Interventional radiology was consulted for embolization.

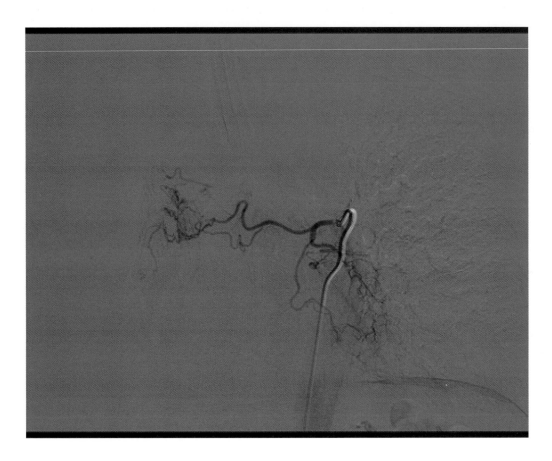

■ Questions

1. Which test would be most helpful prior to angiography?
   A. Serum hemoglobin level
   B. Chest radiograph
   C. Bronchoscopy
   D. Arterial blood gas

2. How many bronchial arteries are typically on the right and on the left?
   A. Three on the right, two on the left
   B. One on the right, two on the left
   C. Two on the right, two on the left
   D. One on the right, three on the left

3. What embolic material is best used for bronchial artery embolization?
   A. Particles
   B. Coils
   C. Dehydrated ethanol
   D. Vascular plug

■ Answers and Explanations

Question 1

C. Correct! Bronchoscopy is helpful in identifying the anatomic source of bleeding and may be useful for therapy as well. Once the side or lobe of bleeding is identified, selective embolization may be performed. Note that active bleeding is rarely identified on angiography.

Other choices and discussion

A. Knowledge of the patient's hemoglobin is useful, but bronchoscopy and possibly angiography may be necessary to control the bleeding regardless of the hemoglobin value.

B. Chest radiograph (or better yet, computed tomography) is useful to help determine the etiology of the bleeding. In this case, the history of cystic fibrosis is provided.

D. Knowledge of the patient's oxygenation is useful, but bronchoscopy and possibly angiography may be necessary to control the bleeding regardless of the oxygenation value.

Other common etiologies of hemoptysis include tuberculosis, lung cancer, bronchiectasis, and aspergillosis. The crucial immediate objective is to identify the anatomic lobe or side of bleeding.

Question 2

B. Correct! Most commonly, there is one bronchial artery on the right and two on the left. This is counterintuitive, as the left lung has two lobes and the right lung has three lobes. These bronchial arteries originate between the T3 and T8 levels. It should be noted that there is significant variation in the origin of the bronchial arteries, with supply potentially coming from intercostal arteries, mammary arteries, and even the thyrocervical trunk.

The other choices are all incorrect.

Question 3

A. Correct! Particulate embolic material is traditionally used for bronchial artery embolization. It allows for vessel occlusion without blocking the origin of the artery. In this way, the same vessel may be catheterized again in the future, should the patient rebleed.

Other choices and discussion

B. Coils are a less robust option for embolization because they do not provide distal occlusion at the site of bleeding. This makes access to the bronchial artery more complicated if the patient bleeds again.

C. Dehydrated ethanol embolization is not traditionally used in the lungs due to its highly noxious nature and the risk of tissue necrosis.

D. Vascular plugs are a less robust option for embolization because they do not provide distal occlusion at the site of bleeding.

Patients with cystic fibrosis are at high risk for having future episodes of bronchial artery hemorrhage.

■ Suggested Readings

Yoon W, Kim JK, Kim YH, Chung TW, Kang HK. Bronchial and nonbronchial systemic arterial embolization for life-threatening hemoptysis: a comprehensive review. Radiographics 2002;22(6):1395–1409

Top Tips

◆ The exact definition of massive hemoptysis is somewhat controversial. A total of 300 to 500 mL of blood per day is a reasonable definition.

◆ A pulmonary artery aneurysm may be a cause of hemoptysis. A pulmonary artery aneurysm is termed a Rasmussen aneurysm.

◆ Every bronchial artery angiogram should be scrutinized for the presence of the anterior spinal artery. This artery supplies the spinal cord. Embolization should not be performed if the anterior spinal artery is within the embolization territory because of the risk of permanent paralysis!

SECTION VI
INTERVENTIONAL IMAGING

Essentials 19

■ Case

A 44-year-old man presents with ascites, abdominal pain, and elevated liver function tests.

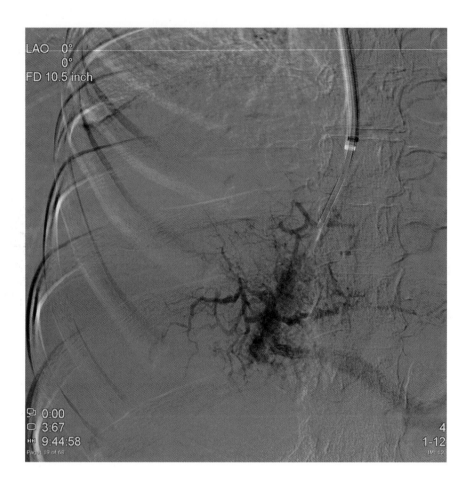

■ Questions

1. Based on the angiographic findings, what is the most likely diagnosis?
   A. Hepatocellular carcinoma
   B. Arterial-portal shunting
   C. Hepatitis C
   D. Budd-Chiari syndrome

2. With respect to the middle hepatic vein, the main right portal vein is located:
   A. Anterior
   B. Posterior
   C. Lateral
   D. Medial

3. When a TIPS is placed to treat bleeding varices, what is the ideal portosystemic venous pressure gradient?
   A. > 12 mm Hg
   B. ≤ 12 mm Hg
   C. ≤ 3 mm Hg
   D. ≥ 15 mm Hg

■ Answers and Explanations

Question 1

D. Correct! This study shows Budd-Chiari syndrome. Budd-Chiari is characterized by thrombosis of the hepatic veins. The treatment beyond medical management is vascular decompression through a transjugular intrahepatic portosystemic shunt (TIPS) procedure, which can be life-saving and preclude the need for transplant.

Other choices and discussion

A. While the patient may have hepatocellular carcinoma, the study shown is from a TIPS procedure and no hepatocellular carcinoma is visualized.

B. This is a hepatic venous study and does not show arterial-portal shunting.

C. While the patient may have hepatitis, this cannot be determined with a hepatic venogram.

Question 2

B. Correct! The right portal vein lies posterior to the middle hepatic vein. A TIPS typically involves connecting the right hepatic vein to the right portal vein. The right hepatic vein is usually the most posterior hepatic vein in the liver and is posterior to the right portal vein. This means that if a needle is placed into the right hepatic vein and aimed anteriorly, it will most likely enter the right portal vein. If the radiologist is in the middle hepatic vein, if he/she aims anteriorly the needle may enter the left portal vein and if he/she aims posteriorly the needle may enter the right portal vein.

The Gore Viatorr stent graft has become the most widely used stent for TIPS placement. The first 2 cm are uncovered for placement in the portal vein, with the remainder of the stent covered to prevent bile leaks or bleeding. This technique has demonstrated increased patency compared to uncovered stents.

The other choices are incorrect.

Question 3

B. Correct! The target gradient for bleeding varices is $\leq$ 12 mm Hg.

Other choices and discussion

A. A gradient > 12 mm Hg would predispose the patient to continued bleeding.

C. A gradient of < 3 mm Hg would help to controlling variceal bleeding, but may put the patient at increased risk for hepatic encephalopathy.

D. A gradient > 15 mm Hg would predispose the patient to continued bleeding.

Normal TIPS ultrasound velocities range from 90 to 190 cm/sec. Evaluation for the direction of flow (which should be toward the liver in the main portal vein and reversed in the left portal vein) and for thrombus in the TIPS should be noted on every TIPS ultrasound. Comparison to prior studies is critical to determine if there is TIPS dysfunction due to the wide variety of appearances of TIPS stents on ultrasound.

Note that the Model for End Stage Liver Disease correlates with the 90-day mortality and can be used to calculate the risk of performing an elective TIPS.

■ Suggested Readings

ACR-SIR-SPR practice parameter for the creating of a Transjugular Intrahepatic Portosystemic Shunt (TIPS). Amended 2014. Acr.org.

Kliewer MA, Hertzberg BS, Heneghan JP, Suhocki PV, Sheafor DH, Gannon PA, Paulson EK. Transjugular Intrahepatic Portosystemic Shunts (TIPS) effects on respiratory state and patient position on the measurement of Doppler velocities. Am J Roentgenol 2000;175:149–152

Top Tips

◆ In patients with traditional anatomy, the right portal vein is *anterior* to the right hepatic vein.

◆ Heart failure, severe coagulopathy, severe liver dysfunction, and hepatic encephalopathy are all relative contraindications to an elective TIPS.

◆ Normal TIPS ultrasound velocities range from 90 to 190 cm/sec.

Essentials 20

■ Case

A 40-year-old man presents with throbbing pain of his right hand. Select image from magnetic resonance angiography is provided.

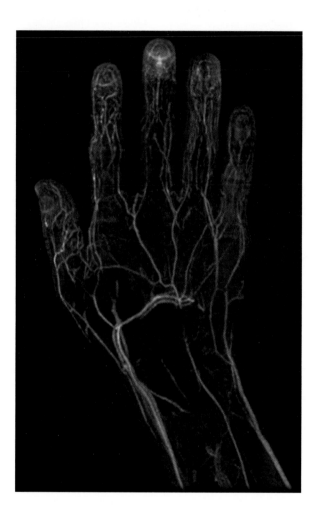

■ Questions

1. What is the most important piece of clinical history needed to make this diagnosis?
   A. Occupational and recreational history
   B. Family history
   C. Medication history
   D. Smoking history
   E. Surgical history

2. All of the following are commonly seen on angiography with this diagnosis EXCEPT?
   A. Stenotic areas
   B. Abrupt cutoff of the vessel
   C. Aneurysm
   D. Corkscrew configuration
   E. Tortuosity of the vessel

3. Which vessel(s) typically primarily supplies the superficial palmar arch?
   A. The radial artery
   B. The ulnar artery
   C. The median artery
   D. The radial and ulnar arteries
   E. The radial, ulnar, and median arteries

■ Answers and Explanations

Question 1

A. Correct! Occupational and recreational history. A history of repetitive trauma is classic for this patient's diagnosis, which is hypothenar hammer syndrome. This patient had a history of playing hockey with repetitive injury to the hypothenar eminence. This repetitive trauma results in intimal hyperplasia with duplication and fragmentation of the internal elastic lamina. Imaging findings include a corkscrew appearance of the distal ulnar artery, abrupt occlusion (as in this case), stenosis, and less commonly, aneurysm formation. This classically occurs in patients with repetitive blunt trauma to the hypothenar eminence, although cases have also been reported after a single injury.

Optimal treatment is not known, given the rarity of the disease. Patients are commonly educated on hand protection, maintenance of a warm environment, and smoking cessation. It has been shown that patients who continue to smoke fail both conservative and invasive treatments. Catheter-based thrombolysis may be pursued. Surgical options include ligation of the ulnar artery (if there is sufficient collateral circulation), direct end-to-end anastomosis, and reconstruction with vein interposition graft.

The other choices are incorrect. Smoking history is important to know when considering treatment, but not to make the diagnosis.

Question 2

C. Correct! Aneurysm may be present, but is much less common with this diagnosis than all of the other provided choices.

With hypothenar hammer syndrome, segmental/digital pressures are helpful in localizing the site of obstruction. Magnetic resonance angiography and computed tomography angiography are helpful both in visualizing the vessels and in excluding alternative etiologies (i.e., bony and soft tissue abnormalities) to explain the patient's symptoms. Catheter-based angiography remains the gold standard and can provide detailed anatomic evaluation of the hand vasculature.

The other choices are incorrect—that is, they are all commonly seen on angiography with this diagnosis.

Question 3

B. Correct! The ulnar artery typically supplies the superficial palmar arch. The superficial palmar arch is considered complete if it supplies all of the fingers and the ulnar side of the thumb. It is considered incomplete if it does not supply the thumb.

Other choices and discussion

A. The distal end of the superficial palmar arch of the ulnar artery communicates with the radial artery in only 34% of cases.

C. The median artery may provide some blood supply to the hand, but this is atypical.

■ Suggested Readings

Blum AG, Zabel JP, Kohlmann R, et al. Pathologic conditions of the hypothenar eminence: evaluation with multidetector CT and MR imaging. Radiographics 2006;26:1021–1044

Swanson KE, Bartholomew JR, Paulson R. Hypothenar hammer syndrome: a case and brief review. Vasc Med 2011;7(2):108–115

Top Tips

◆ Hypothenar hammer syndrome refers to injury to the terminal ulnar artery after it exits Guyon canal. This classically occurs in patients with repetitive blunt trauma to the hypothenar eminence, either related to occupation or recreation.

◆ Patients may present with cold intolerance, pain in the palm, and numbness and color changes in the fingers with sparing of the thumb. Ulceration and gangrene may be present in extreme cases. On physical exam, Allen test is positive.

◆ Hypothenar hammer syndrome shares many common features with thromboangiitis obliterans. Hypothenar hammer syndrome tends to present asymmetrically in the dominant hand, whereas thromboangiitis obliterans tends to present symmetrically, often with lower vessel involvement. Hypothenar hammer syndrome also tends to spare the thumb, unlike thromboangiitis obliterans (when it involves the hand).

Essentials 21

■ Case

A 50-year-old man presents with resistant hypertension and this magnetic resonance angiogram of the renal arteries.

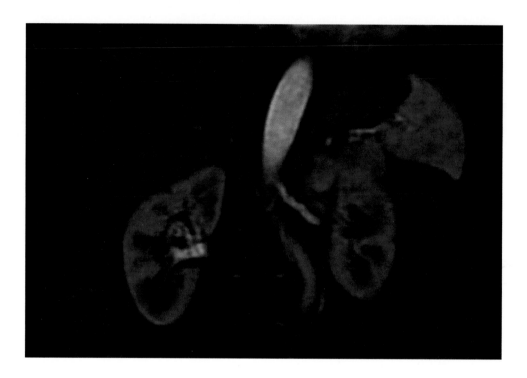

■ Questions

1. What is atypical about this patient's presentation of this disease?
   A. Gender
   B. Age
   C. Presenting sign
   D. Imaging appearance
   E. Location

2. The most commonly affected artery with this condition is?
   A. Carotid
   B. Vertebral
   C. Brachial
   D. Renal
   E. Iliac

3. What is the treatment of choice for a young patient with new onset hypertension resistant to medical treatment and imaging findings suggestive of renal fibromuscular dysplasia ?
   A. Continued medical management
   B. Percutaneous transluminal angioplasty
   C. Primary stent placement
   D. Surgical revascularization
   E. Nephrectomy

■ Answers and Explanations

Question 1

A. Correct! The age, presenting symptom, and imaging findings all point to fibromuscular dysplasia (FMD) as the likely diagnosis. However, females are affected more often than males (3:1).

Other choices and discussion

B. The age in this case is typical for FMD (40 to 60 years old).

C. The presenting sign of hypertension is typical for cases of FMD involving the renal arteries.

D. The imaging shows a classic string of beads appearance, typical for FMD. Note the absence of atherosclerotic plaque. Computed tomography angiography and magnetic resonance angiography are both good modalities to evaluate for FMD, but conventional contrast angiography is the gold standard.

E. Involvement of the renal arteries is typical for FMD.

Question 2

D. Correct! A total of 80% of patients with FMD have renal artery involvement. Involvement of the renal arteries is bilateral in approximately 35% of cases.

There are a variety of imaging appearances of FMD. The classic appearance is seen with the medial fibroplasia subtype, demonstrating the "string of beads" (multifocal areas of stenosis and intervening dilated segments). The intimal fibroplasia subtype manifests as short focal stenoses. The perimedial subtype manifests as long tubular stenoses with fewer dilatations. Adventitial fibroplasia subtypes have also been described. These different subtypes are associated with varying response rates after treatment.

The differential diagnostic considerations of this case appearance include atherosclerotic disease, vasculitis, Marfan's, and Ehlers Danlos. Segmental arterial mediolysis should be considered when there is involvement of the superior mesenteric artery or gastroduodenal artery.

Other choices and discussion

A. Extracranial carotid involvement is the second most commonly involved location.

B. Vertebral arteries (and intracranial carotid) arteries can also be involved, but much less commonly.

C. FMD can involve any artery, but brachial artery involvement is rare.

E. FMD can involve any artery, but iliac artery involvement is rare.

Question 3

B. Correct! Percutaneous transluminal angioplasty is the preferred first-line treatment in young patients with new onset hypertension, especially if the hypertension is resistant to pharmacologic management. Pharmacologic therapy is the first-line therapy for patients with renal FMD and hypertension. If this fails, then percutaneous angioplasty is the preferred treatment. Stent placement is reserved for patients for whom angioplasty is insufficient. Surgical revascularization is needed in rare cases.

Technical success rates for percutaneous angioplasty are > 85%, but strict hypertension cure (defined as blood pressure < 140/90 mm Hg without pharmacologic therapy) is only achieved in 36% of cases. Hypertension cure rates are higher when pharmacologic therapy is continued postintervention. Major complications are less frequent with percutaneous angioplasty than after surgery. Patients should undergo regular surveillance, as the natural history includes new and worsening lesions in up to 40% of cases.

Other choices and discussion

A. Medical management alone is not the treatment of choice. If medical management fails, then percutaneous angioplasty is recommended.

C. Primary stent placement is not recommended, but may be needed if restenosis or dissection occurs after angioplasty.

D. Surgical revascularization may be necessary in some cases.

E. Nephrectomy is not an appropriate treatment for FMD.

■ Suggested Readings

Hickey RM, Nemcek AA. Diagnosis and role of interventional techniques. In Geschwind J-F, Dake MD (eds). Abrams' Angiography. Philadelphia, PA: Lippincott Williams & Wilkins; 2014: 621–622

Varennes L, Tahon F, Grand S, et al. Fibromuscular dysplasia: what the radiologist should know: a pictorial review. Insights Imaging 2015;6(3):295–307

Top Tips

♦ FMD is an idiopathic, nonatherosclerotic, noninflammatory disease that affects small to medium-sized arteries.

♦ Clinical symptoms depend on location and severity of disease. Patients with renal artery involvement may be asymptomatic or present with hypertension. Patients with carotid and vertebral artery involvement may present with headache, dizziness, neck pain, or more serious symptoms including transient ischemic attack or stroke.

♦ Catheter angiography remains the gold standard for diagnosis of FMD due to its high spatial resolution. Computed tomography angiography and magnetic resonance angiography have high specificity but lower sensitivity, and a negative exam does not exclude FMD. Ultrasound can be helpful, with end diastolic velocity ≥ 150 cm/sec, or renal-to-aortic peak systolic velocity ≥ 3.5, suggesting moderate to severe stenosis.

Essentials 22

■ Case

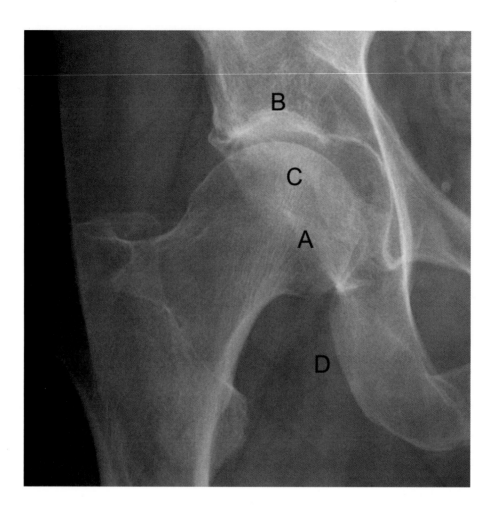

■ Questions

1. Match the letter on the image with the appropriate description of the arterial access site.
   __ Too high
   __ Too low
   __ Ideal access site for retrograde catheterization
   __ Ideal access site for antegrade catheterization

2. What is the ideal skin entry site for retrograde common femoral artery access?
   A. Inguinal fold
   B. Midfemoral head
   C. Upper femoral head
   D. Lower femoral head
   E. Lesser trochanter

3. A 5 French sheath is placed. What is the maximum catheter size that this sheath can accommodate?
   A. 4 French
   B. 4.5 French
   C. 5 French
   D. 5.5 French
   E. 6 French

■ Answers and Explanations

Question 1

B. Too high. Access in this location could lead to intraabdominal bleeding when the access is removed, and it is not easy to hold pressure in this location.

D. Too low. This is likely below the bifurcation of the common iliac artery, and it may be difficult to hold pressure.

A. Ideal access for retrograde catheterization. This access is likely into the common femoral artery in most patients, and pressure may be held against the femoral head to obtain hemostasis.

C. Ideal access for antegrade catheterization. When accessing down the leg, one must access a little higher over the femoral head to have enough "running room" to place a sheath and be able to select the superficial femoral artery.

Question 2

D. Correct! The lower femoral head is the ideal skin entry site for retrograde common femoral artery access.

Other choices and discussion

A. The inguinal fold has a variable relationship to the lower femoral head and is not a good landmark to guide common femoral artery puncture.

B. The midfemoral head is the ideal vessel entry site, not the ideal skin entry site. This is the ideal vessel entry site because the common femoral artery is easily compressed against the femoral head in this location.

C. The upper femoral head is the ideal skin entry site for antegrade common femoral artery access.

E. The lesser trochanter is very low, and the common femoral artery has already bifurcated in many patients at this level.

Lack of adequate hemostasis after the procedure can result in hematoma or hemorrhage. Manual compression should be held for at least 15 minutes. Many practitioners have the leg that was used for access kept straight for a given period of time (often 4 hours for a 4 French sheath, 5 hours for a 5 French sheath, etc.) Vascular closure devices may also be considered, which result in decreased manual compression time, time to mobilization, and time to patient discharge but are not necessarily associated with decreased application rate.

Question 3

C. Correct! 5 French is the maximum catheter size that a 5 French sheath can accommodate. Sheaths are described by their inner diameter versus catheters, which are described by their outer diameter. Catheter size describes the outer diameter in French, where 3F = 1 mm. The French size of sheaths refers to the inner diameter, or the size of catheter that can fit inside the sheath. This means that the actual diameter of the hole created by the sheath is 1.5 to 2F larger than the sheath size.

Other choices and discussion

A. A 5 French sheath can accommodate a larger catheter than 4 French.

B. A 5 French sheath can accommodate a larger catheter than 4.5 French.

D. A 5 French sheath cannot accommodate a catheter larger than a 5 French.

E. A 5 French sheath cannot accommodate a catheter larger than a 5 French.

■ Suggested Readings

Barbetta I, van den Berg JC. Access and hemostasis: femoral and popliteal approaches and closure devices – why, what, when, and how? Semin Intervent Radiol 2014;31(4):353–360

Kaufman JA. Invasive vascular diagnosis. In Mauro MA, Murphy KPJ, Thomson KR, et al (eds). Image-Guided Interventions. Philadelphia, PA: Saunders; 2013: 11–32

Top Tips

◆ Vascular access of the arterial system is accomplished with the Seldinger technique, by which a device is introduced into a blood vessel over a guidewire.

◆ The common femoral artery is the most common access site for angiography. Proper technique, including selection of the appropriate skin entry site, is essential to avoid complications.

◆ To avoid bleeding after the procedure, manual compression for at least 15 minutes is recommended. Keeping the accessed leg straight for several hours post procedure is also helpful.

Essentials 23

■ Case

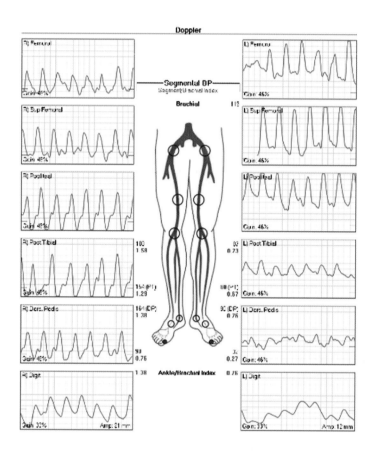

■ Questions

1. What symptoms are expected with an ankle-brachial index (ABI) of 0.5?
   A. The patient likely is asymptomatic.
   B. The patient likely has mild claudication.
   C. The patient likely has moderate claudication.
   D. The patient likely has resting pain.
   E. The patient likely has tissue loss.

2. A falsely elevated ABI may occur in cases of:
   A. Recent exercise
   B. Smoking
   C. Heavily calcified peripheral arteries
   D. Vasculitis
   E. Recent administration of vasodilators

3. A patient comes to the office complaining of mild intermittent leg cramping that improves with rest. Her symptoms do not significantly impact her lifestyle. She has an ABI of 0.8. The next best step is:
   A. Surgical management
   B. Endovascular management
   C. Imaging evaluation
   D. Risk factor modification
   E. Conservative symptom management alone

■ Answers and Explanations

Question 1

C. Correct! Patients with ABI ranging from 0.4 to 0.7 are expected to have moderate claudication. The ABI is a quick, reliable, noninvasive method to assess for peripheral arterial disease. A pneumatic cuff and Doppler ultrasound probe are used to determine the systolic blood pressure at the ankle by assessing the dorsalis pedis and posterior tibial artery pressures bilaterally, and in the arms by assessing the brachial arteries bilaterally. The higher of the dorsalis pedis and posterior tibial artery values is divided by the higher of the brachial artery values to obtain the ratio.

Other choices and discussion

A. The normal range of ABI is 1.0 to 1.2. Less than 0.9 is considered abnormal, but patients may be asymptomatic with mildly abnormal ABI.

B. Patients with ABI ranging from 0.7 to 0.9 have mild disease and may be asymptomatic or may have mild claudication.

D. Patients with an ABI of < 0.3 are expected to have rest pain.

E. Patients with an ABI of < 0.3 are expected to have tissue loss.

Question 2

C. Correct! Because heavily calcified peripheral arteries are difficult to compress, this may result in a falsely elevated value. This most often occurs in diabetic patients with calcific medial sclerosis. In these cases, a toe-brachial index can be a valuable indicator of peripheral disease. A normal toe-brachial index is 0.6 to 0.7 or greater. Pulse volume recordings also remain accurate in patients with non-compressible vessels.

None of the other listed choices falsely elevate the ABI.

Question 3

D. Correct! It is important to address modifiable risk factors to reduce overall cardiovascular morbidity and mortality. Management of risk factors, including smoking, hypertension, hyperlipidemia, and diabetes, is an important part of first-line treatment for vascular disease. Lifestyle modifications, such as maintaining a healthy weight and getting regular exercise, are also important.

Patients with chronic arterial insufficiency may be asymptomatic or may present with intermittent claudication. Additionally, these patients sometimes progress to rest pain, tissue loss, and gangrene. Symptoms occur in the muscle group just distal to the region of arterial stenosis. A thorough history and physical exam is needed. Besides a complete vascular exam documenting diminished or absent pulses, careful examination of the skin for color changes, temperature changes, and hair loss should be performed. Examination for ulcers, including their appearance and location, is also important.

Other choices and discussion

A. Revascularization procedures are generally considered in patients with progressive symptoms or those who are severely limited by their symptoms.

B. See answer A.

C. Due to cost, potential radiation exposure, and potential invasive procedures, imaging evaluation is generally not considered unless a patient requires revascularization.

E. Although symptom management is important, this alone is not sufficient treatment for peripheral arterial disease.

■ Suggested Readings

Brooke BS, Black JH. Clinical vascular exam. In Mauro MA, Murphy KPJ, Thomson KR, et al (eds). Image-Guided Interventions. Philadelphia, PA: Saunders; 2013: 46–53

Kaufman J. Lower-extremity arteries. In Kaufman JS, Lee MJ (eds). Vascular and Interventional Radiology. Philadelphia, PA: Saunders; 2013: 334–364

Weinberg I, Jaff MR. Diagnostic noninvasive evaluations: ultrasound and hemodynamic studies. In Geschwind J-F, Dake MD (eds). Abrams' Angiography. Philadelphia, PA: Lippincott Williams & Wilkins; 2014: 388–401

Top Tips

- An ABI of 1.0 to 1.2 is considered normal. Mild arterial occlusive disease is indicated by ABI values from 0.7 to 0.9. ABI values from 0.4 to 0.7 indicate moderate disease, and severe disease is indicated by values < 0.4. Gangrene is often found with ABI values of < 0.2.

- The absolute pressure is also useful for evaluation. An ankle pressure < 50 mm Hg is suggestive of chronic limb ischemia.

- A segmental limb pressure reduction of > 20 mm Hg from one level to the next or compared to the contralateral segment is considered significant. This measurement may be combined with Doppler waveform analysis at each level to provide information about flow as well as pressure.

Essentials 24

■ Case

A patient with a percutaneous cholecystostomy presents for evaluation.

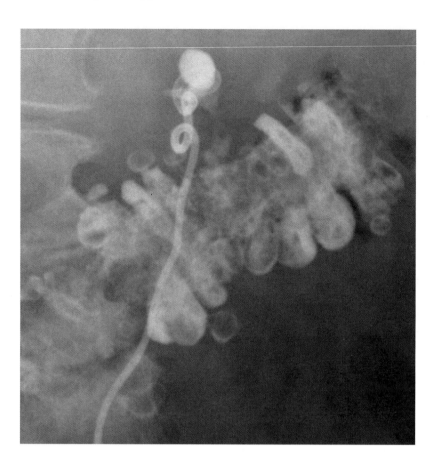

■ Questions

1. Which route is preferred for percutaneous cholecystos-
   tomy placement?
   A. Transgastric
   B. Transpleural
   C. Transhepatic
   D. Transduodenal
   E. Transcolonic

2. What are the Society of Interventional Radiology (SIR)
   guidelines regarding the withholding of aspirin prior to
   cholecystostomy drain placement?
   A. Withhold aspirin for 10 days
   B. Withhold aspirin for 5 days
   C. Withhold aspirin for 3 days
   D. Withhold aspirin for 1 day
   E. No withholding of aspirin recommended

3. What is the pertinent finding on this image?
   A. Cystic duct patency
   B. Gallbladder perforation
   C. Cholelithiasis
   D. Fistula formation
   E. Bile leak

■ Answers and Explanations

Question 1

C. Correct! A transhepatic approach is preferred, which is believed to provide greater catheter stability. Ideally, this approach traverses the bare area of the liver, which ensures that any bile leak that occurs is extraperitoneal. A transperitoneal route is also commonly utilized.

Percutaneous cholecystostomy is placed most commonly to permit gallbladder decompression in the setting of acute cholecystitis in a poor surgical candidate. Occasionally, percutaneous cholecystostomy is also utilized to allow access into the biliary system for stent placement or other biliary intervention. Intravenous antibiotics with gram-negative coverage are often administered, with adjustment of antibiotic coverage after cultures.

The other choices are all incorrect.

Question 2

E. Correct! Percutaneous cholecystostomy tube placement is classified as a moderate risk procedure under SIR guidelines. According to SIR guidelines, aspirin does not need to be withheld for procedures with a moderate risk of bleeding. Other procedures with a moderate risk of bleeding include initial placement of a gastrostomy tube, transabdominal liver biopsy, and intra-abdominal abscess drainage.

There are few contraindications to percutaneous cholecystostomy tube placement. These include the lack of a safe route to the gallbladder and gallbladder tumor that may be seeded by percutaneous access. Coagulopathy is a relative contraindication.

The other choices are all incorrect.

Question 3

D. Correct! Upon injection of the tube, the ascending colon is opacified, confirming a fistula between the gallbladder and the colon. In general, complications of percutaneous cholecystostomy tube placement are rare, and may include bile leak, sepsis, peritonitis, and hemorrhage. Transgression of nearby structures, including pleura and bowel, may also occur, which can result in perforation and fistula formation.

Other choices and discussion

A. The cystic duct is not well visualized on this image.

B. There is no extravasation of contrast into the peritoneum, which would be expected with gallbladder perforation.

C. Cholelithiasis is not seen.

E. Extraluminal contrast is not demonstrated, so there is no evidence of a bile leak.

■ Suggested Readings

Fahrbach TM, Wyse GM, Lawler LP, et al. Percutaneous cholecystostomy. In Mauro MA, Murphy KPJ, Thomson KR, et al (eds). Image-Guided Interventions. Philadelphia, PA: Saunders; 2013: 1008–1013

Patel IJ, Davidson JC, Nikolic B. Consensus guidelines for periprocedural management of coagulation status and hemostasis risk in percutaneous image-guided interventions. J Vasc Interv Radiol 2012;23:727–736

Top Tips

◆ The preferred method of percutaneous gallbladder access is with ultrasound guidance, via either a trocar or with the Seldinger technique. The catheter should be attached to external bag drainage.

◆ In the case of calculous cholecystitis, a tube cholangiogram is performed to assess for patency of the cystic duct prior to removal. Alternatively, the tube may be capped for 48 hours to assess for symptoms. Often, the tube will remain in place until the time of cholecystectomy.

◆ Early postprocedure care includes monitoring of vital signs and symptoms. The tube should be left open to drainage and not capped. The tract is left to mature for 4 to 6 weeks.

Essentials 25

■ **Case**

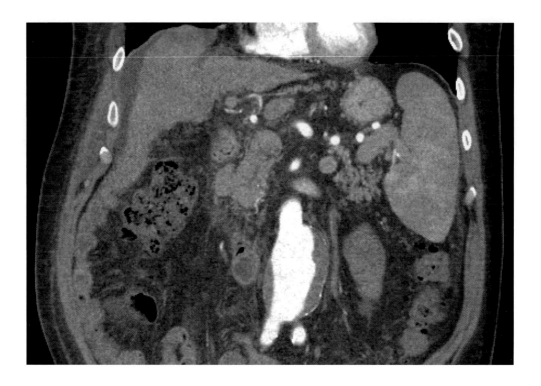

■ **Questions**

1. Which of the following is a typical indication for abdominal aortic aneurysm (AAA) repair?
   A. Presence of an AAA > 4.5 cm
   B. Stable AAA
   C. Growth of an AAA > 0.5 cm in 1 year
   D. Growth of an AAA > 0.5 cm in 6 months

2. Which modality is most likely to underestimate an aneurysm sac size?
   A. Ultrasound
   B. Computed tomography
   C. Magnetic resonance imaging
   D. Conventional angiography
   E. All of the above modalities are similarly accurate

3. Which of the following anatomic considerations is important in planning endovascular repair of an AAA?
   A. Aortic neck length
   B. Aortic neck angulation
   C. Mural thrombus at the aortic neck
   D. Size and tortuosity of the iliac and femoral arteries
   E. All of the above

■ Answers and Explanations

Question 1

D. Correct! Rapid growth of an AAA > 0.5 cm in 6 months is an indication for repair. An infrarenal (below the renal artery takeoff) AAA is defined as an aortic diameter > 3 cm or 50% greater diameter than the adjacent nonaneurysmal aorta. Most AAAs involve the infrarenal aorta, but up to 15% may involve the suprarenal aorta.

Other choices and discussion

A. Presence of an AAA > 5.5 cm is an indication for repair, not 4.5 cm. Repair may be considered in AAAs smaller than 5.5 cm in patients with higher rupture risk (like women). Alternatively, repair may be delayed in older patients who are at higher risk for perioperative mortality.

B. A stable AAA is not usually an indication to repair, unless the size is > 5.5 cm or the patient is symptomatic.

C. Growth of an AAA > 0.5 cm per year is not an indication for repair.

Question 2

D. Correct! Conventional digital subtraction angiography only assesses the patent lumen, cannot assess for mural thrombus, and may underestimate the total aneurysm sac size.

Other choices and discussion

The other choices are all incorrect—that is, they are all capable of accurately measuring aneurysm sac size.

A. Ultrasound is useful for detection and monitoring of an AAA with reasonable estimates of sac size.

B. Computed tomography is excellent at assessing AAA size as well as assessing the aortic neck and access vessels for intervention planning.

C. Magnetic resonance imaging is excellent at assessing aneurysm size, but is limited in evaluation of calcification.

Question 3

E. Correct! All of these factors need to be considered when planning endovascular repair.

The aortic neck is defined as the distance from the lowest renal artery to the beginning of the aneurysmal aorta. A minimum length is needed to ensure proper fixation and sealing of the proximal aspect of the endograft. With current devices, this minimum length is 10 to 15 mm. The aortic neck should be nonaneurysmal.

Angulation of the aortic neck is also important. With current devices, the maximum angulation allowed ranges from 45 to 60 degrees.

The shape of the neck and presence of mural thrombus must also be considered. Another consideration when planning aneurysm repair is the size and tortuosity of the ilio-femoral arteries, to ensure proper sealing of the distal aspects of the endograft. Preservation of one internal iliac artery for pelvic blood flow is recommended. The minimal size of these vessels that can be used depends on the device.

■ Suggested Readings

Vallabhaneni R, Farber MA. Aortic stent-grafts. In Mauro MA, Murphy KPJ, Thomson KR, et al (eds). Image-Guided Interventions. Philadelphia, PA: Saunders; 2013: e97–e103

Yamanouchi D, Matsumura JS. Abdominal aortic aneurysms. In Geschwind J-F, Dake MD (eds). Abrams' Angiography. Philadelphia, PA: Lippincott Williams & Wilkins; 2014: 677–685

Top Tips

- AAAs can be repaired via either open surgical or endovascular techniques. Endovascular approaches result in fewer aneurysm-related deaths when compared to open repair.

- An aneurysm is defined is a focal dilation of at least 50% greater than the width of the normal artery.

- Presence of an AAA > 5.5 cm is an indication for repair.

Essentials 1

■ Case

A 12-year-old male soccer player presents with knee pain.

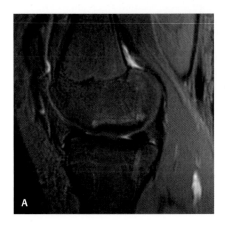 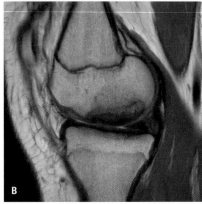 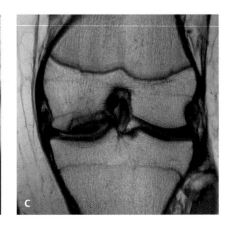

■ Questions

1. What is the diagnosis?
   A. Osteochondritis dissecans
   B. Jumper's knee
   C. Medial collateral ligament rupture
   D. Meniscal tear
   E. Salter Harris type II fracture

2. Which of the following are CORRECT regarding the depicted lesion? (Select ALL that apply.)
   A. Affected patients are typically under the age of 18 years.
   B. Lesions most commonly affect the capitellum.
   C. In the knee, these lesions are most frequently seen within the patella.
   D. The proposed etiology is an injury to an epiphyseal cartilage ossification center.
   E. Surgical treatment options include pinning and osteochondral grafting.

3. Which of the following is(are) a magnetic resonance imaging feature of osteochondritis dissecans instability? (Select ALL that apply.)
   A. Fluid imbibition deep to the lesion
   B. Cortication around the lesion
   C. Fragmentation of the subchondral plate
   D. Displacement or dislocation of the fragment
   E. Bone marrow edema pattern

■ Answers and Explanations

Question 1

A. Correct! Osteochondritis dissecans (OCD) on magnetic resonance imaging appears as a focal well-circumscribed osteochondral lesion at the epiphysis, frequently occurring in the knee at the lateral aspect of the medial femoral condyle. This is also sometimes termed an osteochondral lesion.

Other choices and discussion

B. Jumper's knee is a chronic insertional injury of the proximal attachment of the patellar tendon, presenting as thickening and increased signal within the tendon and bone marrow edema in the adjacent patella.

C. The visualized medial collateral ligament is intact.

D. No meniscal tear is demonstrated.

E. A Salter Harris type II fracture would pass across the growth plate and through the metaphysis. The growth plates and metaphyses in this patient are intact.

Question 2

A. Correct! Patients with OCD lesions tend to be young (under 18 years) and are twice as likely to be male.

D. Correct! Although the exact cause is unknown, OCD is thought to be secondary to an injury of an ossification center in the epiphyseal cartilage.

E. Correct! Surgical treatment options for unstable OCD lesions include microfracture, pinning of the osteochondral lesion, and osteochondral grafting (autograft or allograft).

Other choices and discussion

B. OCD most commonly affects the knee. It can also be seen in the talar dome of the ankle and in the capitellum of the elbow.

C. In the knee, osteochondral lesions are most frequently seen in the lateral aspect of the medial femoral condyle (70%). Lateral condylar lesions are the next most frequent (10 to 20%). Patellar lesions account for 5 to 10% of cases, and trochlear lesions are rarely seen.

Question 3

A. Correct! A T2 hyperintense (fluid intensity or granulation tissue intensity) rim surrounding an OCD lesion suggests instability in adults. However, because osteochondral lesions frequently heal with conservative management in juvenile patients, the criteria are stricter, and this rim must be *fluid* signal. The presence of cysts (even one) surrounding an OCD lesion in an adult is consistent with instability, but in a juvenile patient, the cysts should be > 5 mm in size and multiple in number to suggest instability. But even in the latter scenario, some lesions will go on to heal without surgical intervention.

B. Correct! Low-signal intensity rim or cortication around the lesion suggests instability. This would have a similar appearance to chronic ununited fractures elsewhere in the body, with the low signal cortication seen on the opposing surfaces of both the lesion and the parent bone.

C. Correct! Fragmentation of the subchondral plate suggests instability.

D. Correct! Displacement or dislocation of the fragment suggests instability.

Incorrect choice and discussion

E. A bone marrow edema pattern may be seen within the lesion or the donor site in the setting of an OCD. However, this alone is not a sign of instability.

■ Suggested Readings

Chang GH, Paz DA, Dwek JR, Chung CB. Lower extremity overuse injuries in pediatric athletes: clinical presentation, imaging findings, and treatment. Clin Imaging 2013;37(5):836–846

McKay S, Chen C, Rosenfeld S. Orthopedic perspective on selected pediatric and adolescent knee conditions. Pediatr Radiol 2013;43(Suppl 1):S99–106

Moktassi A, Popkin CA, White LM, Murnaghan ML. Imaging of osteochondritis dissecans. Orthop Clin North Am 2012;43(2):201–211, v–vi

Top Tips

- ◆ OCD lesions are most frequently seen in patients under 18 years and affect males more than females.

- ◆ OCD is most commonly seen in the knee, at the lateral aspect of the medial femoral condyle.

- ◆ Signs of OCD instability on magnetic resonance imaging include a fluid signal rim deep to the lesion, cortication of the fragment and the adjacent donor site, and displacement or dislocation of the lesion.

SECTION VII
MUSCULOSKELETAL
IMAGING

Essentials 2

■ Case

A previously healthy 48-year-old man presents with trauma and right foot pain.

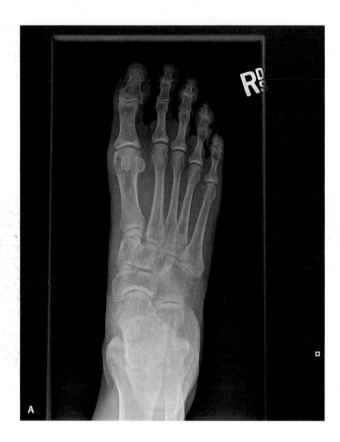
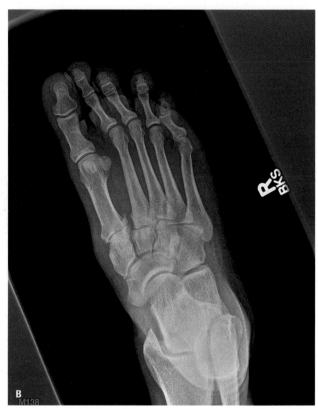

■ Questions

1. Which ONE of the following is the correct diagnosis?
   A. Second metatarsal base fracture
   B. Lisfranc fracture-dislocation
   C. Neuropathic joint
   D. Chopart joint dislocation
   E. Midfoot sprain

2. How many components make up the injury in this case?
   A. One
   B. Two
   C. Three
   D. Four
   E. Six

3. What is the best next step in management for this patient?
   A. Surgical fixation
   B. Closed reduction
   C. Placing the patient in a walking boot
   D. Repeat radiographs in 10 to 14 days
   E. Ultrasound

■ Answers and Explanations

Question 1

B. Correct! This is a Lisfranc fracture-dislocation. Offset of the second tarso-metatarsal (TMT) joint is the result of a Lisfranc ligament injury. The Lisfranc ligament runs from the second metatarsal base to the medial cuneiform. Lisfranc fracture-dislocations are divided into homolateral, in which the first through fifth metatarsals are displaced laterally, and divergent, in which the second through fifth metatarsals are displaced laterally but the first metatarsal is displaced medially. Complete Lisfranc fracture-dislocations involve all five metatarsals. In the test case, the first metatarsal base is fractured and dislocated medially. This is an example of an incomplete divergent Lisfranc fracture-dislocation. Disruption of the Lisfranc ligament typically occurs with midfoot plantar flexion in low impact trauma and with direct force in high impact trauma (i.e., motor vehicle accident).

Other choices and discussion

B. The second metatarsal base is not fractured.

C. This patient has an unremarkable past medical history and presents with an acute injury, making neuropathy unlikely. Note that neuropathy can predispose to a Lisfranc ligament injury. This is often seen in diabetic patients, may be clinically silent, and may result in midfoot arthritis and pes planus.

D. The Chopart joint refers to the calcaneocuboid and talonavicular joints. These are normal in the test case.

E. A midfoot sprain refers to Lisfranc ligament sprain without disruption of the second TMT joint. The test case demonstrates a more serious injury.

Question 2

C. Correct! The Lisfranc ligament has three components: dorsal, interosseous, and plantar. All connect the base of the second metatarsal to the medial cuneiform. The dorsal band is the weakest, explaining the frequent dorsal dislocation of the second metatarsal base with a Lisfranc ligament rupture. Weight-bearing views of the foot are very useful in depicting this dorsal dislocation.

Question 3

A. Correct! A Lisfranc fracture-dislocation or Lisfranc ligament injury that is unstable or displaced can lead to osteoarthritis and midfoot collapse if not surgically repaired in anatomic alignment.

Other choices and discussion

B. The more conservative treatment of closed reduction puts the patient at a greater risk for subsequent morbidity.

C. The more conservative treatment of placing the patient in a walking boot puts the patient at a greater risk for subsequent morbidity.

D. Repeating the radiograph is unlikely to add useful information, as the diagnosis is made on the initial radiographs.

E. Ultrasound may detect a tear of the Lisfranc ligament. However, because the radiograph already shows a Lisfranc fracture-dislocation, ultrasound is not needed. Some surgeons use computed tomography or magnetic resonance imaging for preoperative planning and to assess for additional radiographically occult fractures that can accompany Lisfranc injuries.

■ Suggested Readings

Crim J. MR imaging evaluation of subtle Lisfranc injuries: the midfoot sprain. Magn Reson Imaging Clin N Am 2008;16(1): 19–27

Siddiqui NA, Galizia MS, Almusa E, Omar IM. Evaluation of the tarsometatarsal joint using conventional radiography, CT, and MR imaging. Radiographics 2014;34(2):514–531

Top Tips

- In both homolateral and divergent Lisfranc injuries, the second through fifth metatarsals are displaced laterally. In divergent, the first metatarsal is displaced medially. In homolateral, the first metatarsal is displaced laterally (i.e., remains congruent with the other metatarsals).

- A Lisfranc injury can be easily missed on plain film, especially if the foot is imaged without weight bearing. Weight-bearing views are very important if there is concern for a midfoot injury. Even subtle offset of the second TMT joint suggests a Lisfranc injury.

- The Lisfranc ligament runs from the second metatarsal base to the medial cuneiform.

Essentials 3

■ Case

A 27-year-old woman presents with thumb pain following an acute injury.

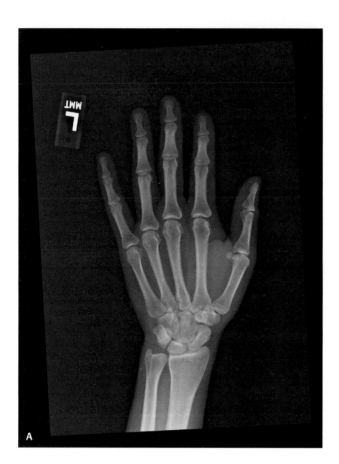

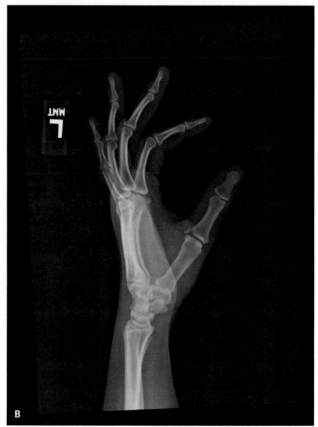

■ Questions

1. Which diagnosis do the radiographs demonstrate?
   A. Ulnar collateral ligament injury
   B. Radial collateral ligament injury
   C. Pulley injury
   D. Extensor tendon injury
   E. Flexor tendon injury

2. Which ONE of the following choices is NOT an appropriate step in the management of the injury shown above?
   A. Magnetic resonance imaging
   B. Surgical fixation
   C. Repeat radiographs with stress views
   D. Conservative management
   E. Ultrasound

3. What is the mechanism of injury in this case?
   A. Hyperadduction
   B. Hyperabduction
   C. Axial loading
   D. Hyperextension
   E. Hyperflexion

■ Answers and Explanations

Question 1

A. Correct! A small bony fragment adjacent to the ulnar base of the thumb proximal phalanx is seen. This indicates an ulnar collateral ligament (UCL) avulsion fracture. This has been classically referred to as a "gamekeeper's thumb," referencing chronic UCL injuries in patients who repetitively broke the necks of small game (rabbits). Today, this injury is most commonly seen with skiers (although "skier's thumb" is considered more of an acute injury by some). The fracture fragment in this case is displaced and rotated. The thumb metacarpophalangeal joint may be in valgus angulation with radial subluxation of the proximal phalanx.

Other choices and discussion

B. The radial collateral ligament attaches to the radial aspect of the proximal phalanx and, if injured, results in an avulsion fragment at that site and/or ulnar subluxation of the proximal phalanx.

C. Pulley injuries rarely result in avulsion fractures and therefore are typically radiographically occult.

D. An extensor tendon injury is not present in the test case. A dorsal avulsion fracture and a fixed flexion deformity could represent an extensor tendon injury.

E. A flexor tendon injury is not present in the test case. A volar avulsion fracture and a fixed extension deformity could represent a flexor tendon injury.

Question 2

C. Correct! Stress views should never be performed in patients with a gamekeeper's thumb, as stress views can actually create a Stener lesion and transform a nonsurgical injury into a surgical injury. A Stener lesion is present when the torn UCL is abnormally displaced over the adductor aponeurosis/adductor pollicus tendon. This alignment will prevent normal ligament healing, and therefore a Stener lesion requires surgical fixation.

Other choices and discussion

A. Magnetic resonance imaging (MRI) is helpful in evaluating the extent of injury to the UCL and in assessing for a possible Stener lesion. A UCL injury can often be very subtle or occult on initial radiographs.

B. Surgical fixation is required in the presence of a Stener lesion. In this case, the displaced and rotated fracture fragment is concerning for the presence of a Stener lesion. This was subsequently proven surgically, as the patient underwent surgical reduction and fixation of the UCL and avulsion fragment.

D. Conservative management (immobilization and pain control) is often sufficient to treat a nondisplaced UCL tear. However, when a Stener lesion is present, or when conservative management has failed, surgical fixation is required.

E. Like MRI, ultrasound is helpful in evaluating the extent of injury to the UCL and in assessing for a possible Stener lesion. Musculoskeletal ultrasound is often a dynamic examination, but for this indication, dynamic imaging should either be avoided or performed very carefully to avoid causing a Stener lesion.

Question 3

B. Correct! The UCL is injured when the thumb undergoes extreme hyperabduction. Gamekeeping, skiing, and break dancing have all been implicated as risk factors.

Other choices and discussion

A. A hyperadduction injury would not injure the UCL. (An injury to the radial collateral ligament would be more likely with that mechanism.)

The other mechanisms would not typically account for an injury to the UCL.

■ Suggested Readings

Clavero JA, Alomar X, Monill JM, Esplugas M, Golano P, Mendoza M, Salvador A. MR imaging of ligament and tendon injuries of the fingers. Radiographics 2002;22:237–256

Hinke DH, Erickson SJ, Chamoy L, Timins ME. Ulnar collateral ligament of the thumb: MR findings in cadavers, volunteers, and patients with ligamentous injury (gamekeeper's thumb). Am J Roentgenol 1994;163:1431–1434

Hirschmann A, Sutter R, Scweizer A, Pfirrmann CW. MRI of the thumb: anatomy and spectrum of findings in asymptomatic volunteers. Am J Roentgenol 2014;202:819–827

Top Tips

- ◆ Gamekeeper's (or skier's) thumb describes a hyperabduction injury to the UCL of the thumb metacarpophalangeal joint. Ultrasound and MRI are both quite useful in this assessment.

- ◆ A Stener lesion occurs when the torn UCL is displaced above the adductor aponeurosis/adductor pollicus tendon. This requires surgical fixation.

- ◆ Radiographic stress views should not be performed, and extreme care should be taken during dynamic maneuvers with ultrasound to avoid causing a Stener lesion.

Essentials 4

■ Case

A 53-year-old man presents with stiffness, neck and back pain, and no other systemic symptoms.

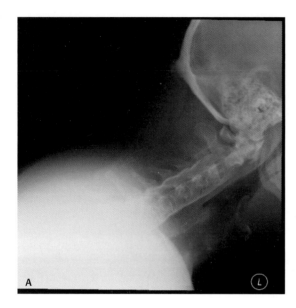

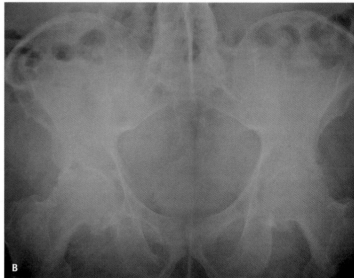

■ Questions

1. Which ONE of the following is the most likely diagnosis?
   A. Psoriatic arthritis
   B. Diffuse idiopathic skeletal hyperostosis
   C. Reactive arthritis
   D. Ankylosing spondylitis
   E. Inflammatory bowel disease arthritis

2. What is the primary site of disease in this disorder?
   A. Bone
   B. Synovial membrane
   C. Enthesis
   D. Cartilage
   E. Ligament

3. What is the most common location of a Romanus lesion?
   A. Cervical spine
   B. Midthoracic spine
   C. Thoracolumbar junction
   D. Lower lumbar spine
   E. SI joints

■ Answers and Explanations

Question 1

D. Correct! The sacroiliac (SI) joints are fused bilaterally, consistent with chronic bilateral sacroiliitis. The cervical spine radiograph shows multilevel thin, bridging syndesmophytes, consistent with a "bamboo spine." This presentation is typical of ankylosing spondylitis, a seronegative spondyloarthropathy with a strong HLA-B27 antigen association. "Seronegative" refers to the absence of rheumatoid factor.

Other choices and discussion

A. Psoriatic arthritis is associated with bulky paravertebral ossification, not thin flowing syndesmophytes, as in the test case. Psoriatic arthritis is commonly associated with asymmetric bilateral sacroiliitis, although in chronic cases, sacroiliitis may become more symmetric.

B. Diffuse idiopathic skeletal hyperostosis is associated with multilevel bulky ossification of the paraspinal ligaments, not thin flowing syndesmophytes. Diffuse idiopathic skeletal hyperostosis is usually considered an incidental finding and is not associated with sacroiliitis, although the SI joints can be fused superiorly by bulky bridging bone, similar in appearance to that seen in the spine.

C. Reactive arthritis (formerly known as Reiter syndrome) is typically associated with asymmetric bilateral sacroiliitis, although in chronic cases, sacroiliitis may become more symmetric. In the spine, reactive arthritis is associated with bulky paravertebral ossification, not thin flowing syndesmophytes.

E. Inflammatory bowel disease is associated with arthropathy, and its radiographic appearance can be similar to that of ankylosing spondylitis. However, because this patient had no gastrointestinal symptoms, inflammatory bowel disease arthritis is unlikely.

Question 2

C. Correct! The enthesis is the primary site of disease in ankylosing spondylitis and represents the connective tissue between a tendon or ligament and bone. Because the SI joints are predominantly lined with fibrocartilage and with very little synovial tissue, these joints can be thought of as entheses, explaining their characteristic involvement in spondyloarthropathies such as ankylosing spondylitis. Chronic inflammation of an enthesis can lead to subsequent ankylosis. Patients with ankylosis are at an increased risk for developing fractures.

Sacroiliitis is usually the first site involved by ankylosing spondylitis. This disease affects the spine and hips, and can also affect the shoulders, knees, hands, and the lung parenchyma (with apical predominant fibrobullous changes).

Other choices and discussion

B. The synovial membrane is the primary site of disease in rheumatoid arthritis, not ankylosing spondylitis.

The other choices are incorrect.

Question 3

C. Correct! The thoracolumbar junction is the most common site of a Romanus lesion. A Romanus lesion is a focal inflammatory erosive area along the anterior superior or anterior inferior margin of a vertebral body and can be seen early in the course of spondyloarthropathies. With magnetic resonance imaging, they show focal short tau inversion recovery hyperintensity during active inflammation. Later, these lesions may become sclerotic as they heal, leading to the "shiny corner" sign. They can also leave behind postinflammatory fatty marrow (without short tau inversion recovery hyperintensity).

Discussion

Regarding the SI joint, there are several mimics of true sacroiliitis. Hyperparathyroidism can cause erosion and mimic bilateral sacroiliitis. Osteitis condensans ilii is not a true sacroiliitis. This refers to benign sclerosis of the ilium as it borders the SI joint. This is often triangular in shape. Diagnosis can be made when this finding is seen with a lack of involvement of the adjacent sacrum and preservation of the SI joint space. This is usually asymptomatic.

Only the lower half of the SI joint represents a true diarthrodial joint. Scrutinize the lower half of the SI joint carefully when assessing for arthropathy.

■ Suggested Readings

Jang JH, Ward MM, Rucker AN, Reveille JD, Davis Jr JC, Weisman MH, Learch TJ. Ankylosing spondylitis: patterns of radiographic involvement—a re-examination of accepted principles in a cohort of 769 patients. Radiology 2011;258:192–198

Kim NR, Choi J-Y, Hong SH, Jun WS, Lee JW, Choi J-A, Kang HS. "MR corner sign": value for predicting presence of ankylosing spondylitis. Am J Roentgenol 2008;191:124–128

Lacout A, Rousselin B, Pelage J-P. CT and MRI of spine and sacroiliac involvement in spondyloarthropathy. Am J Roentgenol 2008;191:1016–1023

Top Tips

◆ Ankylosing spondylitis is associated with symmetric and bilateral sacroiliitis and multilevel bridging syndesmophytes in the spine, leading to ankylosis and the characteristic "bamboo spine" appearance. A spine with ankylosis is at an increased risk of fracture.

◆ Unilateral sacroiliitis is infection until proven otherwise.

◆ Differential diagnoses of bilateral and symmetric sacroiliitis: inflammatory bowel disease, ankylosing spondylitis. Differential diagnoses of bilateral but asymmetrical sacroiliitis: rheumatoid arthritis, gout, psoriatic arthritis, reactive (Reiter arthritis), and osteoarthritis.

Essentials 5

■ Case

A 42-year-old man presents with back pain.

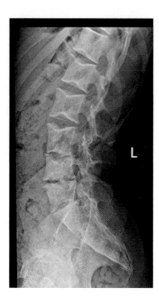

■ Questions

1. Which underlying condition is likely present?
   A. Paget disease
   B. Hyperparathyroidism
   C. Sickle cell disease
   D. Osteopetrosis
   E. Renal osteodystrophy

2. What is the cause of the endplate depression in the test case?
   A. Trauma
   B. Infarction
   C. Infection
   D. Surgery
   E. Hemorrhage

3. Which of the following are musculoskeletal manifestations of sickle cell disease? (Select ALL that apply.)
   A. Osteomyelitis
   B. Growth disturbance
   C. Extramedullary hematopoiesis
   D. Malignancy
   E. Skin ulceration

■ Answers and Explanations

Question 1

C. Correct! The central endplate depression seen in multiple vertebral bodies is typical of sickle cell disease. The biconcave endplates in the test case result in a "fish mouth" appearance. The more characteristic "H shaped" or "Lincoln log" vertebrae may be seen later as the endplate infarcts progress.

Other choices and discussion

A. Paget disease in the spine is characterized by dense sclerosis and overgrowth of the vertebral body.

B. Hyperparathyroidism in the spine produces transverse vertebral body endplate sclerosis, likened to a rugby or "rugger" jersey. If there are superimposed endplate insufficiency fractures, the vertebrae may take on a fish mouth appearance. No endplate sclerosis is present in the test case, however.

D. Osteopetrosis in the spine causes dense vertebral body endplate sclerosis, resulting in a "sandwich" vertebra.

E. Renal osteodystrophy in the spine results in a similar appearance to that of hyperparathyroidism.

Question 2

B. Correct! The vertebral body central endplate depression in sickle cell disease is caused by bone infarcts.

Discussion

Sickle-cell disease is an autosomal recessive condition characterized by abnormally shaped red blood cells. Its impact is extensive throughout the body, and it results in considerable morbidity and mortality. Typical radiographic findings include the vertical "hair-on-end" appearance of the calvarium, H-shaped or "fish-mouth" vertebrae, diffuse osteopenia, and coarsening of the trabeculae in the long bones.

Associated persistence of red marrow in the long bones and additional sites of red marrow reconversion are seen on magnetic resonance imaging. Marrow expansion is also detected on bone scintigraphy. Patients with sickle cell disease are predisposed to both infarcts and osteomyelitis.

Question 3

A. Correct! Patients with sickle cell disease have an increased incidence of osteomyelitis and septic arthritis because of bone infarcts and hyposplenism. Hyposplenism reduces the body's ability to eradicate certain bacteria. Salmonella infections are particularly common with sickle cell patients.

B. Correct! Impaired growth occurs subsequent to bone infarcts, which affect the epiphyses and growth plates.

C. Correct! Although extramedullary hematopiesis occurs more in thalassemia and hemolytic anemias, it can also be seen with sickle cell disease, resulting in osseous expansion and soft tissue masses in the chest, adrenal glands, and skin.

E. Correct! Sickle cell disease causes venous stasis and tissue hypoxia, which produces skin ulceration, particularly over bony prominences.

Incorrect choice and discussion

D. There is no conclusive evidence for an increased risk of musculoskeletal malignancy with sickle cell disease. Renal medullary cancer, a rare and aggressive neoplasm of the kidney, is associated with sickle cell trait.

■ Suggested Readings

Ejindu VC, Hine AL, Mashayekhi M, Shorvon PJ, Misra RR. Musculoskeletal manifestations of sickle cell disease. Radiographics 2007;27(4):1005–1021

Martinoli C, Bacigalupo L, Forni GL, Balocco M, Garlaschi G, Tagliafico A. Musculoskeletal manifestations of chronic anemias. Semin Musculoskelet Radiol 2011;15(3):269–280

Top Tips

- Sickle cell disease predisposes to hematogenous osteomyelitis, and *Salmonella* is the most common pathogen. Prominent red marrow reconversion can be seen in unusual locations, and differentiation from hematogenous osteomyelitis is sometimes difficult.

- Using a patient's younger age and the presence of H-shaped vertebra on a chest radiograph may help to differentiate a sickle cell patient in crisis from a patient with congestive heart failure.

- Sickle cell disease predisposes to multifocal bone infarctions. In the spine, "H-shaped" vertebrae are fairly unique to sickle cell disease, whereas "fish mouth" vertebrae are less specific and can be seen in other conditions including osteoporosis, renal osteodystrophy, and thalassemia.

Essentials 6

■ Case

A 43-year-old woman presents with shoulder pain.

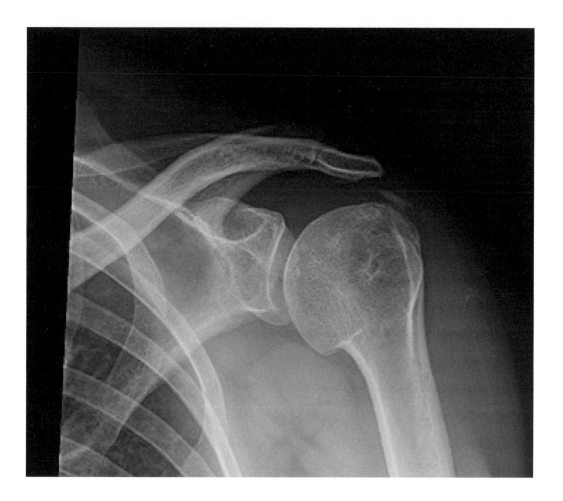

■ Questions

1. Which ONE of the following is the correct diagnosis?
   A. Greater tuberosity fracture
   B. Calcific tendinosis
   C. Frozen shoulder
   D. Humeral head chondroblastoma
   E. Humeral neck fracture

2. Which ONE of these is the MOST common site for the test case finding?
   A. Rotator cuff
   B. Elbow
   C. Knee
   D. Achilles tendon
   E. Thumb

3. Which of the following is(are) true regarding rotator cuff calcific tendinosis? (Select ALL that apply.)
   A. Painful disease is often associated with subdeltoid bursitis.
   B. The main treatment option is surgical resection.
   C. Doppler hyperemia correlates with pain.
   D. There are formative, resting, and resorptive phases.
   E. Calcific deposits can erode into bone.

■ Answers and Explanations

Question 1

B. Correct! There is focal globular soft tissue mineralization in the region of the rotator cuff insertion, consistent with hydroxyapatite crystal deposition, or calcific tendinosis.

Other choices and discussion

A. A greater tuberosity fracture would have bone matrix, not amorphous calcium as is shown in the test case.

C. A frozen shoulder (or adhesive capsulitis) is characterized by thickening and contraction of the joint capsule and synovium of the shoulder. The plain film is typically normal. Magnetic resonance imaging sometimes shows capsular thickening and high signal in the axillary recess, and intermediate signal in the rotator interval.

D. A chondroblastoma is typically a well-defined lucent lesion seen in young patients (younger than age 20 years), localized to the epiphysis of a long bone. The test case demonstrates several small lucent lesions with sclerotic rims in the humeral head. However, these are typical of benign enthesopathic intraosseous cysts.

E. There is no humeral neck fracture. There is a mild humeral head osteophyte formation, which can sometimes mimic a fracture.

Question 2

A. Correct! Calcific tendinosis most commonly affects the shoulders, and in particular the rotator cuff. These calcific deposits may also occur in the wrists, elbows, hands, hips, knees, and feet.

Within the rotator cuff, the distribution breakdown is as follows: supraspinatus (80%), infraspinatus (15%), and subscapularis (5%).

Question 3

A. Correct! Calcific deposits can shed into the overlying subdeltoid bursa, causing inflammation and pain, which may be severe.

C. Correct! Both Doppler hyperemia and subdeltoid bursal distention correlate with pain in calcific tendinosis.

D. Correct! There are formative, resting, and resorptive phases. During the formative phase, calcium crystals coalesce within the tendon to form a calcific focus. During the resting phase, fibrocartilaginous tissue encapsulates the calcific focus. During the resorptive phase, there is spontaneous resorption of the calcium, which generates an inflammatory response that is often characterized by an acute pain syndrome and limited range of motion.

E. Correct! During the resorptive phase, the calcium is shed into the overlying subdeltoid bursa and can erode into bone, causing inflammation. On magnetic resonance imaging, these inflammatory changes can appear very aggressive and raise suspicion for infection or malignancy. Bony erosion can also appear aggressive on computed tomography. Ultrasound and radiographs are recommended for the imaging evaluation of calcific tendinosis, given the typical appearance on these modalities and the relatively low cost.

Other choice and discussion

B. The main treatment is NOT surgical resection. Treatment options for rotator cuff calcific tendinosis include ultrasound-guided aspiration/lavage and subacromial-subdeltoid bursal corticosteroid injection. These have a high treatment success rate. Refractory cases may undergo surgical resection, but this is uncommon.

■ Suggested Readings

Bureau NJ. Calcific tendinopathy of the shoulder. Semin Musculoskelet Radiol 2013;17(1):80–84

Le Goff B, Berthelot JM, Guillot P, Glemarec J, Maugars Y. Assessment of calcific tendonitis of rotator cuff by ultrasonography: comparison between symptomatic and asymptomatic shoulders. Joint Bone Spine 2010;77:258–263

Levy O. Ultrasound-guided barbotage in addition to ultrasound-guided corticosteroid injection improved outcomes in calcific tendinitis of the rotator cuff. J Bone Joint Surg Am 2014;96:335

Top Tips

◆ The most common site of calcific tendinosis (or hydroxyapatite crystal deposition) is the rotator cuff, but this entity can affect other tendons as well, such as the gluteal insertions and the hamstring origins.

◆ Inflammation related to calcific tendinosis can contribute to extreme shoulder pain, prompting a visit to the emergency department or urgent care clinic for evaluation.

◆ Calcific tendinosis eroding into bone can have an aggressive appearance on computed tomography and magnetic resonance imaging, and mimic a malignant bone lesion.

Essentials 7

■ Case

A 56-year-old man presents with anterior knee pain and swelling.

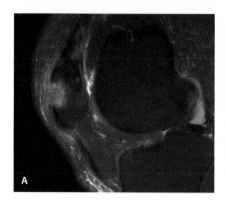
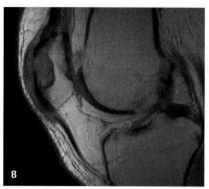
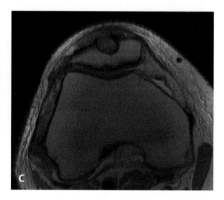

■ Questions

1. Which ONE of the following is the most likely diagnosis?
   A. Gout
   B. Quadriceps tendon tear
   C. Enthesopathy
   D. Rheumatoid arthritis
   E. Osteomyelitis

2. Which of the following is the MOST common site of involvement of this entity?
   A. Hip joint
   B. Medial aspect of the first metatarsal head
   C. Lumbar spine
   D. Radiocarpal joint
   E. Glenohumeral joint

3. Regarding gout, which of the following are correct? (Select ALL that apply.)
   A. Marginal osseous erosions with sclerotic margins and overhanging edges occur late in the disease process.
   B. Sonographic features of gout include joint effusion, as well as echogenic deposits in the joint fluid, the synovium, and/or the cartilage surface.
   C. Tophi are always intra-articular.
   D. Use of urate lowering therapy increases the sensitivity and specificity of dual energy computed tomography (CT) for the diagnosis of gout.
   E. Tophi usually have the typical T1 hypointense, T2 hyperintense appearance of most masses.

■ Answers and Explanations

Question 1

A. Correct! Magnetic resonance images reveal an anterior patellar cortex osseous erosion, with defined sclerotic margins and overhanging edges, giving the appearance of a "rat-bite." The soft tissue material in the bed of the erosion is of intermediate signal. These findings are typical for a gouty tophus.

Other choices and discussion

B. A torn quadriceps tendon at the distal-most insertion on the patella would have the abnormality centered at the tendon (with discontinuity of fibers and intrinsic high signal), rather than centered at the bone, as in this case. If present, a complete quadriceps tendon tear would retract the patella in a distal direction ("patella baja").

C. Patellar enthesopathy is seen as osseous proliferation or spurring at the quadriceps or patellar attachments. It involves inflammation at sites where ligaments, tendons, or joint capsules attach to the bone. Enthesopathy would not be associated with erosions.

D. Erosions associated with rheumatoid arthritis usually occur in the bare areas of synovial joints and do not typically demonstrate the sclerotic margins or overhanging edges seen in gout. Synovitis is the earliest abnormality to appear with rheumatoid arthritis, which is not demonstrated in this case.

E. The lack of an adjacent soft tissue ulcer makes infection less likely than gout. Additionally, an acute infection is unlikely to produce an intraosseous lesion with such well-defined margins. However, infection in soft tissue often affects adjacent bone—for example, direct extension from a foreign body is possible—and infection would be a diagnostic consideration.

Question 2

B. Correct! Approximately 50% of the cases of gout occur at the medial aspect of the first metatarsal head. Gout is found in the ankles (Achilles), feet (intertarsal joints), wrists (carpometacarpal compartment), in entheses around the knees (patellar and popliteus tendons), shoulders, and sacroiliac joints. Bilateral olecranon effusions may be seen and are a clue to the correct diagnosis.

All other choices are incorrect.

Question 3

A. Correct! Marginal osseous erosions with sclerotic margins and overhanging edges occur late in the disease process. Most early presentations of gout have normal plain films.

B. Correct! Sonographic features of gout include joint effusion, as well as echogenic deposits in the joint fluid, the synovium, and/or the cartilage surface. Ultrasound is very sensitive for detecting joint fluid and is also capable of visualizing fine echogenic deposits.

Other choices and discussion

C. Tophaceous deposits are not restricted to intra-articular locations.

D. Dual energy CT has demonstrated a sensitivity and specificity of up to 100% and 95%, respectively, for the diagnosis of gout. However, frequent use of urate lowering therapy may decrease the sensitivity for diagnosing gout with dual energy CT.

E. Tophi have usually do not the typical T1 hypointense, T2 hyperintense appearance of most masses. On magnetic resonance imaging, tophi are usually T1 and T2 isointense and demonstrate prominent enhancement. There may be variable signal, depending on the amount of calcium.

■ Suggested Readings

Girish G, Glazebrook KN, Jacobson JA. Advanced imaging in gout. Am J Roentgenol 2013;201(3):515–525

O'Connor PJ. Crystal deposition disease and psoriatic arthritis. Semin Musculoskelet Radiol 2013;17(1):74–79

Top Tips

◆ The classic radiographic features of gouty erosions are late disease manifestations and include focal intraosseous defects with sclerotic margins and overhanging edges. Because of earlier diagnosis and treatment today, many cases of gout will have a normal radiograph.

◆ With gout, there is preservation of the joint space until late in the disease, unlike osteoarthritis. With gout, there is absence of periarticular demineralization, unlike rheumatoid arthritis.

◆ Tophi on magnetic resonance imaging are variable but often T1 and T2 isointense with prominent enhancement. Dual energy CT is also useful in detecting uric acid crystals and diagnosing gout.

Essentials 8

■ Case

A 45-year-old man presents with knee pain and clicking.

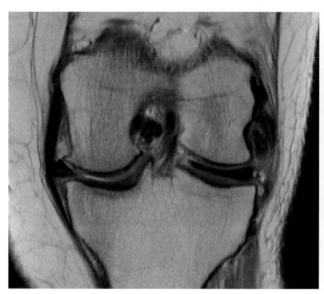 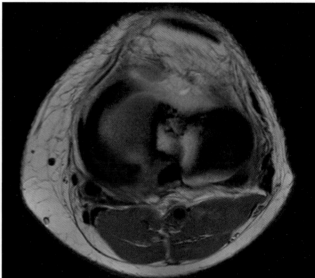

■ Questions

1. Which ONE of the following conditions is both demon-
   strated in this case and predisposes to knee instability?
   A. Osteophytes
   B. Discoid meniscus
   C. Medial collateral ligament tear
   D. Bone bruise
   E. Anterior cruciate ligament tear

2. Regarding this disorder, which of the following are
   correct? (Select ALL that apply.)
   A. Hypermobile
   B. Most frequently affects the lateral meniscus
   C. Acquired condition
   D. Increases the risk of meniscal degeneration
   E. Rarely bilateral

3. Which of the following is(are) correct regarding the
   magnetic resonance imaging (MRI) appearance of a
   discoid meniscus? (Select ALL that apply.)
   A. Demonstrates continuity of the anterior and poste-
      rior horns on three or more contiguous 5-mm thick
      sagittal images
   B. Occupies > 50% of the lateral femorotibial joint
      space
   C. Often demonstrates diffusely increased meniscal
      signal intensity
   D. Presence of a meniscal tear increases the ability of
      MRI to accurately diagnose a discoid meniscus
   E. Arthroscopic treatment may include saucerization
      and debulking

■ Answers and Explanations

Question 1

B. Correct! Discoid meniscus (which is seen in the lateral meniscus of the test case) is thought to represent a multifactorial congenital condition in which the center of the meniscus contains extra meniscal tissue. Despite the extra meniscal tissue, the meniscus is more prone to injury than a normal meniscus. A discoid meniscus may be fully or partially discoid, both of which produce an abnormally thickened and enlarged morphology. A discoid meniscus is often hypermobile, predisposed to injury, and places the patient at an increased risk for knee instability.

Other choices and discussion

A. Osteophytes form as the result of osseous remodeling, typically seen in response to cartilage loss in a joint. If large enough, osteophytes may result in soft tissue impingement or a clicking sensation. Osteophytes would not predispose to joint instability.

C. The medial collateral ligament is slightly thickened, but there is no discontinuity of fibers, no adjacent inflammation, and no evidence for a tear. The thickening in this case may be the result of nonacute altered weight bearing or prior sprain.

D. No obvious bone bruise is present, although fluid-sensitive sequences would be needed to exclude this type of microtrabecular injury. Even if present, a bone bruise would be painful but would not predispose to joint instability.

E. An anterior cruciate ligament tear would predispose the knee to instability, but the anterior cruciate ligament appears intact based on the coronal image.

Question 2

A. Correct! The discoid meniscus is hypermobile and may be devoid of peripheral attachments, predisposing to injury.

B. Correct! The incidence of discoid meniscus is much higher for the lateral meniscus than for the medial meniscus.

D. Correct! There are decreased collagen fibers and loss of normal collagen orientation in a discoid meniscus, and mucoid degeneration is common. Additionally, discoid menisci are more susceptible to injury than normal menisci, as their abnormal shape and thickness results in increased biomechanical stress.

Other choices and discussion

C. Discoid meniscus is a multifactorial congenital condition, not acquired.

E. A discoid meniscus is often bilateral (up to 50%).

Question 3

A. Correct!

B. Correct! This is seen on the coronal images.

C. Correct! Discoid menisci are predisposed to degeneration, which presents as diffuse intrasubstance high signal on MRI.

E. Correct! When discoid menisci are torn or unstable, surgical treatment is considered. Arthroscopic treatment commonly includes saucerization and debulking of the meniscus to restore a normal shape and to stabilize the meniscus, if there is meniscal instability upon probing.

Other choice and discussion

D. The presence of a meniscal tear disrupts the standard meniscal signal and morphology, and somewhat decreases the ability of MRI to accurately diagnose a discoid meniscus.

■ Suggested Readings

Francavilla ML, Restrepo R, Zamora KW, Sarode V, Swirsky SM, Mintz D. Meniscal pathology in children: differences and similarities with the adult meniscus. Pediatr Radiol 2014;44(8):910–925

McKay S, Chen C, Rosenfeld S. Orthopedic perspective on selected pediatric and adolescent knee conditions. Pediatr Radiol 2013;43(Suppl 1):S99–106

Top Tips

- Discoid meniscus most commonly affects the lateral meniscus (incidence ratio is 10:1 for lateral:medial meniscus).

- A total of 2% of the population has a discoid lateral meniscus.

- Discoid menisci are predisposed to degeneration, tear, and subsequent joint instability.

Essentials 9

■ Case

A 13-year-old female dancer presents with persistent heel pain.

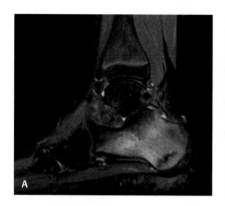 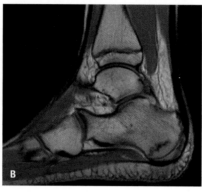 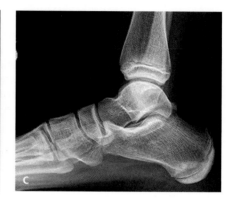

■ Questions

1. Which ONE of the following is the correct diagnosis?
   A. Intraosseous lipoma
   B. Haglund deformity
   C. Achilles tendon tear
   D. Plantar fasciitis
   E. Stress fracture

2. What is the MOST likely mechanism of injury for the test case?
   A. Fall from height
   B. Inversion
   C. Repetitive microtrauma
   D. Forced dorsiflexion
   E. Eversion

3. What is the recommended treatment for the test case?
   A. Curettage and packing
   B. Tendon debridement
   C. Immobilization and rest
   D. Calcaneoplasty
   E. Nonsteroidal anti-inflammatory drugs

■ Answers and Explanations

Question 1

E. Correct! This is a stress fracture. On magnetic resonance imaging (MRI), stress fractures typically present as linear hypointense signal (condensation of trabeculae) with surrounding bone marrow edema. The marrow edema is often intense. Periosteal reaction may be present. Stress reaction is the term used when, in the same clinical scenarios that lead to stress fractures, marrow edema is evident on MRI but no discrete fracture lines are visible.

There are two types of stress fracture. A fatigue fracture is a stress fracture of normal bone undergoing a repetitive load (as in the test case). Fatigue fractures occur in many parts of the body, but are most commonly encountered in the feet, tibia, proximal femur, pelvis, and spine.

An insufficiency fracture is a stress fracture of abnormal bone undergoing a normal or mild load. This is commonly seen in the elderly patient with demineralization. Insufficiency fractures are most often encountered in the spine, pelvis, ribs, as well as many lower extremity subchondral bone locations.

Other choices and discussion

A. An intraosseous lipoma is a benign osteolytic tumor of the bone that has well-defined margins and a central sclerotic nidus on plain film. The calcaneus is the second most common site of this lesion (after the proximal femur). MRI or computed tomography demonstrating fat is diagnostic.

B. Haglund deformity refers to a painful prominence of the posterior superior calcaneus. This is often the result of wearing tight fitting shoes, which leads to retrocalcaneal bursitis.

C. On MRI, tendon tears (including the Achilles tendon) appear as discontinuity of tendon fibers, often occurring in a background of tendinosis.

D. On MRI, plantar fasciitis appears as thickening and high signal of the plantar fascia at the calcaneal origin. This may be associated with edema of the calcaneal marrow and the perifascial soft tissues.

Question 2

C. Correct! Stress (fatigue) fractures occur as the result of low-level stress in bones subjected to repetitive microtrauma. This frequently affects the feet of dancers, long distance runners, and marching military recruits. The most common site of fatigue fracture in the foot is the second metatarsal. The calcaneus is the second most common site. The sesamoid bones and tarsal bones of the foot may also be affected, both of which are often difficult to detect on plain film. Stress fractures are usually treated with immobilization and rest.

Discussion

The other choices are incorrect. Fall from a height, inversion injury, and eversion injury of the foot and ankle potentially result in acute traumatic fractures, not the stress fracture demonstrated in the test case. Forced dorsiflexion of the foot may be associated with an acute Achilles tendon rupture.

Question 3

C. Correct! Stress fractures are usually treated with immobilization and rest.

Other choices and discussion

A. Curettage and packing is used to treat lytic intraosseous lesions.

B. Tendon debridement is performed in cases of tendinopathy that have failed conservative management.

D. Calcaneoplasty is sometimes performed to treat Haglund deformity.

E. Nonsteroidal anti-inflammatory drugs provide some pain relief for stress fracture, but rest and immobilization are needed for fracture healing.

■ Suggested Readings

Goulart M, O'Malley MJ, Hodgkins CW, Charlton TP. Foot and ankle fractures in dancers. Clin Sports Med 2008;27(2):295–304

Oestreich AE, Bhojwani N. Stress fractures of ankle and wrist in childhood: nature and frequency. Pediatr Radiol 2010;40(8):1387–1389

Top Tips

◆ There are two types of stress fracture: A fatigue fracture is the result of a repetitive load injuring a normal bone. An insufficiency fracture is the result of a normal load injuring an abnormal bone.

◆ MRI demonstrates T2 hyperintense signal because of underlying microtrabecular injury. A linear or irregular low signal intensity band corresponding to the fracture line is also often seen. In most patients, the edema on MRI resolves within 6 months.

◆ A subtrochanteric femoral stress fracture in a middle-aged female is a bisphosphonate insufficiency fracture until proven otherwise, and this requires an orthopedic referral, given the propensity for fracture completion.

Essentials 10

■ Case

A 35-year-old man presents with right shoulder pain after falling and feeling a "pop" in his shoulder. He has had similar episodes in the past.

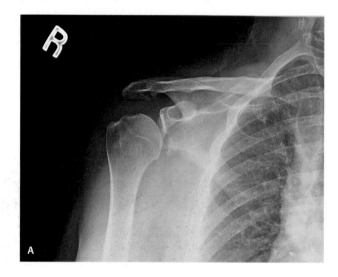

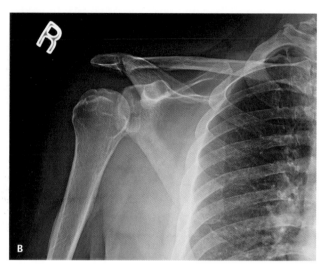

■ Questions

1. What has happened?
   A. Acromioclavicular separation
   B. Distal clavicular osteolysis
   C. Anterior glenohumeral dislocation followed by reduction
   D. Posterior glenohumeral dislocation followed by reduction
   E. Full thickness massive rotator cuff tear

2. In a Latarjet procedure, the area in question is buttressed with a bone graft. From where does this bone graft most commonly originate?
   A. Acromion
   B. Coracoid
   C. Distal fibula
   D. Distal radius
   E. Iliac crest

3. Which ONE of the following is the best modality for diagnosing a postoperative labral tear?
   A. Magnetic resonance imaging (MRI)
   B. MRI arthrogram
   C. Noncontrast CT
   D. Radiograph
   E. Ultrasound

■ Answers and Explanations

Question 1

C. Correct! A bony Bankart lesion (anterior inferior glenoid fracture) and Hill Sachs deformity (posterolateral humeral head impaction fracture) indicate prior anterior glenohumeral dislocation. Most glenohumeral dislocations are anterior, where the humeral head is displaced anteriorly and inferiorly. Hill Sachs fractures occur because of impaction of this portion of the humeral head with the glenoid rim. Computed tomography is sometimes useful in excluding a subtle osseous Bankart.

Other choices and discussion

A. The acromioclavicular joint demonstrates mild degenerative changes but is normally aligned.

B. No erosive changes are seen in the distal clavicle to suggest distal clavicular osteolysis. This entity typically presents as pain localized to the acromioclavicular joint, and is the result of trauma and subsequent resorption of the subchondral bone in the distal clavicle.

D. A posterior glenohumeral dislocation is not seen in this case. Posterior shoulder dislocation represents only 2 to 4% of cases of glenohumeral shoulder dislocation, but is frequently difficult to see on plain film. It is often missed and is a potential cause of malpractice. A posterior shoulder dislocation can be seen with a "trough" sign (also known as the "reverse Hill-Sachs") and a fracture of the posterior glenoid.

E. With a full thickness massive rotator cuff tear, the humeral head might be expected to migrate superiorly and abut the acromion undersurface. That has not occurred in this case.

Question 2

B. Correct! This bone graft most commonly originates from the coracoid. A Latarjet procedure is performed in the setting of glenoid insufficiency. The coracoid and its attached tendons are transferred and fixated to buttress the anterior inferior glenoid rim. Preoperative computed tomography (CT) is often helpful in evaluating the glenoid bone stock and in determining the size of the bony Bankart fragment.

Other choices and discussion

The iliac crest is used (rarely) to buttress the anterior inferior glenoid rim, but the coracoid is much more commonly used in a Latarjet procedure. The other sites are not used.

Question 3

B. Correct! MRI arthrogram is the most accurate modality for diagnosing a labral tear, either pre- or postoperatively. On arthrography, a labral tear can be diagnosed when contrast extends through, or abnormally undercuts, the labrum. The contour of the contrast undercutting the torn labrum is typically irregular. Normal variations of contrast undercutting can occur in the form of a sulcus in the superior labrum or a foramen in the anterior superior labrum. Unlike true tears, these normal variants are typically smooth in appearance, occur in the typical locations listed above, and in the case of the superior sulcus, tend not to extend as deeply or as posteriorly as do true superior labrum anterior posterior tears.

Other choices and discussion

A. Conventional MRI is quite useful in evaluating soft tissues such as the rotator cuff, but is less sensitive than MRI arthrography in evaluating the labrum, especially in the postoperative state.

C. CT is useful in diagnosing bone stock and hardware, but is not accurate in evaluating the postoperative labrum. CT arthrography, on the other hand, can effectively evaluate the labrum in patients who cannot undergo MRI.

D. Radiographs are insensitive for this purpose. They can be useful to exclude dislocation or fracture and to assess hardware position.

E. In the best circumstances, only small portions of the labrum are visible sonographically (usually just the posterior labrum), and ultrasound is especially limited in postoperative labral evaluation.

■ Suggested Readings

Bencardino JT, Gyftopoulos S, Palmer WE. Imaging in glenohumeral instability. Radiology 2013;269(2):323–337

Griffith JF, Antonio GE, Tong CWC, Ming CK. Anterior shoulder dislocation; quantification of glenoid bone loss with CT. Am J Roentgenol 2003;180:1423–1430

Mohana-Borges AVR, Chung CB, Resnick D. MR imaging and MR arthrography of the postoperative shoulder: spectrum of normal and abnormal findings. Radiographics 2004;24:69–85

Top Tips

♦ A total of 50% of all dislocations in the body involve the shoulder. Most of these are anterior dislocations of the glenohumeral joint, but the less common posterior dislocations are often missed on plain film. CT or MRI can be useful for problem cases.

♦ In assessing the labrum, be aware of normal variations within the superior and the anterior superior labrum.

♦ A Hill-Sachs defect is an impaction fracture of the posterolateral humeral head. Be sure to remark on these fractures, even if not acute, as they can "engage" the glenoid rim and result in repeated dislocations.

Details 1

■ Case

A 38-year-old man presents with left knee pain. Radiographs were negative except for a joint effusion. Sagittal and coronal T2-weighted fat-saturated images are shown. Which ONE of the following is the correct diagnosis?

    A. Posterior cruciate ligament rupture
    B. Anterior cruciate ligament (ACL) rupture
    C. Lateral collateral ligament rupture
    D. Medial collateral ligament (MCL) rupture
    E. Iliotibial band rupture

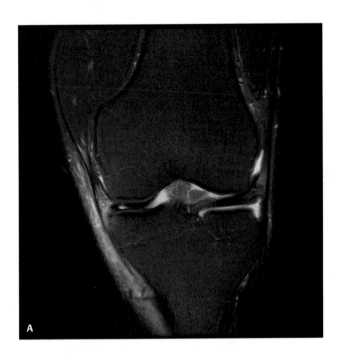 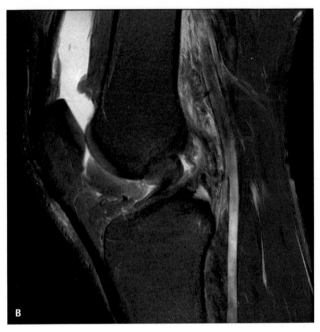

■ The following questions pertain to injury of the ACL.

1. True or False. Magnetic resonance imaging (MRI) is ordered by most orthopedic surgeons in the setting of possible ACL tear for the primary purpose of confirming or excluding the ACL tear.
2. What is the most common mechanism of an ACL injury?
3. On an initial radiograph, what is the most common tibial fracture encountered with this injury?
4. True or False. An impaction fracture of the medial femoral condyle is commonly seen with this injury.

5. Which injuries form the classic O'Donoghue's unhappy triad?
6. True or False. The clinical diagnosis of a posterolateral corner injury is highly accurate.
7. How many bundles comprise the ACL?
8. Which structures can be used in ACL graft reconstruction?
9. What is a cyclops lesion?
10. Name at least two complications more likely to develop if an ACL injury is left unrepaired.

■ Answers and Explanations

B. Correct! The ACL is ruptured. The ACL is composed of dense connective tissue that connects the femur and tibia. It prevents anterior tibial translation relative to the femur.

Other choices and discussion

The other choices are incorrect. The medial collateral ligament is thickened with perifascicular edema, but is not ruptured. The other structures are either normal or not visualized on these images.

Question 1

False. The clinical exam is very accurate in detecting an ACL tear. A good orthopedic surgeon usually doesn't order the test to make the diagnosis. The study is ordered to look for the ancillary findings, like meniscal and other ligamentous injury.

Question 2

An ACL tear is usually caused by a pivot shift injury of the knee. It can also be caused by a direct blow to the knee. The Lachman test is the most sensitive clinical test used to detect an ACL injury. In the Lachman test, the patient is placed supine with the knee bent 20 to 30 degrees. While one hand of the clinician is placed on the thigh, the other hand pulls the tibia anteriorly, assessing for translation relative to the femur. If the ACL is torn, translation occurs.

Question 3

A Segond fracture describes a tibial avulsion of the lateral capsular ligament attachment from the lateral tibial plateau. If this small fracture can be identified on a plain film, there is an extremely high probability of an underlying ACL tear. Posterior tibial plateau impaction injuries (contusions and fractures) are also frequently associated with ACL tears, but these are often only visible with subsequent MRI evaluation.

Question 4

False. An impaction fracture of the *lateral* femoral condyle frequently occurs with an ACL tear. This fracture can be identified on a lateral radiograph by the presence of the deep femoral notch sign, which is an abnormally depressed lateral femoral sulcus (depth > 1.5 mm). Corresponding impaction injury of the posterior tibial plateau is also commonly seen with a pivot shift injury.

Question 5

The classic O'Donoghue's unhappy triad consists of an ACL tear, a medial meniscal tear, and an MCL tear/sprain. In the test case, a complex medial meniscal tear and an intermediate-grade MCL sprain are partially visualized. A tear of the lateral meniscus can also accompany an ACL tear, often occurring near the posterior root attachment.

Question 6

False. The clinical diagnosis of a posterolateral corner injury can be difficult, especially in the setting of additional injuries. Posterolateral corner injury is sometimes associated with an ACL tear and, if missed, chronic instability may result. MRI is accurate in diagnosing posterolateral corner injuries, particularly of the larger components. Components of the corner include the fibular (lateral) collateral ligament, lateral capsule, popliteofibular ligament, popliteus tendon, biceps tendon, as well as the anatomically variable arcuate and fabellofibular ligaments.

Question 7

The ACL is comprised of two bundles: anteromedial and posterolateral. The anteromedial bundle is the stronger of the two and is taut during flexion. A partial ACL tear, or a tear of one bundle, can sometimes occur. Treatment is controversial in this situation. Many believe that tears comprising < 25% of the cross-sectional area of the ligament can be treated conservatively, whereas tears comprising > 50% of the cross-sectional area of the ligament often require surgery, as those tears frequently progress to full-thickness tears.

Question 8

ACL reconstruction is most commonly performed using either a patellar graft or a hamstring graft. The patellar graft is composed of a portion of the patellar tendon with a small bone block on either end. The patellar graft leaves a typical central defect in the proximal patellar tendon that can be seen on MRI. The hamstring graft, often with the gracilis tendon also included, is a soft tissue graft composed of two bundles in an attempt to better mimic the native ACL structure. Hamstring grafts are more frequently used, although neither graft has been conclusively proven to be superior to the other.

Question 9

A cyclops lesion refers to focal arthrofibrosis that forms adjacent to the anterior aspect of the ACL graft near the tibial insertion, and is seen on MRI as a heterogeneous low signal intensity mass. It can lead to impingement, pain, and decreased range of motion. Cyclops lesions occur in approximately 5% of patients with ACL grafts. If symptomatic, they can be treated with arthroscopic excision.

Question 10

Nonsurgical treatment of a complete ACL tear increases the risk of joint instability, with future meniscal tear and premature osteoarthritis as consequences. Surgical reconstruction is typically recommended to prevent these complications. Physical therapy and strengthening exercises can also improve stability in the setting of an ACL tear.

Top Tips

♦ In the setting of trauma, bone contusions in the lateral femoral condyle and the posterolateral tibial plateau are highly suspicious for an associated ACL tear.

♦ In the setting of an ACL tear, if there is edema in the soft tissues of the posterior and lateral knee or a fracture or contusion of the fibular head, consider the possibility of a posterolateral corner injury and carefully evaluate these ligaments and tendons. If missed, this can lead to chronic instability and ACL reconstruction failure.

♦ A Cyclops lesion describes focal arthrofibrosis anterior to the ACL graft. This can cause pain, impingement, and decreased range of motion.

Details 2

■ Case

A 35-year-old man presents with hip pain. Which ONE of the following is the correct diagnosis?
    A. Slipped epiphysis
    B. Osteomyelitis
    C. Normal variant
    D. Avascular necrosis
    E. Labral tear

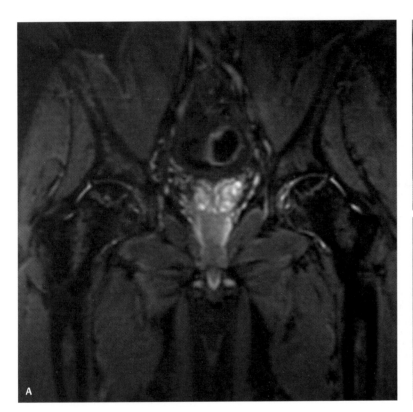

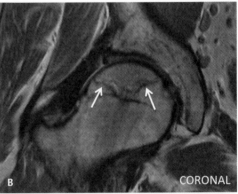

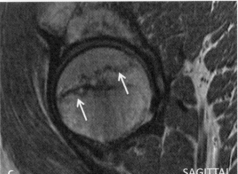

■ The following questions pertain to avascular necrosis.

1. The double line sign is an imaging feature of AVN seen on _____.
2. True or False. Risk factors for AVN include chronic steroid use, alcohol abuse, and trauma.
3. True or False. Disease states such as sickle cell disease, vasculitis, and organ transplantation predispose to AVN.
4. A pediatric hip condition that may progress to AVN is _____.
5. True or False. Subchondral fragmentation and collapse are early imaging features of AVN.

6. True or False. Increased bone density at an otherwise normal joint is one of the earliest radiographic signs of AVN.
7. Surgical treatment options for AVN include _____.
8. "H-shaped vertebral bodies" caused by endplate necrosis are classically described in _____.
9. True or False. AVN is likely caused by interruption of blood supply or impaired perfusion to the affected bone.
10. True or False. The utility of the MRI is only to determine whether AVN is present.

■ Answers and Explanations

D. Correct! Magnetic resonance imaging (MRI) demonstrates the "double line" sign (i.e., inner bright T2 line and outer dark T2 line) at the femoral heads, diagnostic of AVN.

Other choices and discussion

A. The patient is skeletally mature and the epiphyses are not subluxed or dislocated, excluding slipped capital femoral epiphysis (SCFE). SCFE is a relatively common cause of adolescent hip pain. Obesity is a risk factor. SCFE is more commonly found in males than in females, may be bilateral, and is essentially a displaced Salter Harris I fracture.

B. There is no bone marrow edema pattern, cortical destruction, joint effusion, or abscess to raise suspicion for osteomyelitis.

C. Although the abnormality is symmetric, the serpiginous femoral head signal is clearly abnormal.

E. There is no signal or morphologic abnormality within either acetabular labrum to suggest a labral tear, although the sensitivity for detection is decreased without the benefit of joint effusions. Magnetic resonance arthrography can be helpful for the detection of labral tears, as contrast entry into a linear defect in the substance of labrum is consistent with a tear. Contrast entry into the labrum is consistent with a tear. The presence of a sublabral sulcus as a normal variant is debated.

Question 1

The double line sign is an imaging feature of AVN seen on MRI. The inner T2 hyperintense line represents granulation tissue and the outer hypointense line represents sclerotic bone.

Question 2

True. Risk factors for AVN include chronic steroid use, alcohol abuse, and trauma.

Question 3

True. Certain disease states such as hemaglobinopathies, vasculitis, organ transplantation, and pancreatitis predispose to AVN.

Question 4

A pediatric hip condition that may progress to AVN is SCFE. Legg-Calve-Perthes disease is a primary AVN in the pediatric hips.

Question 5

False. Subchondral fragmentation and collapse are late imaging features of AVN.

Question 6

True. Increased bone density at an otherwise normal joint is one of the earliest radiographic signs of AVN. However, radiographs have low sensitivity and specificity for early AVN. MRI is the most sensitive imaging modality to make this diagnosis.

Question 7

Surgical treatment options for AVN include joint replacement and joint-sparing procedures such as core decompression.

Question 8

"H-shaped vertebral bodies" caused by endplate necrosis are classically described in sickle cell disease.

Question 9

True. AVN is likely caused by interruption of blood supply or impaired perfusion to the affected bone.

Question 10

False. MRI in the assessment of AVN gives much more information than simply whether AVN is present. Prognosis and management decisions can be made based on the following: marrow edema in the femoral head and neck, underlying hip arthritis, femoral head flattening, percentage of affected superior surface femoral head, and presence/size of joint effusion.

■ Suggested Readings

Moya-Angeler J, Gianakos AL, Villa JC, Ni A, Lane JM. Current concepts on osteonecrosis of the femoral head. World J Orthop 2015;6(8):590–601

Resnick D, Kransdorf MJ. Bone and Joint Imaging. Philadelphia, PA: W B Saunders Co.; 2005

Zalavras CG, Lieberman JR. Osteonecrosis of the femoral head: evaluation and treatment. J Am Acad Orthop Surg 2014;22(7):455–464

Top Tips

- ◆ Subchondral fragmentation and collapse are late imaging features of AVN.

- ◆ The double line sign is an imaging feature of avascular necrosis seen on MRI.

- ◆ After diagnosing AVN on MRI, include the following in your report: marrow edema in the femoral head and neck, underlying hip arthritis, femoral head flattening, percent of affected superior surface femoral head, and presence/ size of joint effusion.

Details 3

■ **Case**

A 17-year-old female runner presents with acute left hip pain. Which ONE of the following is the correct diagnosis?
   A. Sartorius avulsion
   B. Iliopsoas avulsion
   C. Gluteus medius avulsion
   D. Hamstring avulsion

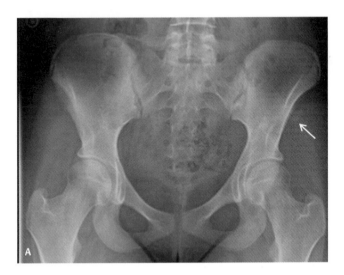

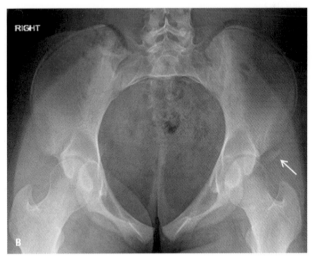

■ **The following questions pertain to avulsion injuries and relevant anatomy.**

1. The rectus femoris originates from the _____.
2. The abdominal muscles insert on the _____.
3. The hip adductor muscles originate from the _____.
4. What is the last apophysis to fuse in the pelvis?
5. Why are pelvic apophyseal injuries common in the adolescent athlete?
6. What is the most common site of apophyseal pelvic injury in adolescents?

7. Avulsion injury at the anterior inferior iliac spine is particularly common in which sports?
8. In a 76-year-old man with a lesser trochanter avulsion fracture, _____ should be excluded.
9. Which populations are at risk for hip abductor tendon injuries?
10. True or False. Avulsion injuries are predominantly restricted to the hip and pelvis.

■ Answers and Explanations

A. Correct! The sartorius tendon originates on the anterior superior iliac spine, which is avulsed on the left in this patient (*arrows*). An avulsion injury occurs when an attached tendon removes a portion of cortical bone from the parent bone during trauma. The ill-defined appearance can mimic a more aggressive process, but the typical locations of avulsion injuries and the leading histories should enable one to make a definitive diagnosis.

Other choices and discussion

B. The iliopsoas inserts on the lesser trochanter.

C. The gluteus medius inserts on the greater trochanter.

D. The hamstring tendons (long head of the biceps femoris, semitendinosus, and semimembranosus) originate at the ischium.

Question 1

The rectus femoris originates with two heads. The direct head originates from the anterior inferior iliac spine, and the reflected head originates between the anterior inferior iliac spine and the superior acetabular rim. Complex partial tears of the muscle can occur as a result of this unique anatomy.

Question 2

The abdominal muscles insert on the iliac crest, superior pubic ramus, and the pubic bone.

Question 3

The hip adductor muscles originate from the superior pubic ramus, pubic body, and inferior pubic ramus. Avulsion injuries at these locations are often due to chronic repetitive stress and may be a cause of athletic pubalgia.

Question 4

The iliac crest apophysis is the last to fuse in the pelvis. The iliac crest apophysis begins to ossify at approximately age 15 and may completely fuse as late as 25 years.

Question 5

The apophyses in the adolescent pelvis may remain unfused into the patient's mid-twenties. The unfused apophysis is the weakest point in the muscle-tendon-bone complex, and is therefore the most susceptible to injury.

Question 6

The most common site of apophyseal pelvic injury in adolescents is the ischial tuberosity. Avulsion injury to the ischial tuberosity at the hamstring origins is often related to soccer, track and field, and other competitive sports.

Question 7

Avulsion injury at the anterior inferior iliac spine is particularly common in kicking sports, such as soccer, rugby, and football.

Question 8

In a 76-year-old man with a lesser trochanter avulsion fracture, malignancy should be excluded. Pelvic avulsion fractures in adult patients should raise suspicion for an underlying pathologic bone lesion.

Question 9

Elderly women > 65 years with underlying hip abductor tendinosis are at risk for tendon injury, either presenting as a partial- or full-thickness tear. Patients with total hip arthroplasty performed via an anterolateral approach are also at risk for hip abductor tear, as this approach requires the incision of the gluteus minimus and gluteus medius.

Question 10

False. Avulsion injuries can occur in many places, including the ankle, foot, hand, and knee. Elbow avulsion injuries can occur in the skeletally immature. Chronic avulsion injuries may leave ossification or calcification at the site of injury.

■ Suggested Readings

McKinney BI, Nelson C, Carrion W. Apophyseal avulsion fractures of the hip and pelvis. Orthopedics 2009;32(1):42

Sanders TG, Zlatkin MB. Avulsion injuries of the pelvis. Semin Musculoskelet Radiol 2008;12(1):42–53

Singer G, Eberl R, Wegmann H, Marterer R, Kraus T, Sorantin E. Diagnosis and treatment of apophyseal injuries of the pelvis in adolescents. Semin Musculoskelet Radiol 2014;18(5):498–504

Top Tips

◆ Nontraumatic avulsion fractures in adult patients should raise suspicion for underlying pathologic bone lesion.

◆ When assessing a plain film cortical bone abnormality, consider whether it could be explained by an avulsion injury. Knowledge of muscle insertions and origins is paramount.

◆ In pediatrics, an asymmetric appearance of an apophysis should raise suspicion for an avulsion injury and/or apophysitis.

Details 4

■ Case

A 10-year-old boy presents with finger pain following basketball injury. Which ONE of the following is the correct diagnosis?

    A. Salter-Harris (S-H) type I
    B. S-H type II
    C. S-H type III
    D. S-H type IV
    E. S-H type V

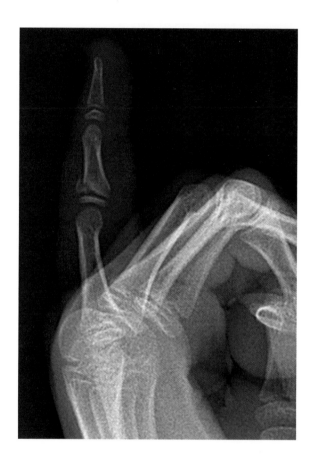

■ The following questions pertain to S-H injuries.

1. Approximately ____% of pediatric fractures involve the physis.
2. According to S-H fracture classification, a fracture involving only the epiphysis and growth plate is a type _____.
3. According to S-H fracture classification, a fracture involving both the epiphysis and metaphysis is a type _____.
4. S-H type _____ fractures have the worst prognosis.
5. True or False. S-H type II fracture is the most common.
6. True or False. S-H type I fracture is considered a crush injury.
7. True or False. S-H type I fracture can only occur if the growth plate is fused.
8. True or False. S-H type IV fractures can result in growth disturbances.
9. True or False. S-H type V fractures can occur as a stress injury.
10. True or False. A Tillaux fracture is a S-H type III fracture.

■ Answers and Explanations

B. Correct! This is a S-H type II fracture. The fracture enters in the plane of the physis and exits through the metaphysis.

The S-H classification is a longstanding and most common classification for pediatric fractures that involve the growth plate. The classification system is important for management and for prognosis, as prognosis worsens as the S-H number increases (1 to 5, with 1 as the best and 5 as the worst).

Question 1

Approximately 15% of pediatric fractures involve the physis.

Question 2

According to S-H fracture classification, a fracture involving only the epiphysis and growth plate is a type III.

Question 3

According to S-H fracture classification, a fracture involving both the epiphysis and metaphysis is a type IV.

Question 4

S-H type V fractures have the worst prognosis. The higher the S-H classification type, the worse the fracture prognosis.

Question 5

True. Type II fractures are the most common. They account for approximately 75% of all physeal fractures.

Question 6

False. A S-H type I is not a crush injury. S-H type I fracture is a separation of the physis, resulting in widening and sometimes epiphyseal slippage (e.g., slipped capital femoral epiphysis). S-H type I is often occult on initial radiograph, only confirmed with healing periosteal reaction on follow up radiograph in 7 to 10 days. Type V fracture is considered a crush injury and is most likely to result in growth disturbance.

Question 7

False. A type I fracture can only occur if the growth plate is *not* fused. All of the S-H fractures occur before complete growth plate fusion.

Question 8

True. S-H type IV fractures can result in growth disturbance. Physeal fractures involving the epiphysis (III and IV) can result in growth arrest. Type IV fractures can result in a physeal bar across the growth plate, which can in turn produce asymmetric growth or deformity.

Question 9

True. Type V fractures can result from a stress injury or repetitive trauma. This is sometimes seen, for example, in gymnastics.

Question 10

True. A Tillaux fracture is a S-H type III fracture. Specifically, this is a fracture through the anterolateral aspect of the distal tibial epiphyses.

■ Suggested Readings

Caine D, DiFiori J, Maffulli N. Physeal injuries in children's and youth sports: reasons for concern? Br J Sports Med 2006;40(9):749–760

Cepela DJ, Tartaglione JP, Dooley TP, Patel PN. Classifications in brief: Salter-Harris classification of pediatric physeal fractures. Clin Orthop Relat Res 2016;474(11):2531–2537

Top Tips

◆ S-H fracture classification describes the patterns of physeal injury. It is useful for prognosis.

◆ S-H type II is by far the most common, accounting for 75% of cases. Keep this fact in mind when trying to categorize a subtle fracture.

◆ Mnemonic SALTR: Type I = **S**lipped; Type II = **A**bove; Type III = **L**ower; Type IV = **T**hrough; Type V = **R**ammed

Details 5

■ Case

A 29-year-old woman presents with a painful enlarging mass in her distal left thigh. Anteroposterior and lateral radiographs, axial postcontrast T1 fat-saturated magnetic resonance imaging (MRI), and technetium 99m-methyl diphosphonate nuclear bone scan are shown. Which ONE of the following is the MOST likely diagnosis?

A. Metastatic breast carcinoma
B. Chondrosarcoma
C. Lymphoma
D. Ewing sarcoma
E. Osteosarcoma

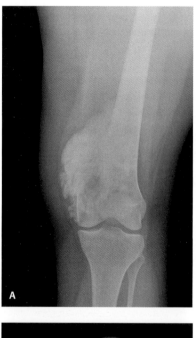

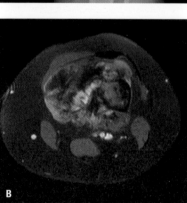

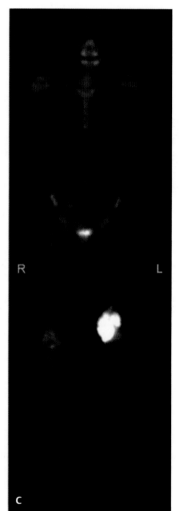

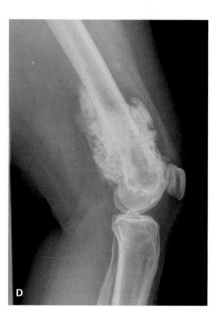

■ The following questions pertain to osteosarcoma.

1. What disease process is associated with the vast majority of secondary osteosarcomas?
2. What is a Codman triangle?
3. What is the most common age of osteosarcoma presentation?
4. How do we define neurovascular encasement on MRI?

5. What is the most common site of metastatic disease in osteosarcoma?
6. What is a skip lesion?
7. What is the most common subtype of surface osteosarcoma?

■ Answers and Explanations

E. Correct! This is an osteosarcoma. Osteosarcoma is the second most common bone malignancy (after multiple myeloma) and frequently arises from the metaphysis or diaphysis of a long bone. It is the most common primary bone malignancy that affects children and adolescents. Most osteosarcomas occur in patients between the ages of 10 and 30, but they can develop in any age, and about 10% occur in patients over 60 years old. Osteosarcoma has a male:female ratio of about 2:1. It is associated with osteoid matrix, which is dense and cloud-like on radiographs. On MRI, the tumor has hypointense signal and enhances heterogeneously. It is associated with focal and often intense uptake on technetium 99m-methyl diphosphonate nuclear bone scan.

Other choices and discussion

A. The large distal femoral mass with extraosseous osteoid matrix is unlikely to represent metastatic breast carcinoma. Breast cancer metastases can be either lytic or blastic, but rarely produce extraosseous osteoid matrix.

B. Chondrosarcoma typically occurs in the fourth or fifth decade of life. In the pelvis and lower extremities, it most commonly involves the iliac wing, but can also involve the proximal or distal femur. It is associated with chondroid (ring and arc) matrix on imaging, which is absent in the test case.

C. Plasmacytoma, a solid mass composed of plasma cells, is associated with multiple myeloma. It is typically lytic and does not produce osteoid matrix. It infrequently occurs in the distal femur.

D. Ewing sarcoma typically occurs in the diaphysis or metaphysis of long bones but is more commonly seen in younger patients (first and second decades). Ewing can present as a large soft tissue mass and periosteal reaction, but it does not produce osteoid matrix.

Question 1

Paget disease is associated with the vast majority of secondary osteosarcomas. Approximately 5% of osteosarcomas are secondary, resulting from malignant transformation of a benign process. The most common benign process associated with the development of secondary osteosarcoma is Paget disease, followed by prior radiation therapy.

Question 2

A Codman triangle describes a triangular shape of periosteal reaction, typically along the margin of an aggressive tumor that "outgrows" the periosteum's ability to contain it. It is commonly seen in osteosarcoma and other aggressive bone lesions.

Question 3

Osteosarcoma has a bimodal age distribution, but the larger peak is centered during the adolescent growth spurt. A second smaller peak occurs in the elderly.

Question 4

Neurovascular encasement by primary bone sarcomas occurs less frequently than with soft tissue sarcomas, with both occurring in < 10% of cases. Encasement is important to identify because of its impact on subsequent resection. High-quality MRI is necessary, but accurate diagnosis of tumor encasement is still sometimes difficult to accomplish, even with the best studies. This is due to several factors, including fascial plane distortion by large tumors and the presence of peritumoral edema. Complete encasement is usually not difficult to establish. Identifying contact > 180 degrees of the circumference of the artery or nerve has been proposed as a cutoff in cases of incomplete encasement, primarily in order to reduce false-positive diagnoses where only neurovascular displacement is present.

Question 5

The lungs are the most common site of metastatic disease. CT is the modality of choice in this assessment. Osteosarcoma can also metastasize to regional lymph nodes. In general, calcified mediastinal nodes and/or calcified lung nodules are almost always benign (the result of prior granulomatous disease), but the much less common metastatic osteosarcoma can look identical.

Question 6

Skip lesions are noncontiguous malignant lesions that occur in the same bone as the primary tumor. MRI, bone scan, and positron emission tomography/CT are all useful in detecting skip lesions.

Question 7

Parosteal osteosarcoma accounts for 65% of surface osteosarcomas. Parosteal osteosarcoma arises from the outer layer of periosteum and usually occurs in the third and fourth decades. It is typically considered a lower-grade malignancy, but can contain focal areas of higher-grade tumor. The radiologic appearance of a parosteal osteosarcoma is typically cloud-like osteoid matrix arising from a juxtacortical location, often with a narrow stalk of attachment to the cortex. Initially, the medullary cavity is uninvolved, but can become invaded by tumor as the lesion grows in size. Prognosis is significantly better with parosteal osteosarcoma than with conventional osteosarcoma, and has a 10-year survival of 80 to 90%.

Top Tips

- For osteosarcoma, MRI is useful in determining the tumor extent, and in determining whether it involves bones, muscles, an adjacent joint, or a neurovascular bundle. This information can affect the resectability of the tumor and must be described in the radiologist's report.

- Because the needle track from biopsy is assumed to be contaminated and will need to be resected during surgery, it is important for the radiologist performing the biopsy to consult with the orthopedic oncologist regarding the biopsy approach.

- Parosteal, periosteal, and high-grade surface osteosarcomas arise from the periosteum and are collectively referred to as surface osteosarcomas. Parosteal osteosarcoma is the most common and has a much better prognosis than conventional osteosarcoma.

Image Rich 1

■ Case

Match the appropriate diagnosis with the provided image.
    A. Rheumatoid arthritis (RA)
    B. Calcium pyrophosphate deposition arthropathy
    C. Erosive osteoarthritis (OA)
    D. Psoriatic arthritis

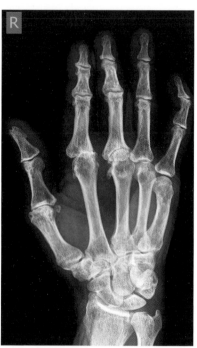

1.

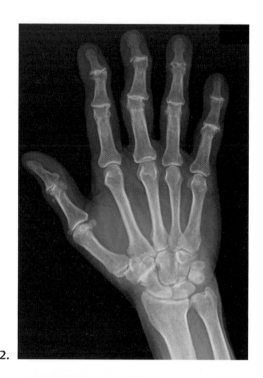

2.

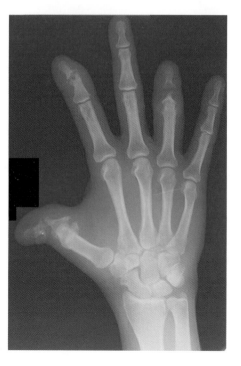

3.

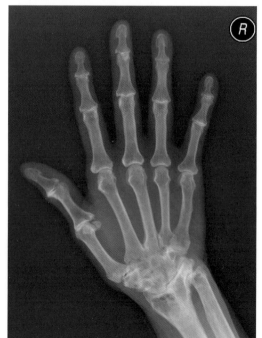

4.

■ Answers and Explanations

1. B. Calcium pyrophosphate deposition arthropathy. Calcium pyrophosphate deposition arthropathy describes calcium pyrophosphate dihydrate deposition in and around joints, provoking an inflammatory response (pseudogout) and subsequent development of degenerative changes. The second and third metacarpophalangeal joints are characteristically involved in the hand, as in this case. The joint spaces are severely narrowed with subchondral cystic changes and "hooked" osteophytes arising from the second and third metacarpal heads. Chondrocalcinosis commonly occurs in the triangular fibrocartilage complex in the wrist (not seen in this case).

2. C. Erosive OA. Erosive OA refers to a subtype of OA that has an additional erosive component. Patients are predominantly female, Rh factor negative, and postmenopausal. Erosive OA has a distal distribution, usually involving the distal interphalangeal (DIP) and/or proximal interphalangeal joints. Central subchondral erosions with productive adjacent bony changes develop. This creates the characteristic "gull wing" appearance. This "gull wing" appearance is seen in the test case (second through fourth DIP joints). Joint space narrowing associated with typical OA is also seen.

Because this entity has an inflammatory component, the symptoms may resemble RA or psoriatic arthritis. With erosive OA, however, systemic symptoms are absent, and the distribution of typical OA is present. In addition, marginal erosions do not occur in erosive osteoarthritis.

3. D. Psoriatic arthritis. Skin psoriasis nearly always precedes the development of psoriatic arthritis. Approximately 10 to 15% of patients with skin psoriasis will go on to develop psoriatic arthritis. The majority of these patients are HLA B-27 positive. Findings of psoriatic arthritis include marginal erosions, productive bony formation ("fluffy periostitis"), and overlying soft tissue swelling ("sausage digit"). These findings are seen in the test case at the second DIP joint. Distribution is typically distal and can be either symmetric or asymmetric, and unilateral or bilateral. Pencil-in-cup deformities may be seen, as in the fourth DIP joint in the test case. In the spine, bulky lateral osteophytes and asymmetric sacroiliitis are characteristic of psoriatic arthritis.

4. A. RA. RA is a chronic inflammatory arthritis primarily affecting synovial tissue. Rh factor is nearly always positive. In the hands and wrists, predominant involvement is seen at the metacarpophalangeal joints and the carpus. Marginal erosions with soft tissue swelling may be seen. Magnetic resonance imaging can detect findings of RA (such as marrow edema and synovitis) earlier than radiographs. In the test case, advanced joint destruction has occurred with carpal remodeling and some carpal auto-fusion, but no osteophytes are present. In larger joints, RA is associated with relatively concentric, severe joint space narrowing. Ultimately, joints affected by RA can undergo secondary osteoarthritis after treatment, which may result in a confusing constellation of imaging findings including osteophytes.

■ Suggested Readings

Helms CA, Vogler JB, Simms DA, Genant HK. CPPD crystal deposition disease or pseudogout. Radiographics 1982;2(1):40–52

Jacobson JA, Girish G, Jiang Y, Resnick D. Radiographic evaluation of arthritis: inflammatory conditions. Radiology 2008;248:378–389

Martel W, Stuck KJ, Dworin AM, Hylland RG. Erosive osteoarthritis and psoriatic arthritis: a radiologic comparison in the hand, wrist, and foot. Am J Roentgenol 1980;134:125–135

Sommer OJ, Kladosek A, Weiler V, Czembirek H, Boeck M, Stiskal M. Rheumatoid arthritis: a practical guide to state-of-the-art imaging, image interpretation, and clinical implications. Radiographics 2005;25:381–398

Steinbach LS, Resnick D. Calcium pyrophosphate dihydrate crystal deposition disease revisited. Radiology 1996;200:1–9

Top Tips

- Erosive OA: DIP and proximal interphalangeal joints with the characteristic "gull wing" appearance.

- Psoriatic arthritis: Combination of marginal erosions, bony proliferative changes, and "sausage digit" swelling. "Pencil-in-cup" appearance can be a late advanced finding.

- RA: Bilaterally symmetric and purely erosive arthritis favoring the carpus and metacarpophalangeal joints. Severe concentric joint space narrowing in affected large joints. Closely analyze the fifth metatarsophalangeal joints in the feet as well.

- Calcium pyrophosphate deposition arthropathy: Second and third metacarpal head "hooked" osteophytes, subchondral cysts, and triangular fibrocartilage complex chondrocalcinosis.

- Remember that secondary OA can be superimposed upon underlying changes from any treated or "burned out" inflammatory arthritis.

Image Rich 2

■ Case

A 16-year-old boy presents with fever, knee pain, and swelling. Match the appropriate letter from within the images with the provided diagnosis.

1. Soft tissue abscess
2. Sinus tract (cloaca)
3. Periosteal reaction
4. Intraosseous abscess
5. Physeal destruction

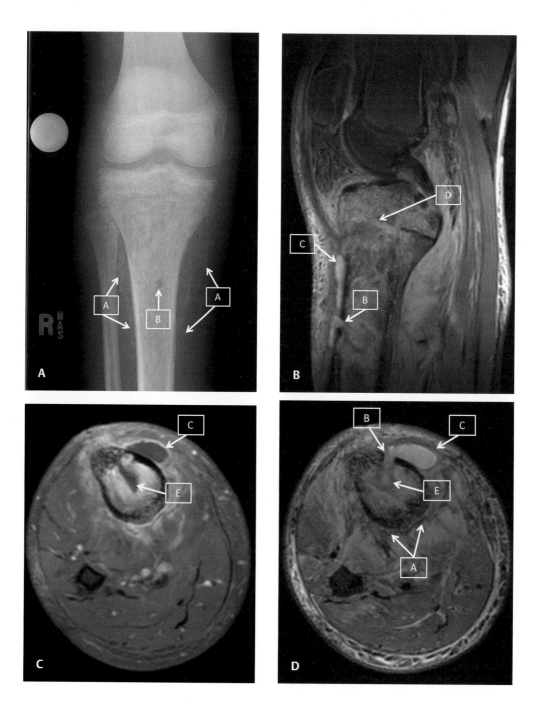

■ Answers and Explanations

1. C

2. B

3. A

4. E

5. D

Discussion

Osteomyelitis can occur as the result of direct spread from a contiguous source (e.g., trauma, fixation hardware, joint implant), vascular insufficiency (peripheral vascular disease), or hematogenous dissemination. The most common inciting organism in osteomyelitis is *Staphylococcus aureus.*

Infants and children are frequently affected via hematogenous spread, and this is primarily seen at the highly vascularized metaphyseal sites. The growth plate in pediatric cases may protect from spread into the epiphysis (although not always, as seen in the test case). In infants, infection may spread across the physis via transphyseal vessels not present in older children. Involvement of the growth plate can lead to growth disturbances and chronic deformity.

Radiographs may be normal in the early stages of acute osteomyelitis. Magnetic resonance imaging is the most sensitive imaging modality and will detect bone marrow edema, soft tissue edema, abnormal tissue enhancement, cortical break-through, and associated abscess.

Radiographs have better sensitivity for the detection of non-acute osteomyelitis than they do with acute osteomyelitis. With subacute and chronic osteomyelitis, radiographs can show cortical destruction, periosteal reaction, and soft tissue thickening. Magnetic resonance imaging in these cases is particularly useful in detecting intraosseous (Brodie) abscesses, subperiosteal abscesses (particularly in the pediatric population), osseous sinus tract (cloaca), and sequestered necrotic bone (sequestrum). The presence of a sequestrum or large abscess should be highlighted in the radiologist's report, as these findings may require surgical intervention.

■ Suggested Readings

Dodwell ER. Osteomyelitis and septic arthritis in children: current concepts. Curr Opin Pediatr 2013;25(1):58–63

Jaramillo D. Infection: musculoskeletal. Pediatr Radiol 2011;41(Suppl 1):S127–134

Lew DP, Waldvogel FA. Osteomyelitis. Lancet 2004;364:369–379

Top Tips

◆ The most common organism in osteomyelitis is *Staphylococcus aureus.*

◆ When a sequestrum or large abscess is present in chronic osteomyelitis, surgical intervention might be necessary.

◆ In the pediatric population, both osteomyelitis and neoplasm (such as Ewing sarcoma or metastases) tend to occur at the highly vascularized metaphysis. Both can have a similar appearance on imaging.

Image Rich 3

■ **Case**

Match the appropriate diagnosis with the provided image.
1. Kohler disease
2. Frieberg infraction
3. Legg Calve Perthes disease
4. Kienbock disease

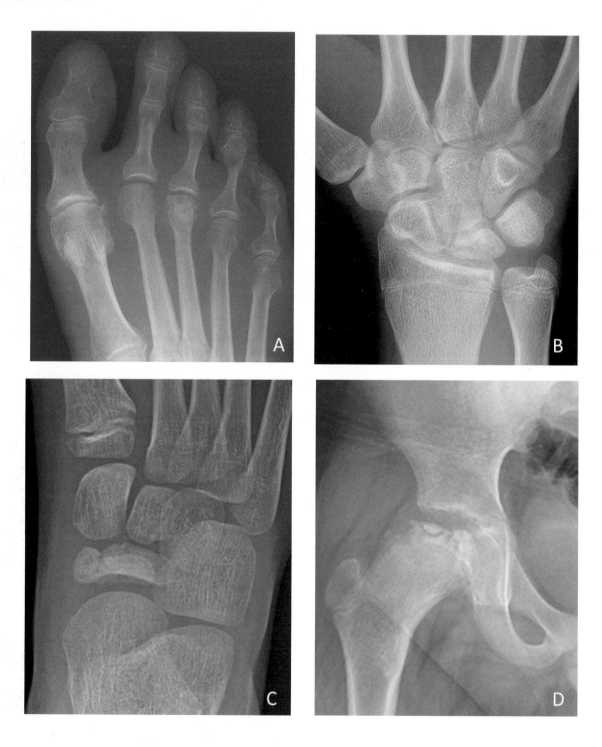

■ Answers and Explanations

1. C

2. A

3. D

4. B

Discussion

These four are all examples of osteochondroses. Osteochondrosis is a term used to describe an aseptic ischemic necrosis of bone, usually affecting the epiphyseal or apophyseal bone. Osteochondroses are commonly seen in the pediatric and young adult population, and they are typically self-limited. However, complications from osteochondroses may occur, including premature growth plate closure, osteochondral bodies, and secondary osteoarthritis.

On X-ray and computed tomography, osteochondroses demonstrate sclerosis, subchondral flattening, and osseous fragmentation. On magnetic resonance imaging, affected bone is T1 and PD hypointense, and marrow edema in the parent bone is commonly seen. The appearance mimics avascular necrosis on imaging.

Osteochondroses of specific bones are commonly eponymous, usually named for the individual that described the disease. Examples of osteochondroses in the upper extremity include Kienbock disease (lunate) and Panner disease (capitellum). In the lower extremity, examples include Legg Calve Perthes disease (capital femoral epiphysis), Kohler disease (tarsal navicular), Sever disease (calcaneal apophysis), and Freiberg infraction (second or third metatarsal head). Scheuermann disease is an osteochondrosis in the spine affecting the ring apophysis. Approximately 40 different osteochondroses have been described, and any epiphysis or apophysis is potentially subject to this pathology. Osgood-Schlatter disease is self-limited fragmentation of the tibial tubercle with soft tissue swelling and thickening at the insertion of the patellar ligament.

The sometimes-used term "osteochondritis" is a misnomer, as there is no inflammation in this process and the cartilage is not primarily affected.

■ Suggested Readings

Brant WE, Helms CA. Fundamentals of Diagnostic Radiology. Philadelphia, PA: Lippincott, Williams & Wilkins; 2007: 1155

Resnick D. Osteochondroses. In Resnick D. Diagnosis of Bone and Joint Disorders. 4th edition. Philadelphia, PA: WB Saunders; 2002: 3686–3741

Top Tips

◆ Osteochondroses usually affect epiphyseal or apophyseal bone and are typically self-limited.

◆ Complications may include premature growth plate closure, osteochondral bodies, and secondary osteoarthritis.

◆ Be aware that the apophysis is the equivalent of an epiphysis, so any pathology affecting one can also affect the other.

Image Rich 4

■ Case

Match the appropriate image with the correct diagnosis.
- A. Osteoid osteoma
- B. Nonossifying fibroma (NOF)
- C. Enchondroma
- D. Unicameral bone cyst

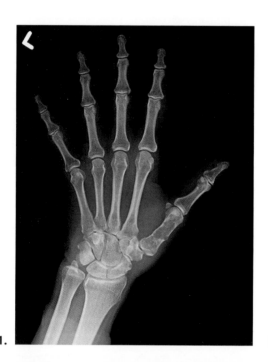

1.

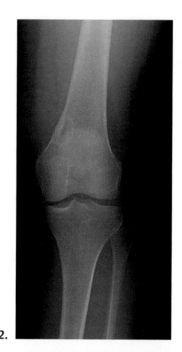

2.

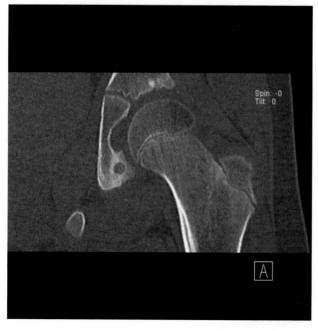

3.

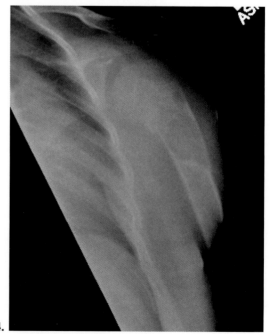

4.

■ Answers and Explanations

1. C. Enchondroma. Enchondroma is a commonly occurring benign lesion composed of hyaline cartilage. It is found most often in the hand, followed by the long bones. It is usually diagnosed in the third and fourth decades as an incidental finding. The typical radiographic appearance of an enchondroma is that of an expansile lytic lesion with a thin sclerotic rim, with or without internal chondroid (ring and arc) matrix. On MRI, an enchondroma appears heterogeneously T2 hyperintense.

Due to the benign nature of this lesion, no treatment is necessary, except in the case of a pathologic fracture (which would then be treated with curettage and fixation). Enchondromatosis is called Ollier disease. The combination of enchondromatosis and soft tissue hemangiomas is called Maffucci syndrome.

It is important to differentiate an enchondroma from a chondrosarcoma. Chondrosarcomas are rare in the hands, which is the most common site for enchondromas. Enchondromas do not usually cause pain (unless fractured), whereas chondrosarcomas usually do cause focal pain. Chondrosarcomas are commonly associated with cortical destruction and a soft tissue mass, whereas enchondromas are not. Sometimes, differentiation is very challenging.

2. B. NOF. NOF, fibroxanthoma, and fibrous cortical defect all describe histologically identical benign fibrous lesions that commonly arise in the metaphysis of long bones. NOF is typically found in children or adolescents. This lesion is seen radiographically as a nonaggressive lytic lesion with a sclerotic rim. It is found in an eccentric, endosteal position within the metaphysis or diaphysis. On magnetic resonance imaging (MRI), NOF is often heterogeneous, T1 hypointense, variably T2 hypointense, and sometimes exhibits heterogeneous mild enhancement. NOF is associated with mildly increased uptake on nuclear bone scan.

No treatment is usually necessary, and biopsy is not recommended as the radiographic appearance is diagnostic. Biopsy may actually be misleading, because scattered giant cells can occur within an NOF. In the case of a pathologic fracture or impending fracture, surgical fixation may occasionally be indicated.

3. A. Osteoid osteoma. Osteoid osteoma is a benign bone-forming tumor that occurs most commonly during the second and third decades. It can be associated with significant pain that is worse at night and relieved by aspirin. On radiographs and computed tomography, it typically presents as a well-defined lucent nidus centered in the bone cortex, often with pronounced surrounding sclerosis and periosteal reaction. On MRI, there is surrounding marrow edema, but the appearance of the nidus is variable, as is the degree of enhancement. An osteoid osteoma is associated with intense uptake on nuclear bone scan. The nidus of an osteoid osteoma is the neoplastic tissue and is rarely larger than 1.5 to 2 cm in diameter, but the surrounding reactive marrow edema and periosteal reaction can cover a larger area (and may also involve the adjacent soft tissues). A total of 10 to 20% of osteoid osteomas occur in the spine, and these are typically localized to the posterior elements. Scoliosis develops in approximately 75% of spinal osteoid osteomas from chronic muscle spasm.

The treatment of choice for osteoid osteoma is image-guided ablation performed under general anesthesia. Ablation is a minimally invasive treatment with a high cure rate and a quick recovery. The natural history of osteoid osteoma is spontaneous regression, and for lesions in locations where there is high potential for complication from ablation or surgical curettage, chronic nonsteroidal anti-inflammatory drug therapy may be the best option.

4. D. Unicameral bone cyst. A unicameral bone cyst is a benign, fluid-filled collection that most commonly develops within the long bones. It appears on radiographs as a geographic lytic lesion with a thin sclerotic rim. The overlying cortex may be scalloped. Pathologic fractures can occur through the lesion, producing a fragment of bone within the cavity known as the "fallen fragment" sign.

Treatment is indicated in the setting of a pathologic fracture (as in this case) or an impending fracture. Surgical curettage is the most common treatment.

■ Suggested Readings

Basile A, Failla G, Reforgiato A, Scavoe G, Mundo E, Messina M, Caltabiano G, Arena F, Ricceri V, Scavoe A, Masala S. The use of microwave ablation in the treatment of osteoid osteomas. Cardiovasc Intervent Radiol 2014;37:737–742

Douis H, Saifuddin A. The imaging of cartilaginous bone tumours. I. Benign lesions. Skeletal Radiol 2012;41:1195–1212

Hetts SW, Hilchey SD, Wilson R, Franc B. Case 110: nonossifying fibroma. Radiology 2007;243:288–292

Murphey MD, Flemming DJ, Boyea SR, Bojescul JA, Sweet DE, Temple HT. Archives of the AFIP. Enchondroma versus chondrosarcoma in the appendicular skeleton: differentiating features. Radiographics 1998;18:1213–1237

Pretell-Mazzini J, Murphy RF, Kushare I, Dormans JP. Unicameral bone cysts: general characteristics and management controversies. J Am Acad Orthop Surg 2014;22:295–303

Rosenthal DI, Hornicek FJ, Torriani M, Gebhardt MC, Mankin HJ. Osteoid osteomas: percutaneous treatment with radiofrequency energy. Radiology 2003;229:171–175

Smith SE, Kransdorf MJ. Primary musculoskeletal tumors of fibrous origin. Semin Musculoskelet Radiol 2000;4(1):73–88

Top Tips

- NOF, unicameral bone cyst, and enchondromas are all benign "don't touch" lesions.

- It is important to differentiate an enchondroma from a chondrosarcoma. Signs of chondrosarcoma may include pain, larger size, cortical destruction, and soft tissue mass.

- Some benign bone lesions, such as NOF and fibrous dysplasia, can have varied and sometimes confusing appearances on MRI. If you encounter an indeterminate primary bone lesion on MRI, always correlate with a radiograph and/or computed tomography, as the diagnosis may become suddenly obvious.

Image Rich 5

■ Case

Match the appropriate tarsal coalition with the provided image.
1. Talonavicular
2. Cubonavicular
3. Calcaneonavicular
4. Subtalar (talocalcaneal)

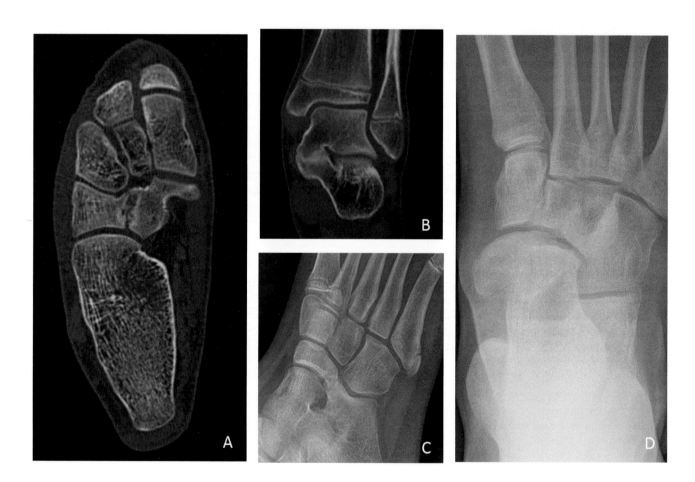

■ Answers and Explanations

1. D

2. A

3. C

4. B

Discussion

These four cases are nice examples of tarsal coalitions. A tarsal coalition is an aberrant union between two or more tarsal bones. Tarsal coalitions may be either osseous (synostosis) or nonosseous. If nonosseous, they may be further categorized as cartilaginous (synchondrosis) or fibrous (syndesmosis). A coalition is nonosseous when there is no bridging bone across the coalition. Nonosseous coalitions in pediatric patients may later ossify, with subsequent skeletal maturity. More than half of the cases of tarsal coalition are bilateral. The most common joints affected are the talocalcaneal (subtalar) and calcaneonavicular joints, which make up approximately 90% of cases.

Altered biomechanics related to a subtalar coalition may cause a pes planovalgus deformity, with flattening of the longitudinal arch and forefoot abduction. Prolonged restriction of motion caused by subtalar coalition may eventually lead to arthrosis of the posterior facet, the midtarsal, and the tibiotalar joints. Nonoperative treatment is commonly the first-line therapy for symptomatic tarsal coalition, but surgical treatment is indicated when conservative measures fail. Surgical options include resection of the coalition and arthrodesis. Although radiographs can sometimes identify or suggest tarsal coalition, computed tomography is the most effective imaging modality in making this diagnosis.

■ Suggested Readings

Lawrence DA, Rolen MF, Haims AH, Zayour Z, Moukaddam HA. Tarsal coalitions: radiographic, CT, and MR imaging findings. HSS J 2014;10(2):153–166

Newman JS, Newberg AH. Congenital tarsal coalition: multimodality evaluation with emphasis on CT and MR imaging. Radiographics 2000;20(2):321–332

Zaw H, Calder JD. Tarsal coalitions. Foot Ankle Clin 2010;15(2):349–364

Top Tips

- ◆ The most common tarsal coalitions are talocalcaneal (subtalar) and calcaneonavicular, which make up approximately 90% of cases. Remember "Non Contrast CT" (navicular-calcaneal, and calcaneal-talar)

- ◆ Tarsal coalitions may be osseous (synostosis) or nonosseous. If nonosseous, they are either cartilaginous (synchondrosis) or fibrous (syndesmosis).

- ◆ Tarsal coalitions are often seen only in retrospect on plain film. For a pediatric patient with a painful foot and ankle and a "normal" plain film, consider reassessing for a tarsal coalition or an osteochondral lesion of the talar dome.

More Challenging 1

■ Case

A 36-year-old woman presents with hip pain.

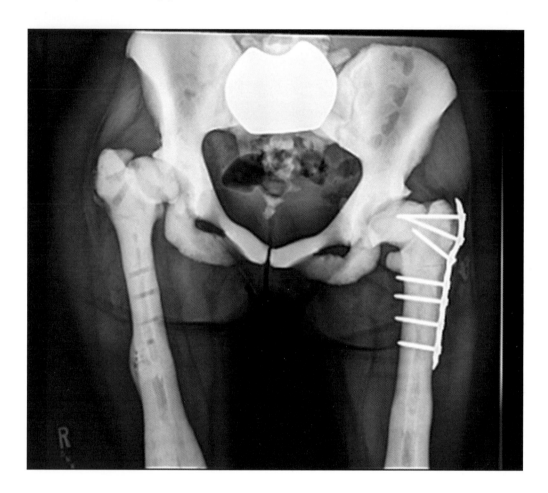

■ Questions

1. The patient's severe diffuse bone sclerosis, combined with a history of sandwich vertebra and pathologic fractures, suggests which ONE of the following diagnoses?
   A. Paget disease
   B. Pyknodysostosis
   C. Osteopetrosis
   D. Renal osteodystrophy

2. Diffuse osseous sclerosis combined with digital subperiosteal resorption, soft tissue calcification, and vertebral endplate sclerosis suggests:
   A. Paget disease
   B. Pyknodysostosis
   C. Osteopetrosis
   D. Renal osteodystrophy

3. Diffuse osseous sclerosis combined with short stature, wormian bones, and delayed closure of the cranial sutures suggests:
   A. Paget disease
   B. Pyknodysostosis
   C. Osteopetrosis
   D. Renal osteodystrophy

■ Answers and Explanations

Question 1

C. Correct! Osteopetrosis is a hereditary condition that results in a markedly dense appearance of bone and obliteration of the medullary canal, and this is seen in the test case. Although the bone appears comparatively dense, it is actually more brittle than normal and is predisposed to frequent fracture. The autosomal recessive form of this disease either results in stillbirth or childhood demise. The autosomal dominant form is less severe and presents later. The radiologic appearance of osteopetrosis has been described as endobone, or "bone-within-bone." The endplate sclerosis in osteopetrosis is thicker and more defined than is typically seen in renal osteodystrophy. In the spine, this has been described as a "sandwich spine."

Other choices and discussion

A. Paget disease is generally found in the elderly. It begins with a lytic phase and progresses to an osteoblastic phase, with the osteoblastic phase resulting in trabecular coarsening, cortical thickening, and bone enlargement. Trabecular coarsening and the typical bone enlargement are not seen in this case. In addition, bone involvement by Paget disease is sporadic and involves either one bone (monostotic) or several bones (polyostotic), but it is not a diffuse skeletal disease.

B. Pyknodysostosis is an autosomal recessive disease that results in hyperostosis that narrows but otherwise spares the medullary canal. Patients present with short stature and other characteristic findings.

D. Patients with renal osteodystrophy most commonly demonstrate osteopenia, but may also exhibit osteosclerosis. However, the osteosclerosis in this case is considerably greater than would be expected in renal osteodystrophy.

Question 2

D. Correct! Patients with renal osteodystrophy most commonly demonstrate osteopenia, but may also exhibit osteosclerosis. Osteosclerosis, combined with vertebral endplate sclerosis ("rugger jersey spine") and subperiosteal resorption along the radial aspect of the middle phalanges, strongly suggests renal osteodystrophy.

Other choices and discussion

A. An individual bone affected by Paget disease may, in some ways, resemble involvement by renal osteodystrophy, but Paget is not a diffuse skeletal disease.

B. Digital subperiosteal resorption and soft tissue calcification are not seen in pyknodysostosis. In addition, the entire vertebral cortex would be sclerotic, not just the endplates.

C. While the "sandwich vertebrae" appearance somewhat resembles the "rugger jersey spine" of renal osteodystrophy, digital subperiosteal resorption and soft tissue calcification are not seen with osteopetrosis.

Question 3

B. Correct! Pyknodysostosis is an autosomal recessive disease that results in diffuse skeletal hyperostosis and narrowed, but not obliterated, medullary canals. The bones are also hypoplastic, resulting in short stature, typical craniofacial anomalies, and distal phalangeal morphology simulating acro-osteolysis. Wormian bones and significantly delayed cranial suture closure are hallmarks.

Other choices and discussion

A. Paget disease affects the elderly and therefore does not alter bone development.

C. Osteopetrosis has no delayed cranial suture closure, no wormian bones, and no bone hypoplasia.

D. Renal osteodystrophy is most commonly osteopenic. However, if a patient exhibits osteosclerosis, none of the other above findings will be present.

■ Suggested Readings

Brant WE, Helms CA. Fundamentals of Diagnostic Radiology. Philadelphia, PA: Lippincott, Williams & Wilkins; 2007: 1163–1167

Ihde LL, Forrester DM, Gottsegen CJ, Masih S, Patel DB, Vachon LA, White EA, Matcuk GR Jr. Sclerosing bone dysplasias: review and differentiation from other causes of osteosclerosis. Radiographics 2011;31(7):1865–1882

Top Tips

◆ Differential diagnoses for diffuse osteosclerosis: renal osteodystrophy, sickle cell disease, myelofibrosis, osteopetrosis, pyknodysostosis, metastatic carcinoma, mastocytosis, Paget disease, athletes, and fluorosis.

◆ Mnemonic for differential diagnosis of diffuse osteosclerosis: **R**egular **S**ex **M**akes **O**ccasional **P**erversions **M**uch **M**ore **P**leasurable **A**nd **F**antastic. Those diagnoses are: renal osteodystrophy, sick cell disease, myelofibrosis, osteoporosis, pyknodysostosis, metastases, mastocytosis, Paget disease, athletes, and fluorosis.

◆ With Paget disease, remember "coarsened trabeculae and thickened cortex."

More Challenging 2

■ Case

Patient 1: A 58-year-old man presents with shoulder pain. Patient 2: A 65-year-old man presents with shoulder pain.

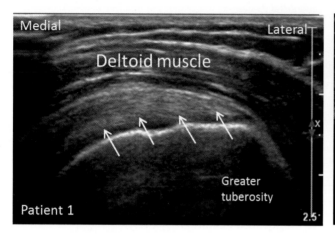

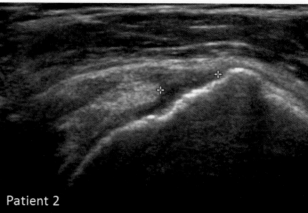

■ Questions

1. What is patient 2's diagnosis?
   A. Subacromial bursitis
   B. Calcific tendinosis
   C. Rotator cuff tear
   D. Proximal humeral fracture
   E. Glenohumeral arthritis

2. What shoulder pathology can be successfully evaluated with ultrasound? (Select ALL that apply.)
   A. Subacromial bursitis
   B. Bankart deformity
   C. Rotator cuff tear
   D. Calcific tendinosis
   E. Biceps tendinopathy

3. Which of these procedures can be successfully performed using ultrasound guidance? (Select ALL that apply.)
   A. Calcific tendinosis aspiration
   B. Bone lesion biopsy
   C. Glenohumeral joint injection
   D. Subacromial bursal injection

■ Answers and Explanations

Question 1

C. Correct! There is a rotator cuff tear. The supraspinatus tendon is torn and retracted from its insertion at the greater tuberosity. Note the normal ultrasound appearance of the supraspinatus tendon in patient 1 (*arrows*).

Other choices and discussion

The other choices are incorrect. The subacromial bursa is not distended. There is no soft tissue mineralization demonstrated in the rotator cuff tendon. No humeral fracture is seen, and the glenohumeral joint is not shown.

Question 2

A. Correct! Fluid distention of the subacromial bursa (bursitis) is easily detected using ultrasound.

C. Correct! Ultrasound has accuracy similar to magnetic resonance imaging in detecting a rotator cuff tear. A minority of institutions with well-trained staff and high-resolution transducers use ultrasound over magnetic resonance imaging as the screening method, when rotator cuff pathology is the main clinical question.

D. Correct! Calcific deposits in the rotator cuff tendons are easily detected using ultrasound.

E. Correct! Biceps tendinosis, tenosynovitis, and tear are well-evaluated using ultrasound.

Other choice and discussion

The other choice is incorrect. A Bankart deformity (injury of the anterior/inferior labrum and glenoid) is poorly evaluated on ultrasound because of its suboptimal location for an acoustical window.

Question 3

A. Correct! Calcific tendinosis aspiration can be readily performed, with ultrasound the preferred modality for this procedure.

C. Correct! The glenohumeral joint is easily accessed for therapeutic injection using ultrasound (usually via a posterior approach).

D. Correct! The subacromial bursa can be accurately targeted for therapeutic injection as well as aspiration using ultrasound guidance.

Other choice and discussion

The other choice is incorrect. Ultrasound evaluates intraosseous lesions poorly and is therefore not useful for bone biopsy purposes.

■ Suggested Readings

Beggs I. Shoulder ultrasound. Semin Ultrasound CT MR 2011;32(2):101–113

Jacobson JA. Shoulder US: anatomy, technique, and scanning pitfalls. Radiology 2011;260(1):6–16

Martinoli C, Bianchi S, Prato N, Pugliese F, Zamorani MP, Valle M, et al. US of the shoulder: non-rotator cuff disorders. Radiographics 2003;23(2):381–401

Top Tips

◆ Rotator cuff insertion tears are well evaluated on ultrasound. Because of its low cost and ready availability, some institutions use ultrasound as the primary screening tool to assess the cuff.

◆ In the shoulder, ultrasound is also useful in the assessment of biceps tendinopathy, subacromial bursitis, and calcific tendinosis.

◆ In patients over 40 years old, the most common causes of shoulder pain include rotator cuff disease, impingement, osteoarthritis, and frozen shoulder.

More Challenging 3

■ Case

A 28-year-old man presents with a history of blue sclera, recurrent fractures since childhood, and chronic bone deformities. Bone density is abnormal. Bilateral lower extremity radiographs are shown.

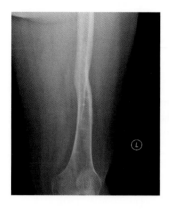 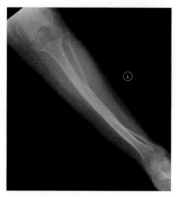 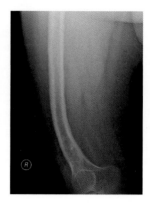 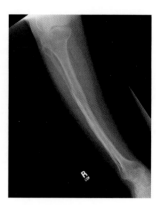

■ Questions

1. Which ONE of the following is the MOST likely diagnosis?
   A. Nonaccidental trauma
   B. Achondroplasia
   C. Neurofibromatosis
   D. Osteogenesis imperfecta
   E. Multiple hereditary exostosis

2. Which subtype of this condition does the patient most likely have? Select the BEST answer.
   A. I
   B. II
   C. III
   D. IV
   E. Either I or IV

3. Which of the following is/are a common treatment for this diagnosis? (Select the BEST answer.)
   A. Bisphosphonate treatment
   B. Chronic corticosteroid treatment
   C. Vitamin D supplementation
   D. A and B
   E. A and C

■ Answers and Explanations

Question 1

D. Correct! This is OI. OI results from a genetic defect in collagen type I production, which leads to multiple fractures. Patients with OI can have blue sclera and hearing loss. Radiographs usually demonstrate osteopenia with chronic fractures and subsequent osseous deformities.

Other choices and discussion

Blue sclera would not be expected with any of the other choices.

A. The bone density is typically normal in nonaccidental trauma.

B. In the lower extremities, an achondroplastic often exhibits metaphyseal flaring and an elongated fibula, which are not present in the test case.

C. Musculoskeletal manifestations of neurofibromatosis can include posterior vertebral scalloping, rib notching/dysplasia, and bowing of the long bones, especially the tibia. Tibial pseudoarthrosis is a well-known potential sequelae of neurofibromatosis. However, blue sclera would not be expected.

E. Multiple hereditary exostoses can cause osseous deformities, but unlike the test case, they would appear as multiple osteochondromas and often present with diaphyseal aclasis (broadened shaft at the end of long bones).

Question 2

E. Correct! OI types I and IV are compatible with a normal lifespan. Given that this patient is 28 years old, he likely has OI type I or type IV.

Other choices and discussion

The other choices are incorrect. OI type II is incompatible with life. OI type III has a high mortality rate in childhood due to numerous fractures and severe deformities.

Question 3

E. Correct! Patients with OI are often treated with both bisphosphonate therapy and vitamin D to improve bone quality. Reduction and surgical fixation may be indicated in some instances for patients with OI presenting with acute fractures.

Other choices and discussion

Chronic steroid treatment is not used in the treatment of OI and, in fact, is discouraged because steroids cause demineralization and further weaken bones.

■ Suggested Readings

Burnei G, Vlad C, Georgescu I, Gavriliu TS, Dan D. Osteogenesis imperfecta: diagnosis and treatment. J Am Acad Orthop Surg 2008;16(6):356–366

Resnick D. Diagnosis of Bone and Joint Disorders. 4th edition. Philadelphia, PA: Saunders; 2002: 4398–4409

Top Tips

◆ It is important to differentiate OI from nonaccidental trauma. Patients with OI typically have decreased bone density.

◆ Treatment for OI involves bisphosphonate and vitamin D supplementation. Disabling bone deformities can be surgically corrected.

◆ OI types I and IV are compatible with a normal lifespan and usually appear normal at birth, presenting with fractures later in life. OI type II is usually fatal in utero, and OI type III has a high mortality rate in childhood.

More Challenging 4

■ Case

A 63-year-old woman presents with left wrist pain.

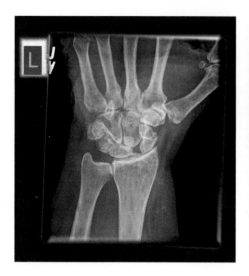 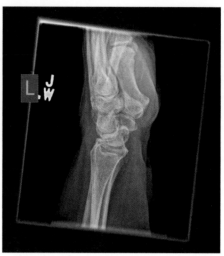

■ Questions

1. Which ONE of the following is the correct diagnosis?
   A. Scaphoid nonunion advanced collapse wrist
   B. Scapholunate advanced collapse (SLAC) wrist
   C. Volar intercalated segmental instability
   D. Midcarpal instability
   E. Perilunate dislocation

2. Which component of the scapholunate ligament is most important in maintaining stability and anatomic alignment?
   A. Volar
   B. Membranous
   C. Dorsal

3. When osteoarthritis involves the wrist, it frequently involves the radiocarpal joint. Which wrist joint is actually the MOST commonly affected?
   A. Lunotriquetral
   B. Distal radioulnar
   C. Capitolunate
   D. Triscaphe
   E. Scapholunate

■ Answers and Explanations

Question 1

B. Correct! This is a case of SLAC wrist. SLAC wrist is a common pattern of malalignment in the wrist that begins with the disruption of the scapholunate ligament. Osteoarthritis occurs first in the radiocarpal joint and subsequently in the capitolunate joint. In the test case, osteoarthritis is present in both the radiocarpal and capitolunate joints.

Dorsal intercalated segmental instability and/or rotation of the scaphoid can also occur, followed eventually by proximal migration of the capitate. Dorsal intercalated segmental instability is present in this case, indicated by dorsal tipping of the lunate, a lunocapitate angle > 30 degrees, and a scapholunate angle > 60 degrees.

Trauma is the most common cause of SLAC wrist. However, findings of SLAC wrist are also found in inflammatory conditions like calcium pyrophosphate deposition disease arthropathy and avascular necrosis of the lunate or scaphoid.

Other choices and discussion

A. Scaphoid nonunion advanced collapse wrist occurs in the setting of a nonunited scaphoid fracture. The subsequent pattern of osteoarthritis and eventual proximal capitate migration is similar to the development of osteoarthritis in a SLAC wrist. No scaphoid fracture is seen in this case.

C. Volar intercalated segmental instability typically occurs with lunotriquetral ligament injury and is not present in this case. Dorsal intercalated segmental instability is present in this case.

D. The lunotriquetral joint is anatomically aligned in this case, making a lunotriquetral ligament injury unlikely.

E. A perilunate dislocation refers to an injury where the capitate is dislocated relative to the lunate, but the lunate articulates normally with the distal radius. This dislocation is not present in the test case.

Question 2

C. Correct! The dorsal band of the scapholunate ligament is the thickest component of the scapholunate ligament and plays the most important role in stabilizing the scapholunate joint. This band is usually well seen on magnetic resonance axial and coronal plane high-resolution images. Complete defects are usually symptomatic.

Other choices and discussion

The volar band of the scapholunate ligament is typically thinner than the dorsal band. It assists in stabilizing the scapholunate joint. The membranous, or interosseous, component contributes little to scapholunate stability. Isolated tears of the interosseous component are often asymptomatic.

The lunotriquetral ligament also has three bands, but the volar band is the most important for stability.

Question 3

D. Correct! The triscaphe joint describes the articulation between the scaphoid, trapezium, and trapezoid, and is the most common location of osteoarthritis in the wrist. The vast majority of osteoarthritis in the wrist occurs in a periscaphoid distribution, predominantly involving the triscaphe and radiocarpal joints.

Other choices and discussion

Osteoarthritis can occur in both the distal radioulnar joint and in the capitolunate joint (in the later stages of SLAC wrist), but these sites are less common than the triscaphe joint for osteoarthritis. The scapholunate joint is not a common location of osteoarthritis.

■ Suggested Readings

Crema MD, Zenter J, Guermazi A, Jomaah N, Marra MD, Roemer FW. Scapholunate advanced collapse and scaphoid nonunion advanced collapse: MDCT arthrography features. Am J Roentgenol 2012;199:W202–W207

Tischler BT, Diaz LE, Murakami AM, Roemer FW, Goud AR, Arndt III WF, Guermazi A. Scapholunate advanced collapse: a pictorial review. Insights into Imaging 2014;5:407–417

Top Tips

- The *dorsal* band is the thickest component of the scapholunate ligament and is most important in providing stability. Its disruption can lead to *dorsal* intercalated segmental instability.

- SLAC wrist is a common pattern of malalignment in the wrist and can also occur in the setting of scapholunate ligament disruption.

- The majority of osteoarthritis in the wrist occurs in a periscaphoid distribution, with the triscaphe joint most commonly involved, followed by the radiocarpal joint.

More Challenging 5

■ Case

A 50-year-old man presents with muscle weakness and acute severe right shoulder pain at rest. No recent injury and no significant past medical history.

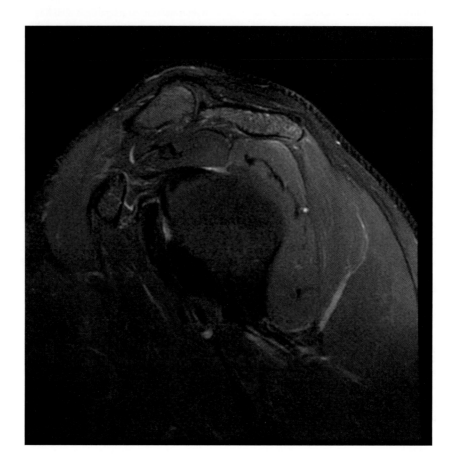

■ Questions

1. Given the location of the abnormal findings, which nerve distribution is likely involved?
   A. Suprascapular nerve
   B. Subscapularis nerve
   C. Axillary nerve
   D. A and C
   E. A and B

2. Which ONE of the following is the correct diagnosis?
   A. Parsonage-Turner syndrome
   B. Inflammatory myopathy
   C. Rotator cuff impingement
   D. Spinoglenoid notch cyst
   E. Nerve compression by fibrous bands

3. Which of the following choices are reasonable next steps in treatment? (Select ALL that apply.)
   A. Pain control using nonsteroidal anti-inflammatory drugs and opioids
   B. Referral for potential surgical decompression
   C. Magnetic resonance imaging of the cervical spine
   D. Physical therapy
   E. Electromyography

■ Answers and Explanations

Question 1

D. Correct! Both the suprascapular and axillary nerves are involved. The infraspinatus, teres minor, and deltoid muscles are edematous. Muscle edema indicates acute denervation. Acute denervation manifests as muscle edema and chronic denervation manifests as muscle atrophy. The suprascapular nerve innervates the infraspinatus muscle, and the axillary nerve innervates the teres minor and deltoid muscles. Therefore, the suprascapular and axillary nerves are both involved.

Other choices and discussion

A. The suprascapular nerve innervates the supraspinatus and the infraspinatus muscles. In the test case, the infraspinatus muscle is edematous, implicating suprascapular nerve involvement. However, teres minor and deltoid muscle edema indicate that another nerve must also be involved.

B. The subscapularis muscle is normal, so the subscapularis nerve is not involved.

C. The axillary nerve is involved, as it innervates the abnormal teres minor and deltoid muscles. However, infraspinatus muscle edema indicates that another nerve must also be involved.

E. The subscapularis muscle is normal, so the subscapularis nerve is not involved.

Question 2

A. Correct! Parsonage-Turner syndrome is a brachial neuritis typically associated with an acute onset of shoulder pain and muscle weakness. It is often suspected to represent a postviral immune response, although not every patient recalls a viral illness. It can also occur after trauma or surgery. Parsonage-Turner characteristically involves multiple nerve distributions, usually involving some combination of the suprascapular, axillary, and subscapularis nerves. The vast majority of cases involve the suprascapular nerve.

Other choices and discussion

B. An inflammatory myopathy is typically associated with an elevation in inflammatory markers (e.g., creatine kinase). It can also be associated with skin changes (rash).

C. Rotator cuff impingement occurs when bone rubs against rotator cuff muscle or tendon during movement, producing irritation. One reason why the supraspinatus is most commonly involved is because of its proximity to an acromioclavicular joint osteophyte or a subacromial spur. Symptoms typically are initially mild and may progress over time. In this case, the sudden onset of pain at rest makes impingement less likely.

D. The spinoglenoid notch connects the supraspinatus and infraspinatus fossae. A cyst within the spinoglenoid notch can occur in association with a posterior or superior labral tear. This sometimes causes impingement of a branch of the suprascapular nerve that innervates the infraspinatus. This can lead to infraspinatus edema and atrophy. However, a spinoglenoid notch cyst would not cause denervation of the teres minor or deltoid muscles.

E. Compression of the axillary nerve by one or more fibrous bands is a possible cause of quadrilateral space syndrome. In this situation, the axillary nerve is compressed as it passes through the quadrilateral space. This can lead to denervation of the deltoid and teres minor muscle, but should not affect the infraspinatus muscle.

Question 3

A. Correct! Parsonage-Turner syndrome can be very painful, especially in the acute phase, and medication with nonsteroidal anti-inflammatory drugs and opioids is often necessary to manage the symptoms.

C. Correct! Before confirming the diagnosis of Parsonage-Turner syndrome, it is important to exclude compression of the cervical nerve roots with magnetic resonance imaging of the cervical spine. The suprascapular, axillary, and subscapularis nerves all arise, at least partially, from the fifth and sixth cervical nerve roots.

D. Correct! Physical therapy can be very helpful to patients with Parsonage-Turner syndrome in preventing muscle atrophy, which often develops from both pain and disuse.

E. Correct! Electromyography can be useful in cases of Parsonage-Turner syndrome to identify the severity of muscle denervation and to identify the muscles involved.

Other choice and discussion

B. Parsonage-Turner syndrome can be very painful and debilitating, but it is typically a self-limited condition that resolves in 1 to 2 years. It is not related to impingement of a muscle, tendon, or nerve, and surgical decompression is NOT indicated.

■ Suggested Readings

Bredella MA, Tirman PF, Fritz RC, Wischer TK, Stork A, Genant HK. Denervation syndromes of the shoulder girdle: MR imaging with electrophysiologic correlation. Skelet Radiol 1999;28(10):567–572

Feinberg JH, Radecki J. Parsonage-Turner syndrome. HSS J 2010;6(2):199–205

Scalf RE, Wenger DE, Frick MA, Mandrekar JN, Adkins MC. MRI findings of 26 patients with Parsonage-Turner syndrome. Am J Roentgenol 2007;189(1):W39–44

Top Tips

◆ Parsonage-Turner syndrome is an idiopathic brachial neuritis related to autoimmune dysfunction following viral infection or injury and typically involves multiple nerve distributions. Edema in several muscles should be a red flag to consider this diagnosis.

◆ In these cases, it is important to rule out other causes of denervation such as a spinoglenoid notch cyst or cervical nerve root compression. Cervical spine magnetic resonance imaging is useful to confirm or exclude proximal pathology causing denervation.

◆ Parsonage-Turner syndrome is usually a self-limited condition that resolves within 1 to 2 years. Supportive treatment such as pain management and physical therapy is often very helpful.

Essentials 1

■ Case

A 6-day-old term neonatal boy presents with an abnormal electroencephalogram following prolonged perinatal resuscitation.

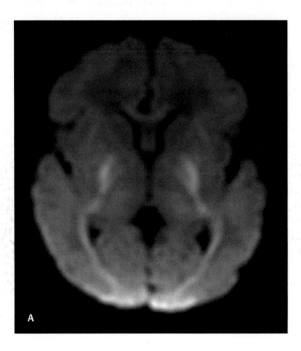

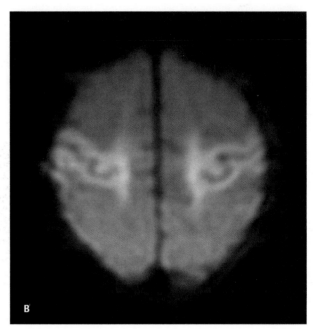

■ Questions

1. What is the MOST likely diagnosis?
   A. Metachromatic leukodystrophy
   B. Severe global hypoxic-ischemic injury
   C. Pantothenate kinase-associated neuropathy
   D. Mitochondrial encephalopathy with lactic acidosis and stroke-like episodes
   E. X-linked adrenoleukodystrophy

2. Which of the following structures is MOST commonly affected in a term neonate when this injury occurs in a partial prolonged manner?
   A. Thalamus
   B. Putamen
   C. Watershed zones (border zones)
   D. Cerebellum
   E. Pons

3. What property of tissue in the central nervous system is responsible for differences in signal intensity on diffusion-weighted imaging?
   A. Axonal cytoskeleton
   B. Myelin sheaths
   C. Fast-axonal transport systems
   D. Intact cell membranes
   E. Osmolality

■ Answers and Explanations

Question 1

B. Correct! This is hypoxic-ischemic injury (HII). Areas of active myelination are most susceptible to ischemic injury in the term neonate. As such, the basal ganglia (particularly the posterior putamina), ventrolateral thalami, hippocampus, dorsal brainstem, corticospinal tracts, and perirolandic regions are most affected by severe HII. In the acute phase, these areas will exhibit restricted diffusion, although normal findings have rarely been reported in the first 24 hours. In the preterm infant, severe HII affects the thalami and brainstem with relative preservation of the basal ganglia and cerebral cortex.

Other choices and discussion

A. Metachromatic leukodystrophy is a lysosomal storage disease that typically presents with symmetric and confluent T2 hyperintense signal in the periventricular white matter. This may have a "tiger-stripe" appearance due to areas of preserved myelination along medullary veins. Given the absence of these findings and the presence of symmetric restricted diffusion involving the basal ganglia, optic radiations, and perirolandic regions in the test case, metachromatic leukodystrophy is incorrect.

C. Pantothenate kinase-associated neuropathy is a type of neurodegeneration with brain iron accumulatio. It has an autosomal recessive inheritance pattern. The classic imaging finding is that of T2 hypointense signal in the globus pallidus with central hyperintensity ("eye of the tiger" sign), which is not present in this case.

D. Typical imaging findings in mitochondrial encephalopathy with lactic acidosis and stroke-like episodes are stroke-like lesions in the cortex that do not conform to a vascular territory. Parietal and occipital cortices are involved most frequently. Other findings include lacunar infarcts and basal ganglia calcifications. These findings are not shown in the test case. Symptoms of mitochondrial encephalopathy with lactic acidosis and stroke-like episodes do not tend to manifest until adolescence.

E. X-linked adrenoleukodystrophy is a peroxisomal disorder seen in male children. Imaging findings include T2 hyperintense signal beginning in the splenium of the corpus callosum and spreading peripherally as the disease progresses. Contrast enhancement is seen in the intermediate zone of the demyelinated area, along the periphery ("leading edge" enhancement). Primary involvement of the deep gray matter and cortices in the test case argues against X-linked adrenoleukodystrophy.

Question 2

C. Correct! During prolonged periods of partial asphyxia in the term neonate, blood is preferentially shunted to the deep gray matter, brainstem, and cerebellum at the expense of the white matter and cortex, resulting in injury to the cerebral watershed or border zones. In the preterm infant, less profound HII results in germinal matrix hemorrhage and deep periventricular white matter injury.

Other choices and discussion

A. The thalamus is generally spared in partial prolonged asphyxia but involved in severe HII. Severe HII in the term neonate also involves the basal ganglia (especially the posterior putamina), ventrolateral thalami, hippocampi, dorsal brainstem, corticospinal tracts, and perirolandic cortices. On the contrary, partial prolonged asphyxia in the term neonate typically affects the watershed areas in the brain.

B. The putamen is generally spared in partial prolonged asphyxia but involved in severe HII.

D. The cerebellum is spared.

E. The pons is spared.

Question 3

D. Correct! Diffusion-weighted imaging generates a map of the apparent diffusivity (measured by apparent diffusion coefficient) of water molecules in their microenvironment. The term "apparent" is used because while the true diffusivity of water is constant, its apparent diffusivity is influenced by its environment. In the brain, intact cell membranes hinder the diffusion of water molecules, giving the appearance that the diffusivity of water in the parenchyma is reduced relative to the diffusivity of water in cerebrospinal fluid. Various pathologies further reduce the apparent diffusivity of water (i.e., cause restricted diffusion, as reflected by bright diffusion-weighted imaging and dark apparent diffusion coefficient signal intensity) with respect to normal brain, including anything causing cytotoxic edema (e.g. infarction), hematomas at certain stages, purulent material (in abscesses), and tumors with high nucleus-to-cytoplasmic ratios.

The other choices are all incorrect.

■ Suggested Readings

Gillard JH, Waldman AD, Barker PB, eds. Clinical MR Neuroimaging: Diffusion, Perfusion, and Spectroscopy. Cambridge: Cambridge University Press; 2005

Huang BY, Castillo M. Hypoxic-ischemic brain injury: imaging findings from birth to adulthood. Radiographics 2008;28:417–439

Osborn AG. Osborn's Brain: Imaging, Pathology, and Anatomy. Philadelphia, PA: Wolters Kluwer/Lippincott Williams & Wilkins; 2012

Top Tips

◆ Severe HII in the term neonate involves the basal ganglia (posterior putamina), ventrolateral thalami, hippocampi, dorsal brainstem, corticospinal tracts, and perirolandic cortices.

◆ Partial prolonged asphyxia in the term neonate often affects the cerebral watershed areas.

◆ Look for symmetric restricted diffusion of the affected areas within 24 hours of the insult.

Essentials 2

■ Case

A 68-year-old man presents with confusion, unstable gait, and slurring of speech.

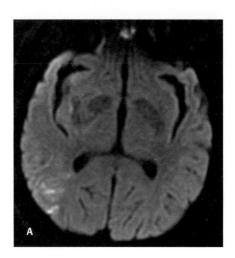
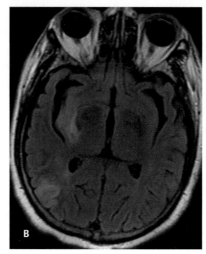
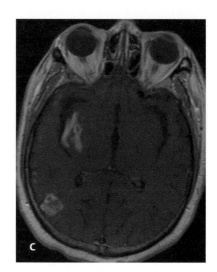

■ Questions

1. What is the MOST likely diagnosis?
   A. Metastatic disease
   B. Invasive fungal infection
   C. Lymphoma
   D. Multifocal glioblastoma
   E. Subacute infarction

2. What is the approximate timeline and pattern of parenchymal enhancement after the injury from the test case occurs?
   A. Enhancement begins at 2 hours, peaks at 2 days, and disappears by 2 weeks
   B. Enhancement begins at 1 day, peaks at 1 week, and disappears by 1 month
   C. Enhancement begins at 2 days, peaks at 2 weeks, and disappears by 2 months

   D. Enhancement begins at 4 days, peaks at 4 weeks, and disappears by 4 months
   E. Enhancement begins at 7 days, peaks at 4 weeks, and disappears by 4 months

3. What is the name for the finding of serpiginous cortical T1 hyperintensity that is often seen with subacute infarcts?
   A. Cortical ribboning
   B. Cortical laminar necrosis
   C. Cortical tram-track sign
   D. Cortical rim sign
   E. Transmantle sign

■ Answers and Explanations

Question 1

E. Correct! This patient has a subacute infarction. The findings of cortical or gyral edema and contrast enhancement in the distribution of a vascular territory (middle cerebral artery territory in this patient) are most consistent with subacute infarction. Parenchymal enhancement is caused by leakage of the contrast agent across the disrupted blood–brain barrier. Enhancement can be gyral (if cortical involvement is present) or generalized or ring-like (if basal ganglia or brainstem involvement is present). It usually begins at the end of the first week following complete infarction and typically disappears by 2 months. However, parenchymal cortical enhancement can also be seen with incomplete infarction, usually occurring between 2 to 4 hours after the ischemia onset and disappearing 24 to 48 hours later. This type of enhancement is postulated to occur from vascular occlusion with very early reperfusion and is associated with a good prognosis. Of note, intravascular (arterial) and meningeal enhancement can be seen with acute infarcts, which are commonly seen and resolve within the first week of a stroke.

Discussion

The other choices are all incorrect. The gyral pattern of enhancement, lack of edema relative to the size of the enhancing lesions on fluid-attenuated inversion recovery imaging, and location of the lesions within a vascular (right middle cerebral artery) territory make metastatic disease, invasive fungal infection, lymphoma, and multifocal glioblastoma unlikely. Note that invasive fungal infections can sometimes cause infarct-like lesions.

Question 2

C. Correct! Enhancement begins at 2 days, peaks at 2 weeks, and disappears by 2 months. The "2-2-2 rule" is a good approximation of the timeline and pattern of parenchymal enhancement following an ischemic event. It typically begins 4 to 7 days after complete infarction but can be seen as early as 1 to 2 days after the event. In the majority of strokes, enhancement is present between 1 week and 2 months, although it can persist for up to 4 months. An alternative diagnosis should be considered if enhancement persists beyond this time. Of note, the presence of early parenchymal enhancement within 6 hours of a stroke predicts a higher risk for hemorrhagic transformation, especially if the stroke is located in the basal ganglia or deep gray matter.

The other choices are all incorrect.

Question 3

B. Correct! Cortical laminar necrosis, or pseudolaminar necrosis, is due to oxygen and/or glucose depletion and mainly affects the third layer of the cerebral cortex, which is the most vulnerable of the six cortical layers to hypoxia and hypoglycemia. The T1 hyperintensity is related to denatured proteins in necrotic cells or fat-laden macrophages, not from calcium or hemoglobin products. This phenomenon is often detected 2 weeks after a stroke and can be seen as early as 3 to 5 days following the event. It typically resolves after 3 months but may persist for more than a year.

Other choices and discussion

A. Cortical ribboning is hyperintensity of the cortex on diffusion-weighted imaging and is a useful diagnostic sign of Creutzfeldt-Jacob disease.

C. Cortical tram-track sign is produced by cortical calcifications due to leptomeningeal vascular anomalies in patients with Sturge-Weber syndrome.

D. Cortical rim sign is useful to distinguish renal infarct from acute pyelonephritis. It denotes continued enhancement of the peripheral cortex of an infarcted kidney because of capsular collateral arteries.

E. Transmantle sign is an imaging feature of focal cortical dysplasia. It is most often found in type 2 focal cortical dysplasia (Taylor-type dysplasia). This dysplasia is characterized by linear T2/fluid-attenuated inversion recovery signal extending from the ventricle to the cortex and represents arrested neuronal migration.

■ Suggested Readings

Allen LM, Hasso AN, Handwerker J, et al. Sequence-specific MR imaging findings that are useful in dating ischemic stroke. Radiographics 2012;32:1285–1297

Karonen JO, Partanen PL, Vanninen RL, et al. Evolution of MR contrast enhancement patterns during the first week after acute ischemic stroke. Am J Neuroradiol 2001;22:103–111

Seth NK, Torgovnick J, Macaluso C, et al. Cortical laminar necrosis following anoxic encephalopathy. Neurol India 2006;54:327

Top Tips

- Remember the "2-2-2" enhancement rule for subacute infarcts: enhancement begins at 2 days, peaks at 2 weeks, and disappears by 2 months.

- Enhancement can be gyral or ring-like. Remember the mnemonic **MAGIC DR** for rim-enhancing brain lesions: **m**etastases, **a**bscess, **g**lioblastoma, **i**nfarct (subacute), **c**ontusion, **d**emyelinating diseases, **r**adiation necrosis.

- Cortical laminar necrosis (or pseudolaminar necrosis), characterized by gyral T1 hyperintensity, is usually seen 2 weeks after infarction but can occur as early as 3 to 5 days after a stroke.

Essentials 3

■ Case

A 50-year-old woman with a history of alcoholism presents with acute alcoholic hepatitis, septic shock, and somnolence.

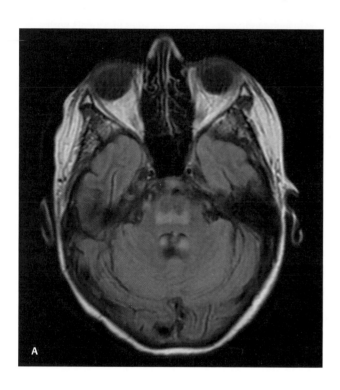

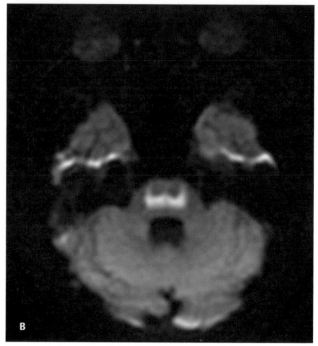

■ Questions

1. What is the MOST likely diagnosis?
   A. Abscess
   B. Acute infarction
   C. Osmotic demyelination syndrome
   D. Posterior reversible encephalopathy syndrome
   E. Glioma

2. The most frequent cause of this disorder is rapid correction of which ONE of the following?
   A. Hyponatremia
   B. Hypokalemia
   C. Hypocalcemia
   D. Hypophosphatemia
   E. Hypomagnesemia

3. Which of the following comprises the clinical symptoms that can be seen from brainstem injury due to osmotic demyelination syndrome (central pontine myelinolysis)?
   A. Quadriplegia, dysarthria, dysphagia, lethargy
   B. Quadriplegia, dysarthria, dysphagia, tremor
   C. Diplopia, dysarthria, dysphagia, tremor
   D. Locked-in syndrome, dysarthria, dysphagia, tremor
   E. Amnesia, dysarthria, dysphagia, tremor

■ Answers and Explanations

Question 1

C. Correct! This patient has osmotic demyelination syndrome (ODS). "Trident-shaped" T2 or T2/fluid-attenuated inversion recovery hyperintense signal sparing the corticospinal tracts and ventrolateral pons, as in the test case, is characteristic of pontine involvement by ODS. Restricted diffusion, which is also seen, indicates the acute phase of disease. While ODS most frequently involves the pons, extrapontine involvement—including the thalamus, basal ganglia, white matter, and rarely, the cerebral cortex—may also be seen.

Other choices and discussion

A. On magnetic resonance imaging, an abscess appears as a central core of T2 hyperintensity and restricted diffusion surrounded by a thin T2 hypointense and enhancing rim. In the above case, while the lesion itself demonstrates T2 hyperintensity and restricted diffusion, the absence of a thin T2 hypointense rim, mass effect, and edema makes this answer choice incorrect.

B. An acute pontine infarct would appear as a focal paramedian lesion exhibiting restricted diffusion. Pontine infarcts result from thrombosis of pontine perforators arising from the basilar artery. Central and symmetric restricted diffusion surrounding the corticospinal tracts in the test case makes pontine infarct unlikely.

D. The central variant of posterior reversible encephalopathy syndrome (PRES), which is an uncommon pattern of PRES, may involve the brainstem, cerebellum, thalamus, and basal ganglia. Pontine involvement may be patchy or diffuse, but sparing of the corticospinal tracts as seen in the test case would not be expected with PRES. The most typical appearance of PRES, occurring in > 90% of cases, is vasogenic edema within the parietal and occipital lobes.

E. The absence of mass effect and the sparing of the corticospinal tracts argue against the diagnosis of glioma.

Question 2

A. **Correct!** The most frequent cause of ODS is rapid correction of hyponatremia. To prevent ODS, hyponatremia should be corrected at a rate of no more than 8 to 12 mmol/L of sodium per day. The rate of rise in plasma sodium concentration should be even lower in patients at higher risk for osmotic demyelination, such as those with chronic alcoholism, cirrhosis, and malnutrition.

Other choices and discussion

B. While concomitant hypokalemia may play a contributory role, the pathogenesis of ODS is secondary to the rapid correction of hyponatremia.

C. Rapid correction of hypocalcemia can contribute to cardiac arrhythmias and is not associated with ODS.

D. Rapid correction of hypophosphatemia can lead to complications such as hypocalcemia, tetany, and hypotension.

E. Hypomagnesemia is incorrect.

Question 3

A. Correct! The clinical manifestations of ODS become apparent 2 to 6 days following the rapid correction of sodium. Symptoms/signs that can be seen with the pontine variant of ODS (central pontine myelinolysis) include anything neurologically related to brainstem injury such as quadriplegia, dysarthria, dysphagia, lethargy, diplopia, and locked-in syndrome. Locked-in syndrome is a condition in which the patient is conscious and awake but globally paralyzed except for the ability to move his or her eyes; this syndrome often results from an acute lesion involving the ventral pons.

Other choices and discussion

The other choices are all incorrect. Whereas quadriplegia, dysarthria, dysphagia, diplopia, and locked-in syndrome can be seen with central pontine myelinolysis due to brainstem involvement, tremor and other movement disorders are typically seen with the extrapontine variant of ODS (extrapontine myelinolysis) affecting the basal ganglia. In addition, amnesia is not usually associated with ODS.

■ Suggested Readings

Howard SA, Barletta JA, Klufas RA, et al. Best cases from AFIP: osmotic demyelination syndrome. Radiographics 2009;29:933–988

Huq S, Wong M, Chan H, et al. Osmotic demyelination syndromes: central and extrapontine myelinolysis. J Clin Neurosci 2007;14;684–688

King JD, Rosner MH. Osmotic demyelination syndrome. Am J Med Sci 2010;339:561–567

Top Tips

- ◆ ODS is most often the result of rapid chronic hyponatremia correction.

- ◆ Common conditions associated with ODS: alcoholism, malnutrition, and liver transplantation.

- ◆ Pontine involvement by acute ODS ("central pontine myelinolysis") appears on magnetic resonance imaging as "trident-shaped" T2 hyperintensity and restricted diffusion in the central pons sparing the corticospinal tracts and ventrolateral pons.

Essentials 4

■ Case

A 55-year-old woman presents with history of rheumatoid arthritis presents with left complete hemianopsia.

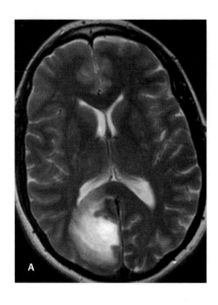
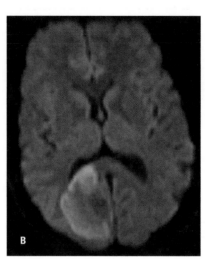
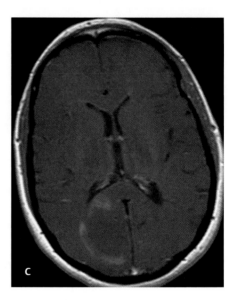

■ Questions

1. What is the MOST likely diagnosis?
   A. Metastasis
   B. Pyogenic abscess
   C. Tumefactive demyelinating lesion
   D. Acute infarction
   E. Hematoma

2. Which pattern of enhancement is MOST characteristic of this process?
   A. Ring enhancement with enhancing nodule
   B. Open ring or incomplete ring enhancement
   C. Thick and irregular ring enhancement
   D. Gyral enhancement
   E. Nodular enhancement

3. Which of the following is an immune-mediated microvascular endothelial disorder characterized by the following clinical triad: encephalopathy, sensorineural hearing loss, and vision impairment?
   A. Multiple sclerosis
   B. Acute disseminated encephalomyelitis
   C. Neuromyelitis optica
   D. Progressive multifocal leukoencephalopathy
   E. Susac syndrome

■ Answers and Explanations

Question 1

C. Correct! This is a tumefactive demyelinating lesion (TDL). TDLs are well circumscribed, exert little mass effect, and produce relatively little surrounding edema for their size. Enhancement is variable but, when present, appears as an incomplete ring of enhancement ("leading edge" enhancement), as in this case. Apparent diffusion coefficient values are elevated (facilitated diffusion) in the lesion as a whole, although peripheral restricted diffusion can be observed, a feature also present in the test case. While the natural progression of TDLs is unknown, a number of studies have reported that most patients with TDLs will be eventually diagnosed with multiple sclerosis (MS) or a neuromyelitis optica spectrum disorder. A subset of patients does not progress to typical MS. The majority of patients with TDLs respond favorably to corticosteroid therapy.

Other choices and discussion

A. The marked hyperintense T2 signal intensity, incomplete rim of restricted diffusion and enhancement, and relative paucity of perilesional edema in this case argues against metastatic disease.

B. The classic appearance of a mature pyogenic abscess is a round mass with a relatively T1 hyperintense and T2 hypointense rim, a complete rim of enhancement that may be thinner along the ventricular side, and a core of T2 hyperintense signal and restricted diffusion representing the walled-off purulent material. Mass effect and surrounding edema is common. In the above case, the lesion demonstrates restricted diffusion along the periphery, making this answer choice unlikely.

D. The test case does not conform to a vascular distribution and is confined to the white matter, making acute infarction unlikely.

E. The imaging appearance of a hematoma varies depending on the age of the hemorrhage. Although the solid clot component of a hematoma can exhibit restricted diffusion, the peripheral pattern of restricted diffusion (and marked T2 hyperintensity of the lesion), as seen in the test case, is not typical of hematoma.

Question 2

B. Correct! An open or incomplete ring of enhancement is most suggestive of a demyelinating process, although enhancement may be variable. The enhancing portion of the lesion is thought to represent the leading edge of demyelination.

Other choices and discussion

A. Ring enhancement with enhancing nodule is more typical of infectious or neoplastic processes. Toxoplasmosis, neurocysticercosis, metastases, and some primary brain tumors can have this appearance.

C. Thick and irregular ring enhancement is more suggestive of a necrotic neoplasm.

D. Gyral enhancement can be seen in the subacute phase of cerebral infarction following reperfusion.

E. Nodular enhancement can be seen in the setting of metastasis, septic emboli, and granulomatous processes.

Question 3

E. Correct! Susac syndrome (retinocochleocerebral vasculopathy) is an immune-mediated microvascular occlusive endotheliopathy. Patients present with the clinical triad of encephalopathy, sensorineural hearing loss, and vision impairment due to branch retinal artery occlusions. Magnetic resonance imaging shows multiple T2 hyperintense lesions in the brain, including the corpus callosum, that can mimic MS. In Susac syndrome, there is involvement of the middle layer of the corpus callosum with sparing of the undersurface, whereas in MS, the undersurface is involved.

Other choices and discussion

A. MS is the most common primary demyelinating disorder of the central nervous system involving the brain and spinal cord. Magnetic resonance imaging demonstrates multiple, usually small, T2 hyperintense plaques that characteristically involve the callososeptal interface with perivenular extension ("Dawson's fingers"). Therefore, white matter spots in the brain that appear ovoid in shape and are oriented perpendicular to the plane of the lateral ventricles should raise the suspicion for underlying MS. The diagnosis of MS itself is based on both clinical and imaging findings, taking into account the Revised McDonald criteria, which characterizes lesions disseminated in space and time, and presence of oligoclonal immunoglobulin-G bands in cerebrospinal fluid.

B. Acute disseminated encephalomyelitis is an immune-mediated demyelinating disorder that can occur weeks following a viral prodrome or vaccination. In contrast to MS, acute disseminated encephalomyelitis is usually a monophasic illness and occurs most frequently in children.

C. Neuromyelitis optica, also known as Devic syndrome, is an immune-mediated demyelinating disease that preferentially involves the optic nerves (optic neuritis) and spinal cord (transverse myelitis).

D. Progressive multifocal leukoencephalopathy is an infectious demyelinating process caused by reactivation of the human polyomavirus JC in immunocompromised patients.

■ Suggested Readings

Dagher AP, Smirniotopoulos J. Tumefactive demyelinating lesions. Neuroradiology 1996;38:560–565

Top Tips

- TDLs are large (> 2 cm) lesions that usually involve the white matter and have little mass effect and edema for their size.

- Open or incomplete ring enhancement and restricted diffusion along the periphery of a lesion are characteristic imaging features of demyelinating lesions.

- Although many patients with TDLs will be eventually diagnosed with MS, a number of patients will not progress to MS.

Essentials 5

■ Case

A 35-year-old woman with migraine history presents with acute onset headache differing in quality from her usual headaches. Magnetic resonance imaging of the brain (not shown) was normal. Magnetic resonance angiography was performed at presentation (left) and at 3-month follow up (right). Erythrocyte sedimentation rate and C-reactive protein levels were normal.

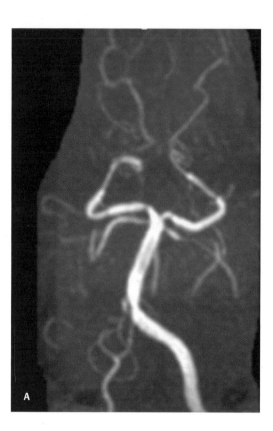
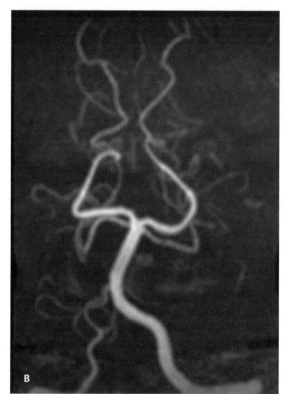

■ Questions

1. What is the MOST likely diagnosis?
   A. Moyamoya disease
   B. Dissection
   C. Reversible cerebral vasoconstriction syndrome
   D. Vasculitis
   E. Atherosclerotic disease

2. What is the MOST common clinical presentation of this disorder?
   A. Thunderclap headache
   B. Seizure
   C. Syncope
   D. Sudden onset focal neurologic deficit
   E. Encephalopathy

3. Most patients with reversible cerebral vasoconstriction syndrome have normal nonvascular brain imaging, although some may have positive findings such as hemorrhage, vasogenic edema, and infarction. These findings BEST overlap with which ONE of the following disorders?
   A. Progressive multifocal leukoencephalopathy
   B. Posterior circulation stroke
   C. Venous sinus thrombosis
   D. Gliomatosis cerebri
   E. Posterior reversible encephalopathy syndrome

■ Answers and Explanations

Question 1

C. Correct! This is reversible cerebral vasoconstriction syndrome (RCVS), also known as Call-Fleming syndrome. RCVS is a clinical and radiographic syndrome manifested by hyperacute onset of severe headache with segmental cerebral arterial vasoconstriction that can affect the anterior and/or posterior circulation(s). The test case clinical presentation of a severe and sudden onset headache with self-limited angiographic findings of multifocal narrowing involving the superior cerebellar and posterior cerebral arteries is typical of RCVS. By definition, the vasoconstriction with RCVS should resolve within 3 months. It occurs most frequently in young to middle-aged adults, and women are more affected than men. While a third of cases may occur spontaneously, a specific trigger can be identified in some patients (e.g., complications of pregnancy such as eclampsia or preeclampsia, postpartum state, and exposure to vasoactive or recreational drugs such as cocaine, cannabis, ecstasy, selective serotonin reuptake inhibitors, nasal decongestants, pseudoephedrine, and migraine medications).

Other choices and discussion

A. Moyamoya disease is a progressive arteriopathy characterized by progressive stenosis of the supraclinoid internal carotid arteries. In Japanese, the name "moyamoya" means "puff of smoke" and describes the appearance of small collateral vessels that form to compensate for arterial occlusions. Involvement of the posterior circulation occurs less frequently, and when it does occur, anterior circulation steno-occlusive disease is also usually present. Unlike RCVS, imaging findings do not resolve on follow up imaging.

B. Dissection would not present as transient and self-limited multifocal narrowing of the bilateral posterior cerebral and superior cerebellar arteries.

D. Imaging findings of central nervous system vasculitis include multisegmental narrowing of the cerebral arteries, and while patients may also present with headache, the headache tends to be more subacute and insidious in onset than in this test case. In contrast to RCVS, imaging findings would not be expected to improve without appropriate treatment. In addition, serum markers of inflammation, such as erythrocyte sedimentation rate and C-reactive protein, are often elevated in patients with vasculitis and not elevated in patients with RCVS.

E. Atherosclerotic vascular narrowing would not resolve at a 3-month follow-up. Furthermore, atherosclerotic vascular disease frequently affects older patients, and there is often the presence of calcified vascular plaques elsewhere. Interestingly, the distribution of atherosclerosis has been shown to differ among races. Extracranial atherosclerosis is more common in Caucasians, whereas intracranial atherosclerosis is more common in non-Caucasians.

Question 2

A. Correct! The most common clinical pvresentation is a thunderclap headache (a severe headache characterized by very sudden onset), occurring in 94 to 100% of patients. This type of headache may wax and wane over minutes to days and may recur over weeks. A thunderclap headache is not entirely specific for RCVS and may also be seen in patients with aneurysmal subarachnoid hemorrhage.

The other choices are all incorrect.

Question 3

E. Correct! Posterior reversible encephalopathy syndrome (PRES), a neurologic disorder that occurs due to the inability of the cerebral circulation to autoregulate in response to insults like acute hypertension, can be seen with or without RCVS. On MRI, PRES most frequently presents as symmetric or asymmetric areas of vasogenic edema in the parietal and occipital lobes, involving the subcortical and cortical locations. However, despite being termed posterior, it can be found in other areas of the brain including the watershed or border zone territories, frontal and inferior temporal lobes, cerebellum, basal ganglia, and brainstem. Other findings include focal parenchymal hemorrhage, microhemorrhage, sulcal subarachnoid hemorrhage, and acute infarction.

Other choices and discussion

A. The imaging findings of classic progressive multifocal leukoencephalopathy are nonenhancing geographic T2 hyperintense lesions with little to no enhancement or mass effect. Lesions involve the subcortical white matter, extend into the deep white matter as the disease progresses, and are asymmetric when multifocal. Hemorrhage and vascular territory infarcts are not typically present with progressive multifocal leukoencephalopathy.

B. While posterior circulation infarcts can occur with RCVS, they are not present in every case. The appearance of hemorrhages in RCVS (when present) is also more similar to posterior reversible encephalopathy syndrome than to hemorrhagic transformation of posterior circulation strokes.

C. Although hemorrhage, edema, and infarction may occur with venous sinus thrombosis, findings related to the latter are usually confined to venous drainage territories and typically not bilateral and symmetric, as may be seen with RCVS.

D. Gliomatosis cerebri is defined by diffuse gliomatous infiltration of at least three lobes of the brain and tends to be more asymmetric than the findings in RCVS. Also, hemorrhage and infarction are typically not present with gliomatosis.

Top Tips

◆ RCVS is a clinical and radiographic syndrome characterized by thunderclap headache, multisegmental cerebral vascular narrowing, normal blood work (erythrocyte sedimentation rate and C-reactive protein), and resolution of imaging findings within 3 months.

◆ RCVS can occur spontaneously or can be precipitated by specific triggers (e.g., drug exposure, pregnancy complications, and postpartum state).

◆ Complications of RCVS include sulcal subarachnoid hemorrhage, intraparenchymal hemorrhage, cerebral infarction, and PRES.

Essentials 6

■ Case

A 66-year-old man presents with vertigo.

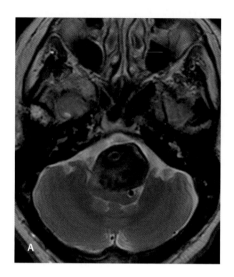
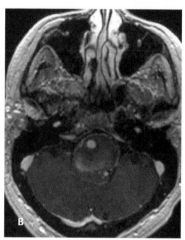
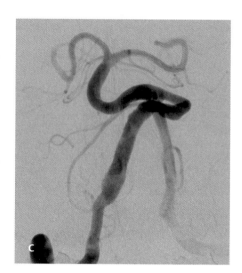

■ Questions

1. What is the MOST likely diagnosis?
   A. Dissecting pseudoaneurysm
   B. Pontine hematoma
   C. Choroid plexus tumor
   D. Medulloblastoma
   E. "Black" epidermoid

2. Which one of the following is LEAST likely to be associated with this disorder?
   A. Tobacco smoking
   B. Hyperlipidemia
   C. Trauma
   D. Extracranial internal carotid artery location
   E. Larger initial pseudoaneurysm size

3. What artifact sometimes seen with nonthrombosed aneurysms is responsible for ghosting in the phase-encoding direction?
   A. Susceptibility artifact
   B. Aliasing artifact
   C. Pulsation artifact
   D. Chemical shift artifact
   E. Gibbs artifact

■ Answers and Explanations

Question 1

A. Correct! This is a dissecting pseudoaneurysm. The large sac surrounding the intracranial segment of the right vertebral artery is consistent with a large pseudoaneurysm (left image). No gadolinium enhancement is seen within the sac on postcontrast T1-weighted image (middle image), indicating that it is largely thrombosed. This is confirmed on digital subtraction angiography (right image). The T1 hyperintensity around the periphery of the sac represents peripheral thrombus. Often, the segment or artery distal to the pseudoaneurysm or irregularly dilated segment is narrowed, and this provides a clue to the presence of a dissection. Carotid and vertebral artery dissections can result in aneurysmal dilation (pseudoaneurysms) at the site of dissection. Depending on the location, they can be fusiform or saccular in morphology. Pseudoaneurysms have the potential to enlarge, rupture, and form thrombus and embolize, leading to transient ischemic attacks and strokes. Treatment strategies are not well established but include medical management with antiplatelet or anticoagulation therapy, surgical intervention, and endovascular stenting.

Other choices and discussion

B. The lesion in this patient is extra-axial and causes mass effect on the pons, rather than arising intrinsically from the brainstem. A pontine hematoma, sometimes caused by hypertension, an underlying tumor, or a vascular malformation, would be centered within the substance of the pons.

C. Choroid plexus tumors (which include World Health Organization grade 1 choroid plexus papillomas, grade 2 atypical choroid plexus papillomas, and grade 3 choroid plexus carcinomas) are avidly enhancing intraventricular tumors. The test case lesion is not enhancing and does not originate from the ventricles.

D. Medulloblastoma is a World Health Organization grade 4 tumor that usually arises in the posterior fossa in children but can also rarely develop in adults. The location of the tumor is dependent on its molecular subgroup: the WNT (wingless) type occurs in the cerebellar peduncle/cerebellopontine angle cistern region, the SHH (sonic hedgehog) type occurs in the cerebellar hemispheres (lateral), and group 3 and group 4 types occur in the midline (fourth ventricle). Unlike medulloblastoma, the test case lesion is an extra-axial process that surrounding the right vertebral artery.

E. "Black" epidermoids have prolonged T1 values and appear "black" on T1-weighted images. They have reduced lipid content with no triglycerides or fatty acids. The presence of restricted diffusion is pathognomonic for an epidermoid, a feature that is not present in the above case.

Question 2

D. Correct! Extracranial internal carotid artery (ICA) location is the least likely of the choices provided. In one retrospective study of traumatic and spontaneous extracranial ICA dissections, dissecting pseudoaneurysms of the extracranial ICA did not grow in 90% of patients.

Other choices and discussion

A. Smoking decreases the activity of alpha-1 antitrypsin, which disrupts connective tissue integrity and results in increased pseudoaneurysm formation and enlargement.

B. Hyperlipidemia contributes to the weakening of vessel walls, promoting formation and growth of pseudoaneurysms.

C. Traumatic dissections have a higher propensity for pseudoaneurysm formation and growth than do nontraumatic and spontaneous etiologies. Traumatic cases of dissection include motor vehicle accidents (leading cause), direct assault, hanging and sporting injuries, and chiropractic neck manipulation.

E. Larger initial pseudoaneurysm size is associated with enlargement.

Question 3

C. Correct! Pulsation artifact. Pulsation of vascular structures can lead to ghosting in the phase-encoding direction. In other words, ghosts of the pulsating vessel appear at constant intervals in the phase-encoding direction. Pulsation artifact can be seen with nonthrombosed aneurysms. Similarly, loss of pulsation artifact may indicate aneurysm thrombosis.

Other choices and discussion

A. Magnetic susceptibility artifact refers to a distortion in the magnetic resonance image, often seen around metallic hardware or dental devices, due to local inhomogeneities introduced by the metallic object.

B. Aliasing artifact, also known as wrap-around artifact, occurs when the field of view is smaller than the body part being imaged. It results in spatial mismapping to the opposite side of the image. This artifact can be minimized or eliminated by oversampling the data, using surface coils, increasing the field of view, and switching the frequency and phase encoding directions.

D. Chemical shift artifact is caused by differences in resonance frequencies of fat and water. It manifests as a bright or dark outline at fat-water interfaces along the edges of an organ or lesion in the frequency-encoding direction. Fat suppression techniques can help to minimize or eliminate chemical shift artifacts.

E. Gibbs or signal truncation artifacts are ripple-like features that occur in areas characterized by abrupt transitions between regions of high and low signal intensity. They are frequently identified on T2-weighted magnetic resonance images of the spine at the interface of the low signal intensity spinal cord with the high signal intensity cerebrospinal fluid, producing a false appearance of hydromyelia.

Top Tips

◆ Think of dissecting pseudoaneurysm when observing an irregular and dilated segment of the vertebral artery and narrowing of the vessel distally.

◆ Treatment for pseudoaneurysms includes medical management with antiplatelet or anticoagulation therapy, surgical intervention, and endovascular stenting.

◆ Presence of pulsation artifact can help to diagnose a nonthrombosed aneurysm; similarly, lack of pulsation artifact can indicate thrombosis of an aneurysm.

Essentials 7

■ Case

A 56-year-old woman presents with occasional left facial tingling and headaches.

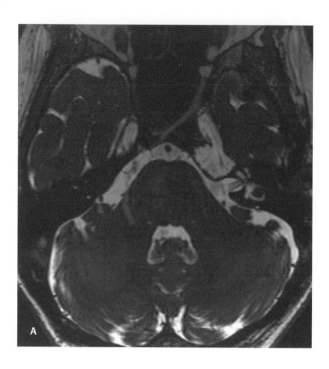

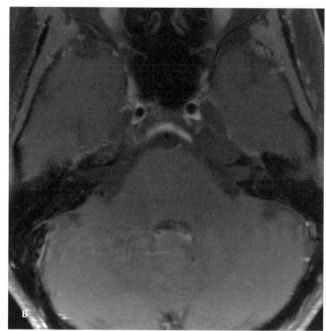

■ Questions

1. What is the MOST likely diagnosis?
   A. Trigeminal schwannoma
   B. Cholesterol granuloma
   C. Congenital cholesteatoma
   D. Petrous apex cephalocele
   E. Petrous apex effusion

2. This lesion represents a/an:
   A. Meningocele
   B. Encephalocele
   C. Mucocele
   D. Epidermoid cyst
   E. Tumor

3. In the vast majority of cases, what is the BEST management for petrous apex cephaloceles?
   A. Nothing
   B. Short-term imaging follow up
   C. Biopsy
   D. Surgical resection
   E. Radiation therapy

■ Answers and Explanations

Question 1

D. Correct! Petrous apex cephalocele is a rare lesion of the petrous apex representing herniation of the posterolateral aspect of Meckel cave into the petrous apex. Characteristic imaging findings of a petrous apex cephalocele include a nonenhancing unilateral or bilateral fluid signal intensity mass, arising from Meckel's cave, with smooth erosion of the bony petrous apex. No enhancement is present in the test case (right image), although enhancement may be present if the gasserian ganglion (trigeminal ganglion) is located within the cephalocele. These lesions are often incidentally identified and are typically asymptomatic. However, if a lesion is symptomatic, surgical intervention is an option.

Other choices and discussion

A. Trigeminal schwannoma is a slow-growing tumor that originates in Meckel's cave. It is typically hyperintense to brain on T2-weighted images and demonstrates prominent enhancement.

B. Cholesterol granuloma is the most common cystic lesion of the petrous apex, often occurring in young to middle-aged patients with a history of chronic otitis media. This lesion is typically hyperintense on T1-weighted images, and there is usually no associated enhancement.

C. Congenital cholesteatoma, also known as an epidermoid cyst, is an intraosseous lesion most frequently found in the petrous apex. It contains keratin and cholesterol. These lesions frequently restrict on diffusion-weighted imaging, a feature that is not present in this case. Congenital cholesteatomas differ from middle ear cholesteatomas, which are typically acquired secondary to perforation or rupture of the tympanic membrane.

E. An effusion can occur in pneumatized petrous apex air cells. Petrous effusions follow fluid intensity on all magnetic resonance imaging sequences and do not usually enhance. Because the test case also involves Meckel's cave, a simple effusion as an answer choice is incorrect.

Question 2

A. Correct! Meningocele. A petrous apex cephalocele can represent either a meningocele or an arachnoid cyst, depending on the presence or absence of a dural lining (which is often difficult to identify on magnetic resonance imaging). A meningocele contains herniated dura and leptomeninges. The wall of an arachnoid cyst is comprised of arachnoid cells that form a translucent and thin membrane.

Other choices and discussion

B. An encephalocele refers to herniated brain elements, which may be dysplastic.

C. A petrous apex mucocele is similar to a mucocele found in the paranasal sinuses. It is caused by postinflammatory obstruction of pneumatized petrous air cells.

D. An epidermoid cyst, also known as a congenital cholesteatoma, is a benign intraosseous lesion most frequently found in the petrous apex.

E. A petrous apex cephalocele does not represent a tumor.

Question 3

A. Correct! Nothing. Petrous apex cephaloceles are asymptomatic, incidental findings in the vast majority of cases and require no further workup or surgical intervention. However, a small percentage of patients do have symptoms, which may include hearing loss, headaches, cerebrospinal fluid otorrhea, trigeminal neuralgia, and meningitis. Symptomatic patients have erosion of the cephalocele into the otic capsule or pneumatized petrous air cells. Surgical intervention should be considered in these cases.

Other choices and discussion

B. No further imaging is necessary for an asymptomatic and incidentally detected petrous apex cephalocele.

C. There is no role for biopsy in a petrous apex cephalocele as magnetic resonance imaging is definitive. In fact, biopsy is contraindicated and can lead to cerebrospinal fluid leaks, seizures, and meningitis.

D. Surgical treatment is only indicated when lesions erode into the temporal bone air cells, producing symptoms. In > 95% of cases, petrous apex cephaloceles are asymptomatic and incidentally detected on imaging.

E. There is no role for radiation in the treatment of petrous apex cephaloceles.

■ Suggested Readings

Moore KR, Fischbein NJ, Harnsberger HR, et al. Petrous apex cephaloceles. Am J Neuroradiol 2001;22:1867–1871

Razek AA, Huang BY. Lesions of the petrous apex: classification and findings at CT and MR imaging. Radiographics 2012;32:151–173

Top Tips

- ◆ Petrous apex cephalocele is a "DO NOT TOUCH" lesion in the vast majority of cases. Most are asymptomatic and incidentally detected.

- ◆ Look for a lesion that is centered outside of the petrous apex, is contiguous with Meckel's cave, and follows fluid signal intensity on all magnetic resonance imaging sequences.

- ◆ Petrous apex cephalocele either represents a meningocele or an arachnoid cyst.

Essentials 8

■ Case

A 74-year-old man with congestive heart failure presents with back pain.

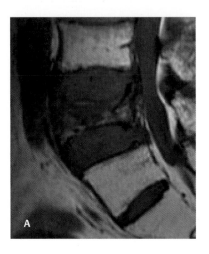 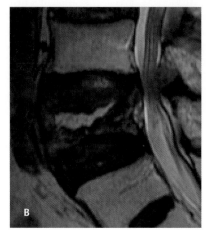 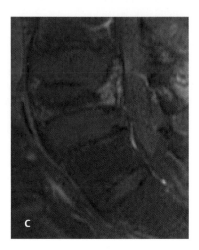

■ Questions

1. What is the MOST likely diagnosis?
   A. Metastasis
   B. Osteomyelitis
   C. Osteonecrosis
   D. Degenerative disease
   E. Chondrosarcoma

2. On histologic analysis, the intravertebral fluid cavity ("fluid" sign) in this disorder represents:
   A. Serous fluid
   B. Blood products
   C. Purulent fluid
   D. Marrow fibrosis and edema
   E. Cerebrospinal fluid

3. Which of the following is the BEST next step in management, IF the test patient experiences chronic and severe pain that is reproducible to palpation at the level of the magnetic resonance imaging findings?
   A. Watchful waiting
   B. Analgesics
   C. Incision and drainage
   D. Vertebroplasty/kyphoplasty
   E. Interbody fusion

■ Answers and Explanations

Question 1

C. Correct! This is osteonecrosis. Osteonecrosis, or avascular necrosis, of the vertebral body is an uncommon phenomenon that occurs as the result of nonunion from postcompression fracture ischemia. "Kummel disease" represents delayed vertebral body collapse, most often involving the anterior segment of the vertebral body, after traumatic or osteoporotic nontraumatic mechanisms. Two classic imaging signs of vertebral osteonecrosis include the "vacuum cleft" sign (gaseous collections within the collapsed vertebral body appearing as very low signal intensity on T1-, T2-, and T2*- weighted images) and the "fluid" sign (fluid cavity appearing as high signal intensity on T2-weighted images and low signal intensity on T1-weighted images). The "fluid" sign located along the superior aspect of a collapsed L5 vertebral body is present in the test case.

Other choices and discussion

A. Lack of a marrow-replacing soft tissue mass argues against metastatic disease.

B. Involvement of the adjacent disc space (discitis) as well as extensive paraspinal soft tissue enhancement would be expected with bacterial osteomyelitis. Epidural and soft tissue abscesses can also be seen with discitis-osteomyelitis.

D. The "fluid" sign (as seen in the test case) is not typical for degenerative change or for any of the other diagnoses.

E. Lack of a characteristic expansile mass argues chondrosarcoma.

Question 2

D. Correct! Histologic analysis of the intravertebral fluid cavity shows reactive marrow fibrosis and edema with a high turnover rate, features indicative of osteonecrosis.

Discussion

The other choices are all incorrect. The fluid cavity does not directly communicate with the spinal canal and, therefore, does not represent cerebrospinal fluid.

Question 3

D. Correct! Aggressive treatment including vertebroplasty or kyphoplasty should be considered when intravertebral fluid is identified on magnetic resonance imaging, as treatment can prevent further collapse of affected vertebral bodies and adjacent levels. The "fluid" sign indicates formation of a cavity between viable bones that will not spontaneously heal and may become nonunited. Vertebroplasty or kyphoplasty is an effective treatment in relieving pain symptoms for patients with compression fractures, particularly those who have tenderness on exam at the level of the fracture.

Other choices and discussion

A. Watchful waiting is insufficient for a symptomatic patient.

B. While administration of analgesics is a key part of conservative management, it may not be enough to curb the patient's symptoms of pain. At this point, more aggressive treatment should be considered.

C. Incision and drainage would be useful for infection, which is not present in the test case.

E. Spinal fusion can certainly be considered for patients with severe intractable pain due to vertebral osteonecrosis. However, the risk of surgery is higher than the risk of vertebroplasty, especially in patients with comorbid illness (like this patient).

■ Suggested Readings

Sanal B, Nas OF, Buyukkaya R, et al. Kummel disease and successful percutaneous vertebroplasty treatment. Spine J 2015;15:e9–10

Yu CW, Hsu CY, Shih TT, et al. Vertebral osteonecrosis: MR imaging findings and related changes on adjacent levels. Am J Neuroradiol 2007;28:42–47

Top Tips

◆ Intravertebral vacuum cleft and fluid signs are highly suggestive of vertebral osteonecrosis or avascular necrosis (Kummel disease).

◆ Appearance of the fluid cavity on imaging represents marrow fibrosis and edema on histopathology.

◆ Vertebroplasty or kyphoplasty is an effective treatment for patients with Kummel disease, particularly if pain is reproducible at the level of fracture on exam.

Essentials 9

■ Case

An 85-year-old man presents with progressive lower extremity weakness, numbness, and pain.

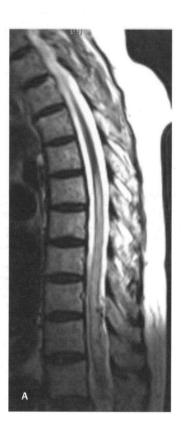
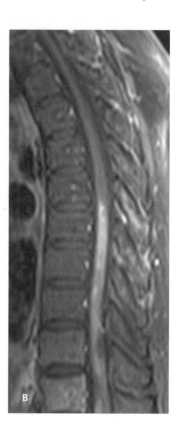

■ Questions

1. What is the MOST likely diagnosis?
   A. Myxopapillary ependymoma
   B. Hemangioblastoma
   C. Spinal cord infarction
   D. Multiple sclerosis
   E. Spinal dural arteriovenous fistula

2. Which of the following describes the typical demographic features of a patient with the disorder in the test case?
   A. Young adult woman presenting with acute myelopathy
   B. Young adult man presenting with slowly progressive myelopathy

   C. Middle-aged woman presenting with acute myelopathy
   D. Elderly woman presenting with acute myelopathy
   E. Elderly man presenting with slowly progressive myelopathy

3. Which ONE of the following treatments has the highest success rate for fistula occlusion?
   A. Watchful waiting
   B. Intravenous steroids
   C. Embolization with liquid polymers
   D. Embolization with polyvinyl alcohol
   E. Surgical management

■ Answers and Explanations

Question 1

E. Correct! This is a spinal dural arteriovenous fistula (SDAVF). Classic magnetic resonance imaging findings of SDAVF (which are also seen in this case) include enlarged perimedullary veins appearing as serpentine signal voids in the subarachnoid space, long segment cord T2 signal abnormality resulting from venous congestion or venous ischemia (left image), and associated enhancement (right image).

The most common type of SDAVF occurs between a radiculomeningeal artery and a radicular vein in the dura adjacent to the spinal nerve root. This results in venous congestion and ischemia in the spinal cord.

Other choices and discussion

A. Myxopapillary ependymomas are World Health Organization grade 1 tumors that arise almost exclusively from the conus medullaris, cauda equina, and filum terminale. The classic appearance is a sausage-shaped mass (which is not present in the test case) causing posterior vertebral body scalloping. The scalloping reflects the tendency for slow growth.

B. Hemangioblastomas are tumors that arise sporadically or in association with von Hippel-Lindau disease. Spinal hemangioblastomas are usually intramedullary in location and appear along the dorsal aspect of the cord. Associated findings include syrinx, cord edema, and prominent vascular flow voids. The lack of a focal enhancing nodule or mass in the test case argues against hemangioblastoma.

C. Imaging findings of spinal cord infarction include hyperintense T2 signal and restricted diffusion centrally within the spinal cord that may have a "snake-eye" or "owl-eye" configuration on axial images. Sudden onset of symptoms (in contrast to the gradual progression of symptoms in the test case) would be expected with spinal cord infarction.

D. Demyelinating plaques associated with multiple sclerosis involve short segments of the spinal cord. Acute demyelinating lesions can enhance and can be associated with some cord swelling. However, the length of cord involvement and the flow voids surrounding the cord in the test case suggest an alternative diagnosis.

Question 2

E. Correct! The classic patient with a SDAVF is an elderly male patient presenting with progressive myelopathy. SDAVFs are acquired lesions, although the exactly etiology is not known.

Discussion

The other choices are all incorrect. A young patient with an acute presentation would be atypical for a SDAVF.

Question 3

E. Correct! Surgical occlusion of the arterialized radicular vein supplied by the shunt is the single most effective treatment for SDAVF. In fact, a recent meta-analysis suggested complete occlusion of the fistula following surgery in 98% of cases. However, in more complex cases, a multimodal approach consisting of embolization and surgery may be needed.

Other choices and discussion

A. Watchful waiting is risky because if left untreated, SDAVFs can cause considerable morbidity with progressive spinal cord symptoms.

B. Intravenous steroids are not used to treat SDAVFs. In fact, there are case reports showing an association between the initiation of intravenous steroid therapy and acute exacerbation of myelopathy in the setting of a SDAVF.

C. Embolization with liquid polymers is an effective treatment for SDAVF, with a success rate between 44 to 100%. However, surgery has an even higher rate of successful fistula occlusion.

D. Embolization with polyvinyl alcohol leads to a higher recurrence rate (as high as 30 to 93%) than embolization with either liquid polymers or surgery.

■ Suggested Readings

Chu BC, Terae S, Hida K, et al. MR findings in spinal hemangioblastomas: correlation with symptoms and with angiographic and surgical findings. Am J Neuroradiol 2001;22:206–217

Krings T, Geibprasert S. Spinal dural arteriovenous fistulas. Am J Neuroradiol 2009;30:639–648

Strowd RE, Geer C, Powers A, et al. A unique presentation of a spinal dural arteriovenous fistula exacerbated by steroids. J Clin Neurosci 2012;19(3):466–468

Top Tips

- SDAVFs are acquired fistulous connections between a radiculomeningeal artery and radicular vein, resulting in venous congestion and venous ischemia in the spinal cord.

- Think of SDAVF in an elderly patient with progressive myelopathy.

- Magnetic resonance imaging findings include dilated perimedullary veins appearing as flow voids along the surface of the cord, cord edema, and enhancement.

Essentials 10

■ Case

A 77-year-old man presents with progressively worsening myelopathy over the last 5 years. Two months ago, he began having worsening left leg numbness, right toe paresthesias, and left foot drop.

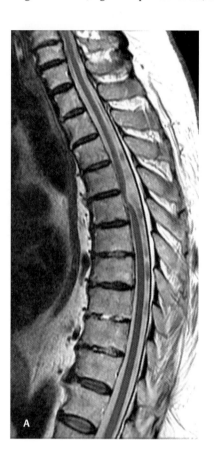
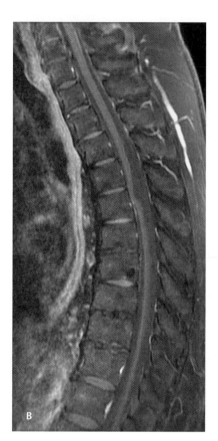

■ Questions

1. What is the MOST likely diagnosis?
   A. Intradural arachnoid cyst
   B. Schwannoma
   C. Thoracic cord herniation
   D. Subdural hematoma
   E. Epidural abscess

2. The test case illustrates a disorder that most frequently occurs at which levels in the spine?
   A. C2–C6
   B. C7–T3
   C. T4–T7
   D. T8–T11
   E. T12–L2

3. What is the MOST common clinical presentation of thoracic spinal cord herniation?
   A. Radiculopathy
   B. Loss of upper extremity pain and temperature sensation
   C. Ascending paralysis
   D. Central cord syndrome
   E. Brown-Séquard syndrome

■ Answers and Explanations

Question 1

C. Correct! This is a thoracic cord herniation. There is focal anterior displacement of the thoracic spinal cord through a dural defect with secondary enlargement of the dorsal subarachnoid space. Unimpeded cerebrospinal fluid (CSF) pulsation artifact dorsal to the cord excludes a space-occupying lesion. Sometimes, conventional magnetic resonance imaging (MRI) demonstrates cord displacement with enlargement of the dorsal subarachnoid space, but can be insufficient at ruling in or ruling out a dorsal intradural extramedullary cystic lesion (e.g. arachnoid cyst, epidermoid cyst, cystic schwannoma), which have similar signal characteristics to CSF. In these cases, high-resolution T2-weighted, diffusion-weighted, and postcontrast imaging may provide more information. Computed tomography myelogram can also be performed to evaluate for a space-occupying lesion, although a filling defect, if one were detected, would be nonspecific without the additional information from MRI. Spinal cord herniation is a rare and likely underdiagnosed but treatable cause of progressive cord myelopathy.

Other choices and discussion

A. T2-weighted images demonstrate unimpeded CSF pulsation artifact posterior to the displaced cord. CSF pulsation artifact is unlikely to be present within an intradural arachnoid cyst as there is minimal flow within the cyst.

B. Unimpeded CSF pulsation artifact dorsal to the cord excludes a space-occupying lesion. In addition, a schwannoma typically demonstrates enhancement, which is not present in this case.

D. Subdural collections in the spine are located in the potential space between the dura mater and the arachnoid mater. The subarachnoid space, not the subdural space, is enlarged in the test case.

E. The images demonstrate focal anterior displacement of the thoracic spinal cord with secondary enlargement of the dorsal subarachnoid space. The epidural space, which is external to the hypointense line denoting the position of the dura, appears normal in this case, arguing against epidural abscess. Abscesses are classically T2 hyperintense, enhance peripherally, and exhibit restricted diffusion.

Question 2

C. Correct! Idiopathic spinal cord herniation most frequently occurs at the T4–T7 level.

The other choices are all incorrect.

Question 3

E. Correct! The most common presentation of idiopathic spinal cord herniation is that of Brown-Séquard syndrome, which is characterized by ipsilateral paralysis, loss of vibratory and position sense, contralateral loss of pain and temperature sensation, or other myelopathic sequelae.

Other choices and discussion

A. Radiculopathy occurs in the setting of nerve root compression.

B. Loss of pain and temperature sensation in the upper extremities, in a cape-like distribution, occurs in the setting of a cervical spinal cord syrinx.

C. Ascending paralysis can occur in the setting of Guillain-Barré syndrome.

D. Central cord syndrome is the most common incomplete spinal cord injury syndrome and most frequently occurs in the setting of acute trauma.

■ Suggested Readings

Carter BJ, Griffith BD, Schultz LR, et al. Idiopathic spinal cord herniation: an imaging diagnosis with significant delay. Spine J 2015;15:1943–1948

Haber MD, Nguyen DD, Li S. Differentiation of idiopathic spinal cord herniation from CSF-isointense intraspinal extramedullary lesions displacing the cord. Radiographics 2014;34:313–329

Parmar H, Park P, Brahma B, et al. Imaging of idiopathic spinal cord herniation. Radiographics 2008;28:511–518

Top Tips

◆ Spinal cord herniation occurs when a portion of the cord herniates through a ventral dural defect. Brown-Séquard syndrome is the most frequent clinical presentation of spinal cord herniation.

◆ Typical imaging features: anterior displacement of the thoracic spinal cord within the thecal sac with enlargement of the dorsal subarachnoid space.

◆ Consider contrast-enhanced MRI with diffusion-weighted imaging and high-resolution MRI, or computed tomography myelography, in cases where a dorsal lesion cannot be excluded on the basis of conventional MRI.

Details 1

■ Case

A 20-year-old man with a history of uncomplicated orthotopic heart transplant for familial dilated cardiomyopathy presents with fever, nausea, and vomiting. What is the MOST likely diagnosis?
    A. Infarction
    B. Lhermitte-Duclos disease
    C. Leptomeningeal metastases
    D. Viral meningoencephalitis
    E. Lymphoma

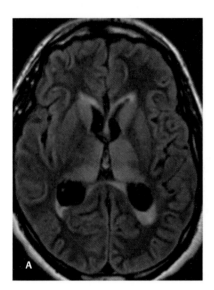 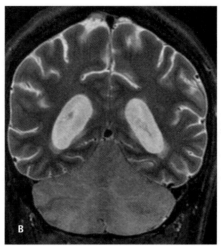 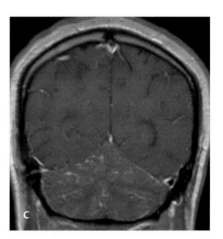

■ The following questions pertain to intracranial infection.

1. What percentage of patients with meningitis have abnormal leptomeningeal enhancement on MRI?
2. True or False. The typical CSF profile for viral infection is as follows: elevated opening pressure, markedly increased white blood cell count (polymorphonucleocyte predominant), low glucose, and elevated protein.
3. West Nile virus is transmitted by _____.
4. What is the treatment of West Nile virus encephalitis?
5. True or False. Herpes encephalitis has a predilection for involvement of the limbic system.
6. In herpes encephalitis, disease is usually [unilateral/bilateral] and [symmetric/asymmetric].

7. What is the treatment for herpes encephalitis?
8. True or False. Herpes VZV has a propensity for infecting immunosuppressed patients (e.g. patients with autoimmune deficiency syndrome) and can cause severe vasculitis in these patients.
9. An immigrant child presents with slowly progressive behavioral changes and ataxia with multifocal white matter disease on MRI. What is the MOST likely diagnosis?
10 True or False. Zika virus is associated with fetal microcephaly and intracranial calcifications.

■ Answers and Explanations

D. Correct! This is viral meningoencephalitis. Magnetic resonance imaging (MRI) findings of viral infection vary and largely depend on specific pathogens. In West Nile virus encephalitis (test case), typical imaging features include T2/fluid-attenuated inversion recovery (FLAIR) hyperintensity involving the basal ganglia, thalami, mesial temporal lobes, brainstem, and cerebellum. Involvement is often symmetric. Diffusion restriction and enhancement may or may not be present. Other viral encephalitides, such as eastern equine encephalitis, Japanese encephalitis, measles, and mumps, can have similar neuroimaging features.

Other choices and discussion

A. In this case, bilateral involvement of the basal ganglia, thalami, and entire cerebellum is not confined to a vascular territory and is, therefore, not consistent with arterial infarction.

B. Lhermitte-Duclos disease is characterized by a diffusely infiltrative lesion involving the cerebellum. It is typically T2 hyperintense and has a thickened, gyriform morphology of the folia, giving the lesion a striated appearance. The nonstriated appearance of the cerebellum, presence of leptomeningeal enhancement along the folia, and bilateral involvement of the basal ganglia and thalami argue against this answer choice.

C. While this case does demonstrate abnormal leptomeningeal enhancement in the cerebellum, the diagnosis of leptomeningeal metastases does not fully explain symmetric T2/FLAIR signal abnormality within the basal ganglia and thalami.

E. Enhancing lesion(s) within the basal ganglia and periventricular white matter that show restricted diffusion are classic imaging findings of primary CNS lymphoma, features that are not present in the test case. On the other hand, secondary CNS lymphoma preferentially involves the skull, dura, and leptomeninges; parenchymal masses also occur but are less common.

Question 1

A total of 50% of patients with meningitis have abnormal leptomeningeal enhancement on MRI. The initial diagnosis of meningitis is based on clinical and laboratory assessment, not on imaging studies. The role of neuroimaging is to confirm the suspected diagnosis of meningitis, to assess for signs of increased intracranial pressure (e.g., brain edema and hydrocephalus) before lumbar puncture, and to assess for complications of meningitis.

Question 2

False. The question details the typical CSF profile for bacterial meningitis (elevated opening pressure, markedly increased white blood cell count (polymorphonucleocyte predominant), low glucose, and elevated protein. Viral infection typically shows normal to elevated opening pressure, increased white blood cell count (lymphocyte predominant), normal glucose (most commonly), and normal to elevated protein.

Question 3

Mosquito bite. West Nile virus is a flavivirus (ribonucleic acid virus) that is arthropod-transmitted (mosquito).

Question 4

Treatment of West Nile virus encephalitis is supportive and may include intravenous hydration, antinausea medication, respiratory support, and seizure management. Currently, there is no vaccine for West Nile virus.

Question 5

True. Herpes encephalitis typically involves the limbic system (medial temporal lobe, insula, subfrontal area, and cingulate gyri), although cerebral convexity and occipital cortex may also become involved.

Question 6

In herpes encephalitis, disease is usually bilateral and asymmetric.

Question 7

The treatment for herpes encephalitis is intravenous acyclovir. Without immediate treatment, herpes encephalitis has a 70% mortality rate. Even with treatment, herpes encephalitis is fatal in one-third of cases. Survivors often have permanent neurologic dysfunction; only a small percentage of survivors (2.5%) return to a normal functional life.

Question 8

True. VZV often affects immunosuppressed individuals and may present as multifocal infarcts due to severe vasculitis. Small vessel vasculitis generally occurs only in the immunocompromised patient.

Question 9

Subacute sclerosing pancephalitis is a postinfectious progressive encephalitis occurring years after measles infection, typically occurring in children and early adolescents. A history of measles occurring before 18 to 24 months of age significantly increases the risk of subacute sclerosing pancephalitis.

Question 10

True. Although 80% of Zika virus infections are asymptomatic, there is growing evidence for the association between Zika virus infections in pregnant women and fetal brain abnormalities such as microcephaly and intracranial calcifications.

Top Tips

- ◆ Think of viral encephalitis for T2/FLAIR signal hyperintensity ($+/-$ restricted diffusion and $+/-$ enhancement) involving the basal ganglia, thalami, mesial temporal lobes, deep white matter, brainstem, and cerebellum.

- ◆ Herpes encephalitis preferentially affects the limbic structures of the brain; specifically, look for bilateral or, less commonly, unilateral involvement of the mesial temporal lobes.

- ◆ Only 50% of patients with meningitis show abnormal leptomeningeal enhancement on MRI.

Details 2

■ Case

A 20-year-old woman presents with dizziness. What hereditary disease is associated with this lesion?
- A. Sturge-Weber
- B. Neurofibromatosis type 2
- C. Osler-Weber-Rendu
- D. Tuberous sclerosis
- E. von Hippel-Lindau (VHL)

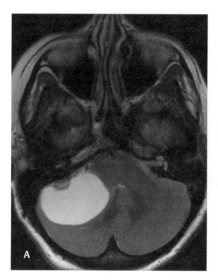 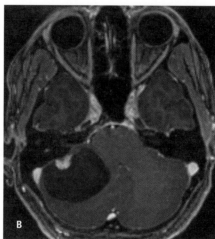 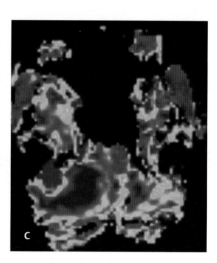

■ The following questions pertain to VHL and hemangioblastomas.

1. What is the most common presenting ophthalmic feature of VHL?
2. True or False. Solitary hemangioblastomas are associated with VHL in an average of 10 to 20% of cases.
3. True or False. A total of 75% of patients with VHL develop endolymphatic sac tumors.
4. Solid hemangioblastomas may secrete _____ and may subsequently produce _____ which generally resolves following tumor resection.
5. True or False. VHL has been linked to mutations on chromosome 3.
6. Hemangioblastoma is classified as a World Health Organization (WHO) grade [1/2/3/4] tumor.

7. True or False. Perfusion imaging with cerebral blood flow maps can be used to distinguish between hemangioblastomas and pilocytic astrocytomas.
8. What is the name of the fluid-filled cavity within the spinal cord that is present in 40 to 60% of VHL patients with spinal hemangioblastomas?
9. Hemangioblastomas of the spinal cord are most commonly [intramedullary, mixed intra- and extramedullary, intradural extramedullary, extradural] in location.
10 True or False. The first line of treatment for cerebellar hemangioblastoma is chemoradiation.

■ Answers and Explanations

E. Correct! VHL is an autosomal dominant syndrome characterized by multiple hemangioblastomas (most frequently arising in the cerebellum); retinal hemangioblastomas; endolymphatic sac tumors; cysts of the kidney, pancreas, liver, and epididymis; renal cell carcinomas; islet cells tumors; pheochromocytomas; and adenomas. Although hemangioblastomas may be cystic, solid, or mixed, the classic appearance is that of a predominantly cystic lesion in the lateral cerebellum with an enhancing and highly vascular mural nodule.

Other choices and discussion

A. Sturge-Weber is a phakomatosis that is characterized clinically by facial "port-wine" stain, seizures, and hemiplegia. Typical imaging findings include pial angiomatosis, cortical "tram-track" calcification, enlarged ipsilateral choroid plexus, hemiatrophy, and Dyke-Davidoff-Masson syndrome (characterized by calvarial hemihypertrophy, enlarged frontal sinuses, and elevated petrous ridge/sphenoid wing), none of which is present in this case.

B. Neurofibromatosis type 2 is a phakomatosis that is transmitted on chromosome 22q12 and is characterized by the **MIS ME** lesions (**m**ultiple **i**nherited **s**chwannomas, **m**eningiomas, and **e**pendymomas). Bilateral vestibular (cranial nerve 8) schwannomas are the pathognomonic lesions of neurofibromatosis type 2.

C. Osler-Weber-Rendu (hereditary hemorrhagic telangiectasia) is an autosomal dominant disorder consisting of mucocutaneous telangiectasias and visceral (primarily brain, lungs, and liver) arteriovenous malformations, none of which is present in this case. One of the most common signs is recurrent epistaxis from sinonasal mucocutaneous telangiectasias.

D. Tuberous sclerosis is a phakomatosis that is characterized clinically by adenoma sebaceum, mental retardation, and seizures. The typical intracranial manifestations of tuberous sclerosis include calcified periventricular subependymal nodules, cortical and subcortical tubers, radial migration lines (linear or wedge-shaped T2/fluid-attenuated inversion recovery hyperintensities that extend from the ventricle to the cortex), and subependymal giant cell astrocytomas, none of which is present in this case.

Question 1

Retinal hemangioblastomas are the most common presenting ophthalmic feature of VHL. Retinal hemangioblastomas are found in 25 to 60% of VHL gene carriers and are multiple and bilateral in approximately 50% of cases. Sight-threatening complications, which tend to be associated with larger angiomas, are due to retinal detachment and hemorrhage.

Question 2

True. A total of 4 to 40% (average of 10 to 20%) of patients with solitary hemangioblastomas have VHL. In contrast, cerebellar hemangioblastomas ultimately develop in over 80% of patients with VHL.

Question 3

False. A total of 15% of VHL patients develop endolymphatic sac tumors.

Question 4

Solid hemangioblastomas may secrete erythropoietin and may subsequently produce polycythemia vera, which generally resolves following tumor resection.

Question 5

True. VHL is transmitted through autosomal dominant inheritance in 20% of cases on chromosome 3p25.

Question 6

Hemangioblastoma is classified as a WHO grade 1 tumor. WHO grade 1 tumors are slow-growing, nonmalignant, and associated with long-term survival. WHO grade 2 tumors can be malignant or nonmalignant and are relatively slow-growing tumors that may potentially recur as higher-grade tumors. WHO grade 3 tumors are malignant and often recur as higher-grade tumors. WHO grade 4 tumors are extremely aggressive malignant tumors.

Question 7

True. The mural nodules in hemangioblastomas are hypervascular and demonstrate elevated cerebral blood flow, whereas pilocytic astrocytomas are avascular masses.

Question 8

A syrinx is the name of the fluid-filled cavity within the spinal cord that is present in 40 to 60% of VHL patients with spinal hemangioblastomas.

Question 9

A total of 60% of hemangioblastomas that occur in the spinal cord are intramedullary, 11% are mixed intra- and extramedullary, 21% are intradural extramedullary, and 8% are extradural. They occur most frequently in the thoracic cord followed by the cervical cord.

Question 10

False. The standard treatment for cerebellar hemangioblastoma is surgical resection and stereotactic radiosurgery, not chemoradiation. Radiosurgery is useful in patients with VHL who have multiple hemangioblastomas or deeply located tumors.

Top Tips

- ◆ Think hemangioblastoma for a cystic mass with a solid, hypervascular, and enhancing mural nodule in the cerebellum.

- ◆ Perfusion imaging with cerebral blood flow maps is useful to show the hypervascular nature of the solid nodule.

- ◆ VHL is characterized by multiple hemangioblastomas; endolymphatic sac tumors; cysts of the kidney, pancreas, liver, and epididymis; renal cell carcinomas; islet cells tumors; pheochromocytomas; and adenomas.

Details 3

■ Case

A 64-year-old man presents with sudden onset left-sided weakness and gaze deviation. In the setting of acute infarct, the perfusion images indicate:

A. No tissue at risk
B. Tissue at risk throughout the entire right hemisphere
C. Tissue at risk in the right middle cerebral artery territory
D. Tissue at risk in the right anterior cerebral artery territory
E. Tissue at risk in the right posterior cerebral artery territory

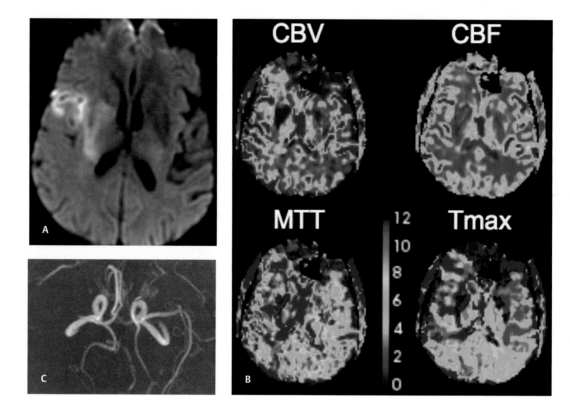

■ The following questions pertain to strokes and associated imaging findings.

1. Mechanical thrombectomy should be performed within ____ hours after symptom onset as a treatment in acute stroke patients with large artery occlusions in the anterior circulation.
2. MTT is the time between _____ and _____.
3. True or False. Normal CBV is approximately 4 to 5 mL/100 g.
4. True or False. Normal CBF in human gray matter is approximately 90 to 100 mL/100 g/min.
5. What is the relationship of CBF, CBV, and MTT expressed as an equation?
6. Following an acute stroke, when does "pseudonormalization" of signal occur on apparent diffusion coefficient (ADC) maps?

7. Fluid-attenuated inversion recovery (FLAIR) images are positive _____ hours after onset of stroke symptoms.
8. When does hemorrhagic transformation usually occur after an acute stroke?
9. Postischemic hyperperfusion is associated with a better prognosis in the [acute/subacute] stage.
10 In patients with acute ischemic strokes, _____ is a term that indicates hyperintense signal of the subarachnoid cerebrospinal fluid space on FLAIR magnetic resonance imaging following gadolinium administration.

■ Answers and Explanations

C. Correct! In the setting of acute infarct, the perfusion images indicate tissue at risk in the right middle cerebral artery territory. The perfusion images show a larger territory of Tmax and mean transit time (MTT) delay relative to the volume of diffusion abnormality in the right middle cerebral artery territory. The findings of diffusion-perfusion mismatch are consistent with tissue at risk or tissue that can potentially be salvaged with thrombolysis techniques. Cerebral blood flow (CBF) and cerebral blood volume (CBV) are reduced in the right basal ganglia region but relatively maintained in the remainder of the middle cerebral artery territory. This indicates the presence of collateral flow and preservation of autoregulatory mechanisms, further supporting the need for urgent mechanical thrombolysis in this patient with an acute occlusion of the right middle cerebral artery (especially since the onset of symptoms was < 6 hours from presentation).

Discussion

The other choices are all incorrect. The extent of Tmax and MTT delay is much larger than the extent of restricted diffusion in this patient, indicating tissue at risk (penumbra). Matched diffusion and perfusion defects, on the other hand, would indicate complete infarction with no tissue at risk.

Question 1

Mechanical thrombectomy should be performed within 6 hours of symptom onset in patients with anterior circulation strokes and only after a patient receives intravenous tissue plasminogen activator. Intravenous tissue plasminogen activator, the only thrombolytic approved by the US Food and Drug Administration for the treatment of ischemic stroke, should be administered within 3 hours (and up to 4.5 hours in eligible patients) after symptom onset.

Question 2

MTT is the time between arterial inflow and venous outflow.

Question 3

True.

Question 4

False. Normal CBF in human gray matter is about 50 to 60 mL/100 g/min. At 35 mL/100 g/min, protein synthesis within neurons halts. Tissue can survive at this oligemic stage if CBF does not decrease any further. At 20 mL/100 g/min, synaptic transmission between neurons is disrupted leading to loss of function of "living" neurons; ischemic tissue at risk is found at this stage. At 10 mL/100 g/min (< 20% of normal values), irreversible cell death (infarction) occurs.

Question 5

CBF (amount of blood per unit time) = CBV (amount of blood)/MTT (time)

Question 6

"Pseudonormalization" of signal occurs on ADC maps at 10 to 15 days. Following an acute stroke, high signal intensity on diffusion-weighted imaging remains for 10 to 14 days. Low signal intensity on ADC remains for 7 to 10 days. Pseudonormalization may then occur at 10 to 15 days. High signal intensity on ADC follows.

Question 7

Six to twelve hours. While diffusion-weighted imaging is typically positive within 6 hours after a stroke, high signal intensity on FLAIR is usually seen after 6 hours.

Question 8

Hemorrhagic transformation usually occurs within the first 24 to 48 hours of an acute stroke. In almost all cases, it is present 4 or 5 days after a stroke.

Question 9

Postischemic hyperperfusion is associated with a better prognosis when it occurs in the acute stage. It occurs from restoration of perfusion pressure to normal values in a vascular territory that has been previously affected by severe ischemia as a result of spontaneous or therapeutic recanalization of an occluded vessel. In the early acute stage, hyperperfusion following ischemia is typically transient and associated with a better prognosis. Hyperperfusion lasting into subacute stages of ischemia is associated with increased edema and hemorrhage and a less favorable prognosis.

Question 10

Hyperintense acute reperfusion marker (HARM) is a term that indicates hyperintense signal of the subarachnoid cerebrospinal fluid space on FLAIR magnetic resonance imaging following gadolinium administration. It is caused by leakage of gadolinium into the subarachnoid space through a disrupted blood–brain barrier and is often found in patients with acute ischemic strokes.

■ Suggested Readings

Allen LM, Hasso AN, Handwerker J, et al. Sequence-specific MR imaging findings that are useful in dating ischemic stroke. Radiographics 2012;32:1285–1297

Kohrmann M, Struffert T, Frenzel T, et al. The hyperintense acute reperfusion markeron fluid-attenuated inversion recovery magnetic resonance imaging is caused by gadolinium in the cerebrospinal fluid. Stroke 2012;43:259–261

Lui YW, Tang ER, Allmendinger AM, et al. Evaluation of CT perfusion in the setting of cerebral ischemia: patterns and pitfalls. Am J Neuroradiol 2010;31:1552–1563

Tomandi BF, Klotz E, Handschu R, et al. Comprehensive imaging of ischemic stroke with multisection CT. Radiographics 2003;23:565–592

Top Tips

◆ Diffusion-perfusion match indicates completed infarct, whereas diffusion-perfusion mismatch indicates tissue at risk (penumbra).

◆ CBV is a good indicator of collateral flow.

◆ Restricted diffusion typically occurs within 6 hours of an acute stroke, whereas FLAIR becomes positive after 6 to 12 hours.

Details 4

■ Case

A 64-year-old asymptomatic woman presents with normal neurologic exam and no prior medical history. What is the MOST likely etiology for this cavernous sinus lesion?
   A. Meningioma
   B. Lymphoma
   C. Inflammatory pseudotumor
   D. Metastasis
   E. Pituitary macroadenoma

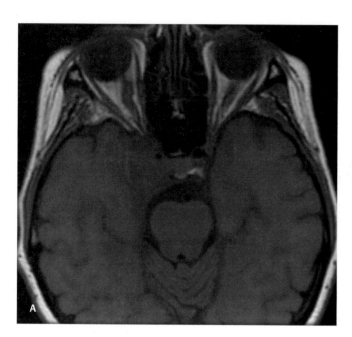
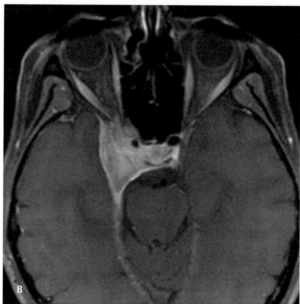

■ The following questions pertain to the cavernous sinuses.

1. Which cranial nerves (CNs) traverse the cavernous sinus?
2. Major efferent venous channels of the cavernous sinus include _____ and _____, the former of which drains into the transverse sinus and the latter of which drains into the internal jugular vein.
3. What are the two most reliable signs of cavernous sinus invasion by pituitary adenoma?
4. True or False. Cavernous sinus meningioma and inflammatory pseudotumor (Tolosa-Hunt syndrome) can be distinguished on imaging by the presence of internal carotid artery narrowing in the former but not in the latter.
5. True or False. Stereotactic radiosurgery is a treatment option for symptomatic cavernous sinus meningiomas.

6. What is the main risk of treating a cavernous sinus meningioma compressing the optic apparatus with stereotactic radiosurgery?
7. Assuming a similar histologic grade, the prognosis of a cavernous sinus meningioma is [better/worse/similar] to the prognosis of a meningioma elsewhere in the brain.
8. Cavernous sinus involvement in infections, particularly bacterial, is usually secondary to _____.
9. True or False. Cavernous sinus thrombophlebitis is a self-limited and easily treatable condition.
10. In head and neck malignancy, perineural spread of tumor to the cavernous sinus usually occurs through which CNs?

■ Answers and Explanations

A. Correct! This is a meningioma. Most cavernous sinus meningiomas arise from the lateral dural wall. They rarely arise within the cavernous sinus itself. In the test case, there is a homogeneously enhancing mass in the cavernous sinus with a characteristic dural "tail" along the tentorium and associated narrowing of the internal carotid artery. The presence of a dural tail and narrowing of the carotid artery are highly suggestive of a cavernous sinus meningioma.

Other choices and discussion

B. Isolated primary cavernous sinus lymphoma is rare. Secondary or metastatic lymphoma involving the cavernous sinus is more common. When present, there is usually evidence of disease elsewhere. Secondary lymphoma also usually involves the dura or leptomeninges. Lymphoma is not typically associated with arterial narrowing, arguing against this answer choice.

C. Tolosa-Hunt syndrome is idiopathic inflammatory pseudotumor involving the cavernous sinus, with the characteristic clinical triad of painful ophthalmoplegia, cranial nerve palsies, and response to corticosteroids. Unilateral involvement is more common than bilateral involvement.

D. Metastases can involve the cavernous sinus by a hematogenous route (seen most frequently with lung and breast cancer) or by perineural spread (seen commonly with head and neck malignancies). Hematogenous metastases usually involve the central skull base and secondarily extend into the cavernous sinus. They are often aggressive and destructive.

E. There is no involvement of the pituitary gland, which would be expected with a pituitary macroadenoma. Pituitary adenomas that extend laterally through the medial dural wall and into the cavernous sinus may surround and encase the internal carotid artery, but they usually do not compromise the lumen.

Question 1

The following CNs traverse the cavernous sinus: oculomotor nerve (CN III), trochlear nerve (CN IV), ophthalmic nerve (V1 branch of CN V), maxillary nerve (V2 branch of CN V), and abducens nerve (CN VI). All of the listed nerves except for the abducens nerve course through the lateral wall of the cavernous sinus. The abducens nerve is located inferolateral to the cavernous segment of the internal carotid artery and medial to the lateral wall of the sinus.

Question 2

Major efferent venous channels of the cavernous sinus include the superior petrosal sinus and inferior petrosal sinus, the former of which drains into the transverse sinus and the latter of which drains into the internal jugular vein.

Question 3

Complete encasement of the internal carotid artery and presence of tumor between the internal carotid artery and the lateral wall of the cavernous sinus are the two most reliable signs of cavernous sinus invasion by pituitary adenoma.

Question 4

False. Narrowing of the internal carotid artery is often seen with both cavernous sinus meningioma and inflammatory pseudotumor (Tolosa-Hunt syndrome).

Question 5

True. Surgical debulking and/or stereotactic radiosurgery are two treatment options in the management of symptomatic cavernous sinus meningiomas.

Question 6

Tumors compressing the optic chiasm, nerves, or tracts should be considered for surgical resection to avoid the risk of radiation-induced optic neuropathy. A 2-mm margin should separate the tumor from the optic tract to allow for safer irradiation.

Question 7

A cavernous sinus meningioma is similar in prognosis to meningiomas elsewhere in the brain, assuming they are of the same histologic grade. However, given its location, cavernous sinus meningiomas are more often associated with CN deficits than are meningiomas in other places. While metastases do occur, they are rare (0.1 to 0.2%). Atypical (World Health Organization grade 2) and malignant (World Health Organization grade 3) meningiomas have higher recurrence and lower 5-year survival rates.

Question 8

Cavernous sinus involvement in infections, particularly bacterial, is usually secondary to direct extension from adjacent sinonasal infections.

Question 9

False. Cavernous sinus thrombophlebitis, which is often a clinical diagnosis, is a rare and potentially lethal condition that is difficult to treat. It is most commonly caused by sphenoid sinusitis due to *Staphylococcus aureus*. The mainstay of therapy is the immediate application of broad-spectrum antibiotics,

Question 10

In head and neck malignancy, perineural spread of tumor to the cavernous sinus usually occurs through the following CNs: maxillary (V2) and mandibular (V3) divisions of the trigeminal nerve (CN V).

Top Tips

- ◆ Dural "tail" and narrowing of the internal carotid artery are highly suggestive features of cavernous sinus meningioma.

- ◆ Lymphoma and pituitary adenomas involving the cavernous sinus do not narrow the internal carotid artery.

- ◆ Inflammatory pseudotumor of the cavernous sinus (Tolosa-Hunt) can mimic cavernous sinus meningioma on imaging, but the clinical presentation is different.

Details 5

■ Case

A 67-year-old afebrile man with poorly controlled diabetes presents with progressive left ear pain and facial weakness. Laboratory analysis revealed normal white blood cell count but elevated erythrocyte sedimentation rate (ESR). What is the MOST likely diagnosis?

    A. Squamous cell carcinoma
    B. Nasopharyngeal carcinoma
    C. Metastasis
    D. Sarcoidosis
    E. Skull base osteomyelitis

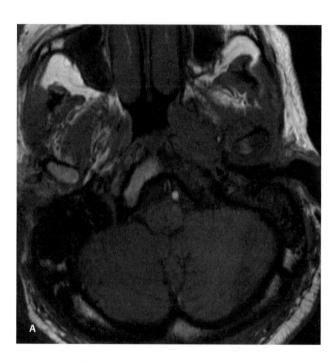 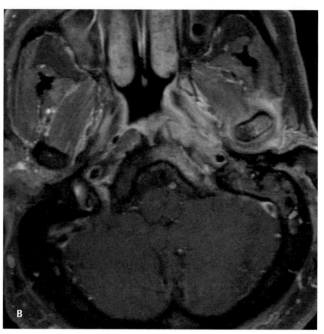

■ The following questions pertain to skull base pathology.

1. What is the most common pathogen found in skull base osteomyelitis arising from otitis externa?
2. What precipitates most cases of atypical central skull base osteomyelitis that occur without otitis externa?
3. True or False. Signs of fever, leukocytosis, and positive blood cultures are classically present in patients with skull base osteomyelitis.
4. True or False. In most cases, contrast-enhanced MRI is definitive for diagnosing skull base osteomyelitis.
5. True or False. Computed tomography and/or MRI are reliable methods to evaluate clinical response to treatment in patients with skull base osteomyelitis.
6. Destruction of anatomic fascial planes on postcontrast MRI is more consistent with [central skull base osteomyelitis/malignancy].

7. Two nuclear medicine scans that can help support the diagnosis of skull base osteomyelitis are _____ and _____ scans.
8. What is the treatment of choice in skull base osteomyelitis?
9. True or False. Complications that can arise as a result of skull base osteomyelitis include cavernous sinus thrombosis, cranial neuropathy, meningitis, and brain parenchymal involvement.
10. Involvement of the [upper/lower] cranial nerves is highly suggestive of clival pathology.

■ Answers and Explanations

E. Correct! This is skull base osteomyelitis. Skull base osteomyelitis is typically initiated by ear infections in older patients with poorly controlled diabetes or other immunosuppressive diseases. Skull base osteomyelitis without precipitating ear infections (atypical skull base osteomyelitis) is much less common. The diagnosis of skull base osteomyelitis should be strongly considered in the background of headaches, cranial neuropathy, elevated ESR, and abnormal clival and/or temporal bone imaging findings. Highly sensitive but nonspecific magnetic resonance imaging (MRI) features include T1 hypointensity and T2 hyperintensity of the marrow as well as marked enhancement of the involved clivus or temporal bone. Surrounding pre- and paraclival soft tissue infiltration with obliteration of normal fat planes is also common. No identifiable mass is usually detected. These features are all present in the test case.

Other choices and discussion

A. Squamous cell carcinoma of the head and neck can mimic skull base osteomyelitis on imaging with similar involvement of the clivus and soft tissues. However, it usually appears as a more focal destructive mass rather than as a diffuse, transpatial, and infiltrative process, as in the test case. No identifiable mass is present in this patient.

B. Although nasopharyngeal carcinoma can be diffusely infiltrative, a discrete and identifiable mucosal mass is frequently identified. No mucosal mass is present in this case.

C. Hematogenous metastasis can involve the skull base and surrounding soft tissues. However, lack of a focal destructive mass and no reported history of a primary malignancy make this answer choice unlikely. In addition, an elevated ESR would not be expected in the setting of a skull base malignancy.

D. Sarcoidosis and other inflammatory/granulomatous diseases can mimic skull base osteomyelitis. However, the diffuse marrow signal abnormality and the contiguous nonnodal soft tissue involvement in the test case is atypical for sarcoid.

Question 1

Pseudomonas aeruginosa is the most common pathogen found in skull base osteomyelitis arising from otitis externa.

Question 2

Paranasal sinus inflammatory disease precipitates most cases of atypical central skull base osteomyelitis that occur without otitis externa. Atypical skull base osteomyelitis that does not begin with otitis externa is much less common and is centered on the central skull base (clivus) rather than the temporal bones. It arises from the paranasal sinusitis in most cases but can also be hematogenous in origin.

Question 3

False. Classic signs of infection such as fever, leukocytosis, and positive blood cultures are frequently absent in typical and atypical skull base osteomyelitis.

Question 4

False. Because the imaging appearance is highly sensitive but nonspecific for skull base osteomyelitis, tissue sampling is often required for definitive diagnosis.

Question 5

False. CT and/or MRI are not reliable methods to evaluate clinical response to treatment in patients with skull base osteomyelitis because imaging abnormalities frequently lag behind the clinical response.

Question 6

Destruction of anatomic fascial planes on postcontrast MRI is more consistent with malignancy. Restoration or "normalization" of fascial plane anatomy on postcontrast MRI is more typical of central skull base osteomyelitis than of malignancy. The appearance of "normal" tissue planes is not usually present with malignancy.

Question 7

Two nuclear medicine scans that can help support the diagnosis of skull base osteomyelitis are technetium bone and gallium scans. Whereas technetium bone scans can be helpful for the initial diagnosis of skull base osteomyelitis, they often remain positive for months following clinical resolution of infection. Gallium scans have also been shown to be a sensitive indicator of infection and are useful in monitoring treatment response and assessing for recurrence, particularly as gallium is absorbed by macrophages and reticuloendothelial cells over a period of 2 or 3 days.

Question 8

Long-term (> 3 months) antimicrobial therapy is the mainstay of treatment in skull base osteomyelitis. Surgical debridement is helpful in patients with more aggressive infection. Strict diabetic control is also very important to prevent exacerbation of infection.

Question 9

True. Complications that can arise as a result of skull base osteomyelitis include cavernous sinus thrombosis, cranial neuropathy, meningitis, and brain parenchymal involvement.

Question 10

Lower. Involvement of the cranial nerve VI and the lower cranial nerves (IX, X, XI, XII) is highly indicative of clival involvement by malignancy or infection.

Top Tips

♦ Strongly suspect skull base osteomyelitis in a diabetic or immunocompromised patient who presents with headaches, lower cranial nerve palsy, elevated ESR, and clival and/or temporal bone imaging abnormalities.

♦ MRI is highly sensitive but nonspecific for skull base osteomyelitis. Tissue sampling is often required for diagnostic confirmation.

♦ On MRI, look for T1 hypointensity and marked enhancement of the clivus and/or temporal bone as well as surrounding transpatial infiltration of the surrounding soft tissues.

Image Rich 1

■ Case

Match the appropriate image with the correct diagnosis.
  A. Cranial nerve (CN) VIII
  B. CN V
  C. CN VI
  D. CN VII

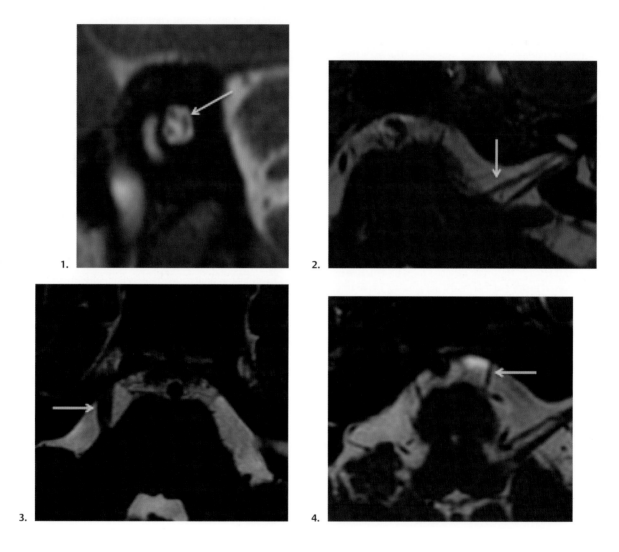

1.

2.

3.

4.

■ Answers and Explanations

1. A. CN VIII (superior vestibular branch). CN VIII, also known as the vestibulocochlear nerve, transmits sound and balance from the inner ear to the brain. The nerve emerges from nuclei located in the superior aspect of the medulla, exits at the pontomedullary junction, and courses through the cerebellopontine angle and into the internal auditory canal (IAC). There, it splits into the cochlear and vestibular nerves. The cochlear branch runs in the anterior-inferior portion of the IAC, whereas the vestibular branches run in the posterior superior and inferior portions of the IAC. This image is a sagittal fast imaging employing steady-state acquisition (FIESTA) of the IAC.

2. D. CN VII (facial nerve). CN VII, also known as the facial nerve, has multiple functions, including controlling the muscles of facial expression, mediating taste for the anterior two-thirds of the tongue, and supplying the parasympathetic fibers to many head and neck ganglia. The nerve exits the pontomedullary junction and courses through the cerebellopontine angle and into the IAC, where it runs in the anterior superior portion of the canal. There are six named segments of the facial nerve: intracranial (cisternal), meatal (intracanalicular), labyrinthine, tympanic, mastoid, and extratemporal. This image is an axial FIESTA of the IAC.

3. B. CN V (trigeminal nerve). CN V, also known as the trigeminal nerve, is responsible for facial sensation and for controlling the muscles of mastication. The nerve exits the lateral pons and courses anterior to the gasserian ganglion in Meckel's cave. From the gasserian ganglion, the nerve trifurcates into three branches: V1 (ophthalmic nerve), V2 (maxillary nerve), and V3 (mandibular nerve). These branches exit the skull base through the superior orbital fissure, foramen rotundum, and foramen ovale, respectively. This image is an axial FIESTA of the IAC.

4. C. CN VI (abducens nerve). CN VI controls the movement of the lateral rectus muscle of the eye. The nerve exits the nucleus from the pons at the pontomedullary junction, courses anteriorly through the prepontine cistern and Dorello's canal and into the cavernous sinus. This image is an axial FIESTA of the IAC.

■ Suggested Readings

Binder DK, Sonne DC, Fischbein NJ, eds. Cranial Nerves: Anatomy, Pathology, Imaging. New York, NY: Thieme; 2010

Grossman RI, Yousem DM, eds. Neuroradiology: The Requisites. Philadelphia, PA: Mosby; 2003

Top Tips

◆ **7-up, coke down**: Mnemonic to remember the positions of CNs VII and VIII within the IAC. CN **VII** lies **superior** in the canal, whereas the **coch**lear branch of CN VIII lies **inferior** in the canal. Both are located in the anterior quadrant of the IAC. The superior vestibular nerve (SVN) and inferior vestibular nerve (IVN), vestibular branches of CN VIII, are in the posterior quadrant.

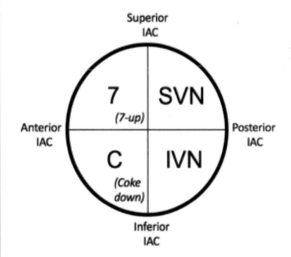

◆ **SO4, LR6**: Mnemonic to remember the major actions of CNs IV and VI. CN IV innervates the **s**uperior **o**blique, and CN VI innervates the **l**ateral **r**ectus muscles of the eye. CN III innervates the rest of the extraocular muscles.

◆ Anatomy of the CNs is best seen on heavily T2-weighted sequences (FIESTA), whereas pathology of the CNs is best seen on postcontrast thin-section T1-weighted and fat-saturated images.

Image Rich 2

■ Case

Match the appropriate image with the correct diagnosis.
  A. Invasive pituitary macroadenoma
  B. Chordoma
  C. Metastasis
  D. Chondrosarcoma

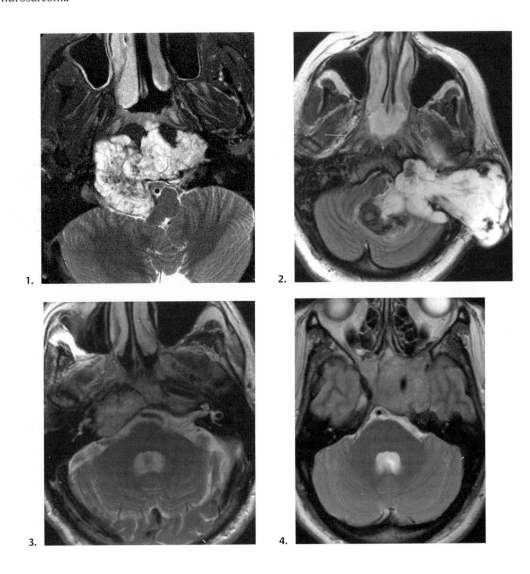

1.   2.   3.   4.

■ Answers and Explanations

1. B. Chordoma. Chordomas are locally aggressive tumors arising from primitive notochord remnants. They commonly occur in the craniovertebral region, usually within the clivus and related to the spheno-occipital synchondrosis. Imaging classically reveals an expansile, destructive, T2 hyperintense, enhancing mass that occurs in the midline. The T2-hyperintense nature of the mass is due to physaliphorous cells, which are large cells with vacuolated cytoplasms.

2. D. Chondrosarcoma. Chondrosarcomas are tumors that arise from cartilage, endochondral bone, or primitive mesenchymal cells in the brain or meninges. These lesions are typically off-midline in location and centered on the petro-occipital fissure. Imaging classically reveals a heterogeneously enhancing, T2 hyperintense mass with characteristic "arc" calcifications and "whorls" of enhancing lines in tumor matrix. In contrast to chordomas, chondrosarcomas have a higher mean apparent diffusion coefficient value ($> 2000 \times 10^{-6}$ mm^2/s) on diffusion-weighted imaging.

3. C. Metastasis. Metastases of the central skull base occur relatively infrequently but are still more common than primary bone lesions. They are usually destructive lytic lesions (although some may be sclerotic) and often have a soft tissue component. The most common primary cancers to metastasize to the skull base are prostate, breast, and lung cancer. Lesions have variable signal intensity on magnetic resonance imaging but usually enhance after gadolinium administration.

4. A. Invasive pituitary macroadenoma. The classification of pituitary adenomas is based on size: microadenomas are < 1 cm and macroadenomas are > 1 cm. Extension of adenomas can occur superiorly into the suprasellar cistern, laterally into the cavernous sinus, and inferiorly through the skull base into the sphenoid sinus and nasopharynx. Most are indolent and histologically benign, although some lesions can grow rapidly and display invasive tendencies, as is seen in this case. Encasement of the internal carotid artery can occur, but the lumen is not typically compromised (in contrast to meningioma or inflammatory pseudotumor). Two reliable signs of cavernous sinus invasion are the complete encasement of the internal carotid artery and the presence of tumor between the internal carotid artery and the lateral wall of the cavernous sinus.

■ Suggested Readings

Laine FJ, Nadel L, Braun IF. CT and MR imaging of the central skull base. Part 2. Pathologic spectrum. Radiographics 1990;10:797–821

Nadarajah J, Madhusudhan KS, Yadav AK, et al. MR imaging of cavernous sinus lesions: pictorial review. J Neuroradiol 2015;42:305–319

Yeom KW, Lober RM, Mobley BC, et al. Diffusion-weighted MRI: distinction of skull base chordoma from chondrosarcoma. Am J Neuroradiol 2013;34:1056–1061

Top Tips

- Look for location, presence of "arcs and whorls," and diffusion signal characteristics to distinguish chordomas from chondrosarcomas.

- Prostate, breast, and lung carcinoma are the most common primary malignancies to metastasize to the central skull base.

- Pituitary adenomas can extend superiorly into the suprasellar cistern, laterally into the cavernous sinus, and inferiorly into the sphenoid sinus and nasopharynx.

Image Rich 3

■ Case

Match the appropriate image with the correct diagnosis.
  A. Primary central nervous system (CNS) lymphoma
  B. Glioblastoma
  C. Oligodendroglioma
  D. Diffuse astrocytoma

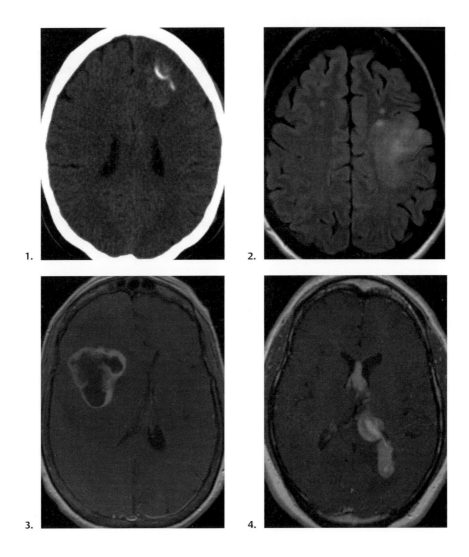

1.

2.

3.

4.

■ Answers and Explanations

1. C. Oligodendroglioma. World Health Organization (WHO) grade 2 oligodendrogliomas are well-differentiated and slow-growing tumors that diffusely infiltrate the cortical and subcortical brain. The classic scenario is that of a middle-aged adult presenting with a partially calcified and heterogeneously enhancing mass in the cortical and subcortical frontal lobe. More aggressive oligodendrogliomas, which are more likely to enhance than low-grade tumors, are termed anaplastic oligodendrogliomas and are WHO grade 3 tumors. IDH1 mutation and co-deletions of chromosomes 1p and 19q are associated with a more favorable prognosis. Relative cerebral blood volumes within oligodendrogliomas are variable and do not necessarily indicate a more malignant lesion (e.g., markedly elevated blood volume has been described with low-grade tumors that have 1p deletions).

2. D. Diffuse astrocytoma. WHO grade 2 diffuse astrocytomas are well-differentiated, expansile, and slow-growing (but infiltrative) tumors that are typically homogeneous, T2 hyperintense, and do not enhance. The presence of enhancement suggests malignant transformation. These tumors can be focal or diffuse and can involve both the white matter and cortex. An IDH1(+), ARTX(+), and MGMT(+) molecular phenotype is associated with a more favorable prognosis. Relative cerebral blood volume in low-grade astrocytomas is relatively lower than in malignant tumors.

3. B. Glioblastoma. WHO grade 4 glioblastoma is the most common primary intracranial neoplasm. It is a highly aggressive and malignant tumor that often has necrosis, microvascular proliferation, and hemorrhage. The prognosis is poor for patients with this tumor, with a mean survival time of approximately 12 months. Primary de novo glioblastomas tend to occur in older patients and are more aggressive than secondary glioblastomas (malignant transformation from a lower-grade tumor), which tend to develop in younger patients. Tumors with MGMT(+) promoter methylation status have better response to chemotherapy (temozolomide). In addition, relatively elevated cerebral blood volume and lower apparent diffusion coefficient values (indicative of higher cellularity) are more characteristic of glioblastomas than of lower-grade tumors.

4. A. Primary CNS lymphoma. Primary CNS lymphoma classically presents as enhancing lesion(s) within the periventricular white matter and basal ganglia that show restricted diffusion. They often involve and can cross the corpus callosum ("butterfly" neoplasm). Of note, other "butterfly" neoplasms include high-grade astrocytoma, glioblastoma, and metastases. Relative cerebral blood volume is mildly elevated in lymphoma but typically much less elevated than in malignant gliomas.

■ Suggested Readings

Al-Okaili RN, Krejza J, Wang S, et al. Advanced MR imaging techniques in the diagnosis of intraaxial brain tumors in adults. Radiographics 2006;26(Suppl 1):S173–189

Grossman RI, Yousem DM, eds. Neuroradiology: The Requisites. Philadelphia, PA: Mosby; 2003

Hartmann M, Heiland S, Harting I, et al. Distinguishing of primary cerebral lymphoma from high-grade glioma with perfusion-weighted magnetic resonance imaging. Neurosci Lett 2003;338:119–122

Hilario A, Ramos A, Perez-Nuñez A, et-al. The added value of apparent diffusion coefficient to cerebral blood volume in the preoperative grading of diffuse gliomas. Am J Neuroradiol 2012;33:701–707

Top Tips

- Imaging features suggestive of higher-grade tumor: large size, mass effect, enhancement, necrosis, hemorrhage, lower apparent diffusion coefficient values, and elevated relative cerebral blood volume.

- IDH1+, 1p19q co-deletions, and MGMT+ molecular status predicts prolonged survival in patients with low-grade and high-grade gliomas.

- "Butterfly" tumor differential: glioblastoma, lymphoma, metastasis.

Image Rich 4

■ Case

Match the appropriate image with the correct diagnosis.
- A. Classic epidermoid cyst
- B. White epidermoid cyst
- C. Vestibular schwannoma
- D. Meningioma

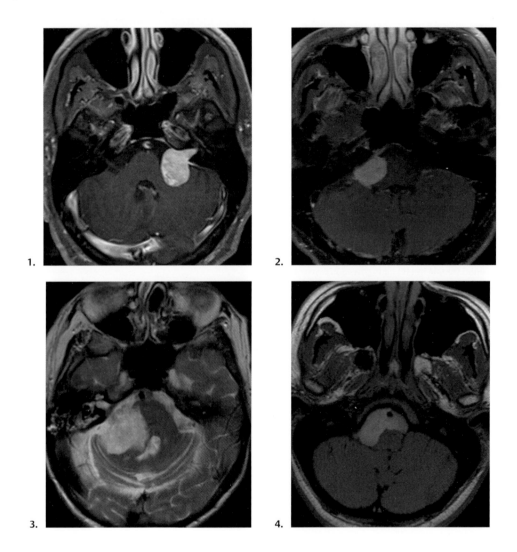

1.

2.

3.

4.

■ Answers and Explanations

1. C. Vestibular schwannoma. A vestibular schwannoma (also known by its misnomer, acoustic neuroma) is a benign tumor of Schwann cells arising from the vestibular division of cranial nerve VIII. Classic imaging features of a vestibular schwannoma are of a well-defined and enhancing mass in the cerebellopontine angle and internal auditory canal with expansion of the porus acusticus. Microhemorrhage, intramural cysts, and associated arachnoid cysts may be present. In contrast to meningiomas, "dural tails" are not usually present. Bilateral vestibular schwannomas are classic lesions of neurofibromatosis type 2.

2. D. Meningioma. A meningioma of the cerebellopontine angle typically presents as a homogeneously enhancing extra-axial mass with a "dural tail." The dural tail, which is typically centered along the posterior wall of the petrous bone and may extend into the internal auditory canal, usually represents reactive change rather than neoplastic infiltration. Calcification within meningiomas is not uncommon. Unlike vestibular schwannomas, meningiomas rarely widen the porus acusticus.

3. A. Classic epidermoid cyst. An epidermoid cyst is a benign congenital lesion that arises from inclusion of ectodermal epithelial elements during neural tube closure. The classic imaging presentation of an epidermoid cyst is a T2 hyperintense mass with cauliflower-like margins and restricted diffusion. It often insinuates itself around nerves and blood vessels in the cerebellopontine angle. Epidermoids do not typically enhance, although thin rim of enhancement may occur. Calcification along the lesion margin may also be present.

4. B. White epidermoid cyst. "White epidermoid," a rare variant of epidermoid cyst, demonstrates high T1 signal. This is due to high lipid content comprised of mixed triglycerides and unsaturated fatty acid residues. A neurenteric cyst, a benign congenital malformation of endodermal origin, can have a similar appearance.

■ Suggested Readings

Chen CY, Wong JS, Hsieh SC, et al. Intracranial epidermoid cyst with hemorrhage: MR imaging findings. Am J Neuroradiol 2006;27:427–429

Grossman RI, Yousem DM, eds. Neuroradiology: The Requisites. Philadelphia, PA: Mosby; 2003

Medhi G, Saini J, Pandey P, et al. T1 hyperintense prepontine mass with restricted diffusion—A white epidermoid or a neurenteric cyst? J Neuroimaging 2015;25:841–843

Top Tips

- Vestibular scwhannomas typically widen the porus acusticus and lack "dural tails," in contrast to cerebellopontine angle meningiomas.

- Look for restricted diffusion in a T2 hyperintense mass to diagnose an epidermoid cyst.

- T1 hyperintensity within a cerebellopontine angle or prepontine lesion may indicate a "white epidermoid" or neurenteric cyst.

Image Rich 5

■ Case

Match the appropriate image with the correct diagnosis.
- A. Plasmacytoma
- B. Hemangioma
- C. Chordoma
- D. Chondrosarcoma

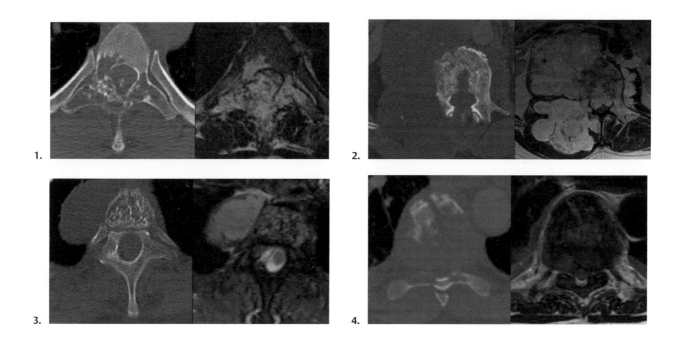

1.

2.

3.

4.

■ Answers and Explanations

1. D. Chondrosarcoma. Chondrosarcoma is the second most common primary nonlymphoproliferative malignancy of the spine in adults, with a peak prevalence between 30 and 70 years of age. The thoracic and lumbar spine are most often involved. At presentation, 15% occur in the vertebral body, 40% occur in the posterior elements, and 45% occur in the vertebral body and posterior elements. Chondrosarcomas typically present on imaging as large, calcified masses with associated bony destruction. Chondroid matrix is best appreciated on computed tomography (CT). Typical magnetic resonance imaging (MRI) features include very high signal intensity on T2-weighted images (due to high water content of hyaline cartilage) and a ring and arcs pattern of enhancement.

2. C. Chordoma. Chordoma is a rare malignancy arising from remnants of the primitive notochord, with peak prevalence in the fifth and sixth decades of life. While chordomas most commonly occur in the sacrococcygeal region, they can also be found in the spheno-occipital region and in vertebral bodies (the latter most commonly involving the cervical spine). Within the spine, chordomas frequently involve the vertebral body and spare the posterior elements. On imaging, these tumors manifest as expansile and destructive masses. Typical MRI features include very high signal intensity on T2-weighted images (due to the presence of characteristic physaliphorous cells) and moderate heterogeneous enhancement. Hemorrhage and proteinaceous material, manifesting as high signal intensity on T1-weighted images, can also be seen.

3. B. Hemangioma. Vertebral hemangiomas are common lesions of the bone. They are composed of thin-walled vessels lined by endothelial cells and infiltrate the medullary space between bony trabeculae. They most commonly occur in the thoracic and lumbar spine. While the majority are seen in the vertebral bodies, some also extend into or occur within the posterior elements. Occasionally, vertebral hemangiomas can increase in size and extend into the spinal canal, resulting in cord compression. Vertical striations or a honeycomb appearance is classic for a hemangioma, manifesting as a "polka-dot" appearance on cross-sectional CT. Typical MRI features include high signal intensity on T1- and T2-weighted images (due to the presence of fat and interstitial edema) and marked enhancement (due to its highly vascular nature). Flow voids are also commonly seen.

4. A. Plasmacytoma. Plasmacytoma is a focal proliferation of malignant plasma cells without diffuse involvement of the bone marrow. A solitary plasmacytoma is an uncommon tumor, occurring in < 10% of patients with plasma cell neoplasms. The majority of patients are older than 60 years of age. Plasmacytomas usually present as a single collapsed vertebral body. They may be purely lytic, mixed but predominantly lytic, or (rarely) sclerotic. On MRI, they typically have low signal intensity on T1-weighted images, high signal intensity on T2-weighted images (although this is variable), and marked homogeneous enhancement.

■ Suggested Readings

Rodallec MH, Feydy A, Larousserie F, et al. Diagnostic imaging of solitary tumors of the spine: what to do and say. Radiographics 2008;28:1019–1041

Top Tips

- Combination of CT and MRI features can help to differentiate between primary osseous tumors of the spine.

- CT: Look for chondroid matrix in chondrosarcoma, bony destruction in chordoma, and honeycomb or polka-dot appearance in hemangioma.

- MRI: Look for very high signal intensity on T2-weighted images for chondrosarcoma and chordoma; high signal intensity on T1-weighted images for hemangioma; and low signal intensity on T1-weighted images for plasmacytoma.

More Challenging 1

■ Case

A 55-year-old woman with a history of glioblastoma (left image). Six months after surgery, radiation, and temozolomide, she presents for follow-up magnetic resonance imaging (middle and right images).

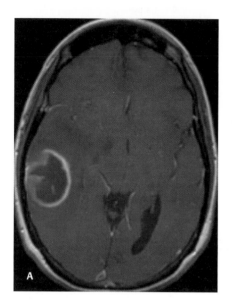
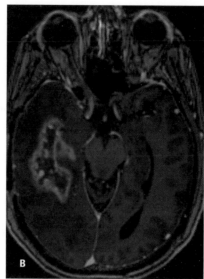
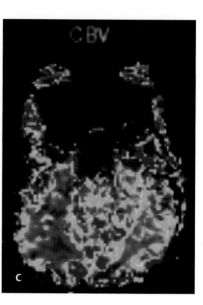

■ Questions

1. What is the MOST likely diagnosis on the 6-month follow up magnetic resonance imaging?
   A. Abscess
   B. Radiation necrosis
   C. Recurrent glioblastoma
   D. Subacute infarction
   E. Tumefactive demyelination

2. From the tracer tissue concentration-time curve, relative cerebral blood volume is represented by the:
   A. Area under the curve
   B. Arterial input function
   C. Height of deconvolved curve
   D. Area under deconvolved curve divided by height
   E. Mean transit time divided by cerebral blood flow

3. Radiation necrosis commonly occurs within which of the following time periods following radiotherapy?
   A. Within 1 day
   B. One day to one week
   C. One week to one month
   D. One to three months
   E. Three months and beyond

■ Answers and Explanations

Question 1

B. Correct! This is most likely radiation necrosis. Differentiation between radiation necrosis and tumor recurrence on follow up magnetic resonance imaging (MRI) is extremely difficult because there is significant overlap in the imaging features of these entities. Features that may favor radiation necrosis over tumor recurrence include conversion from a nonenhancing to an enhancing lesion following radiation, appearance of lesions distant to the primary resection site, involvement of the corpus callosum or periventricular white matter, and a "soap bubble" or "swiss-cheese" appearance of the lesion. Other features that may favor radiation necrosis include: lower relative cerebral blood volume (rCBV) values on perfusion imaging (as seen in the test case) and higher apparent diffusion coefficient (ADC) values (possibly due to vasogenic edema) on diffusion imaging, although lower ADC values (due to gliosis or fibrosis) have also been reported. To further complicate the issue, mixed radiation necrosis and tumor recurrence can coexist. The gold standard for distinguishing radiation necrosis from tumor recurrence is biopsy or resection, which confirmed the diagnosis in the test case.

Other choices and discussion

A. The typical imaging features of a cerebral abscess include smooth or irregular peripheral enhancement, surrounding vasogenic edema, and central restricted diffusion, the latter signifying the presence of purulent material.

C. As detailed in choice B, it is often difficult to differentiate recurrent glioblastoma from radiation necrosis. While the lower rCBV of this lesion suggests radiation necrosis, it would be hard to exclude the possibility of tumor recurrence. Given this dilemma, surgical biopsy of the lesion was performed and revealed treatment necrosis. In order to address the limited capability of MRI to distinguish between the two entities, criteria (Macdonald criteria and Radiological Assessment in Neuro-Oncology criteria) were adopted, although issues surrounding accurate diagnosis remain.

D. Subacute infarction is unlikely given the mass-like appearance of the lesion. Enhancement in subacute infarcts is frequently gyral or cortical, although subcortical and deep parenchymal enhancement may also be seen.

E. Tumefactive demyelinating lesions typically present as incomplete ring-enhancing masses. The thick and irregular wall of the lesion is the test case is not consistent with demyelination.

Question 2

A. Correct! Cerebral blood volume (CBV) represents the volume of blood per unit of brain tissue, measured in mL/100 gm. Measurements of CBV (and cerebral blood flow [CBF]) are semiquantitative or relative because they depend on nonuniform features such as variability between subjects and bolus injection. They are frequently obtained by using an internal standard of reference, such as normal-appearing gray or white matter. Furthermore, rCBV is determined by integrating the area under the tracer tissue concentration-time curve.

Other choices and discussion

B. The arterial input function describes the time-dependent contrast agent input to the tissue of interest. It is required to account for confounding effects of how a bolus of contrast agent arrives to the tissue and to determine and quantify a property of the issue such as CBF.

C. The initial height of the deconvolved tissue concentration-time curve represents CBF. CBF (measured in mL/100g/min) refers to the volume of blood passing through a given amount of brain tissue per unit time.

D. The area under the deconvolved curve divided by the height represents mean transit time (MTT). MTT (commonly measured in seconds) represents the time between arterial inflow and venous outflow, or the time it takes for blood to pass through a given amount of brain tissue.

E. CBV (mL/100 g) = MTT (seconds) × CBF (mL/100 g/min).

Question 3

E. Correct! Radiation necrosis typically presents during the late-delayed phase (3 months to years) following radiotherapy. It often results in endothelial apoptosis and inflammation. The incidence of radiation necrosis is approximately 3 to 24%, and its occurrence is related to treatment duration, radiation dose, and total treated brain volume. Patients may be asymptomatic or they may experience significant neurologic deficits. Treatment interventions such as steroids, bevacizumab, and surgical resection depend on the clinical picture.

Discussion

The other choices are incorrect. Acute and early delayed effects of radiation typically occur within 3 months after initiation of radiation therapy. These early radiation effects are presumably due to vasodilation, disruption of the blood–brain barrier, and edema. Clinical symptoms of headache, nausea, and somnolence are common. Symptoms are typically self-limited and do not necessarily require corticosteroid treatment.

■ Suggested Readings

Shiroishi MS, Castellazzi G, Boxerman JL, et al. Principles of T2*-weighted dynamic susceptibility contrast MRI technique in brain tumor imaging. J Magn Reson Imaging 2015;41:296–313

Tomandi BF, Klotz E, Handschu R, et al. Comprehensive imaging of ischemic stroke with multisection CT. Radiographics 2003;23:565–592

Verma N, Cowperthwaite MC, Burnett MG, et al. Differentiating tumor recurrence from treatment necrosis: a review of neuro-oncologic imaging strategies. Neuro Oncol 2013;15:515–534

Top Tips

◆ Radiation necrosis is typically a late delayed effect of radiation, occurring 3 months to years after radiotherapy.

◆ Differentiation between radiation necrosis and tumor recurrence is difficult; the gold standard is surgical biopsy and/or resection.

◆ MRI features that favor radiation necrosis over tumor are lower rCBV values on perfusion imaging and higher apparent diffusion coefficient values on diffusion imaging.

More Challenging 2

■ Case

A 41-year-old woman presents with new-onset memory difficulties and both simple and partial complex seizures.

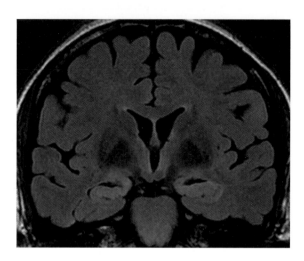
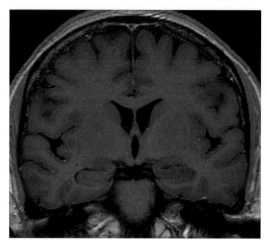

■ Questions

1. Symmetric involvement of the limbic structures is LEAST likely to be found with which of the following?
   A. Paraneoplastic encephalitis
   B. Gliomatosis cerebri
   C. Autoimmune encephalitis
   D. Herpes encephalitis
   E. Status epilepticus

2. What imaging feature seen in the test case is associated with mesial temporal sclerosis?
   A. Hippocampal architectural distortion
   B. Hippocampal atrophy
   C. Hippocampal enhancement
   D. Hippocampal T2/FLAIR hyperintensity
   E. Mammillary body atrophy

3. Of the following autoantibodies that can be found in the serum or cerebrospinal fluid in patients with paraneoplastic syndromes, which is the LEAST likely to be associated with a tumor?
   A. Anti-Hu
   B. Anti-voltage-gated potassium channel
   C. Anti-Ri
   D. Anti-Ma2
   E. Anti-N-methyl-D-aspartate receptor

■ Answers and Explanations

Question 1

B. Correct! Symmetric involvement of the hippocampi without involvement of adjacent lobes is inconsistent with gliomastosis cerebri, which is a diffuse and usually indolent process without predilection for the limbic system. Often, there is expansion of an involved area and T2/fluid-attenuated inversion recovery (FLAIR) hyperintensity affecting multiple contiguous lobes that may or may not involve the corpus callosum. Typically, there is little or no enhancement.

Other choices and discussion

A. In the test case, there is symmetric hyperintense FLAIR signal abnormality of the hippocampi without associated enhancement. This can be seen with paraneoplastic encephalitis, a type of limbic encephalitis that is associated with a systemic cancer and with antibodies against intracellular neuronal antigens. Classic imaging features of limbic encephalitis include T2/FLAIR hyperintensity in the mesial temporal lobes, insula, cingulate gyrus, and inferior frontal white matter. There is also minimal or patchy enhancement and rare diffusion restriction. Bilateral involvement is more frequent than unilateral involvement, and cerebellar atrophy may be seen in cases associated with cerebellar degeneration.

C. Symmetric hippocampal signal abnormality can also be seen with autoimmune encephalitis, another type of limbic encephalitis. While autoimmune encephalitis may or may not be associated with a cancer, the presence of antibodies targeted against cell membrane or synaptic receptors is usually present. Autoimmune and paraneoplastic encephalitis cannot be differentiated based solely on imaging features; the diagnosis often relies on autoantibody detection in serum and/or cerebrospinal fluid.

D. Herpes encephalitis involves the temporal lobes and limbic system, typically in a bilateral and asymmetric pattern. It may be indistinguishable from limbic encephalitis on imaging, although restricted diffusion and hemorrhage are more common features of herpes encephalitis. A key to accurate diagnosis is polymerase chain reaction analysis of the cerebrospinal fluid.

E. Seizures can cause T2/FLAIR hyperintensity of the supratentorial cortex and subcortical white matter but sometimes also involve the hippocampi, corpus callosum, and/or thalami (pulvinar nuclei). Diffusion restriction is common in the acute setting, whereas enhancement (typically gyral or leptomeningeal) is variable. Marked hyperemia on perfusion imaging can be identified on the side of the seizure focus. Systemic workup and follow up imaging may be necessary to differentiate this from herpes or limbic encephalitis.

Question 2

D. Correct! This patient shows symmetric T2/FLAIR hyperintensity of the hippocampi. The classic imaging triad of mesial temporal sclerosis includes abnormal T2/FLAIR hyperintensity of the hippocampus, hippocampal atrophy, and architectural distortion of the hippocampus. Secondary signs include atrophy of the ipsilateral fornix and mammillary body and enlargement of the ipsilateral choroidal fissure and temporal horn. This patient does not have imaging consistent with mesial temporal sclerosis, given the absence of hippocampal atrophy and architectural distortion.

All other choices are incorrect.

Question 3

B. Correct! These antibodies are elevated in patients with autoimmune voltage-gated potassium channel complex encephalitis, one of the most common forms of autoimmune encephalitis. Tumor association is rare. Treatment consists of seizure control and/or immunosuppressive agents.

Other choices and discussion

A. Anti-Hu antibodies are commonly elevated in patients with small cell lung cancer who present with a paraneoplastic syndrome.

C. Anti-Ri antibodies are commonly elevated in patients with small cell lung, breast, or gynecologic cancer who present with a paraneoplastic syndrome.

D. Anti-Ma2 antibodies are commonly elevated in patients with testicular cancer who present with a paraneoplastic syndrome.

E. Anti-N-methyl-D-aspartate receptor antibodies are elevated in patients with anti-N-methyl-D-aspartate receptor encephalitis, which is a highly characteristic neuropsychiatric syndrome with movement disorders, seizures, and autonomic dysfunction. It most commonly occurs in young women and children. Over half of these patients have an associated tumor, most commonly teratomas of the ovaries.

■ Suggested Readings

Dalmau J, Rosenfeld M. Autoimmune encephalitis update. Neuro Oncol 2014;16:771–778

Honnorat J, Antoine JC. Paraneoplastic neurological syndromes. Orphanet J Rare Dis 2007;2:22

Kotsenas AL, Watson RE, Pittock SJ, et al. MRI findings in autoimmune voltage-gated potassium channel complex encephalitis with seizures: one potential etiology for mesial temporal sclerosis. Am J Neuroradiol 2014;35:84–89

Sarria-Estrada S, Toldeo M, Lorenzo-Bosquet C, et al. Neuroimaging in status epilepticus secondary to paraneoplastic autoimmune encephalitis. Clin Radiol 2014;69:795–803

Top Tips

- Limbic encephalitis, which includes paraneoplastic and autoimmune etiologies, is characterized by bilateral (more common than unilateral) involvement of the mesial temporal lobe and adjacent structures.

- Imaging features of limbic encephalitis often overlap with herpes encephalitis and seizure-related changes, making diagnosis largely dependent on systemic workup and/or follow up imaging.

- Longstanding limbic encephalitis with seizures can progress to mesial temporal sclerosis, which is characterized by a classic imaging triad of hippocampal T2/FLAIR signal hyperintensity, atrophy, and architectural distortion.

More Challenging 3

■ Case

A 34-year-old man hit by a car presents with acute cognitive decline, breathing difficulties, rash, and right proximal femoral fracture.

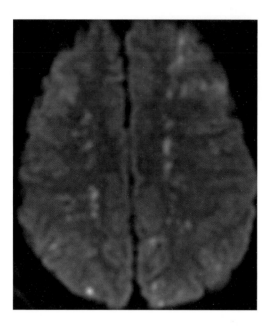 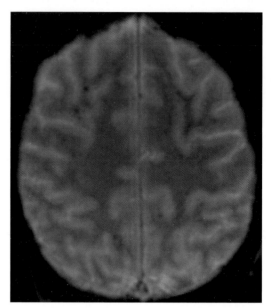

■ Questions

1. What is the MOST likely diagnosis?
   A. Cerebral fat embolism
   B. Traumatic axonal injury
   C. Hypoperfusion
   D. Vasculitis
   E. Metastatic disease

2. What is the classic clinical triad of the disorder presented in the test case?
   A. Neurologic dysfunction, respiratory distress, renal dysfunction
   B. Neurologic dysfunction, respiratory distress, petechial skin rash
   C. Neurologic dysfunction, respiratory distress, cardiac abnormalities
   D. Neurologic dysfunction, renal dysfunction, deep venous thrombosis
   E. Neurologic dysfunction, deep venous thrombosis, anasarca

3. What percentage of patients with traumatic long bone fractures develop clinically significant fat embolism syndrome?
   A. < 5%
   B. 10%
   C. 25%
   D. 50%
   E. 75%

■ Answers and Explanations

Question 1

A. Correct! The most likely diagnosis is cerebral fat embolism. Classic magnetic resonance imaging (MRI) findings of cerebral fat embolism are found in the test case and include multiple, dot-like lesions of restricted diffusion consistent with microembolic infarcts ("starfield appearance") and multiple petechial hemorrhages on gradient-recalled echo or susceptibility-weighted imaging in the brain. These lesions are predominantly found in the bilateral watershed or borderzone territories but can also be seen in the basal ganglia, corpus callosum, and cerebellum.

Fat embolism syndrome is often associated with displaced long bone fractures of the lower extremities, occurring between 12 hours and 3 days after the inciting trauma. It can also occur as a rare complication of sickle cell disease, caused by bone marrow infarcts and necrosis. Fat embolism syndrome with neurologic symptoms is termed "cerebral fat embolism syndrome." Fat emboli can pass through pulmonary capillaries in the absence of shunting lesions and result in systemic embolization, or may be due to a preexisting intracardiac right-to-left or arteriovenous shunt.

Other choices and discussion

B. Cerebral fat embolism syndrome can mimic traumatic axonal injury with the similar features of microhemorrhages and multiple foci of vasogenic and cytoxic edema. Differential considerations of multiple microhemorrhages (hypointense foci on gradient-recalled echo or susceptibility-weighted imaging) in the brain include septic and fat emboli, chronic hypertension, cerebral amyloid angiopathy, cavernous malformations, vasculitis, hemorrhagic diffuse axonal injury, and hemorrhagic metastases. Given the history of trauma, distinguishing cerebral fat embolism from traumatic axonal injury can be challenging based solely on imaging. In this case, the patient's clinical symptoms, presence of a long bone fracture, and lack of other manifestations of traumatic brain injury (e.g., no gross intracranial hemorrhage) make traumatic axonal injury less likely.

C. Hypoperfusion injury can produce bilateral watershed or borderzone infarcts. However, this is not consistent with the patient's history and presentation. Also, the presence of microhemorrhages in the brain would be atypical for hypoperfusion injury.

D. Vasculitis can also produce bilateral watershed or borderzone microinfarcts and microhemorrhages. Angiographic evaluation of the vessels may demonstrate bead-like irregularity, stenosis, and occlusion of small vessels. In this case, however, the patient's clinical presentation, trauma history, and imaging findings are more consistent with cerebral fat embolism syndrome.

E. Metastatic disease typically presents as solitary or multiple enhancing lesions with surrounding vasogenic edema. These features are not present in the test case.

Question 2

B. Correct! The classic clinical triad for fat embolism syndrome includes neurologic symptoms, respiratory distress, and petechial skin rash. Neurologic symptoms vary and can range from a subclinical presentation to seizures and coma. Although full neurologic manifestations usually develop after pulmonary symptoms, neurologic dysfunction may be the only manifestation of fat embolism syndrome. In addition, the number of lesions in the white matter on MRI is correlated with the score on the Glasgow coma scale.

The other choices are all incorrect.

Question 3

A. Correct! Subclinical fat embolism syndrome is extremely common after traumatic long bone fractures, but a clinically significant syndrome occurs in < 5% of cases. Of these patients, 60% have neurologic manifestations (cerebral fat embolism syndrome). In the majority of cases, neurologic function is gradually recovered over days to months, although this condition can be potentially life-threatening, with reported mortality rates ranging from 13 to 87%.

The other choices are all incorrect.

■ Suggested Readings

Bodanapally UK, Shanmuganathan K, Saksobhavivat N, et al. MR imaging and differentiation of cerebral fat embolism syndrome from diffuse axonal injury: application of diffusion tensor imaging. Neuroradiology 2013;55:771–778

Ryu CW, Lee DH, Kim TK, et al. Cerebral fat embolism: diffusion-weighted magnetic resonance imaging findings. Acta Radiol 2005;46:528–533

Simon AD, Ulmer JL, Strottmann JM. Contrast-enhanced MR imaging of cerebral fat embolism: case report and review of the literature. Am J Neuroradiol 2003;24:97–101

Top Tips

- A "starfield" pattern (multiple foci of restricted diffusion throughout the brain, predominantly in the watershed territories) on MRI is characteristic of cerebral fat embolism syndrome.

- Clinical triad for fat embolism syndrome: neurologic dysfunction, respiratory distress, petechial skin rash.

- Cerebral fat emboli are generally associated with traumatic long bone fractures of the lower extremities but can rarely occur as a complication of sickle cell disease.

More Challenging 4

■ Case

A 54-year-old man with hepatitis was found unconscious.

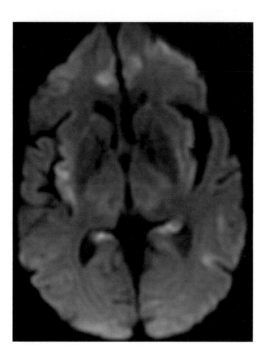

■ Questions

1. What is the MOST likely diagnosis?
   A. Acute hyperammonemic encephalopathy
   B. Hypoglycemia
   C. Hypoxic ischemic encephalopathy
   D. Emboli
   E. Vasculitis

2. Elevation of which metabolite peak on magnetic resonance spectroscopy is most characteristic of this disorder?
   A. Choline (3.22 ppm)
   B. Myo-inositol (3.56 ppm)
   C. N-acetylaspartate (2.02 ppm)
   D. Glx (glutamine and glutamate) (2.1 to 2.55 ppm)
   E. Creatine (3.02 ppm)

3. Which of the following is NOT a treatment for hyperammonemia?
   A. Lactulose
   B. Increase protein intake
   C. Hemodialysis
   D. Increase caloric intake of glucose and lipids
   E. Antiseizure medications

■ Answers and Explanations

Question 1

A. Correct! This patient has acute hyperammonemic encephalopathy. In adults, acute hyperammonemic encephalopathy is often seen in very ill patients with acute hepatic dysfunction leading to prolonged hyperammonemia and brain injury. Imaging features suggestive of acute hyperammonemic encephalopathy are T2/fluid-attenuated inversion recovery hyperintensity and diffusion restriction involving the bilateral insular and cingulate cortices. Involvement of other brain regions such as the subcortical white matter, brainstem, basal ganglia, and thalami are more variable. Sparing of the perirolandic and occipital cortices has also been described.

Other choices and discussion

B. Classic imaging features of adult hypoglycemia are edema and diffusion restriction involving the posterior cortices of the brain (temporal, parietal, and occipital) and basal ganglia. Involvement of the thalami and subcortical and deep white matter is uncommon.

C. Hypoxic ischemic encephalopathy typically manifests as restricted diffusion involving the borderzone territories (more common in injuries that are mild-moderate in severity) and gray matter structures including the basal ganglia, thalami, cerebral cortex, cerebellum, and hippocampi (seen in cases with more severe injury).

D. Embolic infarcts typically occur in multiple vascular distributions involving the terminal cortical branches. Microemboli are also associated with borderzone or watershed infarcts.

E. Given involvement of the bilateral and relatively symmetric insular and cingulate cortices in this case, the diagnosis of vasculitis is unlikely.

Question 2

D. Correct! Elevated glutamine levels can be detected on magnetic resonance spectroscopy (MRS) as Glx, a mixture of glutamine and glutamate (peak between 2.1 to 2.55 ppm on MRS). Increased levels of ammonia in the brain are rapidly metabolized into glutamine; this physiologically demanding process can lead to elevated cellular osmolarity, inflammation, loss of cerebral autoregulation, and cerebral edema. Of note, as most findings on MRS are nonspecific and can be seen with many entities, MRS is not routinely used in clinical practice. However, MRS may be helpful in specific cases, primarily to support and confirm findings on conventional magnetic resonance sequences (e.g., detecting Glx peak in patients with acute hyperammonemic encephalopathy, detecting reduced N-acetylaspartate and creatine and elevated choline peaks in patients with brain tumors or active demyelination, and detecting cytosolic amino acids at 0.9 ppm in patients with a pyogenic or fungal abscess).

Other choices and discussion

A. Choline (peak at 3.22 ppm on MRS) is a component of phospholipid metabolism and is a marker of cellular membrane turnover.

B. Myo-inositol (peak at 3.56 ppm on MRS) is a glial marker located in astrocytes and is a product of myelin degradation.

C. N-acetylaspartate (peak at 2.02 ppm on MRS) is a marker of neuronal and axonal integrity.

E. Creatine (peak at 3.02 ppm on MRS) is a marker of cerebral metabolism.

Question 3

B. Correct! *Restriction* of dietary protein and discontinuation of total parenteral nutrition are parts of the treatment in hyperammonemia, as they are metabolic sources of ammonium.

Other choices and discussion

A. Lactulose therapy helps to reduce ammonia production.

C. Hemodialysis is used to quickly reduce plasma ammonium levels in severe cases.

D. Caloric intake is provided by glucose and lipids in these patients.

E. Antiseizure medications are used in patients with acute hyperammonemia, although the use of valproic acid can exacerbate this condition because serum ammonia levels are increased due to a reduction in urea cycle function.

■ Suggested Readings

Brandao LA, Domingues RC. MR Spectroscopy of the Brain. Philadelphia, PA: Lippincott Williams & Wilkins; 2004

McKinney AM, Lohman BD, Sarikaya B, et al. Acute hepatic encephalopathy: diffusion-weighted and fluid-attenuated inversion recovery findings, and correlation with plasma ammonia level and clinical outcome. Am J Neuroradiol 2010;31:1471–1479

Takanashi J, Barkovich AJ, Cheng SF, et al. Brain MR imaging in acute hyperammonemic encephalopathy arising from late-onset ornithine transcarbamylase deficiency. Am J Neuroradiol 2003;24:390–393

U-King-Im JM, Yu E, Bartlett E, et al. Acute hyperammonemic encephalopathy in adults: imaging findings. Am J Neuroradiol 2011;32:413–418

Top Tips

◆ Think of acute hyperammonemic encephalopathy (a potentially reversible condition) in a patient with liver failure who has brain magnetic resonance imaging showing diffusion restriction involving the bilateral insular and cingulate cortices.

◆ Increased serum ammonia levels can result in increased glutamine/glutamate levels, which can be detected as an elevated Glx peak on MRS.

◆ Differential for cortical restricted diffusion (**MISTI**): **m**itochondrial disorder (MELAS); **i**nfection (meningoencephalitis, Creutzfeldt-Jakob disease), **s**eizure activity, **t**oxic/metabolic, and **i**schemia (arterial infarct, venous infarct, hypoxic ischemic injury).

More Challenging 5

■ Case

A 46-year-old man presents with headache, neck pain, and dysphagia after sustaining a fall from his bed.

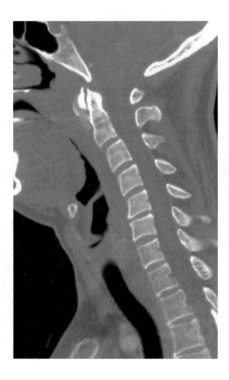
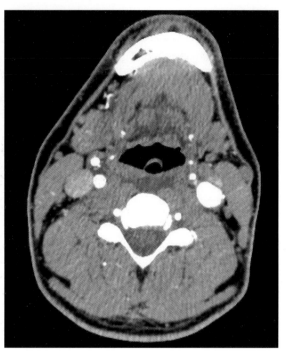

■ Questions

1. What is the MOST likely diagnosis?
   A. Discitis-osteomyelitis with prevertebral abscess
   B. Retropharyngeal abscess
   C. Internal jugular vein thrombosis
   D. Acute calcific tendinitis of the longus colli muscle
   E. Suppurative lymphadenitis

2. What is the treatment for this condition?
   A. Surgical drainage
   B. Intravenous antibiotics
   C. Percutaneous drainage
   D. Nonsteroidal anti-inflammatory drugs
   E. Anticoagulation

3. Deposition of what substance in the superior oblique tendons of the longus colli muscles is responsible for calcific tendinitis?
   A. Hemosiderin
   B. Cholesterol
   C. Monosodium urate
   D. Calcium pyrophosphate
   E. Calcium hydroxyapatite

■ Answers and Explanations

Question 1

D. Correct! This patient has acute calcific tendinitis of the longus colli muscle. Amorphous calcifications of the longus colli tendon (anterior to C1/C2) and the presence of a retropharyngeal effusion are pathognomonic for this entity. In addition, there are no enlarged lymph nodes or destructive bony changes to suggest an infectious process. Patients with acute calcific longus colli tendinitis can present with neck pain, dysphagia, and odynophagia. They may have low-grade fever and a mildly elevated white blood cell count, and there may be a history of recent upper respiratory infection or minor trauma.

Other choices and discussion

A. Discitis-osteomyelitis would show destructive changes centered at the disc space with erosion of the adjacent bony endplates. A prevertebral abscess would enhance peripherally with contrast. In the test case, the vertebral column is intact and there is no enhancement associated with the retropharyngeal fluid collection.

B. While there is a retropharyngeal effusion that symmetrically expands the retropharyngeal space in the test case, there is no peripheral enhancement to suggest an organized or encapsulated abscess. Furthermore, the presence of calcifications anterior to C1 and C2 is not typical of a retropharyngeal abscess.

C. While internal jugular vein thrombosis can cause a retropharyngeal effusion, the veins are patent in the test case.

E. Suppurative lymphadenitis may be associated with a retropharyngeal effusion or abscess. No low-attenuation retropharyngeal lymph nodes are demonstrated on the provided images to support this diagnosis, however.

Question 2

D. Correct! Acute calcific tendinitis of the longus colli muscle is a noninfectious, inflammatory process and can be treated conservatively with nonsteroidal anti-inflammatory drugs.

Other choices and discussion

A. If an abscess were present, surgical drainage could be indicated.

B. Intravenous antibiotics would be administered if infection were present.

C. If an abscess were present, percutaneous drainage could be indicated.

E. There is no indication for anticoagulation in this case.

Question 3

E. Correct! Acute calcific tendinitis of the longus colli muscle is caused by the deposition of calcium hydroxyapatite in the superior oblique tendons of the longus colli muscles.

Other choices and discussion

A. Hemosiderin is incorrect.

B. Cholesterol deposition in the Achilles tendon is associated with the development of xanthomas.

C. Monosodium urate deposition is associated with gout.

D. Calcium pyrophosphate deposition is seen in calcium pyrophosphate deposition disease.

■ Suggested Readings

Eastwood JD, Hudgins PA, Malone D. Retropharyngeal effusion in acute calcific tendinitis: diagnosis with CT and MR imaging. Am J Neuroradiol 1998; 19:1789–1792

Offiah CE, Hall E. Acute calcific tendinitis of the longus colli muscle: spectrum of CT appearances and anatomical correlation. Br J Radiol 2009; 82:e117–e121

Zibis AH, Giannis D, Malizos KN, et al. Acute calcific tendinitis of the longus colli muscle: case report and review of the literature. Eur Spine J 2013;22:S434–438

Top Tips

- Acute calcific longus colli tendinitis is a noninfectious, inflammatory process caused by the deposition of calcium hydroxyapatite in the superior oblique tendons of the longus colli muscles.

- Patients can present with neck pain, dysphagia, odynophagia, low-grade fever, and mildly elevated white blood cell counts.

- Presence of amorphous calcifications in the superior tendons of the longus colli muscle anterior to C1–C3 is pathognomonic for the diagnosis.

Essentials 1

■ Case

The tech brings you a hepatobiliary scan (ordered for acute cholecystitis) to check for completion of the exam. The surgeon is anxious to operate if the patient has acute cholecystitis.

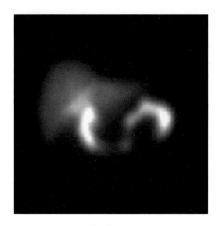

60 minutes

■ Questions

1. Based on the 60-minute image, which ONE of the following is the best next course of action?
   A. Obtain delayed images.
   B. Ask for different views.
   C. Administer water.
   D. Take no action. The study is complete.
   E. Give pharmacologic intervention.

2. Regarding hepatobiliary scintigraphy and cholecystitis, which ONE of the following is correct?
   A. Chronic cholecystitis usually demonstrates delayed gallbladder filling.
   B. Hepatobiliary scanning is less sensitive for the detection of acalculous cholecystitis than it is for calculus cholecystitis.
   C. Enterogastric reflux after cholecystokinin administration implies symptomatic pathology.
   D. The rim sign is typically associated with early stage acute cholecystitis.
   E. If patient has eaten within the last 8 hours, the study should be delayed.

3. Regarding hepatobiliary scintigraphy, biliary dyskinesia, and/or sphincter of Oddi dysfunction, which ONE of the following is correct?
   A. Both cholecystokinin and fatty meal challenge have similar efficacy in diagnosing biliary dyskinesia.
   B. The most physiologic mimic with cholecystokinin infusion is a slow injection over a 3-minute period, followed by 30 minutes of scanning.
   C. An abnormal gallbladder ejection fraction is predictive of a good clinical response to cholecystectomy.
   D. A sphincter of Oddi protocol is used precholecystectomy to determine if sphincterotomy will be needed.
   E. To prevent a false-positive study for acute cholecystitis, morphine should be held prior to hepatobiliary scanning.

■ Answers and Explanations

Question 1

E. Correct! Giving pharmacologic intervention is the best next course of action. (The gallbladder has not filled, so the study is not complete.) The options for confirming filling of the gallbladder include (1) delayed imaging after 3 more hours (total of 4 hours postinjection) or (2) intravenous administration of morphine sulfate followed by 30 additional minutes of imaging. Morphine results in temporary spasm of the sphincter of Oddi (SOD;, facilitating flow through a patent cystic duct into the gallbladder. With either option, if the gallbladder does not fill, the study is positive for acute cholecystitis. Morphine administration permits the most rapid confirmation of acute cholecystitis.

Other choices and discussion

A. Radiotracer overlies both the common bile duct and gallbladder, and it is not clear that the gallbladder has filled. Visualization of the gallbladder confirms patency of the cystic duct and essentially excludes acute cholecystitis. Delayed imaging (performed immediately, 2 to 3 hours later, or even at 18 to 24 hours in the setting of severe hepatocellular dysfunction) is commonly performed when the gallbladder is not seen at 60 minutes. However, as the surgeon is seeking the fastest diagnosis, delayed images are not the best answer.

B. Anterior images are standard. At 60 minutes and with further delay, additional left anterior oblique and right lateral views are usually recommended. However, varying camera positioning at 60 minutes would not clarify the diagnosis in this case.

C. The patient must remain nothing by mouth (NPO) except for water throughout the study to avoid stimulating endogenous cholecystokinin (CCK) and subsequently contracting the gallbladder. Water will not stimulate CCK and helps to clear away unwanted duodenal radiotracer, which better displays the gallbladder. However, giving water would not confirm the diagnosis in this case.

D. The most common indication for a HIDA scan (as in this case) is to assess for acute cholecystitis, and that diagnosis cannot be confirmed at this point.

Question 2

B. Correct! hepatobiliary (HIDA) scanning is less sensitive for the detection of acalculous cholecystitis than it is for calculus cholecystitis. The sensitivity of HIDA scanning for acalculous cholecystitis is 80% (versus 97% for the more "typical" calculus cholecystitis).

Other choices and discussion

A. The HIDA scan is most commonly normal in the setting of chronic cholecystitis, although delayed gallbladder visualization after 1 hour may be seen. In general, scintigraphic evaluation of chronic cholecystitis is less accurate than it is with acute cholecystitis.

C. Enterogastric reflux *before* CCK administration implies symptomatic pathology (bile gastritis). Make sure to look for this often overlooked sign. However, after CCK administration, enterogastric reflux may occur normally and does not need to be reported.

D. The rim sign is seen in 30% of patients with acute cholecystitis. However, this sign is associated with *later stage* acute cholecystitis, including gangrenous cholecystitis.

E. For the prep, remember 4 hours and 24 hours. The patient must be NPO for more than 4 hours (to allow the contracted gallbladder to subsequently relax and distend appropriately), and NPO for less than 24 hours, to prevent excessive stasis.

Question 3

C. Correct! An abnormal gallbladder ejection fraction (GBEF) is predictive of a good clinical response to cholecystectomy. To calculate, GBEF = [(net GB max) − (net GB min)/(net GB max)] × 100.

Other choices and discussion

A. Although fatty food does result in gallbladder contraction, no universally recognized numerical fatty food ejection fraction standards exist.

B. The most physiologic mimic with CCK is a slow intravenous push over 1 hour, generally accomplished with the aid of an injection device. Normal GBEF is ≥ 38%.

D. The SOD protocol is used postoperatively. About 10% of cholecystectomy patients have postoperative pain. SOD dysfunction behaves like a physiologic partial biliary obstruction after cholecystectomy. The SOD protocol scan takes into account numerous data points, collectively determining how well the radiotracer passes into the small bowel.

E. While it is true that narcotics should be held at least three half lives (or approximately 6 hours) prior to HIDA scanning, narcotics do not prevent gallbladder visualization. Narcotics delay bowel visualization through contraction of the SOD, mimicking a functional biliary obstruction.

■ Suggested Readings

Tulchinsky M, Ciak BW, Debelke D, et al. SNM practice guideline for hepatobiliary scintigraphy 4.0. J Nucl Med Technol 2010;38(4):210–218

Top Tips

- Cardiac blood pool activity usually clears rapidly with HIDA scanning (over 5 to 15 minutes). Prominent cardiac uptake still seen at 60 minutes suggests hepatocellular dysfunction.

- The SOD protocol is used in the postcholecystectomy patient with pain to assess for functional delayed biliary clearance.

- False-positive HIDA scan: NPO < 4 hours or > 24 hours, hepatic dysfunction, hyperalimentation, concurrent severe illness, and prior cholecystectomy.

Essentials 2

SECTION IX
NUCLEAR MEDICINE
IMAGING

■ Case

A patient presents with hypercalcemia. Parathyroid scan is shown.

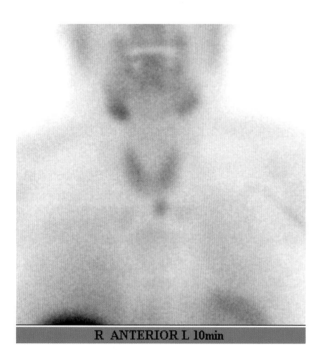
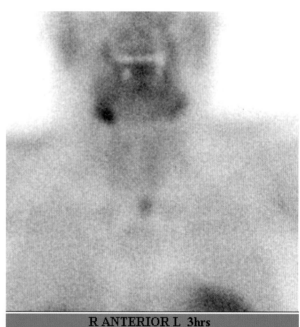

R ANTERIOR L 10min

R ANTERIOR L 3hrs

■ Questions

1. Which ONE of the following is correct?
   A. Standard imaging for this study should include the neck and the entire chest.
   B. This patient almost certainly has both an elevated parathyroid hormone level and an elevated serum calcium level.
   C. The main utility of this sestamibi scan is to differentiate malignancy from primary hyperparathyroidism as the cause of this patient's hypercalcemia.
   D. This patient has a 5 to 10% chance of having more than one parathyroid adenoma.
   E. In the neck, this sestamibi uptake is specific for a parathyroid adenoma.

2. Regarding the treatment for hyperparathyroidism, which ONE of the following correct?
   A. Both medical and surgical treatment in this patient will result in similar outcomes.
   B. If this patient has surgery, his chance of postoperative recurrence is 25%.
   C. The surgeon will likely check intraoperative calcium levels to confirm surgical success.

   D. With newer surgical technique, the need for preoperative scintigraphy has declined.
   E. The parathyroid gland is sometimes surgically implanted into the forearm.

3. Regarding scintigraphy of hyperparathyroidism, which ONE of the following is correct?
   A. The normal parathyroid glands are often seen with sestamibi scintigraphy.
   B. The most common false-negative is a poorly vascularized adenoma.
   C. The most common false-positive is a thyroid adenoma.
   D. Several large studies have demonstrated the benefit of single-photon emission computed tomography over planar imaging.
   E. A positive scintigraphic study must demonstrate a nodule with early increased activity and delayed washout (when compared to the thyroid gland).

■ Answers and Explanations

Question 1

D. Correct! The chance that this patient has more than one parathyroid adenoma is 5 to 10%. Additional adenomas are frequently missed on imaging, often because of their small size. (This study is positive for a parathyroid adenoma.)

Other choices and discussion

A. Standard imaging for this study should include the neck and the *upper* chest. The majority of parathyroid adenomas occur near the thyroid gland, but approximately 5% of adenomas are ectopic, occurring as high as the carotid bifurcation and low as the level of the pericardium. Adenomas may be seen retrotracheal, paracardiac, and rarely intrathyroidal. Imaging of the lower chest is not helpful, however.

B. Although the majority of patients do have concomitant parathyroid hormone (PTH) and serum calcium laboratory abnormalities, about 20% of patients have only one or the other lab abnormality at a time.

C. Malignancy (the second most common cause of hypercalcemia) is associated with suppressed PTH levels, whereas primary hyperparathyroidism (the most common cause of hypercalcemia) has normal or elevated PTH levels. By the time the patient is imaged, the diagnosis of hyperparathyroidism has very likely already been made. The scan is not primarily used to distinguish these entities.

E. Sestamibi is a perfusion agent, and adenomas have high vascularity. However, sestamibi uptake is nonspecific. It has been used with success to identify various malignant masses, including lung cancer, gliomas, and primary bone neoplasms. In addition, thyroid pathology may be seen with sestamibi.

Question 2

E. Correct! The gland is sometimes surgically implanted into the forearm. This is especially the case with hyperplasia surgery, where 3.5 glands are removed.

Other choices and discussion

A. Surgery is the treatment of choice.

B. Treatment is usually curative, although there is a reported 5% recurrence rate. Etiologies of recurrence include ectopic adenoma, failure to diagnose hyperplasia, and a fifth parathyroid gland. Reoperation has a worse outcome and greater morbidity, so it is important to diagnose correctly the first time.

C. The surgeon does measure intraoperative lab values. However, the *PTH* is measured, not the calcium. Success is defined as an intraoperative reduction of PTH by 50%. If that value is not achieved, further surgery is needed.

D. The more extensive standard bilateral neck exploration of the past had a high success rate ($> 90\%$), and the need for preoperative localization for an initial surgery at that time was debated. However, new minimally invasive surgery permits a smaller neck exploration, and the need for preoperative localization has actually increased. Newer techniques lead to less complications and shorter operating room times.

Question 3

C. Correct! The most common false-positive is a thyroid adenoma. Thyroid cancer and parathyroid cancer may also mimic an adenoma on scintigraphy.

Other choices and discussion

A. Normal parathyroid glands are not seen. Visualization suggests pathology.

B. The most common false-negative is a small-sized adenoma. False-negatives may also be seen with a second adenoma or with four-gland hyperplasia.

D. No large studies have convincingly shown that single-photon emission computed tomography (SPECT) is better than planar imaging, although most experienced readers do believe that SPECT helps, especially with localization. One large study did compare early and delayed imaging with planar, SPECT, and SPECT/computed tomography; SPECT/computed tomography early with any type of delayed imaging was the best.

E. Although early increased activity and delayed washout is the most common parathyroid adenoma pattern, variations exist. For example, early washout may also occur. The key to making the diagnosis is to detect any focal perfusion abnormality in a suspicious area. Anatomic correlation is often helpful to confirm that the presumed parathyroid adenoma is not a thyroidal mass.

■ Suggested Readings

Phillips CD, Shatzkes DR. Imaging of the parathyroid glands. Semin Ultrasound CT MR 2012;33(2):123–129

Wong KK, Fig LM, Gross MD, Dwamena BA. Parathyroid adenoma localization with 99mTc-sestamibi SPECT/CT: a meta-analysis. Nucl Med Commun 2015;36(4):363–375

Top Tips

- Hyperparathyroidism etiology: adenoma 85%, hyperplasia 10%, ectopic location of adenoma ($< 5\%$), and carcinoma (rare).

- A negative parathyroid scintigraphic study (in a suspicious clinical setting) should raise concern for multiple gland hyperplasia or small parathyroid adenomas.

- Any focal perfusion abnormality (in a suspicious clinical setting) should be viewed with concern for parathyroid adenoma and anatomically correlated.

Essentials 3

■ Case

Suspected brain death.

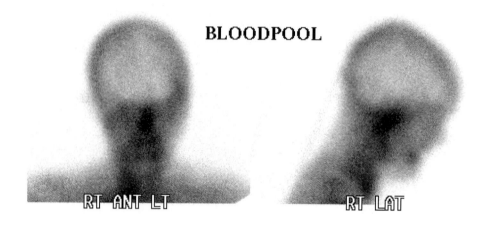

■ Questions

1. Which ONE of the following is correct?
   A. Regardless of the clinical findings, the nuclear test confirms brain death.
   B. Nearly all "almost" brain dead studies (activity restricted to a small portion of the brain) progress to brain death.
   C. If brain flow is seen and the patient condition worsens, the study should be repeated the following day.
   D. Lack of the flow to the brain with brain death is the result of low cardiac output.
   E. The "hot nose" sign is specific for brain death.

2. Regarding the radiopharmaceuticals and the diagnosis of brain death, which ONE of the following is correct?
   A. Agents must be able to cross the blood–brain barrier.
   B. Tc-99m HMPAO and Tc-99m ECD are the preferred agents to diagnose brain death.
   C. A flat line EEG is a good alternative to scintigraphy for confirming brain death.
   D. Peripheral scalp activity precludes the strict diagnosis of brain death.
   E. The size of catheter used for injection must be at least 20 gauge or larger.

3. Regarding seizure workup, which ONE of the following is correct?
   A. The main utility of PET or SPECT of the brain for seizure assessment is to verify seizure activity.
   B. Fludeoxyglucose (FDG) positron emission tomography (PET)/computed tomography (CT) provides a better image than does a SPECT scan, but it is technically less feasible to perform a PET/CT.
   C. Ictal imaging reports a 50% success rate for localization.
   D. Interictal imaging reports a 25 to 30% success rate for localization.
   E. Most patients in the United States receive SPECT imaging prior to seizure resection surgery.

■ Answers and Explanations

Question 1

B. Correct! Patients with minimal perfusion of the brain nearly always progress to complete brain death. However, if any part of the brain is perfused, the study cannot be reported as positive for brain death.

Other choices and discussion

A. The nuclear scan supports the clinical diagnosis of brain death. The important medicolegal point to remember is that brain death is a clinical diagnosis.

C. The radiotracer in the brain persists for up to 48 hours, so next-day imaging is not an option. In general, a brain death study is simple to perform and can be done at the bedside.

D. Brain death results in cerebral edema, which causes increased intracranial pressure and absent intracranial perfusion. On scintigraphy, the diagnosis is made when there is a good injection bolus, good flow in the common carotids approaching the base of skull, but absolutely no flow within the brain.

E. While it is true that the hot nose is often seen with brain death (as a result of shunting from the internal carotid artery to the external carotid artery circulation), this finding is not specific and cannot be used to verify the diagnosis. A hot nose could also be seen, for example, in a patient with an internal carotid artery occlusion but normal brain function.

Question 2

B. Correct! Tc-99m HMPAO and Tc-99m ECD both cross the blood<en dash>brain barrier and are the preferred agents for brain death evaluation. Tc-99m hexamethylpropyleneamine oxime and Tc-99m ECD are easier to interpret than previously used perfusion agents, and they are the radiopharmaceuticals of choice. Unlike diethylenetriamine-pentaacetic acid (DTPA), these radiotracers bind to the cerebral cortex. Static planar images performed shortly after injection demonstrate the lack of brain parenchymal uptake with brain death. The flow images are still important to the diagnosis and act as a safety check in the rare case of an improperly prepared radiopharmaceutical.

Other choices and discussion

A. Although Tc-99m DTPA does not cross the blood–brain barrier, this agent can still be used to diagnose brain death and, in fact, was used for many years for this purpose. DTPA is limited because it cannot bind to the cerebral cortex. However, early flow images that demonstrate perfusion to the brain exclude brain death. As DTPA tracer did not cross the blood–brain barrier, visualizing the transient flow with a bolus injection was necessary. This method was more prone to error. For example, a poor bolus could theoretically cause a false-positive for brain death.

C. A flat line EEG is not an acceptable alternative for confirming brain death. Although this finding is seen with brain death, there are also false-positive causes of flat EEGs, including barbiturates or hypothermia.

D. Peripheral activity in the scalp skin comes from the external circulation, and brain death may still be accurately diagnosed despite this overlying activity. Some investigators have found a rubber band around the skull to be helpful. Other areas of superficial inflammation in the setting of trauma may also show uptake.

E. There is no specific mandated catheter size for the use of brain death assessment by the American College of Radiology or the Society of Nuclear Medicine guidelines. In all cases, a good bolus must be confirmed.

Question 3

B. Correct! The best nuclear imaging available to localize a seizure patient's inciting focus is with FDG PET performed ictal (injection within 2 minutes of the seizure). However, this is extremely impractical to accomplish, given the short half-life of the radiotracer. The next best option is SPECT performed interictal (between periods of seizures). The syringe containing the SPECT agent may be kept nearby when seizure activity is assessed as an inpatient.

Other choices and discussion

A. The vast majority of the time, the clinical diagnosis of seizure activity has already been made at the time of scintigraphy. The main utility of brain PET or SPECT for seizure assessment is localization.

C. Ictal imaging is often challenging to accomplish, but reports an 80 to 90% localization success rate. Increased uptake on PET or SPECT during ictal scanning represents the abnormal focus.

D. Interictal imaging reports a 70% localization success. Decreased uptake on PET or SPECT during interictal scanning represents the abnormal focus.

E. The majority of seizure foci develop in the medial temporal lobe, and this area is often resected with good results. The EEG, the clinical history, and high-resolution epilepsy protocol magnetic resonance imaging identify the pathologic substrate in > 85% of patients. Scintigraphy is only used for problem cases.

■ Suggested Readings

American College of Radiology. ACR Standard for the Performance of Cerebral Scintigraphy for Brain Death. ACR Standards. Reston, VA: American College of Radiology; 1998: 173–175

Top Tips

- Ictal versus interictal. It is "icky" to witness a seizure (ictal). Interictal occurs between those periods.

- For brain death, some experts believe it is a good idea to image the kidneys (to ensure adequate systemic perfusion) and image the injection site (to exclude significant extravasation of radiotracer).

- For brain death, most experts believe that planar imaging suffices, although a minority of institutions use SPECT.

Essentials 4

■ Case

This patient has a possible lower gastrointestinal bleed. Nuclear medicine technetium-99m tagged red blood cell gastrointestinal bleed scan was performed and an image at 30 minutes is shown.

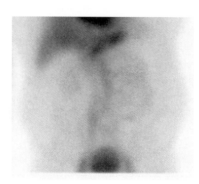

■ Questions

1. Which ONE of the following is correct?
    A. The study is positive for gastrointestinal bleed.
    B. The study is complete and is negative for gastrointestinal bleed.
    C. The best next course of action is immediate catheter angiography.
    D. The activity overlying the central pelvis is likely bladder.
    E. Review of the cine images would probably help greatly in this case.

2. Regarding the technical aspects of gastrointestinal bleed scintigraphy, which ONE of the following is correct?
    A. Sulfur colloid may be used as an alternative agent.
    B. For a study that is clearly positive within the first hour, delayed imaging at 4 to 8 hours is still usually helpful.
    C. Barium within loops of bowel does not pose a problem.

    D. Delayed imaging up to 24 hours is often helpful at localizing the site of bleeding.
    E. If the Ultra tag kit (Mallinckrodt Pharmaceuticals, Dublin, Ireland) is not available, the in vivo method of red blood cell labeling is a good option.

3. Regarding the diagnostic efficacy of gastrointestinal bleed scans, which ONE of the following is correct?
    A. Gastrointestinal bleed scans have 93% sensitivity and 95% specificity.
    B. Gastrointestinal bleeding scintigraphy is of little value unless positive studies are followed with an angiogram.
    C. Diffuse activity in the stomach is usually pathologic.
    D. Nonbowel causes of active bleeding cannot be identified with a tagged red blood cell gastrointestinal bleed scan.
    E. A gastrointestinal bleed scan is of little value for an upper gastrointestinal bleed.

■ Answers and Explanations

Question 1

D. Correct! The activity overlying the central pelvis is likely bladder. The key point is that normal bladder activity (or vascular blush from the penis or uterus) may mask the central lower pelvis assessment.

Other choices and discussion

A. No gastrointestinal (GI) bleed is identified at this point.

B. Although there is no GI bleed seen, the study is not complete. Imaging should be obtained for at least 60 minutes.

C. The best next move is delayed images. If the study becomes positive for GI bleed, catheter angiography might then be indicated. Angiography is not indicated after a negative GI bleed scan.

E. Although review of the cine images is routinely advised, there is no suggestion of even subtle bleeding in the test case. In this particular case, cine would be very unlikely to reveal bleeding.

Question 2

A. Correct! The advantages of the sulfur colloid GI bleed scan include that manipulating the patient's blood is not required and the images themselves suffer less from confounding background uptake. The main disadvantage of the sulfur colloid GI bleed scan is the decreased sensitivity, as sulfur colloid requires even more brisk bleeding for detection. This limitation occurs because the liver and spleen rapidly extract the sulfur colloid (within about 20 minutes), and repeat injections may be required. Numerous comparative studies have confirmed the superiority of tagged RBC scans to sulfur colloid GI bleed scans.

Other choices and discussion

B. A positive study that identifies and localizes the bleed within 1 hour is complete. Further imaging would only serve to delay catheter angiography/other definitive therapy.

C. Barium is not an absolute contraindication, but may cause unwanted photopenic defects.

D. Delayed imaging up to 24 hours is often advised to confirm that a bleed has occurred. However, a 24-hour image is usually not capable of localizing the site of the bleed.

E. When compared to other scintigraphic uses for tagged red blood cells (i.e., multigated acquisition scan, liver hemangioma scan, or splenic scan with heat-damaged red blood cell scan), the GI bleed scan requires the best tag available. This is because free pertechnetate in the stomach and the genitourinary system is quite problematic and often results in false-positive GI bleed scan studies. The in vivo method of labeling RBC or a sulfur colloid scan are options for patients who will not accept the injection of blood.

Question 3

A. Correct! GI bleed scans have 93% sensitivity and 95% specificity for detecting bleeding. This data refers to mid- or lower GI bleeds. The most common site for lower GI bleed is the colon.

Other choices and discussion

B. Even if catheter angiography is not performed, scintigraphy remains useful to make the diagnosis, to stratify risk, and to shape therapy/plan for definitive procedures based on location and rapidity of bleeding.

C. Diffuse activity in the stomach is usually the result of free pertechnetate. By the time scintigraphy is performed, most patients have already had a nasogastric tube placed, which should be able to exclude gastric bleeding. Gastritis could mimic free pertechnetate on a GI bleed scan and is difficult to exclude. Blood is nearly always mobile, so check for movement over time.

D. The radiotracer labels all the blood in the body, so any abnormal accumulation would theoretically be seen. However, bleeding areas that do not reach the GI tract may be more difficult to identify, as the GI tract affords easy visualization through mobility. For example, an active psoas bleed might appear as focal nonmobile accumulation of radiotracer. But keep in mind that tagged RBC scans may be used to detect occult bleeding elsewhere in the body.

E. Although this study is typically performed to assess mid- or lower GI bleeding, the scan is capable of detecting upper GI bleeding. Usually this is not needed, however, as nasogastric lavage is typically performed immediately, followed by endoscopy for suspected upper GI bleed.

■ Suggested Readings

Dam HQ, Brandon DC, Grantham VV, Hilson AJ, Howarth DM, Maurer AH, et al. The SNMMI Procedure Standard/EANM Practice Guideline for Gastrointestinal Bleeding Scintigraphy 2.0 . J Nucl Med Tech 2014;42(4):308–317

Zuckier LS. Acute gastrointestinal bleeding. Semin Nucl Med 2003;33(4):297–231

Top Tips

- The three key criteria for diagnosing an active lower GI bleed on a GI bleed scan include activity outside of the expected anatomic blood pool, a change in intensity of that activity on consecutive images, and movement of that activity.

- When fixed and diffuse gastric activity is seen, consider taking a quick anterior spot neck image. If you see salivary and thyroid uptake, then free pertechnetate must be present, which also explains the gastric activity.

- Distal colonic blood is an exception to the rule of mobility and may not move.

Essentials 5

SECTION IX
NUCLEAR MEDICINE
IMAGING

■ Case

A 51-year-old with multigated acquisition scan prechemotherapy. Current left ventricular ejection fraction is 48%. Previous left ventricular ejection fraction was 58%.

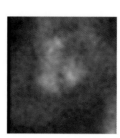

■ Questions

1. Which of the following are possible causes of this decrease? (Select ALL that apply.)
   A. Chemotherapy
   B. Heparin use
   C. Arrhythmia
   D. Technical error, with the region of interest including too much left atrium
   E. Technical error, with left ventricular ejection fraction assessment based on the left anterior oblique view

2. Regarding technetium-99m labeling of red blood cells for multigated acquisition scans, which ONE of the following is the best answer?
   A. The highest possible level of labeling is needed for a multigated acquisition scan.
   B. The Ultra tag kit (Mallinckrodt Pharmaceuticals, Dublin, Ireland) yields 85% labeling efficiency.
   C. To perform the highest yield tag, inject stannous ion, wait 15 minutes, and then inject Tc-99m pertechnetate.
   D. Suboptimal labeling may result from recent blood transfusions, abnormalities of stannous ion preparation, or anemia.
   E. Use of stannous pyrophosphate is optional.

3. Regarding multigated acquisition scanning, which ONE of the following is the best answer?
   A. Multigated acquisition and myocardial perfusion imaging are equally accurate in assessing left ventricular ejection fraction.
   B. Compared to echocardiography, a multigated acquisition scan is more difficult to perform in pulmonary patients.
   C. Oncologists will often alter treatment based on an absolute drop in left ventricular ejection fraction of > 10%.
   D. Left ventricular ejection fraction is the only parameter needed for a good multigated acquisition interpretation.
   E. With a multigated acquisition scan, the left ventricular ejection fraction is calculated as follows: EF = (ES − ED)/ES.

■ Answers and Explanations

Question 1

A. Correct! The most common cardiotoxic medications are used to treat breast cancer and lymphoma. Adriamycin (doxorubicin) results in cumulative toxicity and Herceptin (trastuzumab) results in noncumulative toxicity.

B. Correct! Heparin can reduce labeling efficiency, increase free pertechnetate, increase background activity, and decrease the accuracy of the LVEF. Other problematic medications include some antibiotics, anticonvulsants, antihypertensives, and anti-inflammatory agents.

C. Correct! Arrhythmias can impair the accuracy of a MUGA scan. This scan requires gating with the cardiac cycle, and moderate disturbances in rhythm will cause inaccuracies. For quality control, look for rejected beats. Greater than 10% rejected beats (from preventricular contractions or rapid atrial fibrillation with irregular ventricle response) could cause errors and are a red flag. The time activity curve should look the same at the end as it did at the beginning. Too many rejected beats cause a falloff in counts at the end at a much greater rate.

D. Correct! A common problem with MUGA scanning is un-wanted inclusion of the left atrium in the region of interest. Normally, the left atrium is posterior to the left ventricle, but when the left atrium is enlarged, its counts are included in the calculation, and this falsely lowers the ejection fraction.

Other choice and discussion

E. The left anterior oblique (LAO) is actually the view that is typically used to measure the LVEF. The three standard views for a MUGA include the anterior, the anterior 45-degree oblique (LAO), and the left lateral. The LAO is also known as the "best septal" as it optimally depicts the intraventricular septum and allows for the most accurate view for LVEF calculation.

Question 2

D. Correct! Suboptimal labeling may result from recent blood transfusions, abnormalities of stannous ion preparation, or anemia. To perform a MUGA scan, an exhaustive medication scrutiny is not needed routinely, but if there is a discrepancy in LVEF between serial studies that does not seem to make sense, keep in mind that there is a long list of potential explanations.

Other choices and discussion

A. The highest level of tag is needed for a gastrointestinal bleed scan but not for a MUGA scan. Of course, better tags are always more optimal, but for the majority of MUGA scan patients, adequate tagging is achieved even with the lowest level of efficiency, which is the in vivo method.

B. The Ultra tag kit yields 98% labeling efficiency, "in vivo" yields 80% labeling efficiency, and "modified in vivo" yields 85 to 90% labeling efficiency.

C. To perform the lowest yield tag, inject stannous ion, wait 15 minutes, and then inject technetium-99m pertechnetate. This describes the "in vivo" method. In patients with renal failure or receiving full-dose heparin therapy, the stannous dose may need to be increased.

E. All methods of labeling require stannous pyrophosphate to "pre-tin" the red blood cells, which permits binding of the pertechnetate to the beta chain of the hemoglobin molecule.

Question 3

C. Correct! Oncologists will often alter treatment based on an absolute drop in LVEF of > 10%. Typical oncology management of cardiotoxicity:

- If the patient has a normal baseline LVEF of > 50%: moderate toxicity is defined as a decline of > 10% in absolute LVEF, with a final LVEF of < 50%.
- If the patient has an abnormal baseline LVEF of 30 to 50%: a study is performed before each dose. Doxorubicin is stopped with an absolute decrease in LVEF of 10% or a final LVEF of 30% or less.
- If the patient has an abnormal baseline LVEF of < 30%: medication is not started.

With Adriamycin, one-third of patients develop cardiotoxicity with cumulative doses > 550 mg/m².

Other choices and discussion

A. MUGA is more accurate than myocardial perfusion imaging in assessing LVEF. The basic principle for a MUGA scan is that count rate is proportional to ventricular volume. MUGA and echocardiography are similar in accuracy.

B. Compared to echocardiography, a MUGA scan is easier to perform in pulmonary patients.

D. The following should all be assessed when interpreting a MUGA scan: contractility, global and regional wall abnormalities, cardiac chamber size, and extracardiac pathology such as aneurysm or pericardial effusion. Wall motion abnormalities should also be characterized. Absent wall motion is akinetic, decreased wall motion is hypokinetic, and paradoxical wall motion (seen with aneurysm) is dyskinetic.

E. With a MUGA scan, the LVEF is calculated as follows: $EF = (ED - ES)/ED$. Background activity must first be subtracted from ED and ES counts.

■ Suggested Readings

Skrypniuk JV, Bailey D, Cosgriff PS, Fleming JS, Houston AS, Jarritt PH, et al. UK audit of left ventricular ejection fraction estimation from equilibrium ECG gated blood pool images. Nucl Med Commun 2005;26:205–215

Top Tips

- Physicians checking MUGA scans should confirm a good photopenic septum.
- Falsely elevated LVEF: poor atrial or ventricular separation, falsely high background, ROI at end systole that cuts off a portion of the left ventricle.
- Falsely decreased LVEF: falsely low background leading to insufficient background subtraction, end diastolic ROI that includes a portion of the left ventricle, and end diastolic ROI that includes atrial activity.

Essentials 6

■ Case

Renal scan with Lasix in a 28-year-old patient with left flank pain.

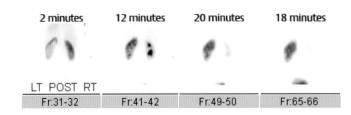

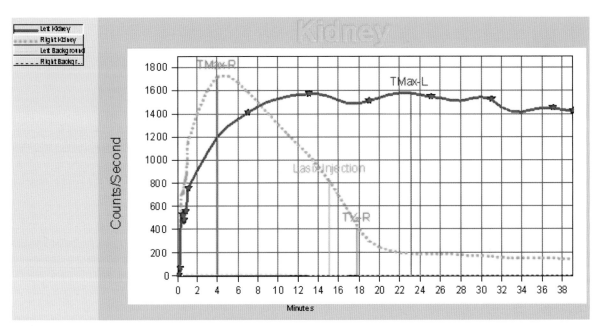

■ Questions

1. Which ONE of the following diagnoses is correct?
   A. Multicystic dysplastic left kidney
   B. Limited study because of poor renal function
   C. Mechanically obstructed left kidney
   D. Dilated, but not mechanically obstructed, left kidney
   E. Essentially normal study

2. Regarding Lasix renal scintigraphy interpretation, which ONE of the following is correct?
   A. A half time ($T\frac{1}{2}$) of > 20 minutes suggests mechanical obstruction.
   B. A $T\frac{1}{2}$ of 15 to 20 minutes is normal.
   C. Lasix scans remain very effective with marked renal dysfunction.

D. Lasix renal scans are particularly accurate in the very young patient.
   E. Unilateral renal obstruction often results in a limited study bilaterally.

3. Regarding technical tips for performing Lasix scintigraphy, which ONE of the following is correct?
   A. Nephrostomy tube patients should have the tube clamped before scanning.
   B. Voiding before the scan is optional.
   C. The standard Lasix dose for all patients is 20 mg.
   D. It is crucial to delay Lasix administration until at least 10 minutes postradiopharmaceutical.
   E. The half time ($T\frac{1}{2}$) should always be calculated after Lasix administration.

■ Answers and Explanations

Question 1

C. Correct! There is poor excretion on the left from the collecting system despite Lasix administration. This is reflected on the time activity curve, with an initial positive slope that remains horizontal. This is the typical appearance of a mechanical obstruction.

Other choices and discussion

A. With multicystic dysplastic kidney, multiple cysts replace part or all of the normally functioning renal tissue. Multicystic dysplastic kidney is found in young children, and the affected kidney has usually either completely regressed or is severely atrophic by adulthood.

B. Although we are not given the patient's serum creatinine, the target-to-background ratio appears satisfactory (i.e., the visual quality of the study is good). In addition, the bladder and collecting systems are promptly seen. These findings suggest normal renal function.

D. If the left kidney was dilated, but not mechanically obstructed, the kidney would be abnormal prior to Lasix, but would promptly excrete after Lasix.

E. At the very least, we can easily see the asymmetry between the kidneys. This is not normal.

Question 2

A. Correct! A $T\frac{1}{2}$ of > 20 minutes suggests mechanical obstruction. After an anatomic study (ultrasound, computed tomography, or magnetic resonance imaging) demonstrates hydronephrosis, the Lasix renal scan is performed to determine the functional significance. (In the past, the invasive Whitaker test was used for this purpose.) Lasix is usually administered after activity is seen in the collecting system. If there is a brisk response to the Lasix, then there is no high-grade mechanical obstruction. Unlike an intravenous pyelogram or computed tomography, the renal scan may be numerically quantified.

Other choices and discussion

B. The $T\frac{1}{2}$ quantifies the rate of excretion from the collecting system. Most nuclear medicine experts believe that a $T\frac{1}{2}$ of < 10 minutes is normal, 10 to 20 minutes is indeterminate, and > 20 minutes is consistent with mechanical obstruction. Some physicians use a $T\frac{1}{2}$ of < 15 minutes as normal.

C. Poor function may render the Lasix challenge nondiagnostic. As a general guideline, creatinine values above 3.0 often result in extremely limited studies.

D. Assessing hydronephrosis in a young child (aged 0 to 2 years) with Lasix scintigraphy may result in a false-positive study because of renal immaturity. Other causes of false-positive studies include partial obstruction, bladder overfilling, renal insufficiency, and longstanding capacious systems.

E. Unilateral renal impairment does not usually cause a rise of serum creatinine, as long as the contralateral kidney is normal. On occasion, acute renal insufficiency does result from unilateral stone-related obstruction, but that is the exception, not the rule.

Question 3

A. Correct! Nephrostomy tube patients should have the tube clamped before scanning. Otherwise, the tracer will be excreted (through the path of least resistance) into the tube. This could mimic "good excretion," even if the collecting system is actually blocked.

Other choices and discussion

B. A distended bladder may cause a false-positive study. Voiding before the scan is standard.

C. A sliding scale of diuretic based on the patient's serum creatinine is helpful in eliciting a response to Lasix. Sliding scale as follows: If the creatinine (Cr) is 1.0, give 20 mg Lasix. If Cr is 1.5, give 40 mg. If Cr is 2.0, give 60 mg. If Cr is 3.0, give 80 mg.

D. The timing of the Lasix administration after the radiopharmaceutical is not critical. In fact, some clinics use the "F-15 renogram," in which the Lasix is actually given 15 minutes *before* the radiotracer is injected.

E. Particularly in healthy patients, the radiotracer may excrete early on, even before Lasix is administered. In those cases, the $T\frac{1}{2}$ should be calculated prior to Lasix administration. Make sure to take the extra step of visually correlating the computer-generated $T\frac{1}{2}$ with the time activity curve.

■ Suggested Readings

Blickman JG, Parker BR, Barnes PD. Pediatric Radiology, The Requisites. Maryland Heights, MO: Mosby Inc.; 2009

Conway JJ. "Well-tempered" diuresis renography: its historical development, physiological and technical pitfalls, and standardized technique protocol. Semin Nucl Med 1992;22:74–84

Top Tips

- Calculate the $T\frac{1}{2}$ at the steepest part of the curve. This is usually after Lasix, but may occur prior to Lasix.

- The region of interest to assess response to Lasix should include the intrarenal collecting system and renal pelvis.

- Camera-based clearance measurements are considered precise, but not necessarily very *accurate*. This means that although the calculated numerical values like glomerular filtration rate and effective renal plasma flow may not be correct, serial studies are useful in determining progression or improvement in disease.

Essentials 7

■ **Case**

A patient with early satiety. Liquid and solid phase gastric emptying studies are shown.

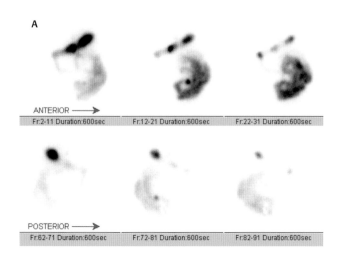

A

ANTERIOR ⟶
Fr:2-11 Duration:600sec   Fr:12-21 Duration:600sec   Fr:22-31 Duration:600sec

POSTERIOR ⟶
Fr:62-71 Duration:600sec   Fr:72-81 Duration:600sec   Fr:82-91 Duration:600sec

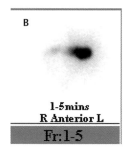

B

1-5mins
R Anterior L
Fr:1-5   Fr:56-60

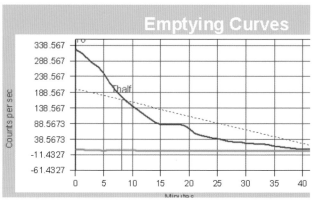

Emptying Curves
338.567
288.567
238.567
188.567   Thalf
138.567
88.5673
38.5673
-11.4327
-61.4327
Courts per sec
0   5   10   15   20   25   30   35   40
Minutes

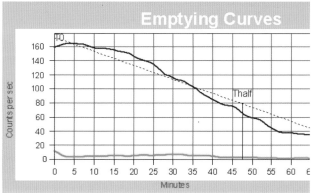

Emptying Curves
160
140
120
100   Thalf
80
60
40
20
0
Courts per sec
0   5   10   15   20   25   30   35   40   45   50   55   60   6
Minutes

■ **Questions**

1. Which ONE of the following is correct?
   A. Curve A is a normal solid phase gastric emptying curve.
   B. Curve B is a normal liquid phase gastric emptying curve.
   C. The actual images offer no diagnostic value.
   D. The normal solid gastric emptying half time is < 90 minutes.
   E. The normal liquid gastric emptying half time is < 23 minutes.

2. Regarding technique of gastric emptying studies, which ONE of the following is correct?
   A. The consensus gastric emptying paper permits the use of any solid food, provided it can be bound to technetium.
   B. Patient positioning affects the rate of emptying.
   C. There is no real downside to performing simultaneous liquid and solid phase imaging using two different radiopharmaceuticals.

   D. A single-headed gamma camera precludes the calculation of a geometric mean.
   E. If a patient eats only half of the meal, but the scan results are normal, the study should simply be reported as normal.

3. Regarding the role of gastric emptying, which ONE of the following is correct?
   A. Scintigraphy can usually differentiate a physiologic from an anatomic cause of delayed emptying.
   B. Gastric retention of > 10% of the meal at 4 hours is abnormal, and this is the single best discriminator of normal and abnormal motility.
   C. It is rare for the 4-hour data to detect delayed emptying that is not already seen at 2 hours.
   D. The downside of the new consensus protocol is that it is more time-consuming and results in less patient throughput than the old way.
   E. As liquid is less sensitive for the detection of delayed gastric emptying, if the solid study is normal, liquid assessment is not necessary.

■ Answers and Explanations

Question 1

E. Correct! The normal liquid gastric emptying half time is < 23 minutes. Although there is no recent consensus paper for liquids, this value is generally considered well established. As liquids normally empty rapidly, a liquid study should only require a maximum of 30 minutes of continuous imaging.

Other choices and discussion

A. Curve A is a normal liquid phase gastric emptying curve. Normally, a liquid curve is monoexponential. The larger the volume, the faster the emptying.

B. Curve B is a normal solid phase gastric emptying curve. Normally, a solid curve is biphasic. Solid emptying begins with a lag phase of 5 to 20 minutes (for grinding food into small particles). Then, the curve becomes linear.

C. The actual images are useful for quality control, a limited anatomic assessment, and to exclude reflux or aspiration.

D. A multispecialty consensus paper was established in 2008 with the following criteria: 1 hour > 10% emptying is normal; 2 hours > 40% emptying is normal; 4 hours > 90% emptying is normal; emptying > 70% at 1 hour is rapid. (Prior to the 2008 consensus, a half time of < 90 minutes was commonly used as normal.) Gastric motility scintigraphy is the gold standard for assessing the rate of gastric emptying.

Question 2

B. Correct! Emptying occurs from fastest to slowest, as follows: standing, then sitting, and then supine. Per the 2008 consensus, upright position imaging is preferred, but either upright or supine positioning is acceptable.

Other choices and discussion

A. The consensus protocol specifies the meal, which includes a low-fat egg white (or egg substitute) meal, toast, jam or jelly, and water. Alternative methods as requested by referring services may be performed and reported, but the conclusions are less clear, as these do not follow the consensus methods. Images are obtained at 0, 1, 2, and 4 hours.

C. There are several downsides to performing simultaneous liquid and solid phase imaging. From a mechanical perspective, the liquid will make the solid "less solid," and the solid will make the liquid "less liquid." Additionally, because of differing photopeaks, there may be downscatter (or even upscatter). Indium-111 has 171 and 247 keV photopeaks, whereas technetium-99m has a 140 keV photopeak. Advantages of dual simultaneous scintigraphy include both patient convenience and the ability to perform delayed intestinal scintigraphy (because of the indium tracer), which has recently become somewhat more popular.

D. The geometric mean with anterior and posterior images is best obtained with dual-headed cameras but can also be obtained with sequential anterior and posterior single-headed camera images.

The geometric mean is the most commonly used and the most accurate method of count calculation in nuclear medicine and is the square root of the (counts anterior × counts posterior).

E. If less than the whole meal is ingested, a disclaimer should be included in the report.

Question 3

B. Correct! Gastric retention of > 10% of the meal at 4 hours is abnormal, and this is the single best discriminator of normal and abnormal motility.

Normal limits for gastric retention are as follows. Lower limits (a lower value suggests rapid emptying): 0.5 hour: 70%; 1 hour: 30%. Upper limits (a higher value suggests delayed emptying): 1 hour: 90%; 2 hours: 60%; 3 hours: 30%; 4 hours: 10%.

Note that "retention" is just another way to view the same findings of "percent emptied," described in question 1.

Other choices and discussion

A. The strength of the gastric emptying study is the ability to identify and quantify the delayed emptying. The weakness is the lack of anatomy. If indicated, endoscopy may be needed.

C. The 4-hour image picks up 30% more delayed gastric emptying than does the 2-hour image alone. Of note, the test can be stopped at 2 hours if normal 4-hour values are achieved.

D. The new protocol is more efficient than the old protocol. Multiple (five or six patients) can be imaged during this time, and this can help with scheduling.

E. In the past, liquid assessment was considered less sensitive. That is now known to be false. A total of 30% of patients' delayed gastric emptying will only be detected with liquid gastric emptying.

■ Suggested Readings

American College of Radiology. ACR–SPR practice parameter for the performance of gastrointestinal scintigraphy. Revised 2015. Accessed June 2016. http://www.acr.org/~/media/26E5C0B4D8C2471FA7229E7B3B25DFF2.pdf

Top Tips

♦ Because liquid gastric emptying is typically rapid, small bowel overlap may erroneously "delay" gastric emptying time, and the images should be inspected to exclude this possibility.

♦ A patient with a percutaneous endoscopic gastrostomy tube may have a gastric emptying study performed directly through the percutaneous endoscopic gastrostomy tube.

♦ The best method for gastric emptying assessment utilizes anterior and posterior imaging with a geometric mean calculation.

Essentials 8

■ Case

A 44-year-old presents with right shoulder pain.

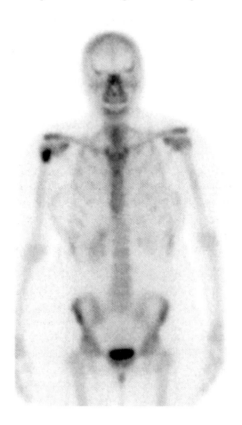

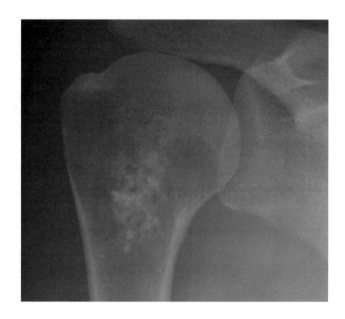

■ Questions

1. Which ONE of the following is the most likely diagnosis?
   A. Bone infarct
   B. Sclerotic metastasis
   C. Enchondroma
   D. Low-grade chondrosarcoma
   E. Benign cyst status post therapy

2. Regarding bone scan and bone lesions on plain film, which ONE of the following is correct?
   A. Bone islands are always normal on bone scan.
   B. Bone scans are usually normal in patients with multiple myeloma.
   C. The main utility for a bone scan in the assessment of a bone lesion is to determine the grade of malignancy.
   D. Lack of bone scan uptake for a sclerotic or chondrous lesion strongly suggests benignity.
   E. One benign bone lesion that is often very hot on bone scan is a nonossifying fibroma.

3. Regarding bone scintigraphy, which ONE of the following is correct?
   A. Progression of metastatic disease is best differentiated from the "flare phenomenon" on bone scan by demonstration of new lesions.
   B. Isolated sternal uptake in patients with breast cancer is very likely benign.
   C. Bilateral axillary uptake is usually clinically insignificant.
   D. Cardiac uptake could not result from a recent Cardiolyte (Lantheus Medical Imaging, Inc., Billerica, MA) study as the two tests use different photopeaks.
   E. Bone scan is more sensitive for lytic bone metastases than for sclerotic bone metastases.

■ Answers and Explanations

Question 1

D. Correct! This is a low-grade chondrosarcoma. The plain film suggests either enchondroma or low-grade chondrosarcoma. With chondrosarcoma, the plain film may appear aggressive, with deep endosteal scalloping, lytic components, pathologic fracture, and soft tissue extension (none of which are demonstrated in this case). However, the bone scan shows intense uptake, and significant bone scan uptake with a chondroid lesion should always raise concern for an aggressive process.

Other choices and discussion

A. Although chondroid lesions and infarcts may be difficult to differentiate from each other on plain film, the test case depicts "rings and arcs." This is typical of a chondroid lesion and would not be seen with an osteoid-forming process. Infarcts often have well-defined sclerotic and serpiginous borders. On bone scan, infarcts demonstrate mild to moderate uptake, unless imaged very early in the disease (rare), in which case a photopenic defect is seen.

B. The intensity of uptake on bone scan in the test case is typical of a sclerotic metastatic lesion, but the unifocality, coupled with the plain film findings of a chondroid lesion, makes metastasis less likely.

C. The plain film findings do support a chondroid lesion, but the bone scan findings would be atypical for an enchondroma. Benign bone lesions (such as enchondromas) typically have little or no bone scan uptake. A total of 20% of enchondromas demonstrate mild uptake, and a very small percent of enchondromas do demonstrate more intense uptake.

E. Bone cysts do occur in the metaphysis and may undergo treatment with curettage and bone grafting, but are commonly seen in the first and second decades. Untreated bone cysts show little if any peripheral uptake. Had there been surgery with bone chips, some uptake on bone scan might be seen, but intense uptake would be unlikely.

Question 2

D. Correct! Lack of uptake for a sclerotic or chondroid lesion is very reassuring for benignity. Moderate uptake is indeterminate. Intense uptake is concerning for an aggressive process, although benign lesions may occasionally show intense uptake.

Other choices and discussion

A. Bone islands (enostosis) are normal compact bone within cancellous bone. These may be confused on plain film with metastases or osteosarcoma, and bone scan can be very helpful in distinguishing, as bone islands are typically not avid on bone scan. However, a small percentage of biopsy proven bone islands have demonstrated mild activity on bone scan.

B. Many myeloma lesions are normal on bone scan. However, the majority of patients with myeloma will have at least one area of abnormal uptake on whole body bone scan.

C. The main utility for a bone scan in the assessment of a bone lesion is (1) to determine the degree of uptake (which is often helpful in distinguishing benign from malignant) and (2) to assess for multifocality. The whole body assessment is a great strength of the bone scan.

E. Nonossifying fibroma is typically not very avid on bone scan. Three benign bone lesions known to have high uptake on bone scan include fibrous dysplasia, osteoid osteoma, and giant cell tumor.

Question 3

A. Correct! The flare phenomenon reflects healing, but presents on bone scan as increased osteoblastic activity at metastatic sites after initiation of treatment. This can last for 6 months. Flare can cause pain, which adds confusion. Computed tomography shows corresponding healing sclerosis. Demonstration of new lesions is helpful in suggesting progression of disease (rather than flare).

Other choices and discussion

B. Isolated sternal uptake in a patient with breast cancer is usually the result of metastatic disease. One study of 34 patients with breast cancer and isolated sternal uptake showed that 76% of those lesions representing metastases.

C. Ipsilateral axillary uptake on the side of injection is nearly always clinically insignificant. However, bilateral axillary uptake warrants further evaluation. Various pathologies including metastatic disease, lymphoma, and granulomatous disease may cause accumulation of radiotracer in lymph nodes.

D. Cardiac uptake on a bone scan could result from a recent Cardiolyte study as both studies use technetium-99m as the radiopharmaceutical.

E. Bone scan is more sensitive for sclerotic bone metastases than for lytic bone metastases. The opposite is true for bone lesions on fludeoxyglucose positron emission tomography/computed tomography, which is more sensitive for lytic lesions.

■ Suggested Readings

Frank JA, Ling A, Patronas NJ, et al. Detection of malignant bone tumors: MR imaging vs scintigraphy. Am J Roentgenol 1990;155(5):1043–1048

Top Tips

- ◆ Rib uptake in a patient with a known malignancy has a 10 to 20% chance of representing metastatic disease.

- ◆ Anterior rib end uptake is usually benign (posttraumatic). Linear rib uptake is more concerning for neoplasm.

- ◆ Although > 50% of myeloma lesions are not visible with bone scan, 75% of patients with multiple myeloma have an abnormal bone scan.

Essentials 9

■ Case

A patient 5 days status post laparoscopic cholecystectomy now presents with symptoms concerning for a biliary leak. Hepatobiliary scan image at 60 minutes is provided.

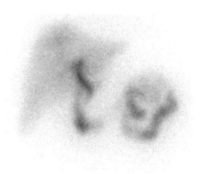

■ Questions

1. Which ONE of the following is true?
   A. Leak is confirmed.
   B. Leak is excluded.
   C. Cholecystokinin is indicated to stimulate a potential leak.
   D. Biliary leaks often respond well to conservative management.
   E. If present, a biliary drain should remain unclamped during the study.

2. Regarding single photon emission computed tomography, which ONE of the following is correct?
   A. It usually takes about 30 minutes to complete.
   B. It cannot be performed on radiopharmaceuticals with suboptimal imaging characteristics, such as I-131 NaI or In-111 WBC.
   C. The technologist must change the camera head to perform single photon emission computed tomography.
   D. At least two heads are required to perform single photon emission computed tomography.
   E. Single photon emission computed tomography/ computed tomography is a software upgrade that facilitates fusion.

3. Regarding scintigraphy and liver lesions, which ONE of the following is correct?
   A. On hepatobiliary scan, visualization of a focal liver lesion is highly suggestive of malignancy.
   B. Tagged red blood cell scan for liver hemangiomas is a very accurate test.
   C. Tagged red blood cell scan for splenic hemangiomas is not a very accurate test.
   D. The only liver lesion that is visible on a sulfur colloid scan is focal nodular hyperplasia.

■ Answers and Explanations

Question 1

D. Correct! Biliary leaks often respond well to conservative management. When interpreting the study, the size of the leak should be estimated (small or large) and the presence or absence of bile duct obstruction should be noted.

Other choices and discussion

A. No leak is seen.

B. Leak is not excluded at this point. Additional 2- to 4-hour delayed imaging is recommended prior to excluding a leak. Patient-positioning maneuvers (i.e., decubitus views) are also helpful in increasing the test sensitivity.

C. Cholecystokinin (CCK) is not indicated to stimulate a potential leak. CCK increases the production and subsequent secretion of bile. Although it is true that administering CCK would probably increase the sensitivity of the test, the downside of increasing the volume of unwanted free bile into the peritoneum outweighs the upside.

E. Bile flow will follow the path of least resistance. An unclamped biliary drain will permit flow into the tubing and the bag, leaving less for the potential site of leak. Thus, an unclamped drain could result in a false-negative leak study. Remember that if a drain is present, it should be clamped during the study.

Question 2

A. Correct! Single photon emission computed tomography (SPECT) usually takes about 30 minutes to complete.

Other choices and discussion

B. The lower count rates and the less optimal image quality seen when imaging with agents such as I-131 NaI or In-111 WBC do pose a challenge in performing quality SPECT. However, in select cases, it is exactly those limitations that mandate taking the extra step of trying SPECT in order to obtain a diagnostic image.

C. The standard camera head does not usually need to be changed to perform SPECT. SPECT is most commonly used with cardiac scans, brain scans, parathyroid scans, cases of back pain including failed back surgery, and oncologic scans including Octreotide and Prostascint. SPECT may occasionally help problem solve with other scans including HIDA scans.

D. Two heads are most commonly used for SPECT, but a single head or three heads are viable options. One study compared the results of single- and double-headed scans for myocardial SPECT. The study determined that of the 426 patients, the single head was actually superior in terms of specificity, but the double head was superior in terms of sensitivity and shorter acquisition time. The authors concluded that double head was preferred.

E. SPECT/computed tomography (CT) is an entirely separate imaging machine that permits nearly simultaneous scanning of both SPECT and CT. It has built-in fusion, similar to modern PET/CT scanners. Lower levels of fusion software are also available, at a much cheaper price, for use with separate SPECT and CT scanners. Software fusion solutions offer less precision than dedicated hardware fusion machinery.

Question 3

B. Correct! Tagged red blood cell (RBC) scan for liver hemangiomas is a very accurate test. A study from 2008 showed a sensitivity of 95% and a specificity of 98% for hepatic hemangiomas. The smallest lesion detected in this study was 0.8 cm. Larger lesions are easier to see and characterize. The typical appearance of a hepatic hemangioma on a tagged RBC scan is a hot spot within the liver on the delayed image.

Other choices and discussion

A. On hepatobiliary scan (HIDA), visualization of a focal liver lesion is not specific. Focal nodular hyperplasia, hepatic adenoma, and hepatocellular carcinoma all contain hepatocytes and may all be visualized on HIDA scans. Neither hemangiomas nor metastases is seen on HIDA.

C. Tagged RBC scan for splenic hemangiomas is a very accurate test. Although this has been studied less extensively, there are multiple reports of splenic hemangiomas following the same scintigraphic pattern as liver hemangiomas on tagged RBC scintigraphy. Hemangiomas are the most common benign masses of the spleen.

D. Although focal nodular hyperplasia is the most commonly seen mass on a sulfur colloid scan, hepatic adenomas may also demonstrate some uptake.

■ Suggested Readings

Bucerius J, Joe AY, Lindstaedt I, Manka-Waluch A, Reichmann K, Ezziddin S, et al. Single- vs. dual-head SPECT for detection of myocardial ischemia and viability in a large study population. Clin Imaging 2007;31(4):228–233

Mettler FA, Guiberteau MJ. Chapter 8. In: Essentials of Nuclear Medicine Imaging. 5th edition. Philadelphia, PA: Saunders; 2006: 203–242

Top Tips

◆ Ultrasound and CT can demonstrate fluid in the gallbladder fossa and in the right upper quadrant. HIDA can confirm that the fluid is biliary.

◆ Many bilomas resolve spontaneously. If needed, treatment may include percutaneous drainage, sphincterotomy, and stenting.

◆ Patients with bile leaks may present with gastrointestinal laboratory abnormalities, abdominal pain, nausea, vomiting, fever, jaundice, and increased biliary drainage. However, some patients with bile leaks are asymptomatic and have normal lab values.

Essentials 10

■ Case

A 140-pound patient presents with chest pain. Stress and rest portions of a myocardial perfusion imaging study are submitted.

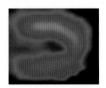 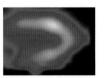

Stress   Rest

■ Questions

1. Which ONE of the following is the most likely diagnosis?
   A. Fixed infarct in the inferior wall
   B. Breast attenuation artifact
   C. Left bundle branch block artifact
   D. Reversible ischemia in the inferior wall, likely right coronary artery distribution
   E. Reversible ischemia, but myocardial perfusion imaging cannot estimate the vascular distribution

2. Statistical methods like Bayes theorem define the optimal patient population for selection of certain diagnostic tests. To diagnose coronary artery disease, which patient would benefit the most from a myocardial perfusion scan?
   A. A 27-year-old woman with shortness of breath. No prior medical history.
   B. A 61-year-old man with chest pain. No prior medical history.
   C. A 65-year-old man with chest pain. Previous myocardial infarction and 50 pack-year smoking history.
   D. A 34-year-old woman with intermittent chest pain. History of asthma.

3. Regarding radiopharmaceuticals used for myocardial perfusion imaging, which ONE of the following is correct?
   A. Sestamibi is hydrophilic and diffuses freely in and out of the myocardial cell.
   B. Myoview (GE Healthcare, Little Chalfont, United Kingdom; tetrofosmin) is similar to Cardiolyte (Lantheus Medical Imaging, Inc., Billerica, MA; sestamibi) but has more delayed liver clearance.
   C. After extraction, thallium undergoes redistribution in a continual exchange between myocardial cell and vascular blood pool.
   D. Advantages of thallium over sestamibi include superior image quality and lower effective radiation dose.
   E. Gating cannot be performed with thallium because of prohibitively low counts.

■ Answers and Explanations

Question 1

D. Correct! There is a reversible defect centered in the inferior wall.

Other choices and discussion

A. There is an inferior wall defect on the stress images that is not seen on the rest images. The defect reverses. An infarct would remain fixed.

B. Breast artifact typically occurs in large breasted women and usually remains fixed. (Less commonly, the defect may "reverse" if the patient positioning changes between stress and rest imaging.) This commonly seen fixed artifact occurs in the anterior and lateral walls.

C. A left bundle branch block defect is typically seen in the septum. It is accentuated by an elevation in heart rate and is therefore more pronounced with exercise testing (rather than with pharmacologic testing). This artifact may be fixed or reversible. One clue on the cine images is paradoxical septal motion, which is sometimes seen in these patients.

E. Although myocardial perfusion imaging is a physiologic test, anatomic distributions correlate reasonably well with defect locations, and these distributions should be suggested in reports. As general guidelines, the left anterior descending feeds the septum and anterior walls, the left circumflex feeds the lateral and inferior lateral walls, and the right coronary artery feeds the inferior septum and the inferior walls of the left ventricle.

Question 2

B. Correct! The epidemiology of patient B places him into an intermediate pretest probability for having the disease. A patient with an intermediate probability of coronary artery disease (CAD) is the most optimal candidate for a myocardial perfusion scan (when performed to diagnose disease).

Other choices and discussion

A. The patient in choice A is very unlikely to have the disease, and a positive scan would most likely represent a false-positive.

C. The patient in choice C has a very high chance of having the disease, and the myocardial perfusion scan would probably add little in the diagnosis of CAD. A positive scan would be expected, whereas a negative scan would most likely represent a false-negative.

D. The patient in choice D is very unlikely to have the disease, and a positive scan would most likely represent a false-positive.

Question 3

C. Correct! This thallium redistribution is advantageous for viability assessment. With normal myocardium, thallium (a potassium analog) clears in 3 hours. In ischemic states, uptake is delayed and reduced and clearance is slow. Rubidium, an agent used for cardiac positron emission tomography perfusion, is a thallium analog and behaves in a similar fashion.

Other choices and discussion

A. Sestamibi is *lipophilic* and is *fixed* in the mitochondria of myocardial cells. Because it is largely fixed in the heart, there is flexibility between the time of injection and the time of scanning. This is useful in the emergency setting, but problematic when assessing viability.

B. Tetrofosmin has more rapid liver clearance than does sestamibi and requires slightly less delay before scanning. This permits a faster throughput of patients compared to sestamibi patients. Nonetheless, sestamibi is more commonly used in the United States.

D. Advantages of *sestamibi over thallium* include superior image quality and lower effective radiation dose. Technetium-99m sestamibi and technetium-99m tetrofosmin have largely replaced thallium because of superior image quality and lower effective radiation dose. Thallium imaging begins sooner than technetium-based imaging, and should start as soon as the patient's heart rate has returned to baseline levels.

E. Thallium does have lower counts and gating is often not performed. However, numerous studies have validated that gating can be successfully performed with thallium. Gating is more challenging and somewhat less accurate and less precise with thallium than it is with technetium-based imaging.

■ Suggested Readings

Gibbons RJ, Balady GJ, Beasley JW, et al. ACC/AHA Guidelines for Exercise Testing. A report of the American College of Cardiology/American Heart Association Task Force on Practice Guidelines (Committee on Exercise Testing). J Am Coll Cardiol 1997;30(1):260–311

Top Tips

◆ A dual isotope protocol uses both thallium and technetium. This combines rapid throughput with the opportunity to assess viability.

◆ Patients with severe CAD may benefit from sublingual nitroglycerin administered several minutes prior to the pharmacologic administration. This can increase the sensitivity for detecting perfused tissue.

◆ Dose infiltration reduces the amount of available radiotracer and may result in artifacts, masking real defects.

Details 1

■ Case

A patient presents with back pain. Which ONE of the following is the best diagnosis?
   A. Discitis
   B. Multiple myeloma
   C. Metastatic disease
   D. Traumatic sequelae
   E. Postoperative change

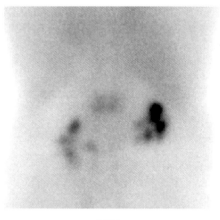
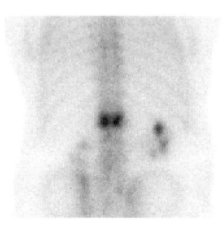

FLOW   POOL   3-HOUR DELAY

Flow, pool, and 3-hour delay.

■ The following questions pertain to bone scintigraphy.

1. In hyperparathyroidism, the typical pattern of extraosseous uptake is found in which organs?
2. True or False. Uptake within pleural fluid or ascites usually means underlying exudate.
3. A "superscan" is less commonly seen today than it was 20 years ago because of _____.
4. The "flare" phenomenon, sometimes seen after cancer treatment, usually lasts _____.
5. True or False. Ipsilateral axillary uptake (on the same side as the injection) is usually benign.
6. Significant free pertechnetate with technetium-99m (Tc-99m) methylene diphosphonate (MDP) leads to excessive uptake in the _____.

7. The highest target-to-background ratio with Tc-99m MDP is seen at ____ hours.
8. What percent of bone loss/turnover is needed for detection with bone scan?
9. Patients with prostate cancer with prostate-specific antigen levels < 10 ng/mL have a ____% chance of having osseous metastatic disease.
10. Approximately 70% of uncomplicated fractures normalize on bone scan by _____.

■ Answers and Explanations

A. Correct! This is a case of discitis. The typical appearance of discitis on bone scan is three-phase increased activity centered at the disc and affecting the adjacent vertebral body endplates. Although three-phase uptake is not a specific finding, the distribution of two contiguous levels in the spine makes a disc-based process (infection) much more likely than a bone-based process. With discitis, the bone is secondarily affected.

Other choices and discussion

Choices B, C, and D are not disc space based. Choice E could involve contiguous levels, but the intensity of uptake seen here would raise a strong concern for infection.

Question 1

In hyperparathyroidism, extraosseous uptake is found in the stomach, lungs, and kidneys.

Question 2

True. Uptake within pleural fluid or ascites on bone scan is usually exudative (and is usually malignant).

Question 3

A "superscan" is less commonly seen today than it was 20 years ago because of improved equipment. A "superscan" is a bone scan with diffuse osseous metastases that may be missed on initial inspection because of the extensive and relatively homogeneous malignant uptake throughout the bones. Because nearly all of the radiotracer is taken up in the bones on a superscan, one clue is the invariably poor visualization of the kidneys. Today, better image quality results in better resolution, and it is now easier to see the subtle metastatic inhomogeneity. Thus, a true "superscan" is less common.

Question 4

The "flare" phenomenon, sometimes seen after cancer treatment, usually lasts up to 6 months. The "flare" phenomenon, with increased intensity on bone scan in known metastatic lesions, indicates a favorable response to treatment. At the same time that the "flare" appears on bone scan, both sclerosis on computed tomography and subjective complaints of pain may increase (resulting in further diagnostic confusion).

Question 5

True. Ipsilateral axillary uptake (on the same side as the injection) is almost always a benign finding and does not need further workup. However, contralateral axillary uptake must be considered pathologic until proven otherwise.

Question 6

Significant free pertechnetate with Tc-99m MDP leads to excessive uptake in the thyroid, stomach, and salivary glands.

Question 7

The highest target-to-background ratio with Tc-99m MDP is seen at 6 to 12 hours. However, scanning is performed earlier to decrease scan times and to optimize patient convenience.

Question 8

A 5% bone loss is needed for detection with bone scan, versus the 50% bone loss needed for detection with plain film.

Question 9

Patients with prostate cancer with prostate-specific antigen levels < 10 ng/mL have a < 1% chance of having osseous metastatic disease.

Question 10

Approximately 70% of uncomplicated fractures normalize on bone scan by 1 year. A total of 95% normalize by 3 years. More complex fractures may persist longer.

■ Suggested Readings

Brenner AI, Koshy J, Morey J, Lin C, DiPoce J. The bone scan. Semin Nucl Med 2012;42(1):11–26

Choong K, Monaghan P, McLean R, et al. Role of bone scintigraphy in the early diagnosis of discitis. Ann Rheum Dis 1990;49(11):932–934

Ouvrier MJ, Vignot S, Thariat J. [State of the art in nuclear imaging for the diagnosis of bone metastases]. Bull Cancer 2013;100(11):1115–1124

Wong DC. Malignant ascites visualized on a radionuclide bone scan. Australas Radiol 1998;42(3):246–247

Top Tips

◆ In adults, 50% of the radiotracer localizes to bone, but in children, that number increases to 75%. That is why pediatric studies look better and why imaging of children at 2 hours is feasible.

◆ Marrow-based or lytic metastatic disease is often occult on bone scan.

◆ Regarding a joint prosthesis, a negative bone scan generally excludes a complicating process. But if activity is seen, determining the significance is difficult, as many uncomplicated prostheses show uptake.

Details 2

■ Case

A liver-spleen scan has been performed. Which ONE of the following is the most likely diagnosis?
   A. Normal
   B. Focal nodular hyperplasia
   C. Colloid shift
   D. Splenosis
   E. Space-occupying lesion

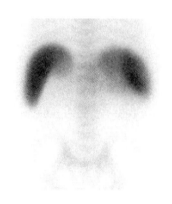

Posterior

■ The following questions pertain to liver-spleen scans.

1. True or False. Colloid shift is a specific finding for irreversible hepatic impairment.
2. True or False. A major problem with liver-spleen scans is that the test only assesses Kupffer cells, which comprise < 10% of liver cells, and therefore the scan doesn't really reflect most liver pathology.
3. True or False. Any marrow uptake seen on a liver spleen scan is abnormal.
4. True or False. Single-photon emission computed tomography (SPECT) is very helpful in assessing colloid shift.
5. True or False. Focal increased uptake in the liver is often seen with a variety of liver neoplasms, including hepatocellular carcinoma and metastases.
6. True or False. With severe colloid shift, pulmonary uptake may be seen.
7. True or False. Uptake with a sulfur colloid scan in a renal transplant may be seen with rejection.
8. True or False. Fatty livers are always normal on a liver-spleen scan.
9. True or False. Splenic scintigraphy is only possible with sulfur colloid.
10. True or False. If the spleen is anatomically present but not seen with scintigraphy, this is termed "functional asplenia."

■ Answers and Explanations

C. Correct! The distribution of radiotracer is abnormal. This is consistent with colloid shift. The uptake of the radiotracer reflects the distribution of hepatic perfusion and functioning reticuloendothelial cells in the liver (Kupffer cells) and spleen. The normal distribution is to the liver (80 to 90%), spleen (10%), and bone marrow (5%).

Other choices and discussion

A. Too much marrow and splenic uptake are seen for this to be normal. The test case findings are consistent with colloid shift. Normally, either no marrow or only very faint marrow uptake is seen.

B. No hepatic mass is seen. Focal nodular hyperplasia retains variable amounts of hepatocytes and Kupffer cells, and may be hot, cold, or of the same intensity as the adjacent liver on a sulfur-colloid scan.

D. There is homogenous activity in the spleen, and there are no additional unexplained areas of activity on the scan to suggest splenosis.

E. There are no definite cold defects to suggest a space-occupying lesion. In the past, liver-spleen scanning was relied upon to detect space-occupying malignant liver lesions. Anatomic imaging has replaced liver-spleen scanning for that purpose.

Question 1

False. Colloid shift is a nonspecific finding and may be due to hepatocellular dysfunction (cirrhosis, passive congestion, chemotherapy), infection (hepatitis, mononucleosis, sepsis), or marrow activation. Patients with diffuse hepatic metastatic disease may also have colloid shift.

Normally, activity in the spleen is equal to or less than that of the liver. Most readers use visual inspection, but if quantification is desired, a spleen-to-liver ratio (based on the posterior image) of > 1.5:1 is abnormal.

Question 2

False. While it is true that Kupffer cells comprise < 10% of the liver mass, these cells adequately reflect most hepatic pathology. Liver-spleen scans are a good barometer of the overall state of the liver.

Question 3

False. Mild marrow uptake is often seen in normal patients. The typical dose for a liver-spleen scan is 5 mCi. Recall that when significantly higher doses of the same radiotracer are injected (20 mCi), routine bone marrow imaging is possible.

Question 4

False. SPECT should be used to assess focal splenic or hepatic masses. However, SPECT is not really needed for colloid shift evaluation, which is determined by viewing the relative distribution of radiotracer in the liver, spleen, and marrow.

Question 5

False. Most space-occupying hepatic lesions are represented by cold defects on liver-spleen scans (if they are large enough to be seen). Focal nodular hyperplasia has the unique characteristic of retaining Kupffer cells and may sometimes demonstrate increased or normal uptake on liver-spleen scans. Rarely, adenomas may also accumulate radiotracer.

Question 6

True. With severe hepatic dysfunction, colloid shift may be seen in the lungs and kidneys.

Question 7

True. This finding may occur after the episode of rejection and does not necessarily indicate acute rejection.

Question 8

False. A fatty liver has a variable appearance on a liver-spleen scan, ranging from normal to diffusely decreased hepatic uptake and colloid shift. For problem liver cases where there is a question of a "mass" versus focal fatty infiltration, sulfur colloid scanning with SPECT may help to confirm normal tissue.

Question 9

False. In addition to imaging with sulfur colloid, the spleen may be selectively assessed with a technetium-99m heat-damaged red blood cell scan. The liver will not be seen with this technetium-99m heat-damaged red blood cell scan. However, disadvantages to this method in comparison to liver-spleen scanning include more steps in preparation and required manipulation with subsequent reinjection of the patient's blood.

Question 10

True. If the spleen is anatomically present but not seen with scintigraphy, this is termed "functional asplenia." The differential diagnoses of functional asplenia include sickle cell anemia (through repeated infarctions), postoperative splenic hypoxia, lupus, aggressive chronic hepatitis, and graft versus host disease.

■ Suggested Readings

Williams S. Liver-spleen imaging—radiopharmaceuticals & technique: Tc-sulfur colloid: (Dose: 5mCi). Aunt Minnie.com. April 3, 2002. Accessed June 2016. http://www.auntminnie.com/index.asp?sec=ref&sub=ncm&pag=dis&ItemID=55289

Top Tips

- ◆ When interpreting a liver-spleen scan, use the posterior view to compare the relative intensities of the spleen and liver.

- ◆ In addition to assessing colloid shift on a liver-spleen scan, make sure to carefully review the images to exclude an incidental mass.

- ◆ Vascular pathologies (superior vena cava syndrome and Budd-Chiari syndrome) occasionally result in focal increased activity on liver-spleen scans because of alterations in perfusion.

Details 3

■ **Case**

This patient has normal thyroid function laboratory tests and is asymptomatic. Which ONE of the following is correct?

    A. The patient has a hyperfunctioning goiter.

    B. The best treatment is observation.

    C. The best treatment is radioiodine therapy.

    D. The chance of any of these thyroid nodules representing cancer is greater than the chance for a person who has a single nodule.

    E. Differentiate a hyperfunctioning gland from a euthyroid gland based only on scintigraphic images is usually very easy.

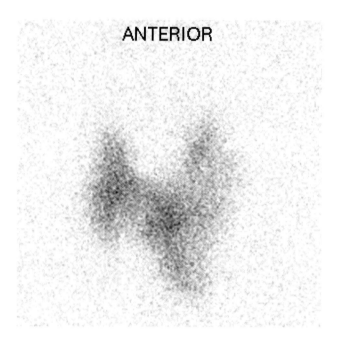

ANTERIOR

■ **The following questions pertain to endocrine scintigraphy.**

1. True or False. Warm nodules are never malignant.

2. True or False. Substernal goiters are best imaged with technetium-99m (Tc-99m) pertechnetate.

3. True or False. A patient currently taking antithyroid medication is an absolute contraindication to a pertechnetate or iodine thyroid scan.

4. True or False. Tc-99m pertechnetate is often recommended for thyroid scintigraphy in the pediatric population because it offers the least radiation exposure.

5. True or False. Cold thyroid nodules that represent well-differentiated thyroid cancer do not retain thyroid function.

6. True or False. Fluorodeoxyglucose (FDG) positron emission tomography (PET)/computed tomography (CT) has higher sensitivity for the detection of well-differentiated thyroid carcinoma than does radioiodine.

7. True or False. Thyroglossal duct cysts often contain functioning thyroid tissue that can be demonstrated with thyroid scintigraphy.

8. True or False. An FDG PET/CT scan is most sensitive for detecting thyroid cancer when the thyroid-stimulating hormone is elevated.

9. True or False. Diffuse hepatic activity on a postablation radioiodine scan is very likely benign.

10. True or False. Normal variant radioiodine activity has been seen in all of the following areas: perspiration, hematoma, inflammatory lung disease, normal gallbladder, and skin wounds.

■ Answers and Explanations

B. Correct! The best treatment is observation. The patient is euthyroid and asymptomatic. No treatment is indicated.

Other choices and discussion.

A. The patient does not have a hyperfunctioning goiter. The labs are normal.

C. In the asymptomatic patient, therapy is typically not indicated. However, note that radioiodine therapy for nontoxic goiters is not unreasonable and is often performed in Europe. Careful studies have confirmed a consistent reduction in thyroid volume after a single dose of therapy.

D. The chance of a thyroid cancer among the nodules in a multinodular gland is less than that for a person with a single thyroid nodule.

E. Differentiating a hyperfunctioning gland from a euthyroid gland based only on the scintigraphic images is not always easy. Diagnosing hyperfunctioning on the images requires suppression, which can be somewhat subjective. For example, windowing of the images can dial suppression in or out. Correlation with the radioiodine uptake and the laboratory values is very helpful.

Question 1

False. Warm nodules can be malignant. Hot nodules (hyperfunctioning with suppression of the rest of the gland) have a < 1% chance of malignancy. However, warm and cold nodules have a greater risk of malignancy. Warm nodules are those that are at least as intense as adjacent thyroid tissue, but without suppression of that tissue.

Question 2

False. High mediastinal blood pool with Tc-99m pertechnetate limits its usefulness for substernal goiter. I-123 NaI is generally considered the best choice, as it offers lower radiation than does I-131 NaI. Some nuclear medicine specialists prefer I-131 NaI.

Question 3

False. While it is true that antithyroid medication is a well-known contraindication, the endocrinologist may want to assess thyroid function while the patient is on therapy.

Question 4

True. For example, Tc-99m pertechnetate may be used to assess lingual thyroid or neonatal hypothyroidism.

Question 5

False. Well-differentiated thyroid cancer cold nodules are cold because they have relatively less function than adjacent normal tissue. However, they retain some function, which is why this tissue can be successfully treated with larger doses of radioiodine.

Question 6

False. FDG PET/CT is most useful when the well-differentiated thyroid carcinoma has become poorly differentiated. It is also useful in anaplastic, Hurthle cell, and medullary thyroid carcinomas. Iodine scans and FDG PET-CT are complementary.

Question 7

False. Thyroglossal duct cysts are typically nonfunctioning.

Question 8

True. The same is true with iodine scintigraphy.

Question 9

True. This commonly seen finding does not correlate with thyroglobulin levels or functioning metastatic disease.

A radioiodine scan normally has physiologic activity in the salivary glands, thyroid (if present), stomach, bowel, urinary bladder, and breasts.

Question 10

True. Like most scintigraphic studies, radioiodine scans are physiologic, not anatomic, and the findings should be correlated with the physical exam and radiologic imaging, as needed.

■ Suggested Readings

Gharib H, Papini E, Valcavi R, Baskin HJ, Crescenzi A, Dottorini ME, et al. American Association of Clinical Endocrinologists and Associazione Medici Endocrinologi medical guidelines for clinical practice for the diagnosis and management of thyroid nodules. Endocr Pract 2006;12(1):63–102

Meier DA, Kaplan MM. Radioiodine uptake and thyroid scintiscanning. Endocrinol Metab Clin North Am 2001;30:291–313

Oh JR, Ahn BC. False-positive uptake on radioiodine whole-body scintigraphy: physiologic and pathologic variants unrelated to thyroid cancer. Am J Nucl Med Mol Imaging 2012;2(3):362–385

Sarkar SD. Benign thyroid disease: what is the role of nuclear medicine? Semin Nucl Med 2006;36,185–193

Top Tips

- Although whole-body radioiodine scans are usually straightforward to interpret, areas of false positive activity sometimes arise. Single-photon emission computed tomography or single-photon emission computed tomography/computed tomography correlation may help with problem cases.

- Nodules smaller than 1 cm are difficult to characterize with thyroid scintigraphy.

- FDG PET/CT and radioiodine scans are complementary in thyroid cancer assessment. Radioiodine is better for well-differentiated tumor, whereas FDG PET/CT is better for poorly differentiated tumor.

Details 4

■ Case

A patient presents with painful right knee, status post right knee replacement 2 years ago and swelling for 2 months. (Left knee is asymptomatic and was replaced 5 years ago.) Regarding this patient and prosthesis scintigraphy, which ONE of the following is the BEST answer?

A. The study is essentially normal.
B. The pattern of increased activity around the joint is reliable in differentiating loosening from infection.
C. Uptake after 1 year in this prosthesis is abnormal and highly suspicious for loosening or infection.
D. A negative bone scan generally excludes a prosthesis-related complicating process.
E. If a white blood cell (WBC) scan is performed next and it shows periarticular uptake, then infection is almost certainly present.

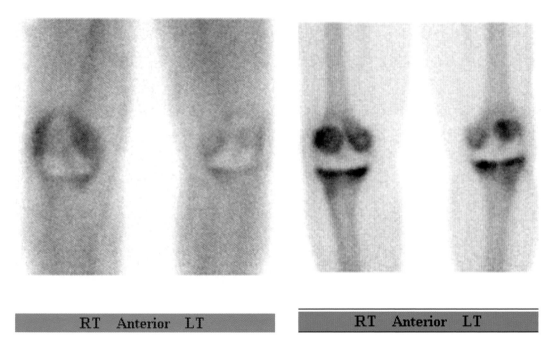

Pool   Three-hour delay

■ The following questions pertain to bone scintigraphy.

1. True or False. Metabolic disease cannot be differentiated from widespread metastatic disease on a bone scan.
2. True or False. Both Paget's disease and fibrous dysplasia are often very hot on bone scan.
3. True or False. Osteoporosis is often detectable on bone scan.
4. True or False. Bone scan is useful in determining when surgery on myositis ossificans is indicated.
5. True or False. Single-photon emission computed tomography (SPECT) can be performed anywhere in the body for a bone scan, without problem of unwanted artifact.

6. True or False. Bone scan in the setting of a vertebral body compression fracture is useful for planning vertebroplasty or kyphoplasty.
7. True or False. Both painful osteoblastic and osteolytic metastases may be treated with beta emitters Strontium-89 or Samarium-153.
8. True or False. WBC activity in Charcot joints is highly specific for infection.
9. True or False. The most common appearance for a septic joint on a bone scan is a normal study.
10. True or False. A cold defect may be seen in the very young pediatric age group in the setting of osteomyelitis.

■ Answers and Explanations

D. Correct! When assessing the painful prosthesis, a negative bone scan is generally reassuring in excluding a complicating process. Note the pitfall that chronic osteomyelitis may occasionally cause a false negative, however.

Other choices and discussion.

A. There is moderately intense periarticular uptake. This study is not normal.

B. Although it was initially thought that focal activity represented loosening while diffuse activity represented infection, there is actually significant overlap, and the distribution of activity is not very helpful in distinguishing these two processes.

C. Prosthesis scintigraphy of the knee is often problematic, when positive. More than 50% of all femoral components and 75% of all tibial components show periprosthetic uptake > 12 months after replacement. In this case, there is abnormal uptake bilaterally, and the activity on the symptomatic right knee is concerning. At surgery, infection was confirmed on the right.

E. Uptake on a WBC scan is either the result of infected material or compressed normal marrow. This would need to be further correlated with a sulfur colloid marrow scan. If the marrow scan uptake is concordant with the WBC scan uptake, then the combined scans are negative for infection.

Question 1

False. Compared to metastatic disease, the uptake with metabolic bone disease is more uniform, extends into the distal appendicular skeleton, and often demonstrates intense calvarial and mandibular uptake. Sometimes, extraosseous uptake from abnormalities with calcium and phosphorus metabolism result in activity in the lungs, stomach, and kidneys.

Question 2

True. Paget's disease often demonstrates intense focal activity on bone scan. Paget's is usually a longstanding disease found in the older population. The pelvis, skull, spine, and long bones are typical areas of distribution. Fibrous dysplasia may demonstrate similarly intense uptake. Fibrous dysplasia is usually found in a younger population.

Question 3

False. Uncomplicated osteoporosis has a normal appearance on bone scan. Bone scan is useful to detect the insufficiency fractures that often develop in the osteoporotic patient.

Question 4

True. Surgery is performed to preserve joint mobility, and myositis ossificans is likely to recur if surgery is performed before the lesion has matured. Serial bone scanning helps with this determination. Mature lesions demonstrate decreasing activity on all three phases, when compared to prior studies.

Question 5

False. Bladder artifact from SPECT is a common source of error in the pelvis. This is caused, in part, from changing bladder activity over time. Improving technical factors have somewhat decreased this problem. Besides SPECT, bone scan evaluation of the pelvis also benefits from optimal planar scintigraphy. This includes optimal voiding, use of catheterization if needed, delayed images, and multiple additional views, include tail-on-detector view and lateral views.

Question 6

True. Increased uptake at the compression fracture on bone scan is highly predictive of a positive clinical response to percutaneous treatment. SPECT/computed tomography is now being used at some centers, with incremental improvement over standard planar imaging.

Question 7

True. A recent positive bone scan is required beforehand. Most patients referred for this treatment have sclerotic lesions on anatomic imaging, but if the patient's lytic lesions elicit significant response on bone scan, these patients may be treated as well.

Question 8

False. Abnormal WBC uptake is seen in both infected and noninfected Charcot joints. Abnormal uptake on WBC that is not seen on bone scan (or is much more hot than on bone scan) is positive for infection.

Question 9

False. In the majority of cases, there is mild activity in a periarticular distribution, best seen on the early images. A normal study is possible, however, and the test should not be used to exclude a septic joint.

Question 10

True. A cold defect, with or without mild peripheral activity, may be seen in the very young pediatric age group in the setting of osteomyelitis. This occurs if the increased pressure impairs the circulation, and this has been termed "cold osteomyelitis." This is uncommon.

■ Suggested Readings

Love C, Marwin SE, Palestro CJ. Nuclear medicine and the infected joint replacement. Semin Nucl Med 2009;39:66–78

Shehab D, Elgazzar AH, Collier BD. Hetertopic ossification. J Nucl Med 2002;43:346–353

Top Tips

- Prosthesis scintigraphy is often challenging. An interval change in bone scan is very useful in diagnosing pathology. Some orthopedic surgeons order a baseline bone scan 6 months after surgery for this reason.

- If a bone scan performed for a painful prosthesis is positive and infection is a concern, the best next move is to obtain both WBC and sulfur colloid scans.

- When a three-phase bone scan for questioned osteomyelitis shows considerable soft tissue uptake at 3 hours, a 24-hour delayed image can improve clearance and increase test specificity.

Details 5

■ Case

A patient presents with glioblastoma multiforme (GBM). The first magnetic resonance imaging (MRI) and positron emission tomography (PET) scan were taken 1 month postoperatively. The second MRI and PET were taken 5 months postoperatively. The patient has completed chemotherapy and radiation therapy, and now has increasing symptoms. Which ONE of the following is the most likely diagnosis?

    A. Recurrent GBM
    B. Pseudoprogression
    C. No active disease
    D. Radiation necrosis

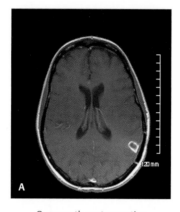

One month post operative

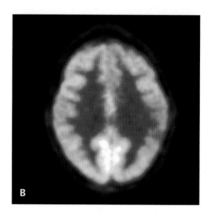

One month post operative

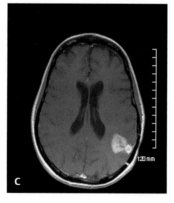

Five months post operative

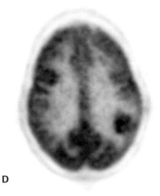

Five months post operative

■ The following questions pertain to brain scintigraphy.

1. True or False. Focal decreased FDG uptake in the brain is extremely unlikely to represent a viable brain mass.
2. True or False. Focal increased FDG uptake in the brain is almost certainly neoplastic.
3. True or False. For primary brain tumors, FDG uptake tends to correlate directly with tumor grade.
4. True or False. Dedicated brain FDG PET/CT compares favorably to MRI in the assessment of brain metastases.
5. True or False. Unlike PET, SPECT of the brain is not useful in differentiating scar from recurrent neoplasm.
6. True or False. Most patients with Parkinson have abnormal dopamine transporter (DAT) scans.
7. True or False. A negative DAT scan essentially excludes Parkinson disease.
8. True or False. DAT scans are of somewhat limited use because of poor intraobserver agreement.
9. True or False. Hot spot amyloid imaging for dementia has proven superior to the standard FDG PET/CT evaluation for dementia.
10. True or False. It is appropriate in select high-risk patients to perform screening or asymptomatic PET brain scanning for dementia.

■ Answers and Explanations

A. Correct! The patient most likely has recurrent GBM. The enhancing tissue on MRI is concordant with the increased uptake on fluorodeoxyglucose (FDG) PET/computed tomography (CT). Distinguishing between progression of disease, pseudoprogression, and radiation necrosis remains difficult with imaging, and a combination of modalities are often needed to reach the best conclusion. A recent meta-analysis found moderate accuracy for FDG PET/CT in detecting glioma recurrence, with a combined sensitivity of 77% and a specificity of 78% for any glioma histology.

Other choices and discussion

B. The timing of the presentation argues against pseudoprogression. Pseudoprogression generally occurs from several weeks to 3 months following treatment. The new symptoms also make pseudoprogression less likely, as the majority of patients with pseudoprogression are asymptomatic. In patients with GBM who undergo chemotherapy and radiation therapy, 28 to 66% develop pseudoprogression. Increased enhancement on postgadolinium T1 and enlargement on fluid sensitive sequences are seen on MRI.

C. There is increased activity at the postsurgical site, so the study is not normal. With recurrence, do not expect the entire lesion to demonstrate pathologic uptake; sometimes only the periphery of the abnormal tissue will show uptake.

D. Radiation necrosis is the most difficult diagnosis to exclude. Radiation necrosis presents 3 months to 3 years after treatment. The overall aggressive histology of the original tumor should always raise concern for possible recurrent disease. Often multimodality imaging, including FDG PET/CT combined with advanced MRI (perfusion MRI, magnetic resonance spectroscopy, and diffusion-weighted imaging/diffusion tensor imaging) are necessary in this evaluation.

Question 1

False. Many brain neoplasms do not demonstrate significantly increased FDG uptake, and some even demonstrate decreased uptake. The differential diagnosis of focal decreased FDG uptake in the brain includes low-grade neoplasm, encephalomalacia/infarction, and atrophy. An interictal seizure focus also causes decreased activity.

Question 2

False. In addition to tumor, the differential diagnosis of focal increased brain activity includes neoplasm (particularly higher grade), encephalitis, and ictal seizure focus.

Question 3

True. Low-grade gliomas are similar in activity to that of white matter, whereas high-grade gliomas are increased in activity relative to white matter. GBM is usually very hot. The location of FDG uptake can be useful in directing the site of biopsy.

Question 4

False. More than 50% of brain metastases are not seen on FDG PET/CT. In part, this is secondary to high background normal brain activity.

Question 5

False. Both PET and SPECT are useful in the differentiation of scar from recurrent neoplasm. Note that the standard radiopharmaceuticals used for imaging of brain death and seizure assessment are not the agents of choice for brain mass characterization. With SPECT, thallium and sestamibi are used for brain mass characterization.

Question 6

True. A DAT scan (I-123 ioflupane) is reasonably sensitive in diagnosing the movement disorder of Parkinson disease. A total of 78% of patients with Parkinson disease have abnormal scans.

Question 7

True. The excellent negative predictive value is arguably the greatest strength of the DAT scan. A negative exam virtually excludes Parkinson. DAT scan is derived from cocaine. There are several challenges with a DAT scan. Many medications can interfere with the test. Because it is derived from cocaine, this medication is an FDA schedule II controlled substance. Finally, because a DAT scan uses radioiodine, the thyroid gland must be blocked before administering the agent.

Question 8

False. DAT scans have very good intraobserver variability. A normal study shows high striatal uptake. An abnormal study shows decreased uptake in the posterior striatum that migrates anteriorly.

Question 9

True—slightly. A large recent meta-analysis showed that amyloid imaging was slightly superior to FDG PET/CT in the detection of Alzheimer dementia (sensitivity 91% versus sensitivity 86%).

Question 10

False. The appropriate use criteria task force from 2013 spells out that even the high-risk asymptomatic patient does not warrant scanning. There are no data to indicate that solely based on risk factors (i.e., APOE genotype and/or family history), the prognosis, course of disease, or greater certainty of diagnosis is aided with amyloid PET imaging.

■ Suggested Readings

Fink JR, Muzi M, Peck M, Krohn KA. Continuing education: multi-modality brain tumor imaging – MRI, PET, and PET/MRI. J Nucl Med 2015;56(10):1554–1561

Top Tips

◆ To assess for recurrent glioma with PET/CT, look at the periphery of the postoperative bed. Then directly correlate that activity with the enhancing portions on the MRI.

◆ Most common causes of dementia: Alzheimer, 50 to 60%; dementia with Lewy bodies, 15 to 25%; frontotemporal dementia, 15 to 25%.

◆ Differential diagnoses of focal decreased FDG brain uptake: low-grade neoplasm, encephalomalacia/infarction, atrophy, and interictal seizure focus.

Image Rich 1

■ Case

Match the ventilation/perfusion (V/Q) scan with the probability of acute pulmonary embolism.
- A. Low probability
- B. High probability
- C. Very low probability
- D. Intermediate probability

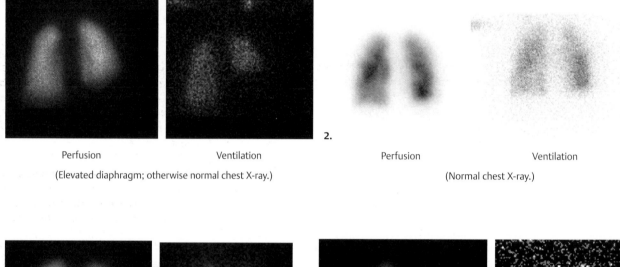

1.

Perfusion   Ventilation

(Elevated diaphragm; otherwise normal chest X-ray.)

2.

Perfusion   Ventilation

(Normal chest X-ray.)

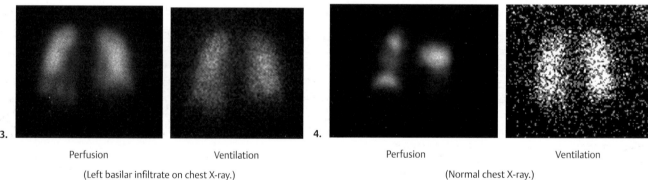

3.

Perfusion   Ventilation

(Left basilar infiltrate on chest X-ray.)

4.

Perfusion   Ventilation

(Normal chest X-ray.)

■ Answers and Explanations

1. C. Very low probability. (Nonsegmental decreased right base perfusion corresponding to elevated diaphragm.)

Prospective investigation of pulmonary embolism (PE) diagnosis (PIOPED) data showed high probability (> 80% risk for PE), intermediate probability (20 to 80% risk for PE), low probability (< 20% risk for PE), and normal. Very low probability (< 10% risk) was added later.

Pleural effusion categorization is debated. In PIOPED, a small but significant acute pleural effusion (less than one-third of the lung) is intermediate probability. However, in more recent classifications, a large pleural effusion of greater than one-third of the lung is very low probability.

With PIOPED, small defects cannot be added together to increase the probability.

2. A. Low probability. (Several small matched defects with normal chest radiograph [CXR].)

There are several accepted V/Q interpretation criteria schemes. This explains, in part, why many physicians have trouble confidently interpreting these scans.

A large defect is > 75% of a segment. A moderate defect is 25 to 75% of a segment. A small defect is < 25% of a segment.

Pulmonary emboli typically extend to the lung periphery. Normally perfused lung surrounding a defect is termed the "stripe" sign and is very unlikely to represent an acute pulmonary embolism.

3. D. Intermediate probability. (Moderate matched perfusion and radiographic defect at the left lung base. The ventilation is more normal than the perfusion at this site.)

With all classifications, moderate and large defects are added together. Moderate sized defects count as "1/2" and large defects count as "1." At least two large mismatched defects, or an additive combination of moderate and large defects totaling at least 2, is high probability.

Probability for triple-matched defects depends upon their location. A triple-matched defect in the lower lung zone is intermediate probability, and a triple-matched defect in the mid- or upper lung zones is low probability.

Modified PIOPED was shown to be more accurate than the original PIOPED criteria. Later, modified PIOPED II criteria changed the reporting to three choices: positive, negative, and nondiagnostic. Prospective investigation study of acute pulmonary embolism diagnosis and modified prospective investigation study of acute pulmonary embolism diagnosis criteria use perfusion and CXR only (no ventilation).

4. B. High probability. (Several large mismatched defects with normal CXR).

With a high clinical suspicion and a high probability scan, there is a > 95% risk for PE. With a low clinical suspicion and a low probability scan, there is a < 5% risk for PE.

Perfusion-only scintigraphy is still very useful in PE assessment. In fact, several interpretation schemes do not use ventilation in their criteria.

All interpretations refer to acute PE. Chronic PE may or may not resolve on V/Q.

Some key points about PIOPED:

- High probability: Two or more large mismatched (V/Q) segmental defects

- Intermediate probability: Two moderate or one large mismatched (V/Q) defect; difficult to characterize as high or low

- Low probability: Any number of small Q defects. Matched (V/Q) defects with CXR negative. Q defect much smaller than CXR defect.

■ Suggested Readings

Miniati M, Pistolesi M, Mariani C, Di Ricco G, Formichi B, Prediletto R, et al. Value of perfusion lung scan in the diagnosis of pulmonary embolism: Results of the prospective investigative study of acute pulmonary embolism diagnosis (Pisa-PED). Am J Respir Cri Care Med 1996;154:1387–1393

Parker JA, Coleman RE, Grady E, et al. SNM practice guideline for lung scintigraphy 4.0. 2011. Accessed July 2016. http://www.snm.org/guidelines

Sostman HD, Miniati M, Gottschalk A, et al. Sensitivity and specificity of perfusion scintigraphy combined with chest radiography for acute pulmonary embolism in PIOPED II. J Nucl Med 2008;49:1741–1748

Top Tips

- High probability, very low probability, and normal scans are very useful to the clinician. Studies that are intermediate or low probability generally need further evaluation.

- Ventilation is not always necessary for a diagnostic study.

- The best candidate for a V/Q scan has a normal CXR. If the CXR is abnormal, consider computed tomography angiogram of the chest.

Image Rich 2

■ Case

Match the bone scan with the correct description.
- A. Artifact from recent study
- B. Benign bone lesion
- C. Nonviable tissue
- D. One cause of rapid demineralization

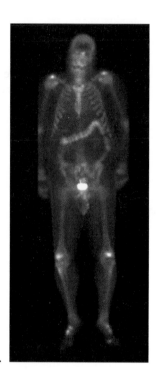

1.

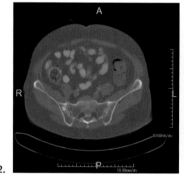

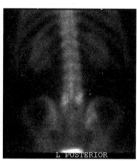

2.

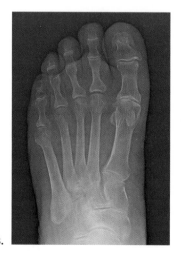

3.

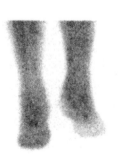

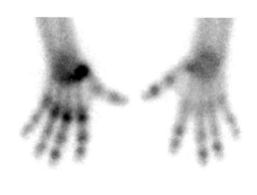

4.

■ Answers and Explanations

1. A. Artifact from recent study. This is a case of bowel uptake seen on bone scan, and this is the result of a recent sestamibi (myocardial perfusion) study. The bone scan should not have been performed within 48 hours of the sestamibi scan. Sestamibi is excreted through the bowel, and the technetium half-life is 6 hours. After 48 hours, the tracer would have been essentially gone. Other considerations in this case of bowel uptake on bone scan include wrong tracer and radiopharmaceutical impurity.

2. B. Benign bone lesion. This is a case of a bone island in the medial right iliac bone that takes up bone scan radiotracer. Typically, a bone island (enostosis) is not avid on bone scan. Rarely, bone islands show some uptake on bone scan. They may also grow. Both of these facts contribute to occasionally making the correct diagnosis more difficult. The main differential is sclerotic metastatic disease.

3. C. Nonviable tissue. This is a case of absent perfusion to the distal toes on the left. This patient had gangrenous toes. Uptake on bone scan requires both adequate flow and metabolism. Osteomyelitis cannot be assessed, although it was present in this case. Another consideration for absent or nearly absent visualization of the toes is attenuation from overlying heavy bandage material. The farther the tracer is from the camera and the more material that it needs to pass through, the lower the resulting counts.

4. D. One cause of rapid demineralization. This is a case of chronic regional pain syndrome (CRPS), and this is one cause of rapid demineralization. CRPS (formerly reflex sympathetic dystrophy) manifests as pain and vasomotor disturbances out of proportion to what might have been very mild trauma.

Bone scan is the imaging study of choice for CRPS. Both osteoporosis on plain film and marrow and soft tissue edema on magnetic resonance imaging support the diagnosis, but neither is as sensitive or specific as is three-phase bone scan. Based on recent consensus criteria, sensitivity and specificity for the diagnosis of CRPS with three-phase bone scan are 80% and 72%, respectively.

Early on, the affected area is clinically swollen and warm. Later, in the irreversible stage, the area is cold and atrophic. The bone scan reflects these clinical findings. Classic bone scan findings early in the disease include diffusely increased flow and pool with increased periarticular activity on delay. Later in the course of the disease, the flow and pool may be decreased compared to the normal tissue. Many variations have been described. Children with CRPS often have normal bone scans.

■ Suggested Readings

Coleman RE, Mashiter G, Whitaker KB, Moss DW, Rubens RD, Fogelman I. Bone scan flare predicts successful systemic therapy for bone metastases. J Nucl Med 1988;29:1354–1359

Kwon HW, Paeng JC, Nahm FS, Kim SG, Zehra T, Oh SW, et al. Diagnostic performance of three-phase bone scan for complex regional pain syndrome type 1 with optimally modified image criteria. Nucl Med Mol Imaging 2011;45(4):261–267

McAfee JG, Reba RC, Majd M. The musculoskeletal system. In Wagner HN Jr, Szabo Z, Buchanan JW, eds. Principles of Nuclear Medicine. 2nd ed. Philadelphia, PA: Saunders, 1995; 986–1012

Top Tips

◆ The classic bone scan appearance of CRPS (diffuse periarticular uptake at all joints in the affected area) is often absent. Sometimes only a portion of the affected joint is abnormal on bone scan. Remember that any asymmetric uptake that is unexplained by focal arthropathy or fracture should be viewed with concern for CRPS, in the correct clinical setting.

◆ Make sure that bandage material is removed for a bone scan, particularly when the clinical question is osteomyelitis. This will remove the overlying attenuating bandage and also remove what might be a radiotracer-soaked bandage.

◆ A good rule of thumb is to wait five half-lives before concluding that the radiotracer is essentially gone.

Image Rich 3

■ Case

Match the images with the correct nuclear whole body scan.
   A. I-131 radioiodine scan
   B. In-111 OctreoScan
   C. Tc-99m HMPAO labeled leukocyte scan
   D. In-111 MIBG scan

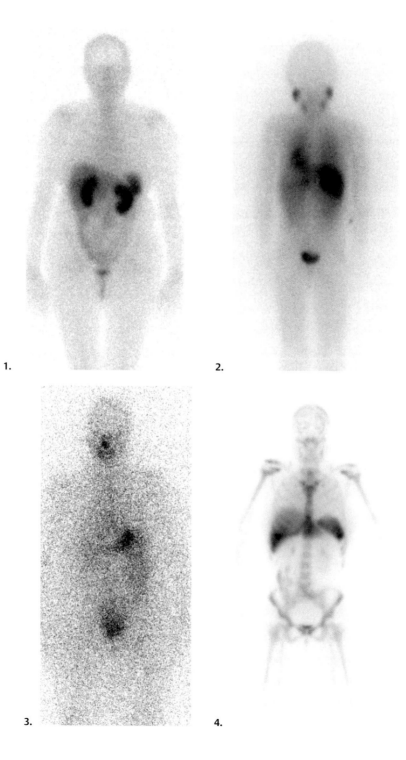

1.

2.

3.

4.

■ Answers and Explanations

1. B. In-111 OctreoScan. Normal uptake can be seen in the liver, spleen, bowel, urinary bladder, pituitary, thyroid, kidneys (cortex and collecting system), and occasionally the gallbladder. Bowel uptake is uncommon at 4 hours but is usually seen at 24 and 48 hours. Bone uptake is abnormal.

Octreoscan is most commonly used to evaluate adrenal medullary tumors (pheochromocytoma, neuroblastoma and ganglioneuroma), GEP (gasteroenteropancreatic) tumors, carcinoid tumors, and occasionally medullary carcinoma of the thyroid. A variety of other tumors demonstrate variable uptake.

2. D. In-111 MIBG (metaiodobenzylguanidine) scan. Normal uptake is seen in the liver, spleen, lungs, salivary glands, skeletal muscles, and myocardium. Since the tracer is excreted in the urine, the bladder and urinary tract show intense uptake. Normal adrenals may be seen in up to 75% with I-123 MIBG. Activity may also be seen in the nasal mucosa, gallbladder, and uterus. In pediatrics, brown fat may be seen. May see faint thyroid despite blocking agent. Bone uptake is abnormal.

MIBG indications are very similar to those of Octreoscan.

3. A. I-131 NaI (radioiodine) scan. Normal uptake is seen in the stomach, salivary glands, urinary bladder and bowel. Normal uptake is typically also seen in the thyroid (absent in this case).

4. C. Tc-99m (hexamethylpropyleneamine oxime) HMPAO (white blood cell) WBC scan. Normal uptake is seen in the spleen, liver, marrow, kidneys, and urinary bladder. Excretion is both renal and hepatobiliary, so gallbladder visualization is not uncommon. The colon is generally seen after one hour. Diffuse lung uptake begins to dissipate at four hours.

Indium-111 WBC (for comparison, not shown). Normal uptake is seen in the liver, spleen, and bone marrow. Indium WBC scanning is less available than Tc-99m WBC scanning, but has the advantage of less normal confounding activity. In-111 WBC has no normal bowel or GU uptake.

Leukocyte preparation for WBC scans. Approximately 50 mL of blood is needed for adults. Smaller volumes are needed for pediatric patients, with a minimum of 10–15 mL. The final preparation is predominantly composed of radiolabeled granulocytes, lymphocytes, and monocytes, but there are also 10 to 20% platelets and erythrocytes.

False-positive leukocyte activity may be seen at sites of mild inflammation, intravenous catheters, nasogastric tubes, drainage tubes, tracheostomies, colostomies, healing fracture sites, and noninfected hematomas. Low-grade uptake may be seen in renal transplants. Active gastrointestinal bleeding or swallowed cells may be mistaken for bowel inflammation.

■ Suggested Readings

Hansen M. Scintigraphic evaluation of neuroendocrine tumors. Appl Radiol 2001;30(6):11–17

Love C, Palestro CJ. Altered biodistribution and incidental findings on gallium and labeled leukocyte/bone marrow scans. Semin Nucl Med 2010;40(4):271–282

Palestro CJ, Brown ML, Forstrum LA, Greenspan BS, McAfee JG, Royal HD, et al. Society of Nuclear Medicine procedure guideline for 99mTc-exametazime (HMPAO)-labeled leukocyte scintigraphy for suspected infection/inflammation. 2004. Accessed July 2016. http://interactive.snm.org/docs/HMPAO_v3.pdf

Palestro CJ, Brown ML, Forstrum LA, McAfee JG, Royal HD, Schauwecker DS, et al. Society of Nuclear Medicine procedure guideline for In-111 leukocyte scintigraphy for suspected infection/inflammation. 2004. Accessed July 2016. http://interactive.snm.org/docs/Leukocyte_v3.pdf

Top Tips

◆ Modify Tc-99m hexamethylpropyleneamine oxime WBC protocols based on the clinical question. For abdominal pathology, obtain additional images before 1 hour. For fever of unknown origin, obtain images at 4 hours. For pulmonary pathology, obtain images after 4 hours. For musculoskeletal infections and for the assessment of vascular graft or shunt infection, obtain images after 4 hours.

◆ There is a high false-negative rate for vertebral osteomyelitis with leukocyte scanning (30 to 50%). Use gallium for this indication.

◆ Be careful with the adrenals on I-123 MIBG scans, as mild adrenal activity is often normally seen. Intense or asymmetric activity is more concerning.

Image Rich 4

■ Case

Match the images with the correct nuclear thyroid scan.
- A. This condition responds well to radioiodine treatment.
- B. This radiotracer eliminates the problem of a discordant nodule.
- C. This benign finding may be confused with viable cancer.
- D. This artifact will not be seen with a pinhole collimator.

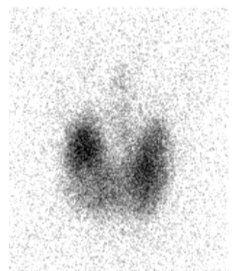

1.

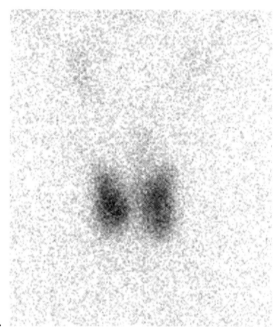

2.

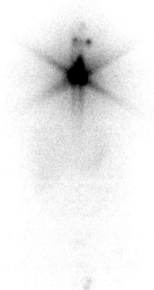

3.

4.

■ Answers and Explanations

4. A. This condition responds well to radioiodine treatment. This is an example of a toxic nodular goiter. A total of 10% of autonomously functioning nodules become toxic. Hyperthyroidism is more likely to occur when nodules grow > 2.5 cm. These nodules tend to respond well to radioiodine therapy.

2. B. This radiotracer eliminates the problem of a discordant nodule. This is a normal I-123 NaI scan. With thyroid scintigraphy, a cold nodule might represent cancer, whereas a hot nodule on a radioiodine scan essentially excludes cancer. Note that even though a cold nodule might be malignant, the majority of cold nodules are benign.

A discordant nodule is one that is hot on a Technetium-99m (Tc-99m) (pertechnetate) scan, but is cold on a 24-hour I-123 NaI scan. The significance of a discordant nodule is that a small percent of these represent cancer. A discordant nodule arises from either reduced organification of iodine or from rapid turnover of organified iodine.

Scanning with I-123 NaI assesses all phases of thyroid function, including trapping, organification, coupling, hormone storage, and secretion.

3. D. This artifact will not be seen with a pinhole collimator. This is a star artifact. This results from septal penetration of high-energy I-131 rays through the collimator septa. This is often seen when a medium-energy collimator (rather than a high-energy collimator) is used for I-131 thyroid imaging. A star artifact makes interpretation of the head and neck difficult.

Because a pinhole collimator has only a single hole, septal penetration is not possible, and a star artifact is not seen with pinhole collimation.

1. C. This benign finding may be confused with viable cancer. This is a case demonstrating swallowed radiotracer within the esophagus. This may be mistaken for thyroid cancer. Having patients rinse with a glass of water prior to the scan often minimizes this artifact.

On whole-body radioiodine scans, radiotracer is normally found in the thyroid, choroid plexus, salivary glands, nasopharynx, stomach, bowel, female breasts, urinary tract, and occasionally in the nasal mucosa.

Note: Unlike the radioiodine scans, a Tc-99m pertechnetate scan (not shown) is the only one that is administered with an intravenous injection. The iodine agents used for thyroid imaging are administered orally.

For pertechnetate, imaging is performed following a 15- to 30-minute delay. Compared to I-123 NaI, Tc-99m pertechnetate is cheaper, takes less time to complete, is trapped but not organified, and results in overall poorer image quality when the uptake is low.

Pertechnetate is the preferred thyroid imaging agent when:

- The patient cannot take oral medication.
- The patient is taking a thyroid-blocking agent such as propylthiouracil. This is because propylthiouracil blocks the organification of iodide following thyroid uptake but will not interfere with the trapping of pertechnetate.
- The evaluation is to assess neonatal congenital hyperthyroidism.

■ Suggested Readings

Intenzo CM, dePapp AE, Jabbour S, Miller JL, Kim SM, Capuzzi DM. Scintigraphic manifestations of thyrotoxicosis. Radiographics 2003;23:857–869

Lind P, Kohlfurst S. Respective roles of thyroglobulin, radioiodine imaging, and positron emission tomography in the assessment of thyroid cancer. Semin Nucl Med 2006;36(3):194–205

Ozcan Kara P, Gunay EC, Erdogan A. Radioiodine contamination artifacts and unusual patterns of accumulation in whole-body I-131 imaging: a case series. Intl J Endocrinol Metab 201412(1):e9329.

Robbins RJ, Schlumberger MJ. The evolving role of 131I for the treatment of differentiated thyroid carcinoma. J Nucl Med 2005;46:28S–37S

Shulkin BL, Shapiro B. The role of imaging tests in the diagnosis of thyroid carcinoma. Endocrinol Metab Clin North Am 1990;19:523–541

Top Tips

- A hot or warm nodule on a pertechnetate scan needs further workup because cancer is not excluded.
- A subset of hyperthyroidism cases demonstrate "rapid turnover," where the uptake is elevated at 4 hours but normalizes at 24 hours. For this reason, uptake values are usually obtained at both the optional early (4 to 6 hours) and the mandatory delayed (24 hours) times.
- Accurate uptake values are obtained with radioiodine but not with Tc-99m pertechnetate. Normal radioiodine uptake values are 10 to 35% at 24 hours and 6 to 16% for 4-hour uptake. Use these numbers somewhat loosely, as they vary regionally.

Image Rich 5

■ Case

Which of the following findings on positron emission tomography (PET)/computed tomography (CT) are at least moderately worrisome for cancer?

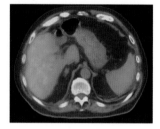

1. Adrenal update and CT

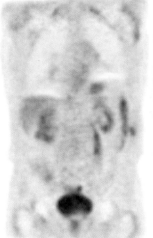
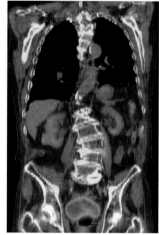

2. Renal mass uptake and CT

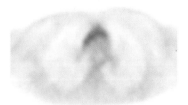

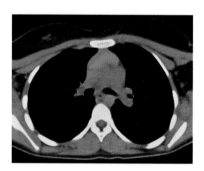

3. Thymic uptake and CT

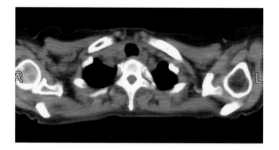

4. Thyroid uptake and CT

■ Answers and Explanations

1. Mild focal adrenal uptake. Not very worrisome.

Mild activity is seen in the right adrenal, with an SUV max of 2.3. This low level of uptake is usually benign. Adenomas generally show an uptake of < 3.1, or less than or equal to liver. Both lipid-rich and lipid-poor adenomas show similar SUVs on fludeoxyglucose (FDG) PET/CT. A total of 3% of benign adenomas have an SUV higher than that of liver.

Myelolipoma is a benign adrenal mass that shows variable uptake. Myelolipomas usually have SUV values less than liver, but on occasion may show high uptake. These masses have macroscopic fat, and fat is well known to sometimes demonstrate prominent FDG uptake.

As in other parts of the body, the size of the tissue assessed is important in lesion characterization. Absent uptake for small adrenal masses (< 10 mm) may be indeterminate. Conversely, even mild uptake in a small nodule with a high-risk patient—for example, one with lung cancer—is worrisome. This is especially true if there is an interval change.

Meta-analysis suggests that visual assessment may be at least as good as SUV measurement in diagnosing disease.

The take home point is that most of the time, adrenal masses can be accurately characterized as either benign or malignant with PET/CT, and further advanced imaging is usually not needed.

This was a case of benign adrenal tissue, which was confirmed on serial imaging.

2. Renal mass with moderate activity. Worrisome.

The mass in the right kidney shown here is FDG-avid. FDG has a limited role in characterizing renal masses, because of variable uptake.

Cysts do not show uptake. Complex cysts may or may not show uptake. Solid renal masses may or may not show uptake. Both benign and malignant masses have variable uptake.

Although lack of activity in a renal mass is encouraging, it is generally accepted that malignancy cannot be ruled out using this parameter alone. Additional considerations include that excreted FDG can mimic tissue uptake, as can misregistration artifact. Although a non-FDG-avid renal cell carcinoma on a PET/CT may be quite subtle, radiologists are still responsible for the noncontrast portion of the study.

This case was an incidental renal cell carcinoma that was FDG-avid.

3. Diffuse thymus uptake. Somewhat worrisome.

Diffuse uptake is seen in the thymus. Key considerations in differentiating benign from malignant include anatomic morphology, age of the patient, knowledge of underlying disease processes, and relationship to recent illness or cancer treatment.

Increased uptake in the thymus is seen in up to 75% of pediatric patients after chemotherapy. Homogeneous uptake after treatment, with no uptake prior to treatment, suggests hyperplasia. Intense or heterogeneous uptake coupled with suspicious CT findings needs further workup. Uptake is common in pediatric patients and may also be seen fairly often in patients as old as their late twenties. One study reported a 44-year-old patient with benign thymic uptake.

Thymic masses and mean SUV max values. Researchers have found that the SUV max mean of thymic hyperplasia is 1.1, of thymoma is 2.1, and of thymic carcinoma is 7.0. Normal hyperplasia after chemotherapy may reach an SUV of 3.8.

Differentiating hyperplasia from active malignant disease is particularly difficult with Hodgkin lymphoma, where up to 70% of thoracic cases actually have thymic involvement. Intense activity and irregular morphology are red flags that neoplasm may be present. As an isolated finding in lymphoma, despite imaging, thymic uptake may require biopsy.

This was a case of a young patient with Hodgkin lymphoma in presumed remission following recent chemotherapy. Serial follow up after this study showed improvement on both the PET and CT (without any additional treatment), suggesting that the tissue had represented benign hyperplasia.

4. Focal thyroid uptake. Worrisome.

Focal uptake is seen in the right lobe thyroid.

One very large PET/CT meta-analysis (which included 125,754 patients) demonstrated focal thyroid uptake in 1.6% of patients. Of those, 36% were malignant.

It is generally considered that diffuse uptake is probably benign, representing either thyroiditis or normal variation. However, malignant exceptions exist. These include lymphoma, metastatic disease, and the typical worrisome focal uptake that is obscured by overlying diffuse benign thyroid activity.

Standard uptake value (SUV) in focal thyroid nodules. In the same large study, SUVs of the focal uptake lesions were calculated. The mean SUV for benign lesions was 4.8 ± 3.1 and for malignant lesions was 6.9 ± 4.7. There was a trend for higher values with malignant lesions, but there was significant overlap.

The take home points are that focal uptake warrants further evaluation, whereas symmetric uptake is usually benign, but still deserves careful scrutiny.

Some refer to incidentally discovered neoplasms on PET/CT as "PAIN": PET-associated incidental neoplasm.

At surgery, this was found to represent papillary thyroid cancer.

■ Suggested Readings

Boland GW, Dwamena BA, Jagtiani Sangwaiya M, Goehler AG, Blake MA, Hahn PF, et al. Characterization of adrenal masses by using FDG PET: a systematic review and meta-analysis of diagnostic test performance. Radiology 2011;259(1):117–126

Dong A, Cui Y, Wang Y, Zuo C, Bai Y. 18F-FDG PET/CT of adrenal lesions. Am J Roentgenol 2014;203(2):245–252

Ferdinand B, Gupta P, Kramer EL. Spectrum of thymic uptake at 18F-FDG PET. Radiographics. 2004;24(6):1611–1616

Kochhar R, Brown RK, Wong CO, Dunnick NR, Frey KA, Manoharan P. Role of FDG PET/CT in imaging of renal lesions. J Med Imaging Radiat Oncil 2010;54(4):347–357

Top Tips

◆ Focal FDG uptake in the thyroid warrants ultrasound correlation. Diffuse uptake is most likely benign.

◆ Diffuse thymic uptake may be either benign or malignant. The interpretation must consider more than just the imaging findings.

◆ Visual assessment of many de novo lesions on PET/CT has a similar accuracy to SUV measurement assessment. If it looks hot, it is hot.

More Challenging 1

■ Case

A premenopausal woman presents with newly diagnosed stage T1 breast cancer. Lymphoscintigraphy images are provided.

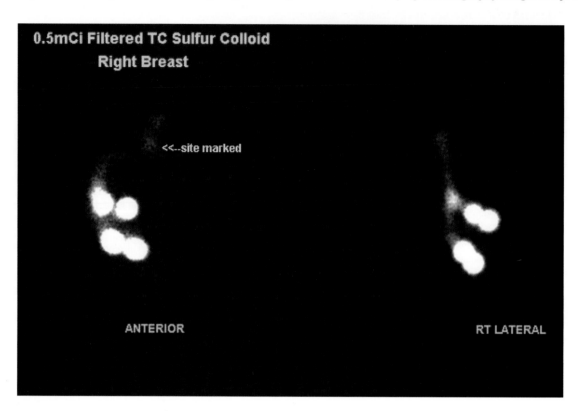

■ Questions

1. Which ONE of the following is correct?
   A. This study fails to identify a sentinel node.
   B. The surgeon will most likely use an intraoperative probe.
   C. All patients with breast cancer should have preoperative sentinel node localization.
   D. The most common radiotracer injection site (for breast cancer) is intratumoral.
   E. If this sentinel node is pathologically negative for neoplasm, the likelihood of metastatic breast cancer in this patient remains 15%.

2. Regarding lymphoscintigraphy technique, which ONE of the following is correct?
   A. Using intraoperative methylene blue with lymphoscintigraphy adds accuracy and sensitivity.
   B. Among superficial injection techniques for breast cancer, subareolar is the proven best.
   C. Lymphoscintigraphy use for oncology is restricted to melanoma and breast cancer.

   D. Pregnancy is a contraindication to radiotracer sentinel lymph node biopsy.
   E. If there is no visible tracer migration, there has probably been a technical error.

3. Regarding lymphoscintigraphy, which ONE of the following is correct?
   A. Patients with positive sentinel lymph nodes go onto axillary lymph node dissection, and patients with negative sentinel lymph nodes are spared axillary lymph node dissection.
   B. The intensity of uptake within a node correlates very well with the likelihood of that node representing a sentinel lymph node.
   C. Surgery personnel involved with lymphoscintigraphy should routinely wear radiation badges.
   D. Gentle mixing of the syringe prior to injection may cause a poor tag and is contraindicated.
   E. Using the smallest particles possible is advantageous, as that permits rapid radiotracer transit.

SECTION IX
NUCLEAR MEDICINE
IMAGING

Answers and Explanations

Question 1

B. Correct! Following the injection, imaging is optional (but strongly suggested). Marking the presumed sentinel node(s) with indelible ink on the patient's skin is also optional. However, using an intraoperative probe by the surgeon is mandatory.

Other choices and discussion

A. This study *does* identify a sentinel node. There is linear accumulation of radiotracer extending from the periareolar injection site to the axilla, where there is a discrete focus of more intense localized activity. This is a sentinel node. The sentinel nodes are the regional nodes that directly drain the primary tumor and are the first nodes to receive lymph-borne metastatic nodes.

Even if the images had failed to show this activity, no conclusion regarding the presence or absence of a sentinel node could be drawn until the intraoperative probe was used.

C. Not all patients with breast cancer should have preoperative sentinel node localization.

Some stages and scenarios of breast cancer are clearly indicated, whereas other scenarios are controversial or not indicated. Established areas for sentinel lymph node (SLN) biopsy include T1 or T2 tumor, ductal carcinoma in situ with mastectomy, older age, obesity, prior to preoperative systemic therapy, and male breast cancer. Inflammatory breast cancer is not recommended. The remaining scenarios are debated.

D. The most common radiotracer injection site (for breast cancer) is periareolar.

However, deep peritumoral and/or intratumoral injections are also acceptable injection sites.

If the goal is axillary staging, superficial periareolar injection may be preferred to deep peritumoral or intratumoral injection. If the goal is to stage extra-axillary nodal basins in addition to regional disease, a deep injection near the tumor site is advised. The methods are complementary, and some institutions use both.

E. The false-negative rate of lymphoscintigraphy for breast cancer ranges from 0 to 3%—that is, the likelihood that the patient has metastatic breast cancer is 0 to 3%. A negative study is very reassuring. However, a negative lymphoscintigraphy study for melanoma is not as reassuring. One paper looking at 1313 melanoma patients determined that the false-negative rate for melanoma SLN assessment was 14.4%.

Question 2

A. Correct! Using intraoperative methylene blue with lymphoscintigraphy adds accuracy and sensitivity. Methylene blue is injected shortly before the surgery. The lymphatic channels turn blue at 5 to 15 minutes and washout at 45 minutes.

Other choices and discussion

B. Options for a superficial injection include subdermal, intradermal, periareolar, and subareolar injection sites. There is no clearly superior method. Multiple studies confirm that the method of injection does not significantly affect the results.

C. Lymphoscintigraphy is most commonly used for melanoma and breast cancer.

However, recently, lymphoscintigraphy use has increased for gynecologic cancers.

D. Pregnancy is not a contraindication to radiotracer SLN biopsy. Nursing mothers should suspend breastfeeding for 24 hours.

E. In a small percentage of patients, tracer migration will not be detected during imaging or even intraoperatively. This does not represent a technical error. The significance of preoperative scintigraphic nonvisualization is not known.

Question 3

A. Correct! Patients with positive SLNs go onto ALND, and patients with negative SLNs are spared ALND. No change in patient outcomes has been shown when comparing these two strategies.

Other choices and discussion

B. The intensity of uptake does not consistently correlate with the likelihood of a given node representing a SLN. Having said that, note that many SLNs are quite hot, and it has been shown that removing all hot axillary nodes does lead to fewer false-negative SLN biopsies.

C. Because exposures in SLN procedures are very low, surgery personnel do not need routine radiation exposure monitoring. The choice to monitor personnel who are involved with a high number of SLN procedures is left to the discretion of the individuals and local standards.

D. Radiocolloid particles are suspended and may settle, if left untouched for a few minutes. Gentle rotation of the syringe prior to injection ensures good mixing of the particles and is *recommended*.

E. The optimal particle size of colloids is a compromise between particles small enough for fast migration, yet big enough for optimal retention in lymph nodes.

Technetium-99m filtered sulfur colloid is the most commonly used agent for lymphoscintigraphy in the United States. Technetium-99m Lymphoseek (Navidea Biopharmaceuticals, Inc., Dublin, Ireland), approved by the US Food and Drug Administration in 2013, has recently gained popularity. Lymphoseek does not depend on particle size. Instead, uptake depends upon dextran-mannose receptors on the surface of macrophages. Several studies have demonstrated that Lymphoseek performs at least as well as sulfur colloid.

Suggested Readings

Society for Nuclear Medicine. The SNM procedure guideline for general imaging 6.0. 2010. Accessed May 2016. http://interactive.snm.org/docs/General_Imaging_Version_6.0.pdf

Top Tips

- A negative SLN biopsy for breast cancer is very reassuring (i.e., offers a very high negative predictive value).
- There are several potential injection methods, but studies show that results do not vary substantially, regardless of the technique employed.
- Radionuclide lymphoscintigraphy can also be used as a noninvasive method for diagnosing extremity lymphedema.

More Challenging 2

■ Case

A 29-year-old woman with a recent history of severe respiratory infection now presents with clinical symptoms of hyperthyroidism. Her free T4 is elevated and her thyroid-stimulating hormone is decreased. You are presented with her I-123 NaI scan.

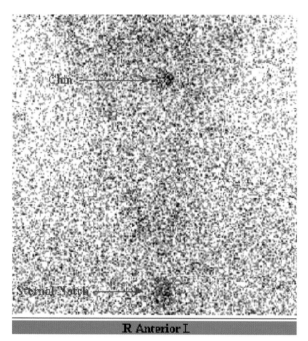 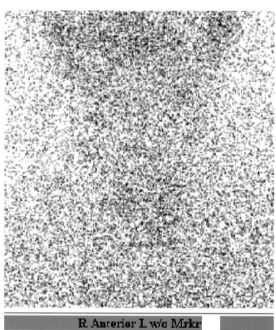

6-Hour Image: RAIU of 1.3%

■ Questions

1. Which ONE of the following is the most likely diagnosis?
   A. Thyrotoxicosis factitia
   B. Nontoxic multinodular goiter
   C. Subacute thyroiditis
   D. Grave disease
   E. Recent intravenous contrast administration

2. Regarding thyrotoxicosis, which ONE of the following is the best answer?
   A. With both toxic multinodular goiter and toxic adenoma, the radioiodine uptake is usually markedly elevated.
   B. An elevated radioiodine uptake with a homogeneously bulbous gland is diagnostic of Grave disease.
   C. In all cases of thyrotoxicosis, the thyroid-stimulating hormone is suppressed.
   D. Struma ovarii might be considered in the setting of biochemical and clinical hyperthyroidism with a poorly visualized thyroid gland by scintigraphy.
   E. There is no difference between thyrotoxicosis and hyperthyroidism.

3. Regarding Grave disease and scintigraphy, which ONE the following is the best answer?
   A. The main utility of the radioiodine uptake and scan is to determine the radioiodine dose for treatment of Grave disease.
   B. Generally, patients should wait 2 months following radioiodine treatment before attempting pregnancy.
   C. Detection of thyrotropin receptor antibodies is diagnostic of Grave.
   D. Radioiodine treatment may improve preexisting thyroid ophthalmopathy.
   E. The radioiodine uptake is invariably elevated at 6 and 24 hours with Grave disease.

■ Answers and Explanations

Question 1

C. Correct! This is a case of subacute thyroiditis. An injured gland with subacute thyroiditis functions poorly and demonstrates very minimal uptake on scintigraphy. Subacute thyroiditis is often seen postpartum or post upper respiratory infection. It is usually self-limited.

Other choices and discussion

A. Medications than decrease iodine uptake in the thyroid gland (such as off-label use of Synthroid) may result in both the scintigraphic and reported laboratory findings of the test case (i.e., thyrotoxicosis factitia). However, given the clinical history, this is not the most likely diagnosis.

B. A nontoxic multinodular goiter would have normal radioiodine uptake (10 to 35%), rather than markedly decreased uptake.

D. With Grave disease, the gland should be well visualized, somewhat bulbous, and the radioiodine uptake (RAIU) should be elevated, not decreased.

E. Iodinated contrast acts as a competitive inhibitor, with thyroid scan and uptake results similar to that of thyrotoxicosis factitia and early subacute thyroiditis.

Question 2

D. Correct! Struma ovarii is a rare teratomatous ovarian tumor that contains hyperfunctioning thyroid tissue, resulting in thyrotoxicosis. Because of the thyrotoxicosis, the thyroid gland should be suppressed and poorly seen with scintigraphy. Other pelvic tumors may also uncommonly cause thyrotoxicosis. For example, hydatidiform moles and choriocarcinomas both secrete human chorionic gonadotropin, which is a thyroid stimulator, and result in thyrotoxicosis.

Other choices and discussion

A. With both toxic multinodular goiter and toxic adenoma, the RAIU is usually upper limits of normal or mildly elevated. This is in distinction from Grave disease, which usually has a greater degree of radioiodine elevation.

B. An elevated radioiodine uptake with a homogeneously bulbous gland is the typical presentation of Grave. However, there are mimics. In particular, during the recovery phase of subacute thyroiditis there may be a "rebound" phenomenon, demonstrating diffusely increased activity in the thyroid.

C. "Thyroid-stimulating hormone (TSH)-induced thyrotoxicosis" is the term used for a pituitary adenoma overproducing TSH, resulting in clinical hyperthyroidism, an elevated free T4, and an elevated TSH. This is the only cause of thyrotoxicosis with an elevated TSH.

E. Thyrotoxicosis is defined as hypermetabolism secondary to an elevated circulating thyroid hormone. Hyperthyroidism, on the other hand, refers to thyrotoxicosis resulting from a hyperfunctioning thyroid gland. Examples of thyrotoxicosis not caused by a hyperfunctioning thyroid gland include subacute thyroiditis, struma ovarii and thyrotoxicosis factitia.

Question 3

C. Correct! This laboratory information is especially useful in the diagnosis of pregnant patients, as radioiodine is absolutely contraindicated with pregnancy. Detection of thyrotropin receptor antibodies is diagnostic of Grave, and most patients with Grave have these antibodies.

Other choices and discussion

A. The main utility of the radioiodine uptake and scan is to differentiate the etiology of the hyperthyroidism. Specifically, is the gland itself hyperfunctioning (Grave, toxic adenoma, toxic multinodular goiter), or is the gland normally functioning but either temporarily injured or unable to receive the feedback because of a blocking agent?

The scan is also useful to demonstrate a possible superimposed cold nodule. If detected, this must be worked up to exclude malignancy prior to radioiodine therapy.

Dosage for Grave treatment is typically 5 to 15 mCi. Dosage may be determined by RAIU and gland size, but comparative studies between calculated and empiric doses do not demonstrate a difference in outcomes.

B. After the initial treatment with radioiodine, a small but significant percentage of patients will require another dose, and this may not be adequately determined for 6 to 12 months following treatment. In addition, potentially harmful radiation changes occur in the sperm and eggs immediately subsequent to radiation treatment.

For these reasons, it is recommended to delay pregnancy for 6 to 12 months after radioiodine therapy.

D. Radioiodine use in patients with ophthalmopathy is somewhat controversial, as this treatment may actually exacerbate the ocular findings. Despite this controversy, radioiodine is still usually considered the treatment of choice.

E. In patients with markedly increased synthesis and turnover, the 6-hour value is elevated but the 24-hour value is normal. This is known as rapid iodine turnover, and is a subtype of Grave.

■ Suggested Readings

Eisenberg B, Arrington ER, Haygood TM, Kelsey CA. Thyroid scintigraphic patterns, radioactive iodine uptake, and Nuclear Regulatory Commission guidelines for radioiodine use. In: Eisenberg B, eds. Imaging of Thyroid and Parathyroid Glands: A Practical Guide. New York, NY: Churchill Livingstone; 1991: 51–57

Top Tips

- Be careful when treating "Grave" with radioiodine, as rebound subacute thyroiditis may look identical with scintigraphy. Use the clinical scenario to differentiate these two possibilities.

- Regarding medications that block radioiodine uptake and the time needed to hold each before attempting scintigraphy, remember the "4, 6, 2, 4, 6" rule. Need to wait 4 days for propylthiouracil, 6 days for methimazole, 2 weeks for T3 supplement, 4 weeks for T4 supplement, and 6 weeks for iodinated contrast.

- Frequency of thyrotoxicosis etiologies: Grave 70%, thyroiditis 20%, toxic adenoma 5%, toxic multinodular goiter 5%, others < 1%.

More Challenging 3

■ Case

A patient presents with a carcinoid tumor. Images from a nuclear scan provided.

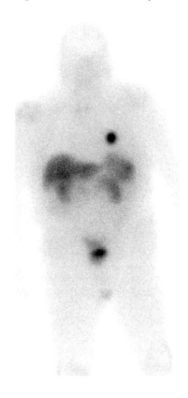

■ Questions

1. Which ONE of the following is correct?
   A. Somatostatin treatment may be continued prior to this scan.
   B. The most sensitive time for OctreoScan tumor detection is 4 hours postinjection.
   C. The subtle thyroid uptake seen here is abnormal and suspicious for medullary thyroid carcinoma.
   D. Tumors that are typically somatostatin-avid include pheochromocytoma, carcinoid, and neuroblastoma.
   E. There are very few causes of false positive activity on an OctreoScan.

2. Regarding metaiodobenzylguanidine scanning, which ONE of the following is correct?
   A. Metaiodobenzylguanidine has considerably greater sensitivity than OctreoScan for the detection of neuroblastoma.
   B. Many medications interfere with metaiodobenzyl-guanidine, somewhat limiting the scan utility.
   C. If the tumor diagnosis is already known, demonstrating uptake with metaiodobenzylguanidine or OctreoScan adds little to patient management.

   D. No special premedication regimen is required prior to metaiodobenzylguanidine scanning.
   E. If the OctreoScan scan is negative, there is no reason to perform a metaiodobenzylguanidine scan for the purpose of localizing a neuroendocrine tumor.

3. Regarding ProstaScint (Aytu BioScience, Inc., Englewood, CO), which ONE of the following is correct?
   A. ProstaScint is more useful for the initial staging of prostate cancer than it is for detecting metastatic disease.
   B. ProstaScint has much lower efficacy than bone scan for detecting osseous metastases.
   C. ProstaScint, OctreoScan, and metaiodobenzylguanidine are all monoclonal antibodies.
   D. If the patient has a human antimouse antibody reaction history, future ProstaScint studies are contraindicated.
   E. Activity in the prostate on ProstaScint after hormone or radiation treatment is a suspicious finding for active malignant disease.

■ Answers and Explanations

Question 1

D. Correct! There is high somatostatin avidity with adrenal medullary tumors (pheochromocytoma, neuroblastoma, and paraganglioma), with an overall sensitivity of > 85%. There is also high avidity for carcinoid tumors, with a sensitivity of 86 to 95%. Gastroenteropancreatic neuroendocrine tumors have variable avidity, ranging from 25 to 60%. (These formerly included terms such as gastrinoma, insulinoma, vasoactive intestine polypeptide-secreting tumors, and glucagonoma. The World Health Organization has more recently classified them as low grade, intermediate grade, and high grade.) Medullary carcinoma of the thyroid has reasonable OctreoScan avidity, with a sensitivity of 50 to 75%. Uptake may also be seen with meningioma, Merkel cell tumor of the skin, pituitary adenoma, and small cell lung cancer.

Other choices and discussion

A. Somatostatin treatment must be withheld prior to an OctreoScan, as the scan uses a radiolabeled-somatostatin analogue. The length of withdrawal depends upon the half-life of the therapeutic agent (at least 1 day for standard agents and 4 to 6 weeks for slow-release formulations).

B. The most sensitive time for OctreoScan tumor detection is 24 hours postinjection, and that is when images are routinely obtained. Four-hour and 48-hour images are also often performed. Lack of physiologic bowel activity is an advantage of the 4-hour images, but the low tumor-to-background ratio at 4 hours results in decreased sensitivity.

C. The thyroid uptake seen here is diffuse, mild, and probably clinically insignificant. Medullary thyroid carcinoma is often somatostatin-avid. However, focal (rather than diffuse) uptake would be expected. Thyroid uptake seen on an OctreoScan is usually benign.

E. False-positive activity on an OctreoScan may be seen with autoimmune disease, bacterial pneumonia, granulomatous disease, postirradiation inflammation, nasopharyngeal infection, and at recent surgical and colostomy sites.

Question 2

B. Correct! Many medications interfere with MIBG, somewhat limiting the scan utility. The list of potential interfering medications is vast, including over-the-counter decongestants, many cardiac medicines, and some antidepressants.

Other choices and discussion

A. Metaiodobenzylguanidine (MIBG) and OctreoScan have similar efficacy in the detection of neuroblastoma, carcinoid, and pheochromocytoma. MIBG is an analogue of noradrenaline and guanethidine. Imaging with I-123 MIBG is optimal at 24 hours. Delayed imaging up to 48 hours is also sometimes utilized.

C. Even if the tumor diagnosis is already made, demonstrating uptake with MIBG or OctreoScan is useful for treatment planning. These scans are less used to diagnose and more used to localize tumor and to confirm uptake, which affects treatment planning.

Patients with somatostatin receptor-positive tumors and with MIBG-avid tumors are more likely to respond to peptide receptor radionuclide therapy and MIBG radionuclide therapy, respectively.

D. MIBG is bound to radioactive iodine, which means that the thyroid gland must be blocked prior to administering the dose of MIBG. This is typically performed with super saturated potassium iodide or Lugol solution. For I-123 MIBG, the blockade should begin 1 day prior to the injection and continued for 1 or 2 days. For patients with an iodine allergy, potassium perchlorate is an alternative.

E. Because MIBG and OctreoScan have different mechanisms of uptake, they may be used as a complementary means in the evaluation of these entities. If the OctreoScan scan is negative, an MIBG scan may still prove positive.

Question 3

B. Correct! ProstaScint is not great at detecting bone metastases.

Other choices and discussion

A. ProstaScint is better at detecting metastatic prostate cancer than it is for initial staging.

C. ProstaScint is a monoclonal antibody. Octreoscan is a neuropeptide. MIBG is a guanethidine analog.

D. Human antimurine antibodies (HAMAs) are found in 5 to 8% of patients after injection, and most resolve within a few months. HAMA may falsely elevate prostate-specific antigen and may result in altered distribution, causing increased activity in the liver.

E. After treatment, long-term nonspecific and benign diffuse prostate fossa uptake may be seen.

■ Suggested Readings

Balon HR, Brown TL, Goldsmith SJ, et al. The SNM practice guideline for somatostatin receptor scintigraphy 2.0. J Nucl Med Technol 2011;39(4):317–324

Raj GV, Partin AW, Polascik TJ. Clinical utility of 111indium-capromab pendetide immunoscintigraphy in the detection of early, recurrent prostate carcinoma after radical prostatectomy. Cancer 2002;94(4):987–996

Top Tips

◆ Thyroid-blocking agents are needed for iodine-based radiotracers (that are not specifically trying to image the thyroid).

◆ Tumors actually within the adrenal glands may be difficult to see on an OctreoScan because of high adjacent renal activity. For these patients, MIBG may be preferred.

◆ Patients with iodine allergies may safely take radioiodine, as the amount of iodine administered is miniscule.

More Challenging 4

■ Case

A 52-year-old woman presents with chest pain and query for coronary artery disease. Technetium myocardial perfusion imaging was performed.

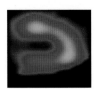
Stress

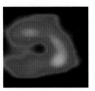
Rest

■ Questions

1. This case demonstrates which ONE of the following?
   A. An example of the most common indication for this test
   B. Transient ischemic dilatation
   C. A limited examination, as the lung-to-heart ratio is not provided
   D. Balanced ischemia
   E. Reverse redistribution

2. Regarding cardiac positron emission tomography, which ONE of the following is correct?
   A. The half-life of the fluorine used for fluorodeoxyglucose is 11 minutes.
   B. N-13 ammonia is used to assess cardiac metabolism.
   C. Rubidium-82 chloride runs the risk of strontium safety issues.
   D. Cardiac positron emission tomography is satisfactorily performed using either treadmill or pharmacologic stress.
   E. Cardiac single photon emission tomography is superior to positron emission tomography for coronary artery disease detection.

3. Regarding myocardial perfusion imaging, which ONE of the following is correct?
   A. Patients who are unable to elevate their left arm cannot have a myocardial perfusion imaging single photon emission tomography study.
   B. Single photon emission tomography myocardial summed scores are comprised of 17 standardized segments.
   C. Electrocardiogram changes seen with pharmacologic and exercise stress are typically of equal significance.
   D. Withholding caffeine for a scheduled treadmill sestamibi stress study is unnecessary.
   E. The patient is midway through the stress portion of the stress test and the monitoring equipment (electrocardiogram, blood pressure, heart rate) fails. The patient is in no apparent distress and wants to continue. It is reasonable to continue under careful observation.

■ Answers and Explanations

Question 1

E. Correct! Reverse redistribution means that the rest image perfusion defects are worse than the stress image perfusion defects. In this case, the rest anterior wall is worse than the stress anterior wall. (The inferior wall is also abnormal, but this is fixed.) Reverse redistribution was first described with thallium, but is also seen with technetium MPI. Its etiology is debated. One known cause is varying the overlying soft tissue position between rest and stress imaging. Overall, reverse redistribution does not indicate ischemia.

Other choices and discussion

A. Determining the presence or absence of disease is the reason for this test patient's scan. However, myocardial perfusion imaging (MPI) is now performed less frequently to actually diagnose disease, and more frequently to determine prognosis, risk stratification, and patient management for known patients with coronary artery disease (CAD). Patients with normal stress perfusion have a better prognosis than do those with abnormal perfusion. Patients with more severe perfusion defects have higher mortality rates than do those with less severe perfusion defects.

B. TID refers to left ventricle chamber dilation seen on stress that improves on rest. TID is a poor prognostic finding. TID typically demonstrates a dilated chamber seen with either exercise or pharmacologic stress. Persistent dilatation is abnormal and suggests multivessel disease.

C. The examination is not limited, even though the lung-to-heart (L/H) ratio is not reported. A normal L/H ratio is 0.5 or less. An abnormally elevated L/H ratio reflects left ventricle dysfunction, congestive heart failure, or three-vessel CAD. This is a somewhat useful sign, but it has been better validated with thallium. Typically, the L/H ratio is not reported with technetium-based products.

D. Balanced ischemia, which refers to multivessel disease, may result in a falsely negative study. One limitation of exercise (compared to pharmacologic stress) is that with exercise, only the most severe lesion is sometimes detected.

Question 2

C. Correct! Rubidium is produced from a strontium-82/Rb-82 generator. The half-life of the Sr-82 parent is 25 days. A new generator is needed each month. Strontium safety issues are very rare with rubidium use, but there have been several reports of "strontium breakthrough" that resulted in excessive radiation exposure.

Rubidium is an analog of potassium, has a short half-life of 76 seconds, produces images that are superior in quality to single photon emission tomography (SPECT), and has less attenuation effect and subdiaphragmatic scatter than do SPECT images.

Other choices and discussion

A. Positron emission tomography (PET) half-lives: O-15 2 minutes (110 seconds); N-13 10 minutes; C-11 20 minutes; F-18 110 minutes; (PET half-lives—2, 10, 20, 110).

B. N-13 ammonia is used for perfusion, not metabolism. For PET, the main cardiac radiotracers include N-13 ammonia and Rb-82 for perfusion, and F-18 fluorodeoxyglucose for metabolism/viability.

D. Cardiac PET uses only pharmacologic (rather than exercise) stress because of the short half-life and because the images are actually acquired during the stress testing. This differs from that of SPECT testing, which allows a break between the exercise stress and the image acquisition.

E. PET has both higher sensitivity and specificity (92% and 85%, respectively) than does SPECT (85% and 80%, respectively) for CAD detection. PET also has higher spatial resolution than SPECT and is better for obese patients. The same interpretation criteria are used for cardiac perfusion PET as for cardiac perfusion SPECT.

Question 3

B. Correct! SPECT myocardial summed scores are commonly comprised of 17 standardized segments. The 17-segment model was developed and endorsed by many professional associations, including the American Heart Association and the American Society of Nuclear Cardiology. It has replaced the older 20-segment model as the standard. The summed stress score is obtained by adding the individual scores from the 17 segments during stress. Normal is < 4, mildly abnormal is 4 to 8, moderately abnormal is 9 to 13, and severely abnormal is > 13.

Other choices and discussion

A. Patients who cannot lift up their left arm can still have an MPI SPECT study. The patient's left arm is usually positioned upward for scanning, but this is not the only option.

C. Electrocardiogram changes observed with pharmacologic stress testing should not be dismissed, but correlate much less well with ischemia than do electrocardiogram changes seen during exercise.

An advantage of exercise over pharmacologic stress is the addition of functional information. The general rule of thumb for most cardiologists is that if the patient is able to exercise adequately, he or she should.

D. While it is true that an exercise test will not be affected by caffeine, a small but significant percentage of exercise cases are converted to pharmacologic stress on the day of the study. Thus, many institutions require withholding caffeine, just in case.

Caffeine is held for 12 to 24 hours and theophylline is held for 48 hours. In all cases of MPI, patients are kept nothing by mouth for 4 to 6 hours.

E. Failure of monitoring equipment is an absolute indication to stop the test.

■ Suggested Readings

American Society of Nuclear Cardiology. Updated imaging guidelines for nuclear cardiology procedures, part 1. J Nucl Cardiol 2001;8(1):G5–G58

Top Tips

◆ Look for TID, which is often associated with severe and extensive CAD.

◆ The key points for MPI cine assessment include excluding motion artifact, excluding an unexpected mass, and noting possible explanations for attenuation artifact (such as large breasts).

◆ Apical thinning is most commonly clinically insignificant.

More Challenging 5

■ Case

A patient with breast cancer with isolated osseous metastases. Conventional fluorodeoxyglucose positron emission tomography/computed tomography showed resolution of activity in sclerotic lesions (not shown). F-18 sodium fluoride positron emission tomography/computed tomography performed to assess the bones, shows persistent uptake in the same sclerotic lesions. In addition, some sclerotic lesions have enlarged. Shown are images from the F-18 sodium fluoride positron emission tomography/computed tomography scan.

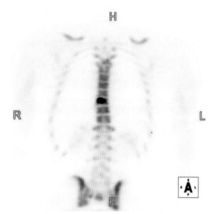
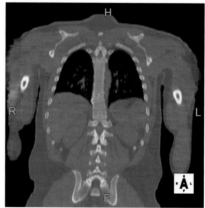
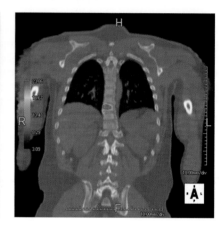

■ Questions

1. Which ONE of the following is the BEST answer?
   A. The bone findings almost certainly represent active disease.
   B. As is seen with a standard bone scan, fluorodeoxyglucose positron emission tomography/computed tomography has the problem of the "flare phenomenon" with treated bone lesions.
   C. F-18 sodium fluoride positron emission tomography/computed tomography can usually easily differentiate treated osseous disease from progression.
   D. Lab value correlation is of little value in assessing bone lesions.

2. Regarding F-18 sodium fluoride bone positron emission tomography/computed tomography, which ONE of the following is the BEST answer?
   A. The glucose level must be checked.
   B. Standard uptake value reporting is standard for treatment follow up.
   C. This scan is more sensitive than a standard bone scan for the detection of bone metastases.
   D. The problem with arthritis and other causes of false-positive uptake is rarely seen with this scan.
   E. The degree of uptake is very useful in differentiating benign from malignant bone lesions.

3. A patient about to be injected for fluorodeoxyglucose positron emission tomography/computed tomography has a serum glucose of 240 mg/dL. Which ONE of the following is the best answer?
   A. This patient is at risk for a false-positive study.
   B. One reasonable course of action is to wait several hours prior to injection.
   C. One reasonable course of action is to administer insulin followed by an immediate fluorodeoxyglucose injection.
   D. The patient's heart is much more likely to be hot than is a heart scanned when the serum glucose is 100 mg/dL.
   E. Scanning is probably still reasonable despite an elevated glucose.

■ Answers and Explanations

Question 1

B. Correct! Flare happens with fluorodeoxyglucose (FDG) positron emission tomography (PET)/computed tomography (CT), too. Osteoblastic flare means an increase in activity in metastatic bone lesions when there is otherwise stable or resolving disease in other lesions. Flare is benign. Distinguishing flare from isolated osseous metastatic disease can be challenging.

Other choices and discussion

A. The bone findings probably represent treated disease. The prior FDG activity within the bone lesions has resolved. Uptake on F-18 sodium fluoride (NaF) PET/CT by itself is not specific and does not alter this diagnosis.

MD Anderson criteria for bone metastases complete response include complete sclerotic fill in of lytic lesion, normalization of bone density on radiograph or CT, normalization of signal intensity on magnetic resonance imaging, or normalization of tracer uptake on skeletal scintigraphy.

C. Both treated disease and progression can show uptake on F-18 NaF PET/CT. This uptake is not specific.

D. Correlation with tumor markers and alkaline phosphatase is often extremely helpful in determining metastatic disease. Working closely with the oncology service for problem cases is mutually beneficial.

Question 2

C. Correct! This scan is more sensitive than a standard bone scan for the detection of bone metastases. Think of this scan as a really good bone scan. F-18 NaF has two-fold higher uptake in bone than does methylene diphosphonate and is therefore more sensitive to bone pathology. In addition, coupling the scan with tomographic images adds specificity. Similar to that of a standard bone scan, uptake is dependent upon regional blood flow and new bone formation.

Other choices and discussion

A. The glucose level does not need to be checked, as this PET scan does not use a glucose analogue. For prep, the patient should be well hydrated and should void prior to the scan.

B. Standard uptake value (SUV) reporting is not the standard for treatment follow up. Use of quantitative indices such as SUV has not been validated, and their value in clinical studies is undefined. When dictating, the SUV may be used for descriptive purposes, but the value should not be used to render a specific diagnosis.

D. The same causes of false-positive uptake seen on conventional bone scan (e.g., arthritis) are seen on the F-18 NaF PET-CT. However, the CT correlation is very helpful in determining the cause.

E. In general, the degree of uptake does not differentiate benign from malignant bone lesions.

Question 3

B. Correct! For a mild glucose elevation, this action may solve the problem.

Other choices and discussion

A. This patient is at risk for a false-*negative* study. Elevated serum glucose undergoes competitive inhibition with the injected radiotracer, which decreases uptake in cancerous lesions. Many institutions reschedule if the serum glucose is > 200 mg/dL.

C. Insulin decreases serum glucose uptake and causes an increase in muscular uptake. This decreases uptake in cancerous lesions. However, insulin is sometimes useful. Newer studies describe successful insulin protocols for diabetic patients with elevated glucose.

Regarding the test answer choice, if insulin is given, FDG should be injected at least 60 (and preferably 90) minutes postinjection, not immediately.

D. It is difficult to predict the cardiac uptake based on glucose levels. Cardiac uptake in the fasting oncology patient is nonuniform and unpredictable. Length of fasting and blood glucose levels do not appear to consistently correlate with the degree of cardiac uptake.

E. Most centers will either reschedule or try to lower the glucose, but doing the scan with an elevated glucose is not recommended.

■ Suggested Readings

Even-Sapir E, Metser U, Mishani E, Lievshitz G, Lerman H, Leibovitch I. The detection of bone metastases in patients with high-risk prostate cancer: 99mTc-MDP Planar bone scintigraphy, single- and multi-field-of-view SPECT, 18F-fluoride PET, and 18F-fluoride PET/CT. J Nucl Med 2006;47:287–297

Jadvar H, Desai B, Conti PS. Sodium 18F-fluoride PET/CT of bone, joint, and other disorders. Semin Nucl Med 2015;45:58–65

Segall G, Delbeke D, Stabin MG, Even-Sapir E, Fair J, Sajdak R, et al. SNM practice guideline for sodium 18F-fluoride PET/CT bone scans 1.0. J Nucl Med 2010;51(11):1813–1820

Top Tips

◆ Brown fat uptake is more likely when there is a lower outdoor temperature and in patients who are younger, female, and have a lower body mass index. Warming the patient prior to injection helps. Benzodiazepine use is debated, but may be indicated for head and neck cancers.

◆ The SUV is a relative measurement that is based on several variables, including the injected dose and the patient body weight. Heavier patients have somewhat higher SUVs than do lighter patients.

◆ An F-18 NaF PET/CT is a really good bone scan. It is better than a standard bone scan for osteoblastic lesions. However, FDG PET/CT is better at osteolytic lesions.

Essentials 1

■ Case

A 6-month-old boy presents with abnormal head shape.

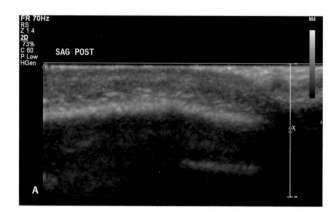

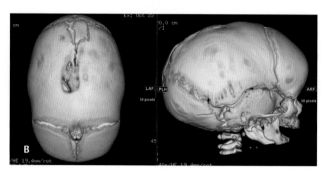

■ Questions

1. Which ONE of the following is NOT a secondary cause of these findings?
   A. Shunted hydrocephalus
   B. Rickets
   C. Sickle cell anemia
   D. Microcephaly
   E. Prenatal polyhydramnios

2. Which disorder is often confused with asymmetric posterior positional plagiocephaly?
   A. Unilateral lambdoid synostosis
   B. Bilateral coronal synostosis
   C. Sagittal synostosis
   D. Metopic synostosis
   E. Multiple suture synostosis

3. Which ONE of the following disorders is NOT commonly associated with craniosynostosis?
   A. Apert syndrome
   B. Crouzon syndrome
   C. Neurofibromatosis type 1
   D. Thanatophoric dysplasia

■ Answers and Explanations

Question 1

E. Correct! This is an example of craniosynostosis, premature fusion of the cranial sutures, as demonstrated by the surface-rendered computed tomography. Screening ultrasound image also demonstrates premature bony fusion represented by the solid hyperechoic calvarium in the expected location of the posterior sagittal suture. External compressive prenatal forces (prenatal constraint) may be a cause. Thus, *oligohydramnios* is a risk factor for premature closure of the cranial sutures, not polyhydramnios.

Other choices and discussion

A. Shunted hydrocephalus can cause secondary craniosynostosis. Inadequate intracranial pressure/inadequate separating forces on the patent sutures can cause premature closure.

B. Metabolic imbalance can cause secondary craniosynostosis. The exact mechanism is not well understood, but the mineral deficiencies in rickets delay vascularization of the growth plates and result in disorganization of chondrocytes and accumulation of osteoid at the metaphysis. Similarly, other calcium metabolic disorders are linked to premature cranial suture closure, including hypophosphatemia, vitamin D deficiency, renal osteodystrophy, and hypercalcemia.

C. Hematologic diseases that cause bone marrow hyperplasia are associated with premature cranial suture closure.

D. Microcephaly can cause secondary craniosynostosis. Similar to shunted hydrocephalus, inadequate intracranial pressure/inadequate separating forces on the patent sutures can cause premature closure.

Question 2

A. Correct! Unilateral lambdoid synostosis causes posterior plagiocephalic head shape, which is similar to the positional molding caused by infants who spend the majority of laying time on their backs. This latter phenomenon is also known as "flat head syndrome." The incidence is estimated to be 1 in 100 infants, but the true incidence may be even greater to due campaigns to prevent sudden infant death syndrome such as "back to sleep" and "face up to wake up." The difference between posterior plagiocephaly caused by positional molding and true unilateral lambdoid synostosis is crucial, as the former is treated conservatively with helmet therapy, while the latter is corrected surgically.

Other choices and discussion

B. Bilateral coronal synostosis causes brachycephaly. This head shape is characterized by a shortened anteroposterior dimension ("brachy" is the Greek root meaning short), resulting in a towering head shape.

C. Sagittal synostosis causes scaphocephaly. This head shape is characterized by an elongated anteroposterior dimension resulting in a boat-shaped head ("scapho" is the Greek root meaning boat). This head shape is also known as dolichocephaly.

D. Metopic synostosis causes trigonocephaly.

E. Severe multisuture synostosis causes a cloverleaf-shaped head. This is associated with multiple disorders.

Question 3

C. Correct! Neurofibromatosis type 1 can cause an abnormal head shape, but this is secondary to sphenoid dysplasia rather than craniosynostosis. In fact, sphenoid dysplasia is one of the many diagnostic criteria for neurofibromatosis type 1.

Other choices and discussion

A. Apert syndrome is an autosomal dominant disorder that is characterized by bilateral coronal suture craniosynostosis, midface hypoplasia, hypertelorism, and syndactyly. It is due to mutations in the fibroblast growth factor receptor 2 gene.

B. Crouzon syndrome is also an autosomal dominant disorder caused by mutations in the fibroblast growth factor 2 gene. However, this syndrome is typically characterized by multiple sutural synostoses. When severe, it manifests as a cloverleaf skull. Syndactyly is not typical in Crouzon syndrome.

D. Type 2 thanatophoric dysplasia is typically caused by a new, sporadic, dominant mutation in the fibroblast growth factor receptor 2 gene. The typical skull manifestation results in a cloverleaf skull due to severe multiple suture craniosynostosis.

■ Suggested Readings

Dover MS. Abnormal skull shape: clinical management. Pediatr Radiol 2008;38(Suppl 3):S484–S487

Peitsch WK, Keefer CH, LaBrie RA, Mulliken JB. Incidence of cranial asymmetry in healthy newborns. Pediatrics 2002;110:e72

Sze RW, Parisi MT, Sidhu M, et al. Ultrasound screening of the lambdoid suture in the child with posterior plagiocephaly. Pediatr Radiol 2003;33:630–636

Top Tips

◆ Multidetector computed tomography with three-dimensional reformations is the gold standard for imaging diagnosis of craniosynostosis.

◆ Targeted high-frequency ultrasound is an effective screening tool.

◆ Craniosynostosis can be primary or secondary. Secondary causes include microcephaly, overshunted hydrocephalus, hematologic conditions that cause marrow hyperplasia, and calcium metabolic disorders such as rickets.

Essentials 2

■ **Case**

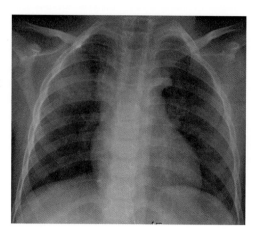

■ **Questions**

1. Why does this type of pneumonia occur more often in children than in adults?
   A. Different bacteria are present in the two populations.
   B. The collateral airways are underdeveloped in children.
   C. The immune system in children organizes the infection differently than in adults.
   D. Clinical symptoms in children present earlier than in adults, resulting in the detection of the atypical rounded appearance more often.

2. Which of the follow features can help differentiate other disease processes from the disorder featured in the test case? (Select ALL that are correct.)
   A. Multiplicity
   B. Air-fluid level
   C. Calcification
   D. Bony erosion of underlying ribs

3. What is the most common pulmonary metastatic lesion in children?
   A. Wilms tumor
   B. Neuroblastoma
   C. Osteosarcoma
   D. Ewing sarcoma
   E. Medulloblastoma

■ Answers and Explanations

Question 1

B. Correct! This is rounded pneumonia (PNA). The collateral pathways of air circulation (channels of Lambert and pores of Kohn) are incompletely developed in children under the age of 8 years. As bronchopneumonia infection attempts to spread, the lack of collateral pathways creates a rounded appearance.

Other choices and discussion

A. Most commonly, *Streptococcus pneumoniae* is responsible for rounded PNA in children. This pathogen is also common in adult community-acquired PNA.

C. It is not the immune system, but rather the anatomic variance, that creates rounded PNA.

D. The timing of symptoms is similar in adults and children, and this is not responsible for rounded PNA.

Question 2

A. Correct! Round PNA is typically solitary. Multiple lesions are more likely to result from other infections (such as fungal) or metastasis.

B. Correct! Air-fluid levels are unusual in round PNA, but can be seen with lung abscess, necrotizing PNA, or an infected bronchogenic cyst.

C. Correct! Calcifications are not present in round PNA, but can be present in thoracic neuroblastoma, fungal infection, pulmonary carcinoid, hamartomas, or osteosarcoma metastasis.

D. Correct! When a thoracic mass is seen in conjunction with rib erosion or soft tissue spread, neuroblastoma should be suspected. Bony involvement is not present in pneumonia.

Question 3

A. Correct! Wilms tumor is the most common primary neoplasm to spread to the lungs. Note that metastatic pulmonary masses are much more common than primary pulmonary malignancies in children.

Other choices and discussion

B. Neuroblastoma pulmonary metastases are rare, and when present, portend a poor prognosis. More commonly, neuroblastoma metastases occur in the bone.

C. Osteosarcoma pulmonary metastases are the second most common cause of pediatric pulmonary metastases, after Wilms tumor. This metastatic lesion can also present with a spontaneous pneumothorax.

D. Although the lung is the most common site of the metastasis for Ewing sarcoma and for many other sarcomas in childhood, it is not the most common cause of metastasis to the lungs.

E. The most frequent of spread of metastasis for medulloblastoma is through the cerebrospinal fluid. Lung metastasis is uncommon.

■ Suggested Readings

Dishop MK, Kuruvilla S. Primary and metastatic lung tumors in the pediatric population: a review and 25-year experience at a large children's hospital. Arch Pathol Laboratory Med 2008;132:1079–1103

Kim Y-W, Donnelly LF. Round pneumonia: imaging findings in a large series of children. Pediatric Radiology 2007;37:1235–1240

SECTION X
PEDIATRIC IMAGING

Top Tips

◆ Round PNA is seen in children < 8 years of age due to underdevelopment of collateral air pathways. If the typical clinical presentation of PNA is present, then no further imaging is required at the time of diagnosis.

◆ Follow up imaging can be considered after an appropriate course of antibiotics, especially if symptoms do not improve.

◆ Metastases are much more common than primary tumors of the lung in children. Wilms tumor is the most common pediatric pulmonary metastatic lesion.

Essentials 3

■ **Case**

An incidental finding in an asymptomatic pediatric patient.

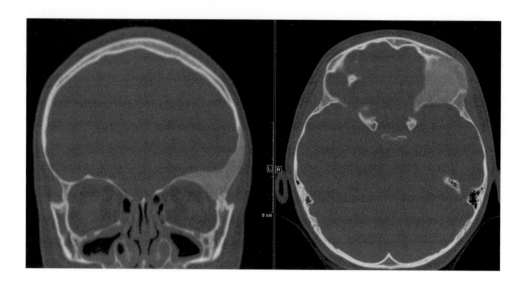

■ **Questions**

1. Which ONE of the following imaging features is most characteristic of this bone finding?
   A. Ground glass appearance of the matrix
   B. Involvement of multiple bones
   C. Cortical destruction
   D. T2 hyperintensity
   E. Ring and arc appearance of the matrix

2. Which ONE of the following entities is characterized by polyostotic fibrous dysplasia, endocrine dysfunction, and cutaneous hyperpigmentation?
   A. Jaffe-Campanacci syndrome
   B. Cherubism
   C. Mazabraud syndrome
   D. McCune-Albright syndrome

3. Although early Caffey disease can be confused with fibrous dysplasia, cortical involvement and periostitis are typically not seen in fibrous dysplasia. Which ONE of the following is a feature of Caffey disease?
   A. Most common site of involvement is the mandible
   B. Patients are asymptomatic
   C. Occurs in children > 6 months of age
   D. Epiphyses are involved
   E. Manifestations usually persist past 2 years of age

■ Answers and Explanations

Question 1

A. Correct! This is fibrous dysplasia (FD). A ground glass matrix with expansion of the marrow space is the most characteristic finding in FD. Computed tomography is the preferred modality to evaluate suspected cases of FD.

Other choices and discussion

B. Although FD can be polyostotic, this is not a defining characteristic. In fact, the majority of cases of FD are monostotic.

C. Cortical destruction is an aggressive feature and should not be present in FD (which is a benign nonaggressive entity).

D. The fibrous component of FD causes T2 hypointensity, not hyperintensity.

E. A ring and arc internal matrix is characteristic of cartilaginous lesions, not FD.

Question 2

D. Correct! These features best describe McCune-Albright syndrome. The endocrine dysfunction is typically precocious puberty, and the hyperpigmentation results in café au lait spots.

Other choices and discussion

A. Jaffe-Campanacci syndrome is characterized by multiple nonossifying fibromas, not by FD. Other features of this entity include café au lait spots and hypogonadism.

B. Cherubism is defined by autosomal dominant FD of the bilateral jaw.

C. Mazabraud syndrome consists of polyostotic FD and intramuscular myxomas.

Question 3

A. Correct! The mandible is the most common location for Caffey disease.

Other choices and discussion

B. Patients with Caffey disease are typically symptomatic. There is a classic triad of fevers, irritability, and soft tissue swelling.

C. Although there have been case reports of Caffey disease in older children, it typically occurs in children < 6 months of age.

D. The cortical hyperostosis spares the epiphysis in Caffey disease.

E. Caffey disease symptoms usually resolve 6 to 12 months after initial presentation. There are rare cases of persistent or protracted courses, but these are atypical.

■ Suggested Readings

Belsuzarri TAB, Araujo JFM, Melro CAM, et al. McCune-Albright syndrome with craniofacial dysplasia: clinical review and surgical management. Surg Neurol Int 2016;7(Suppl 6):S165–S169

Shandilya R, Gadre KS, Sharma J, Joshi P. Infantile cortical hyperostosis (caffey disease): a case report and review of the literature—where are we after 70 years? J Oral Maxillofacial Surg 2013;71:1195–1201

SECTION X
PEDIATRIC IMAGING

Top Tips

- A ground glass appearance on computed tomography is most characteristic of FD.

- McCune-Albright syndrome consists of polyostotic FD, precocious puberty, and café au lait spots.

- Caffey disease occurs in symptomatic children who are < 6 months of age, commonly involves the mandible, and is manifested radiographically by periosteal reaction that spares the epiphysis.

Essentials 4

■ Case

A patient presents with a history of hip dysplasia.

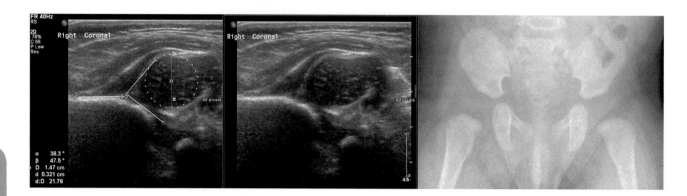

■ Questions

1. What are the normal alpha angle and femoral head coverage?
   A. Greater than 60 degrees and 40%
   B. Greater than 60 degrees and 50%
   C. Greater than 30 degrees and 40%
   D. Greater than 30 degrees and 50%

2. Which ONE of the following is a risk factor for hip dysplasia?
   A. Cephalic presentation
   B. Family history of hip dysplasia
   C. Polyhydramnios
   D. Male sex
   E. Arm deformity

3. What are the criteria for functional immaturity of the hips?
   A. Age < 12 weeks, alpha angle 50 to 60 degrees, and femoral head coverage of 40 to 50%
   B. Age < 12 weeks, alpha angle 40 to 60 degrees, and femoral head coverage of 40 to 50%
   C. Age < 16 weeks, alpha angle 50 to 60 degrees, and femoral head coverage of 35 to 50%
   D. Age < 16 weeks, alpha angle 40 to 60 degrees, and femoral head coverage of 35 to 50%

■ Answers and Explanations

Question 1

B. Correct! An alpha angle > 60 degrees and femoral head coverage of > 50% are normal for patients who are > 12 weeks old. On radiographs, the acetabular angle is the complementary angle to the alpha angle on ultrasound, and thus the normal acetabular angle should be < 30 degrees. This patient has developmental dysplasia of the hip.

Question 2

B. Correct! Family history is a risk factor for developmental dysplasia of the hips.

Other choices and discussion

A. Breech presentation is a risk factor for developmental dysplasia of the hips.

C. Oligohydramnios is a risk factor for developmental dysplasia of the hips.

D. Female sex is a risk factor for developmental dysplasia of the hips and thought to be due to increased sensitivity to the maternal hormone relaxin.

E. Foot deformity, not arm deformity, is a risk factor for developmental dysplasia of the hips.

Question 3

A. Correct! In children < 12 weeks old, laxity of the hip is allowable. This phenomenon is called functional immaturity of the hips and is secondary to maternal estrogen influence and increased ligamentous laxity. In these cases, the alpha angles are between 50 to 60 degrees and the femoral head coverage between 40 and 50%. Up to 90% of cases identified by ultrasound will normalize upon follow up. Thus, a follow up examination is suggested in 4 to 6 weeks.

■ Suggested Readings

Roof AC, Jinguji TM, White KK. Musculoskeletal screening: developmental dysplasia of the hip. Pediatric Annals 2013;42: e238–e244

US Preventive Services Task Force. Screening for developmental dysplasia of the hip: recommendation statement. Pediatrics 2006;117:898–902

SECTION X
PEDIATRIC IMAGING

Top Tips

◆ The normal alpha angle of the hip on ultrasound is > 60 degrees, and the normal femoral head coverage is > 50%.

◆ Children who are < 12 weeks old may have increased laxity of the hips and can normally have a slightly lower alpha angle and femoral head coverage (50 degrees and 40% coverage). This is called functional immaturity of the hips.

◆ Ultrasound is the preferred modality for evaluating the hip before the age of 6 months. Once there is significant ossification of the proximal femoral epiphyses, then radiographs are required.

Essentials 5

■ Case

A patient presents with a history of acute unilateral pelvic pain.

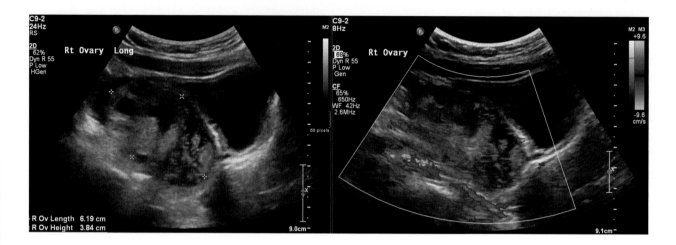

■ Questions

1. Which ONE of the following is the BEST predictor of ovarian torsion?
   A. Lack of arterial Doppler waveforms
   B. Unilateral enlarged ovarian size and volume
   C. Medialization of the ovary
   D. Peripherally displaced follicles
   E. Presence of an ovarian mass

2. Which ONE of the following does NOT predispose female pediatric patients to the disorder presented in this test case?
   A. Ovarian mass
   B. Ovarian cyst
   C. Maternal hormonal stimulation
   D. Hydrosalpinx
   E. Large body habitus

3. Which ONE of the following is the BEST predictor of *testicular* torsion?
   A. Lack of intraparenchymal vascular flow
   B. Unilateral enlarged testicular size and volume
   C. Medialization of the testicle
   D. Microlithiasis
   E. Presence of an intratesticular mass

■ **Answers and Explanations**

Question 1

B. Correct! A unilaterally enlarged ovary is the best indicator of torsion. Asymmetry correlating to the clinical side of symptoms is also an important indicator of torsion. Some studies have described an ovarian length > 5 cm or a volume > 20 mL as sensitive markers of ovarian torsion in children.

Other choices and discussion

A. Although at first glance the absence of arterial waveforms might seem like the most intuitive answer, Doppler findings in cases of ovarian torsion are highly variable, ranging from normal venous and arterial waveforms to completely absent or reversed waveforms. This is a result of the dual blood supply of the ovaries (uterine and ovarian arteries), timing of presentation, and potential intermittent nature of ovarian torsion. Therefore, the presence of intraparenchymal vascular flow (venous or arterial) does not exclude ovarian torsion.

C. Medialization of an ovary is an important secondary sign of torsion, but it is not as sensitive as ovarian size. Medialization refers to twisting of the vascular pedicle, which secondarily displaces the ovary toward the uterus.

D. Peripheral displacement of ovarian follicles is an important secondary sign of torsion, but it is not as sensitive as ovarian size. This finding is due to parenchymal edema/vascular engorgement, which displaces the follicles outward.

E. An ovarian mass predisposes the vascular pedicle to twist, as the mass can act as a fulcrum for the torsion. However, ovarian torsion does not require the presence of a mass, and even when present, concurrent masses are not as sensitive for the detection of ovarian torsion as unilateral ovarian enlargement.

Question 2

E. Correct! There is no correlation between a large body habitus and ovarian torsion.

Other choices and discussion

A. An ovarian solid mass can act as a fulcrum for torsion.

B. An ovarian cyst can act as a fulcrum for torsion.

C. Hormonal stimulation causes ovarian enlargement, which can predispose the ovary to torsion. This is one cause of fetal ovarian torsion.

D. Hydrosalpinx is associated with up to 9% of cases of ovarian torsion.

Question 3

A. Correct! In contrast to ovarian torsion, the most sensitive sign of testicular torsion is lack of parenchymal flow. This is due to a single source of vascular supply. Intermittent testicular torsion should be suspected when there is initial lack of parenchymal flow with subsequent positive parenchymal flow during an ultrasound examination. Evaluation of the spermatic cord is also important, as swirling of the cord or vascular engorgement are sensitive signs for intermittent testicular torsion as well.

Other choices and discussion

B. Although an enlarged testicle is often seen in torsion, it is not as sensitive as lack of intraparenchymal flow. In addition, an enlarged testicle can also be associated with orchitis and testicular neoplasia.

C. Change in the position of the testicle has not been reported as a sign of testicular torsion.

D. Microlithiasis has not been shown to be predictive of testicular torsion. However, there is an association of microlithiasis with germ cell tumor. If microlithiasis is isolated, then no further imaging workup is required. Follow up should be suggested only in patients with an increased risk of germ cell tumor, including personal or family history, maldescent or undescended testes, orchiopexy, or testicular atrophy.

E. Presence of an intratesticular mass does increase the risk of testicular torsion. An abnormally high attachment of the tunica vaginalis results in a bell clapper deformity, which allows the testicle to freely rotate in the scrotum and predisposes to testicular torsion.

■ **Suggested Readings**

Munden MM, Williams JL, Zhang W, et al. Intermittent testicular torsion in the pediatric patient: sonographic indicators of a difficult diagnosis. Am J Roentgenol 2013;201:912–918

Ngo A-V, Otjen JP, Parisi MT, et al. Pediatric ovarian torsion: a pictorial review. Ped Radiol 2015;45:1845–1855

Richenberg J, Belfield J, Ramchandani P, et al. Testicular microlithiasis imaging and follow-up: guidelines of the ESUR scrotal imaging subcommittee. Eur Radiol 2015;25:323–330

Ringdahl E, Teague L. Testicular torsion. Am Fam Physician 2006;74:1739–1743

Waldert M, Klatte T, Schmidbauer J, et al. Color doppler sonography reliably identifies testicular torsion in boys. Urology 2010;75:1170–1174

**SECTION X
PEDIATRIC IMAGING**

Top Tips

◆ An enlarged ovary in the setting of acute unilateral pediatric pelvic pain represents ovarian torsion until proven otherwise.

◆ Absence of ovarian vascular flow is unreliable in the diagnosis of ovarian torsion. This is partially due to a dual blood supply from the ovarian and uterine vessels.

◆ In contrast to ovarian torsion, lack of vascular flow is the most reliable sign of testicular torsion. Detection prior to 6 hours has a good salvage rate.

Essentials 6

■ Case

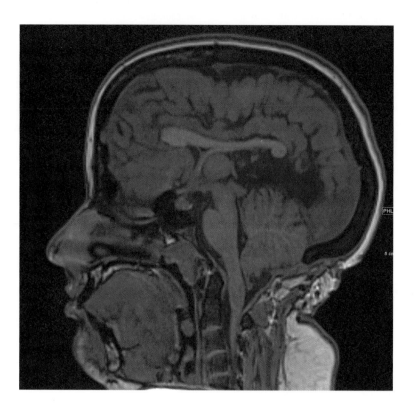

■ Questions

1. Which ONE of the following is characteristic of this entity?
   A. Large posterior fossa
   B. Flattening of the tectum
   C. Tonsillar herniation
   D. Small massa intermedia
   E. Vermian hypoplasia

2. Which ONE of the following prenatal signs does NOT suggest this entity?
   A. Lemon sign
   B. Strawberry sign
   C. Myelomeningocele
   D. Elevated alpha-fetoprotein
   E. Banana sign

3. Which ONE of the following is NOT associated with syringomyelia?
   A. Chiari 1 malformation
   B. Chiari 2 malformation
   C. Scoliosis
   D. Klippel-Feil syndrome
   E. Leukemic involvement of the spine

■ Answers and Explanations

Question 1

C. Correct! This image is characteristic of Chiari malformation type 2, with inferior cerebellar tonsillar herniation, beaked tectum, small posterior fossa, and large massa intermedia. Tonsillar herniation is the most characteristic feature of Chiari malformations. Inferior cerebellar tonsillar herniation > 6 mm below the foramen magnum in symptomatic patients is considered abnormal.

Other choices and discussion

A. The features of Chiari malformation type 2 include a small (not a large) crowded posterior fossa. A large posterior fossa can be seen in Dandy Walker malformations and other associated entities.

B. In Chiari 2, the configuration of the tectum is often beaked, not flattened. This represents fusion of the midbrain colliculi, which are directed posteriorly and invaginate into the cerebellum.

D. A large massa intermedia, which is an interthalamic adhesion (situated above the tectum and midline), is characteristic of Chiari 2 malformation.

E. Vermian hypoplasia is most commonly associated with Dandy Walker malformations. Herniation of the vermis is seen in Chiari 2 malformations, but the vermis is not hypoplastic in these cases.

Question 2

B. Correct! The "strawberry" sign is most commonly associated with trisomy 18. The strawberry sign refers to a flattened occiput and a pointed anterior calvarium. These are associated with hypoplasia of the occipital and frontal bones, causing brachycephaly.

Other choices and discussion

A. The "lemon" sign refers to a biconcave appearance of the frontal bones due to the open neural defect of the spine associated with Chiari 2 malformation. It is rarely seen in fetuses > 24 weeks, secondary to decreased pliability of the calvarium and increased hydrocephalus.

C. By definition, Chiari 2 malformation contains an open neural tube defect, most commonly a myelomeningocele.

D. Elevated maternal alpha-fetoprotein is best evaluated at 15 to 20 weeks of gestation. When elevated, it is suggestive of an open neural tube defect (a prerequisite component of Chiari 2, as discussed above) and should be correlated with the 20-week prenatal ultrasound screening examination. In addition to open neural tube defects, an elevated alpha-fetoprotein is also associated with ventral abdominal wall defects.

E. On axial imaging of the fetal posterior fossa, the "banana" sign represents crowding of the posterior fossa. Specifically, the cerebellar hemispheres form a banana shape as they wrap around the brainstem. This is due to downward herniation of those elements secondary to a tethered cord and an open neural tube defect.

Question 3

E. Correct! Leukemic involvement of the spine affects the bone marrow but not the cord itself.

Other choices and discussion

A and B. Syringomyelia (as known as syrinx) is a cystic spinal cord cavity that is not contiguous with the central cord canal and is due to alterations of cerebrospinal fluid (CSF) flow. Both Chiari 1 and 2 malformations can cause syringomyelia. A screening magnetic resonance imaging examination of the spine should be performed to rule out a syrinx at initial diagnosis of a Chiari malformation.

C. Scoliosis is not a cause for syringomyelia. However, many studies suggest that scoliosis develops in the presence of a syrinx. It is postulated that abnormal intramedullary pressure in the spinal cord causes interference with the postural tonic reflexes. Up to 82% of children with a syrinx will have scoliosis.

D. Klippel-Feil syndrome can cause alterations of CSF flow similar to that of severe scoliosis. In addition, skull and upper cervical spine fusion anomalies associated with the syndrome can also alter CSF flow, mimicking the dynamics of a Chiari malformation.

■ Suggested Readings

Atalar MH, Salk I, Egilmez H. Classical signs and appearances in pediatric neuroradiology: a pictorial review. Polish J Radiol 2014;79:479–489

Driscoll DA, Gross SJ. Screening for fetal aneuploidy and neural tube defects. Genetics in Med 2009;11:818–821

Eule JM, Erickson MA, O'Brien MF, et al. Chiari I malformation associated with syringomyelia and scoliosis: a twenty-year review of surgical and nonsurgical treatment in a pediatric population. Spine 2002;27:1451–1455

Kagawa M, Jinnai T, Matsumoto Y, et al. Chiari I malformation accompanied by assimilation of the atlas, Klippel-Feil syndrome, and syringomyelia: case report. Surgical Neurol 2006;65:497–502

Top Tips

◆ Chiari 1 malformation is peg-like in configuration, and the cerebellar tonsillar herniation below the foramen magnum measures 6 mm or greater in symptomatic patients. A screening spinal imaging study should be performed to evaluate for the presence of a syrinx upon initial diagnosis of a Chiari 1 malformation.

◆ Chiari 2 malformation is always associated with an open spinal defect, most commonly a lumbosacral myelomeningocele.

◆ The "lemon" and "banana" signs represent prenatal sequelae of a Chiari 2 malformation.

Essentials 7

■ Case

A patient presents with a history of congenital pulmonary abnormality.

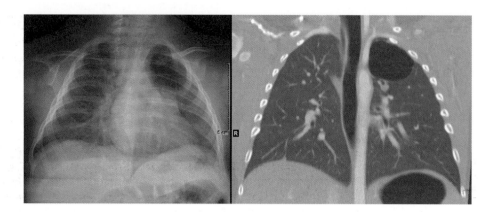

■ Questions

1. Which of the following features differentiate pure congenital pulmonary airway malformation from pulmonary sequestration?
   A. Cystic lung disease
   B. Most commonly occurs in the left upper lobe
   C. Lack of systemic arterial supply
   D. Solid component
   E. None of the above

2. Which ONE of the following is NOT helpful in differentiating between intralobar and extralobar sequestration?
   A. Venous drainage
   B. Arterial supply
   C. Typical age of presentation
   D. Pleural investment

3. Which ONE of the following presents as a solid lung lesion?
   A. Bronchial atresia
   B. Congenital lobar overinflation
   C. Diaphragmatic hernia
   D. Type 3 congenital pulmonary airway malformation
   E. Type 1 pleuropulmonary blastoma

■ Answers and Explanations

Question 1

C. Correct! The test case demonstrates a cystic lesion within the left upper lobe, without aberrant systemic arterial supply or internal lung markings, most consistent with a purely macrocystic congenital pulmonary airway malformation (CPAM). Pure CPAM lesions should not contain a systemic arterial supply, but instead should have a pulmonary artery supply. This is in contradistinction to pulmonary sequestrations that always have a systemic arterial supply and no airway connection. Hybrid CPAMs are lesions with airway connections and systemic arterial supply.

Other choices and discussion

A. Both CPAM and sequestrations can contain cystic components. Type 1 CPAMs are macrocystic, whereas type 2 CPAMs contain smaller cysts.

B. A distinct pattern of lobar involvement has not been described in CPAM. Pulmonary sequestration is typically seen in the lower lobes, with the left side more often involved than the right. The left upper lobe is most commonly affected in congenital lobar overinflation, followed by the right middle lobe, and then the right upper lobe.

D. Solid components can be present in both CPAMs and sequestrations.

Question 2

B. Correct! Arterial supply does not help differentiate between intra- and extralobar sequestration, as both have a systemic arterial supply.

Other choices and discussion

A. Intralobar sequestration typically has pulmonary venous drainage, whereas extralobar sequestration drains systemically.

C. Intralobar sequestration typically presents in later childhood with recurrent pneumonias in the same location. Extralobar sequestration typically presents in the prenatal/neonatal period.

D. Extralobar sequestration has a separate pleural investment, whereas intralobar sequestration shares the pleural investment with the adjacent normal lung. This difference is usually not evident radiographically.

Question 3

D. Correct! Microcystic CPAM (type 3) presents as a solid mass, not a lucent lesion, as is seen in type 1 and 2 lesions (macrocystic and small cysts, respectively).

Other choices and discussion

A. Interruption of a bronchus with hyperlucent lung distally is most characteristic of bronchial atresia. Oftentimes, mucous can fill the interrupted bronchus, creating a "finger in glove" appearance.

B. Congenital lobar hyperinflation is the end result of airway insult and is represented by dilated alveoli. When imaged early in life, these may present as opaque consolidations. However, the opaque appearance is due to incomplete clearance of fluid, and with serial imaging, there will be eventual clearance to a hyperlucent, air-filled lung.

C. Although fluid within herniated bowel can have a solid appearance, some gas is typically present. Thus, this choice is excluded. In fact, gas in herniated bowel can often mimic a lucent lung lesion.

E. Pleuropulmonary blastomas have variable appearances in the chest, including lucent lesions. They are categorized by intralesional components. Air-filled lucent lesions are type 1. Cystic lesions with variable solid components are type 2. Solid lesions with mass effect are type 3.

■ Suggested Readings

Biyyam DR, Chapman T, Ferguson MR, et al. Congenital lung abnormalities: embryologic features, prenatal diagnosis, and postnatal radiologic-pathologic correlation. Radiographics 2010;30:1721–1738

SECTION X PEDIATRIC IMAGING

Top Tips

◆ Radiographically, there are three types of CPAMs: macrocystic, small cysts, and microcystic/solid.

◆ Pulmonary sequestrations have an arterial systemic supply and lack communication to the airways.

◆ Intralobar sequestrations have pulmonary venous drainage, whereas extralobar sequestrations have systemic venous drainage. Intralobar sequestrations often present with recurrent same-site pneumonia.

Essentials 8

■ Case

A patient presents with a history of trauma.

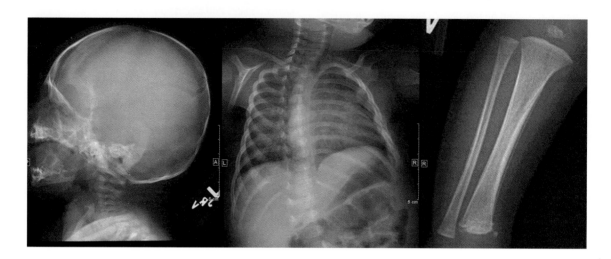

■ Questions

1. Which ONE of the following is consistent with nonaccidental trauma?
   A. Metaphyseal fraying
   B. Diffuse osteopenia
   C. Widening of the physis
   D. Metaphyseal corner fracture

2. The proposed mechanism for a classic metaphyseal lesion is which of the following?
   A. Isolated avulsion fracture at the corner of the metaphysis
   B. Compressive axial force along the axis of the metaphysis
   C. Transmetaphyseal disruption of the trabeculae of the primary spongiosa due to shear or bending forces
   D. Direct perpendicular force to the axis of the diaphysis creating propagation of the fracture through the metaphysis

3. After detection of a classic metaphyseal lesion, what is the next BEST step for the radiologist?
   A. Urgent call to the referring physician, and request a skeletal survey.
   B. Call to the on-call social worker.
   C. Report the findings as usual, as most clinicians understand what a classic metaphyseal lesion signifies.
   D. Call law enforcement.

■ Answers and Explanations

Question 1

D. Correct! This is case of nonaccidental trauma (NAT), with a skull fracture of the parietal bone, multiple healing bilateral posterior rib fractures, and a corner metaphyseal fracture of the distal tibia. Corner metaphyseal fractures are essentially diagnostic of NAT, while all of the remaining listed choices are characteristic of rickets instead. There is some minor controversy on whether healed rickets can have a similar appearance to the metaphyseal corner fracture, aka classic metaphyseal lesion (CML), but if the other listed features of rickets are absent, the CML remains highly suspicious for NAT.

Question 2

C. Correct! As stated above, CML is a transmetaphyseal fracture due to shear or bending forces through the primary spongiosa.

Other choices and discussion

A. Although CML is also known as a metaphyseal corner fracture, it represents more than simply an avulsion injury. The CML is also known as a bucket handle fracture, which more accurately describes the transmetaphyseal fracture course.

B. Compressive forces at the metaphysis are classically associated with a Salter-Harris V fracture of the physis. These fractures are rare.

D. Direct perpendicular force to the axis of the diaphysis can cause transverse fractures or fractures with a butterfly segment. If they do extend to the metaphysis, a CML should not be present.

Question 3

A. Correct! CMLs are strongly associated with child abuse, and in 95% of the cases, an additional traumatic injury is present. A skeletal survey is an effective way of identifying additional osseous injuries in this vulnerable population and has been shown to detect another fracture in up to 87% of the cases.

Other choices and discussion

B. Although a social work consultation is appropriate, this is not the primary responsibility of the radiologist. The urgent call to the referring clinician will prompt this social work evaluation.

C. As stated above, a CML is highly suspicious for NAT, and the responsibility of conveying the seriousness of this finding belongs to the radiologist.

D. Although law enforcement may need to become involved, this decision should be made by the clinicians and social workers after a complete evaluation is performed.

■ Suggested Readings

Thackeray JD, Wannemacher J, Adler BH, et al. The classic metaphyseal lesion and traumatic injury. Ped Radiol 2016;46(8):1128–1133

Wood BP. Commentary on "a critical review of the classic metaphyseal lesion: traumatic or metabolic?" Am J Roentgenol 2014;202:197–198

Top Tips

◆ CML, also known as a metaphyseal bucket handle or corner fracture, is highly suspicious for NAT.

◆ When a CML is detected, direct communication should be made to the referring physician, and a skeletal survey should be performed.

◆ Radiographic findings of rickets include diffuse osteopenia, fraying or cupping of the metaphysis, and widening of the physis.

Essentials 9

■ Case

A pediatric patient with a history of seizures.

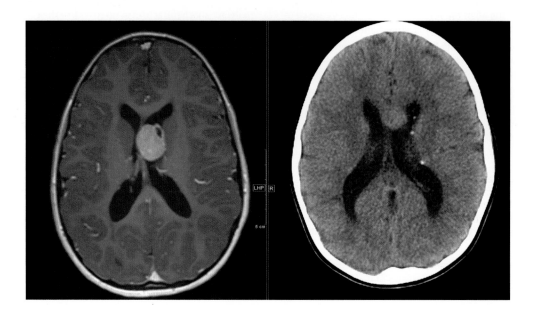

■ Questions

1. Which ONE of the following is MOST characteristic of tuberous sclerosis complex?
   A. Subcortical tubers
   B. Band heterotopia
   C. Cardiac lipomas
   D. Bone cysts
   E. Posterior fossa hemangioblastoma

2. Adenoma sebaceum (angiofibromas of the skin), subependymal nodules, bone islands, and cardiac rhabdomyomas associated with tuberous sclerosis complex are categorized as which of the following?
   A. Malignant tumors
   B. Hamartomas
   C. Teratomas
   D. Dysplasias

3. How can subependymal nodules best be differentiated from subependymal giant cell astrocytomas on imaging?
   A. Size
   B. Location
   C. Calcification
   D. Contrast enhancement
   E. Magnetic resonance spectroscopy

■ Answers and Explanations

Question 1

A. Correct! This is a case of tuberous sclerosis complex (TSC), with multiple calcified subependymal nodules on computed tomography and an enhancing subependymal giant cell astrocytoma on magnetic resonance imaging. TSC consists of the classic clinical triad of seizures, mental retardation, and adenoma sebaceum. Subcortical tubers are one of the hallmarks of TSC. The tubers are scattered through the brain parenchyma and are both T1 and T2 hyperintense prior to myelination, but become T1 hypointense after myelination.

Other choices and discussion

B. Subependymal nodules are characteristic of TSC, are generally distributed in a similar fashion in the germinal matrix, and are most conspicuous in the caudothalamic grooves. Although these are considered heterotopias (subependymal type), they are a separate entity from band heterotopias.

C. Up to 80% of the cases of TSC have intracardiac rhabdomyomas, not lipomas. Oftentimes, multiple rhabdomyomas are present. Thus, a diagnosis of multiple intracardiac rhabdomyomas is very suggestive of TSC.

D. Bone islands, not bone cysts, can be seen in TSC. These benign sclerotic osseous lesions typically have an axial rather than an appendicular distribution.

E. Posterior fossa hemangioblastomas are associated with Von Hippel-Lindau syndrome, not TSC. Other important manifestations of TSC include lymphangioleiomyomatosis in the lungs and angiomyolipomas in the kidneys.

Question 2

B. Correct! Hamartomas are lesions of normal tissue in abnormal locations. All of the sequelae of TSC listed can be considered hamartomas.

Other choices and discussion

A. None of the listed lesions are malignant. Subependymal nodules are benign but can transform into giant cell astrocytoma, a low-grade benign tumor.

C. Teratomas are masses that contain components derived from all three primitive germ cell layers.

D. Dysplasia is a process in which normal cells undergo change to a premalignant stage (as in cervical dysplasia). The listed sequelae of TSC do not have malignant potential and thus do not fit this definition.

Question 3

E. Correct! Magnetic resonance spectroscopy is the most specific indicator of subependymal giant cell astrocytomas (SEGAs), demonstrating high choline-to-creatine and low N-acetylaspartate-to-creatine ratios with SEGAs but not with subependymal nodules. When spectroscopy is not available, the combination of all imaging characteristics should be used to help differentiate SEGAs from subependymal nodules

Other choices and discussion

A. Size alone is not a good discriminator of SEGAs. SEGAs are slow-growing, low-grade tumors originating from subependymal nodules. Some studies have suggested that lesions > 1 cm should raise suspicion for SEGA.

B. All SEGAs are intraventricular, and a majority of SEGAs occur near the foramen of Monro. However, location alone is not diagnostic of SEGAs, as subependymal nodules can also occur near the foramen of Monro.

C. Most (90%) of subependymal nodules will calcify by adulthood. However, prior to adulthood, the lack of calcification is not specific for either SEGAs or subependymal nodules.

D. All SEGAs will demonstrate contrast enhancement. However, subependymal contrast enhancement is variable, ranging from 30 to 80%. Thus, enhancement is not a good discriminator of SEGAs.

■ Suggested Readings

Carvalho Neto A de, Gasparetto EL, Bruck I. Subependymal giant cell astrocytoma with high choline/creatine ratio on proton MR spectroscopy. Arquivos de neuro-psiquiatria 2006;64:877–880

Manoukian SB, Kowal DJ. Comprehensive imaging manifestations of tuberous sclerosis. Am J Roentgenol 2015;204:933–943

Mühler MR, Rake A, Schwabe M, et al. Value of fetal cerebral MRI in sonographically-proven cardiac rhabdomyoma. Ped Radiol 2007;37:467–474

Top Tips

◆ TSC is a hamartomatous disease manifested by skin angiofibromas, subependymal nodules, intracardiac rhabdomyomas, and bone islands.

◆ Other important features of TSC include lymphangioleiomyomatosis of the lungs and renal angiomyolipomas.

◆ SEGAs can be differentiated from their precursor subependymal nodules by a size > 1 cm, contrast enhancement, lack of calcification, predilection for regions near the foramen of Monro, and high choline-to-creatine and low N-acetylaspartate-to-creatine ratios.

Essentials 10

■ Case

A patient presents with an abdominal mass and elevated catecholamines.

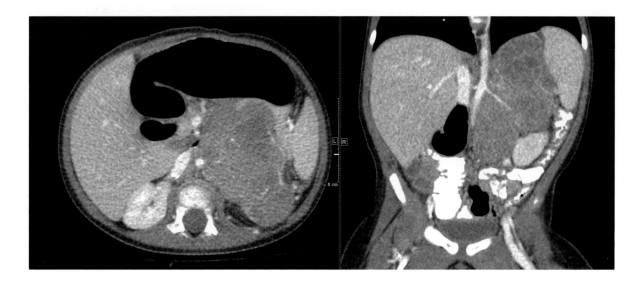

■ Questions

1. Which of the following features does NOT help differentiate adrenal neuroblastoma from Wilms tumor?
   A. Intratumoral calcification
   B. Size
   C. Shape
   D. Bone metastasis
   E. Lung metastasis

2. The new imaged-based International Neuroblastoma Risk Group staging system takes into account image-defined risk factors, rather than surgical findings. Which ONE of the following is a considered a major image-defined risk factor?
   A. Single body compartment involvement
   B. Ascites
   C. Pleural effusion
   D. Encasement or invasion of vascular structures
   E. Abutment to the airway

3. Which imaging modality is BEST to follow up neuroblastoma?
   A. Technetium-99m methyl diphosphonate bone scan
   B. I-123 metaiodobenzylguanidine scan
   C. Fluorodeoxyglucose positron emission tomography/computed tomography
   D. Whole-body magnetic resonance imaging
   E. Computed tomography of the chest, abdomen, and pelvis

■ Answers and Explanations

Question 1

B. Correct! This is a case of neuroblastoma. The images show an irregularly shaped abdominal mass with punctate calcifications. This mass lifts the aorta (seen on the axial computed tomography [CT] image) and encases a branch of the aorta (seen on the coronal CT image). Tumor size is not a good discriminator for neuroblastoma and Wilms tumor. Both can be small or occupy most of the abdomen.

Other choices and discussion

A. Intratumoral calcifications are much more common in neuroblastoma than in Wilms tumor.

C. As a general rule, Wilms tumor grows in a radial fashion, creating a rounded ball-shaped mass that exerts mass effect. On the other hand, neuroblastoma is a "softer" mass and will insinuate between structures, creating a more irregular shape.

D. Bone metastases are much more common in neuroblastoma than in Wilms tumor.

E. Lung metastases are rare in neuroblastoma and are much more common in Wilms tumor.

Question 2

D. Correct! Vascular encasement or invasion is considered a major image-defined risk factor (IDRF). Greater than 50% circumferential encasement qualifies as a major IDRF. In the new INRG staging system, tumor in one body compartment without vital organ involvement is staged as L1. L2 tumors involve one or more major IDRFs. Tumors are staged as M if distant metastases are present. As in the old classification, there is a special stage, MS, signifying improved prognosis in children < 18 months of age. These MS tumors have metastases confined to the skin, liver, and bone marrow. Keep in mind that the bone marrow metastases in MS tumors should only be present on biopsy, and must be negative by iodine metaiodobenzylguanidine (I-123 or I-131 MIBG) imaging.

Other choices and discussion

A. Body compartments in the International Neuroblastoma Risk Group staging system include the neck, chest, abdomen, and pelvis. Involvement of more than one compartment is considered a major IDRF.

B. Ascites should be noted in the findings when staging for neuroblastoma, but it is not considered a major IDRF.

C. Similar to ascites, pleural effusion should be noted in the findings when staging for neuroblastoma, but it is not considered a major IDRF.

E. Simple abutment of the airway does not constitute a major IDRF. Abutment *and* compression is required for inclusion of a major IDRF.

Question 3

B. Correct! Only when the initial tumor is not avid on an I-123 metaiodobenzylguanidine (MIBG) scan (5 to 10% of cases) are other modalities used to follow up neuroblastoma.

Other choices and discussion

A. Nuclear medicine bone scans are not required for staging of neuroblastoma. The majority of neuroblastomas are MIBG-avid. Additionally, MIBG scans are more sensitive and can detect lesions that are not positive on bone scan.

C. Fluorodeoxyglucose positron emission tomography is not as sensitive as an MIBG scan for bone metastases. MIBG single photon emission CT scans can also be performed, if additional anatomic detail is needed after the planar images are reviewed.

D. Whole-body magnetic resonance imaging has not shown to be more sensitive than MIBG for the follow up of neuroblastoma.

E. Although the initial diagnosis may be made by CT, it is not an ideal modality to follow up MIBG-avid neuroblastoma, as follow up with I-123 MIBG scans alone gives much less radiation exposure than performing both scans, and MIBG is more sensitive for osseous metastasis.

■ Suggested Readings

Davidoff AM. Neuroblastoma. Semin Ped Surg 2012;21:2–14

McCarville MB. Imaging neuroblastoma: what the radiologist needs to know. Cancer Imaging 2011;11:S44

Monclair T, Brodeur GM, Ambros PF, et al. The international neuroblastoma risk group (inrg) staging system: an inrg task force report. J Clin Oncol 2009;27:298–303

Sharp SE, Parisi MT, Gelfand MJ, et al. Functional-metabolic imaging of neuroblastoma. Q J Nucl Med Mol Imaging 2013;57:6–20

Top Tips

- When compared to Wilms tumor, an abdominal neuroblastoma more commonly presents with intratumoral calcifications, an insinuating irregular shape, encasement of major structures, and bone metastases.

- Staging of neuroblastoma relies on imaging and is categorized based on distant metastases and the number of anatomic compartments involved.

- A separate MS staging category for neuroblastoma is used for patients < 18 months of age who have metastases confined to the liver, skin, and bone marrow. These patients have a relatively better prognosis when compared to stage M cases.

Details 1

■ Case

A patient with a history of viral encephalitis. Which ONE of the following is TRUE regarding cytomegalovirus (CMV) encephalitis?

    A. Periventricular calcification is atypical.
    B. Cortical dysplasia can result from the infection.
    C. Periventricular cysts are not associated with the infection.
    D. Corpus callosal malformation is diagnostic.

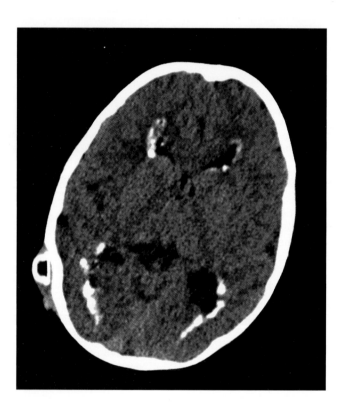

■ The following questions pertain to CMV infection and intracranial imaging.

1. Which sequence is most useful in detection of early herpes simplex viral (HSV) encephalitis?
2. Maternal exposure to cat excreta places the fetus at risk for which encephalitis?
3. Although maternal diabetes is not associated with a known encephalitis, it is associated with what other neural axis diseases?
4. Manifestations of congenital CMV, such as delayed myelination, are dependent upon what factor?
5. Periventricular cysts in congenital CMV represent what disease process?
6. True or False. Congenital CMV is associated with congenital sensorineural hearing loss.
7. True or False. On neonatal ultrasound of the brain, lenticulostriate vasculopathy is diagnostic of congenital CMV infection.
8. Germinal matrix hemorrhage that causes ventricular dilation with intraventricular involvement, but lack of parenchymal extension, is what grade by sonographic evaluation?
9. What sonographic window may be helpful in improved evaluation of the posterior fossa in neonates?

■ Answers and Explanations

B. Correct! One of the important causes of cortical dysplasia is CMV infection. In fact, congenital CMV infection is associated with agyria, pachygyria, polymicrogyria, and schizencephaly. This test case is an example of CMV infection.

Other choices and discussion

A. Periventricular calcification can be striking on computed tomography and is seen in up to 70% of intracranial CMV infections. However, these calcifications are nonspecific and can be seen in many other entities such as other TORCH infections and ischemic or toxic encephalitis.

C. Periventricular cysts are sometimes seen in congenital CMV. These can be visualized in pre- and postnatal sonography of the brain.

D. Although CMV infection can cause parenchymal dysplasias including hippocampal malformation, corpus callosal malformation is not associated with nor diagnostic for CMV infection. The characteristic configuration of the hippocampus in congenital CMV is vertical, instead of the normal horizontal arrangement.

Question 1

Diffusion-weighted imaging is the most useful sequence in the detection of early HSV, as it can reveal cortical involvement earlier than standard magnetic resonance imaging (MRI) sequences. Cortical involvement of HSV encephalitis will present as edema on standard MRI sequences (T1 hypointense, T2 hyperintense, and fluid-attenuated inversion recovery hyperintense). There may be patchy cortical and meningeal enhancement. However, these findings on standard MRI do not present as early as restricted diffusion.

Question 2

Maternal exposure to cat excreta can cause congenital toxoplasmosis, a protozoan infection. The fetal infection occurs across the placenta. The calcification in the brain parenchyma is more random than is seen in congenital CMV. Normocephaly is present in CMV infection, whereas microcephaly is present in toxoplasmosis.

Question 3

Maternal diabetes is associated with caudal regression syndrome, anencephaly, and spina bifida.

Question 4

Manifestations of congenital CMV are dependent on the gestational age at the time of the infection. Perinatal infection typically results in delayed myelination. Evaluation of age-appropriate myelination can be vastly aided by a myelination atlas. Prenatal infections can cause lissencephaly with a small cerebellum (gestational age of 18 weeks or younger), cortical gyral abnormalities (18 to 24 weeks of gestation), and periventricular cysts (third trimester).

Question 5

Periventricular cysts in congenital CMV represent leukomalacia.

Question 6

True. Congenital CMV is associated with congenital sensorineural hearing loss.

Question 7

False. Although lenticulostriate vasculopathy can be seen in congenital CMV infection, it is not a specific sign in isolation. There are many other causes of lenticulostriate vasculopathy including other TORCH infections, chromosomal abnormalities, maternal diabetes, and hypoxic conditions.

Question 8

Ventricular dilation with intraventricular involvement, but lack of parenchymal extension, is Grade 3. Grade 1 hemorrhage is confined to the germinal matrix without ventricular dilation. Grade 2 hemorrhage extends to the ventricles, without hydrocephalus. Grade 4 hemorrhage is defined by intraparenchymal extension.

Question 9

The mastoid or posterolateral fontanelle can aid in improved visualization of the posterior fossa in neonates.

■ Suggested Readings

Jelacic S, de Regt D, Weinberger E. Interactive digital MR atlas of the pediatric brain. Radiographics 2006;26:497–501

Lanari M, Capretti MG, Lazzarotto T, et al. Neuroimaging in CMV congenital infected neonates: how and when. Early Hum Dev 2012;88:S3–S5

Maayan-Metzger A, Leibovitch L, Schushan-Eisen I, Soudack M, et al. Risk factors and associated diseases among preterm infants with isolated lenticulostriate vasculopathy. J Perinatol 2016;36(9):775–778

Okanishi T, Yamamoto H, Hosokawa T, et al. Diffusion-weighted MRI for early diagnosis of neonatal herpes simplex encephalitis. Brain Dev 2015;37:423–431

Papile LA, Burstein J, Burstein R, et al. Incidence and evolution of subependymal and intraventricular hemorrhage: a study of infants with birth weights less than 1,500 gm. J Pediatr 1978;92:529–534

Top Tips

- ◆ Periventricular calcifications in a neonate should prompt evaluation for infectious causes such as TORCH infections.
- ◆ Diffusion-weighted imaging is the most sensitive sequence for detection of intracranial HSV infection.
- ◆ Lenticulostriate vasculopathy is nonspecific, but can be present in TORCH infections.

Details 2

■ Case

A 2-year-old presents with elevated alpha fetoprotein (AFP). Which ONE of the following statements regarding pediatric liver masses in general is TRUE?

  A. Unlike hepatoblastoma, childhood hepatocellular carcinoma (HCC) does not typically lead to an elevated AFP.
  B. Focal nodular hyperplasia (FNH) has an increased incidence in children with a history of prior chemotherapy.
  C. Infantile liver hemangiomas are present at birth.
  D. Mesenchymal hamartomas in the liver are typically solid and malignant.
  E. Undifferentiated embryonal sarcomas of the liver typically lead to an elevated AFP.

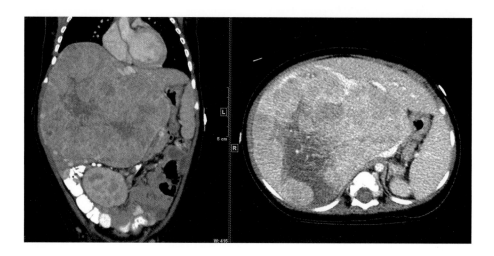

■ The following questions pertain to pediatric hepatic masses.

1. Other than AFP, which additional tumor marker is elevated in hepatoblastoma?
2. What percentage of hepatoblastomas contain calcification?
3. True or False. Hepatoblastomas typically present as homogenous hypoechoic masses.
4. What is the most common site of hepatoblastoma metastases?
5. What imaging feature helps distinguish tumor thrombus from bland thrombus?
6. What is the classic enhancement pattern of an infantile hepatic hemangioma?
7. Aside from FNH, what other solid hepatic mass can present with a central scar?
8. What gadolinium agent is preferred when evaluating for FNH?
9. When multiple hepatic masses are present, the differential should expand to metastasis. What is the most common primary tumor that metastasizes to the liver in children?

■ Answers and Explanations

B. Correct! An important risk factor to remember in cases of FNH is prior exposure to chemotherapy. When this clinical history is present in the setting of a liver mass with a central scar, the diagnosis of FNH should be strongly suspected.

Other choices and discussion

A. The test case images show a large hepatic mass in a young child. With the provided history (elevated AFP in a patient < 4 years old), this hepatic mass is consistent with a hepatoblastoma. However, HCC (a rarer childhood hepatic tumor) can also lead to an elevated AFP level, in both adult and pediatric cases. Note also that the AFP value is a useful marker for follow up purposes.

C. Congenital hemangiomas, within the liver or elsewhere, are present at birth.

D. Mesenchymal hamartomas, within the liver or elsewhere, are not malignant. They consist of benign cells that occur in an abnormal location. Liver hamartomas usually contain a predominant cystic component with variable soft tissue nodules.

E. Undifferentiated embryonal sarcomas of the liver typically do not lead to an elevated AFP. There have been case reports, but this is rare.

Question 1

Although an elevated AFP in the setting of a liver mass for a child < 4 years of age is essentially diagnostic of hepatoblastoma, an elevated beta human chorionic gonadotropin is also occasionally elevated in these tumors. Afflicted children can present with precocious puberty secondary to the elevated human chorionic gonadotropin levels.

Question 2

Up to 50% of hepatoblastomas demonstrate internal calcification.

Question 3

False. The sonographic appearance of a hepatoblastoma is typically heterogeneous, particularly if calcifications are present. Hypoechoic areas often represent regions of tumor necrosis.

Question 4

The lungs are the most common site of hepatoblastoma metastases.

Question 5

Contrast enhancement helps distinguish tumor thrombus from bland thrombus, as tumor thrombus tends to enhance.

Question 6

The classic enhancement pattern of an infantile hepatic hemangioma is peripheral nodular arterial enhancement with progressive centripetal fill-in on delayed imaging.

Question 7

Like FNH, fibrolamellar HCC can have a central scar. Fibrolamellar HCC is found in adolescents and young adults and typically presents as a large hepatic mass in a noncirrhotic liver. The central scar can demonstrate calcification. It demonstrates hyperenhancement on the arterial phase with washout on subsequent phases.

Question 8

Gadoxetate disodium (aka Eovist) is recommended for FNH evaluation. Eovist is a hepatobiliary contrast agent that is partially excreted by hepatocytes. The hepatobiliary phase (approximately 20 minutes after administration) will demonstrate persistent enhancement in cases of FNH, in contrast to hepatic adenomas, which will appear hypointense on this delayed phase.

Question 9

Neuroblastoma is the most common primary tumor to cause hepatic metastasis in children.

■ Suggested Readings

Chung EM, Lattin GE, Cube R, et al. From the archives of the AFIP: pediatric liver masses: radiologic-pathologic correlation. Part 2. Malignant tumors. Radiographics 2011;31(2):483–507

Das CJ, Dhingra S, Gupta AK, et al. Imaging of paediatric liver tumours with pathological correlation. Clin Radiol 2009;64: 1015–1025

Putra J, Ornvold K. Undifferentiated embryonal sarcoma of the liver: a concise review. Archives Path Laboratory Med 2015;139: 269–273

Ricafort R. Tumor markers in infancy and childhood. Pediatr Review-Elk Grove 2011;32:306

**SECTION X
PEDIATRIC IMAGING**

Top Tips

◆ Consider hepatoblastoma in children with a heterogenous liver mass who are < 4 years old. In an older patient with preexisting liver disease, HCC is more common.

◆ Correlation with AFP is helpful because it is elevated in hepatoblastoma and HCC.

◆ Consider FNH in children exposed to chemotherapy, particularly if the classic central scar is present.

Details 3

■ Case

A patient presents with a history of right lower quadrant abdominal pain. Which ONE of the following combination of sonographic signs has the best sensitivity and specificity profile for appendicitis?
 A. Outer diameter > 7 mm, and single wall thickness > 4 mm
 B. Outer diameter > 9 mm, and single wall thickness > 1.7 mm
 C. Outer diameter > 9 mm, and single wall thickness > 4 mm
 D. Outer diameter > 7 mm, and single wall thickness > 1.7 mm

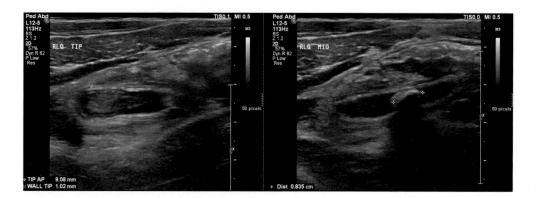

■ The following questions pertain to pediatric appendicitis and other causes of right lower quadrant pain.

1. How often are appendicoliths seen in cases of acute appendicitis?
2. Name at least three secondary sonographic signs of appendicitis.
3. True or False. Enlarged right lower quadrant mesenteric lymph nodes without evidence of appendicitis is diagnostic of mesenteric adenitis.
4. The sonographic target or pseudo-kidney sign is consistent with ileocolic intussusception. What imaging signs predict reduction failure by contrast enema?
5. How often are pathologic lead points present in cases of ileocolic intussusception?

6. A Meckel diverticulum can act as a pathologic lead point in children. What are the "rules of 2" for a Meckel diverticulum?
7. What radiotracer is used for a Meckel scan, and what is its mechanism of uptake?
8. What pharmacologic agents can be used to increase the sensitivity of a Meckel scan?
9. What is the most common complication of a Meckel diverticulum in young children?

■ Answers and Explanations

D. Correct! In a large series with surgical correlation, the most sensitive and specific measurements for acute appendicitis were an outer diameter > 7 mm and single wall thickness > 1.7 mm. The test case is an example of a patient with appendicitis.

Question 1

Appendicoliths are seen in 10 to 20% cases of acute appendicitis.

Question 2

Secondary sonographic signs of appendicitis: adjacent echogenic fat, appendiceal wall hyperemia, enlarged lymph nodes, echogenic free fluid, or loculated fluid.

Question 3

False. Enlarged mesenteric lymph nodes can be present in many alternative diagnoses other than appendicitis. These include, but are not limited to, gastroenteritis, lymphoma, intussusception, and inflammatory bowel disease. Mesenteric adenitis is a clinical diagnosis of exclusion. In addition to the enlarged lymph nodes, thickened or inflamed bowel may be present in mesenteric adenitis.

Question 4

The "dissection" sign and trapped fluid within the intussusceptum are two findings that predict reduction failure by contrast enema. The dissection sign occurs when the contrast material (either air or water-soluble enteric contrast) is interposed between the intussusceptum and the intussuscipiens. Fluid trapped within the intussusception is also associated with a decreased rate of successful reduction. Clinically, when symptoms have been present for > 48 hours, the success rate of reduction also decreases.

Question 5

Pathologic lead points are present in 25% cases of ileocolic intussusception. The incidence of pathologic lead points in cases of intussusception increases as children get older. In fact, a large surgical series demonstrated that pathologic lead points accounted for 5% of cases in patients from 0 to 11 months of age, and up to 60% of cases in patients from 5 to 14 years old.

Question 6

Meckel diverticula are typically located 2 feet from the ileocecal valve, contain at least two types of mucosa, occur in 2% of the population, and are symptomatic before the age of 2.

Question 7

Technetium-99m pertechnetate is used for Meckel. This radiotracer accumulates in ectopic gastric mucosa that is typically present in the diverticulum.

Question 8

Pentagastrin, ranitidine or cimetidine, and glucagon have all been used to increase the sensitivity of a Meckel scan.

Question 9

Gastrointestinal bleeding is the most common complication of Meckel diverticula in young children. In adolescents, gastrointestinal obstruction becomes more common, making it the second most common complication of Meckel diverticula.

■ Suggested Readings

Barr LL, Stansberry SD, Swischuk LE. Significance of age, duration, obstruction and the dissection sign in intussusception. Pediatr Radiol 1990;20:454–456

Blakelock RT, Beasley SW. The clinical implications of non-idiopathic intussusception. Pediatr Surg Int 1998;14:163–167

Fishman MC, Borden S, Cooper A. The dissection sign of nonreducible ileocolic intussusception. Am J Roentgenol 1984;143:5–8

Goldin AB, Khanna P, Thapa M, et al. Revised ultrasound criteria for appendicitis in children improve diagnostic accuracy. Pediatr Radiol 2011;41:993–999

Levy AD, Hobbs CM. From the archives of the AFIP: Meckel diverticulum: radiologic features with pathologic correlation. Radiographics 2004;24:565–587

Ntoulia A, Tharakan SJ, Reid JR, et al. Failed intussusception reduction in children: correlation between radiologic, surgical, and pathologic findings. Am J Roentgenol 2016;207(2):424–433

Top Tips

◆ A noncompressible appendix measuring > 7 mm in diameter with a thickened wall measuring > 1.7 mm is highly suggestive of acute appendicitis.

◆ Idiopathic intussusception occurs in young children, usually < 3 years of age. If this entity occurs in an older child, remember to exclude a pathologic lead point.

◆ The Meckel diverticulum "rules of 2" include at least two types of mucosa (most commonly ectopic gastric mucosa), and this is why a technetium-99m pertechnetate scan is sensitive in the diagnosis.

Details 4

■ Case

A patient presents with a history of bilious emesis. Which of the following is the definitive workup for a child with bilious emesis?

    A. Ultrasound

    B. Fluoroscopic contrast upper gastrointestinal (GI)

    C. Low-dose computed tomography

    D. Fast T2 magnetic resonance imaging such as a half-Fourier-acquired single-shot turbo spin echo sequence

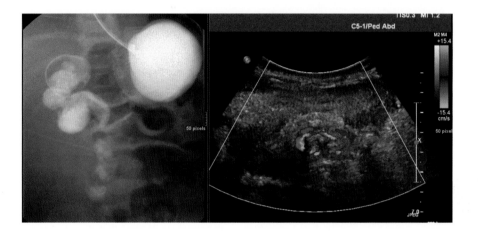

■ The following questions pertain to pediatric right upper quadrant pathology.

1. What are the criteria for proper position of the ligament of Treitz or the DJJ?

2. If on a fluoroscopic upper GI the DJJ is equivocal or borderline, what can the radiologist do to further evaluate for possible malrotation?

3. In what percent of malrotation cases is the cecum abnormally positioned?

4. Midgut volvulus can present radiographically as a "double bubble." What is the differential diagnosis for this appearance?

5. What genetic anomaly is associated with duodenal atresia?

6. What mathematical term is a helpful memory aid for the abnormal measurements on ultrasound for hypertrophic pyloric stenosis (HPS)?

7. True or False. HPS most commonly affects Caucasian male newborns.

8. What is the best position of the child to sonographically evaluate HPS?

9. What is the best way to differentiate pyloric spasm from HPS?

■ Answers and Explanations

B. Correct! Fluoroscopic upper GI is the diagnostic exam of choice when malrotation is to be excluded. It is a specific exam with reported false-negative rates of 3 to 6%. In the test case, the fluoroscopic image demonstrates malrotation. The duodeno-jejunal junction (DJJ) is to the right of the spine in a corkscrew configuration, suggestive of concurrent volvulus, and this is confirmed with sonography.

Other choices and discussion

A. Although abnormal mesenteric vessel orientation has been associated with malrotation, it is not diagnostic. In some instances, a "swirl" or "whirlpool" sign can be detected, which represents the volvulus of the mesenteric root (as is seen in the test case's ultrasound image). Some have suggested that a retroperitoneal course of the third portion of the duodenum on ultrasound (between the superior mesenteric artery and the aorta) can help to exclude malrotation. However, there are instances where the duodenum takes this retroperitoneal course, but malrotation is still present. Thus, sonography is currently not the standard of care for patients present with bilious emesis.

C. Computed tomography is not the definitive workup for a child with bilious emesis.

D. Magnetic resonance imaging is not the definitive workup for a child with bilious emesis.

Question 1

The duodenum should take a retroperitoneal course toward the spine on the lateral projection. The DJJ should be located at least as far left as the left pedicle of the spine, and at the level of the duodenal bulb.

Question 2

If a fluoroscopic upper GI is equivocal or borderline for malrotation, perform a small bowel follow through to document the position of the cecum. A broad mesentery between the DJJ and cecum decreases the risk of midgut volvulus.

Question 3

The cecum is abnormally positioned in 80% of malrotation cases.

Question 4

The "double bubble" represents dilation of both the stomach and the duodenal blub. The differential for this appearance includes duodenal atresia, duodenal web or stenosis, duodenal mass, annular pancreas, and superior mesenteric syndrome.

Question 5

Trisomy 21 is associated with duodenal atresia.

Question 6

Pi or 3.14. Abnormal pyloric muscle thickness is > 3 mm, and abnormal pyloric channel length is > 14 mm. Channel lengths > 16 mm are more specific, but even more important than channel length is real-time evaluation of channel opening during the examination.

Question 7

True. HPS most commonly affects Caucasian male newborns.

Question 8

To sonographically evaluate HPS, place the child right side down. This allows fluid to pool at the antrum and gas to move away from the area of interest.

Question 9

Cine sequences are the best way to differentiate HPS from pyloric spasm. Both may have abnormal measurements of pyloric diameter and channel length, but only pyloric spasm will allow gas and fluid to pass the pylorus during cine sequences.

■ Suggested Readings

Applegate KE, Anderson JM, Klatte EC. Intestinal malrotation in children: a problem-solving approach to the upper gastrointestinal series. Radiographics 2006;26:1485–1500

Hernanz-Schulman M. Pyloric stenosis: role of imaging. Pediatr Radiol 2009;39:134–139

Karmazyn B, Cohen MD. Based on the position of the third portion of the duodenum at sonography, it is not possible to confidently diagnose malrotation. Pediatr Radiol 2015;45:138–139

Yousefzadeh DK. The position of the duodenojejunal junction: the wrong horse to bet on in diagnosing or excluding malrotation. Pediatr Radiol 2009;39:172–177

Top Tips

- In infants presenting with bilious emesis, a fluoroscopic upper GI is the preferred diagnostic test. The duodenum should take a retroperitoneal course, and the DJJ should be at the level of the duodenal bulb and at least as far left as the left pedicle of the spine.

- The "double bubble" appearance is most commonly associated with duodenal atresia, but does have a differential diagnosis, which includes midgut volvulus, duodenal web or mass, and annular pancreas.

- Pi or 3.14 is a useful memory aid for the abnormal measurements in HPS (muscular thickness > 3 mm and channel length > 14 mm). However, more important than channel length is real-time evaluation of pyloric channel opening.

Details 5

■ Case

Which ONE of the following is NOT a part of the Weigert Meyer rule?
  A. Upper pole obstruction
  B. Lower pole reflux
  C. Lower pole ureteral insertion inferomedially on the bladder
  D. Ectopic ureteral association with a ureterocele

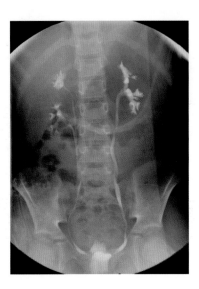

■ The following questions pertain to pediatric genitourinary disease.

1. True or False. Primary megaureter is the result of an aganglionic ureteric segment.
2. True or False. Congenital ureteropelvic junction obstruction is commonly secondary to extrinsic compression (e.g., a crossing vessel).
3. Which ONE of the following diseases is NOT associated with a distended urinary bladder and hydronephrosis?
   A. Megacystis microcolon intestinal hypoperistalsis syndrome
   B. Prune belly syndrome
   C. Posterior urethral valves
   D. Urachal diverticulum
4. Which of the following disease entities is LEAST likely to mimic multicystic dysplastic kidney on imaging?
   A. Fetal hydronephrosis
   B. Autosomal dominant polycystic kidney disease
   C. Autosomal recessive polycystic kidney disease
   D. Multilocular cystic nephroma
5. Posterior urethral valves arise from:
   A. Wolffian duct remnant
   B. Müllerian duct remnant
   C. Stricture of the posterior urethra
   D. Muscular web

6. Which of the following examinations should be performed after a male patient's first urinary tract infection (UTI)?
   A. Renal ultrasound
   B. Abdominal radiograph
   C. Voiding cystourethrogram
   D. Radionuclide cystography
7. What is the highest degree of VUR depicted in the test case?
   A. Grade 1
   B. Grade 2
   C. Grade 3
   D. Grade 4
   E. Grade 5
8. In what age group is VUR most common?
   A. Zero to two years
   B. Three to six years
   C. Seven to eleven years
   D. Twelve to twenty-one years
9. True or False. Periureteral injections for minimally invasive correction of VUR can mimic distal ureteral calculi.

■ Answers and Explanations

C. Correct! The Weigert Meyer rule is used to describe the typical presentation of a duplicated renal collecting system with two separate ureters, as is seen in our case of bilateral vesicoureteral reflux (VUR). Each ureter has its own orifice and insertion on the urinary bladder. The upper renal moiety has an ectopic insertion inferior and medial to the normally positioned lower renal moiety insertion. The upper pole moiety typically also has an associated ureterocele which, if present, can lead to obstruction of the upper pole moiety. In addition, the lower pole moiety is typically associated with VUR.

Question 1

False. Obstructive primary megaureter is secondary to an adynamic segment of distal ureter causing obstruction proximal to this segment. This has often been termed "Hirschsprung's disease of the ureter." However, this is somewhat of a misnomer, as it has not been proven that lack of ganglion cells within the ureteral wall is the cause of the adynamic segment.

Question 2

False. Congenital ureteropelvic junction obstruction is usually not secondary to extrinsic compression. Cases that are secondary to extrinsic compression from a crossing vessel are less common and typically present later in life. In the neonatal period, this is usually an intrinsic phenomenon, which is likely related to abnormal muscle or nerve fibers.

Question 3

D. Correct! Urachal diverticulum is in the spectrum of congenital urachal remnant abnormalities. The most common anomaly is patent urachus, followed by urachal cyst. The urachal remnant can fail to obliterate at its attachment with the urinary bladder, with the remainder becoming obliterated. This results in a vesicourachal diverticulum, which is not commonly associated with hydronephrosis.

Question 4

C. Correct! Autosomal recessive polycystic kidney disease commonly presents with innumerable small renal cysts, often too small to be resolved on ultrasound. The multiple interfaces of adjacent small cysts lead to echogenic kidneys bilaterally, which are typically enlarged secondary to the numerous cysts.

Question 5

A. Correct! Posterior urethral valves arise from Wolffian duct remnant. The thick membranous tissue at the level of the verumontanum (which causes the posterior urethral "valve") is of Wolffian duct origin.

Question 6

A. Correct! Following the guidelines put forth by the American Academy of Pediatrics, renal ultrasound is the test of choice following a febrile UTI in a child, regardless of gender. If no abnormalities are identified, then no further imaging is warranted.

Question 7

C. Correct! Grade 3 reflux is characterized as extension into the ureter and kidney with mild calyceal dilation (best demonstrated in the left kidney in this case).

Question 8

A. Correct! VUR is most common in the newborn to age 2 group. A large portion of patients outgrow VUR by puberty.

Question 9

True. Injection of Dextranomer-hyaluronic acid (Deflux; Salix Pharmaceuticals, Rochester, NY) can eventually calcify and mimic distal ureteral stones. Careful review of the patient's chart should be performed prior to the diagnosis of distal ureteral calculi, especially in children with a history of VUR.

■ Suggested Readings

American Urological Association. Management and screening of primary vesicoureteral reflux in children: AUA guideline. 2010. https://www.auanet.org/common/pdf/education/clinical-guidance/Vesicoureteral-Reflux-a.pdf

Berrocal T. Anomalies of the distal ureter, bladder, and urethra in children: embryologic, radiologic, and pathologic features. Radiographics 2002;22:1139–1164

Kraus SJ. Genitourinary imaging in children. Pediatr Clin North Am 2001;48:1381–1424

Meyer JS. Primary megaureter in infants and children: a review. Urol Radiol 1992;14:296–305

Roberts KB. Urinary tract infection: clinical practice guideline for the diagnosis and management of the initial UTI in febrile infants and children 2 to 24 months. Pediatrics 2011;128:595–610

Yankovic F, Swartz R, Cuckow P, et al. Incidence of Deflux® calcification masquerading as distal ureteric calculi on ultrasound. J Pediatr Urol 2013;9(6, Part A):820–824

Top Tips

◆ In duplicated collecting systems, the Weigert Meyer rule states that the upper pole ureter has an ectopic insertion (inferomedially) and may also be obstructed secondary to a ureterocele.

◆ First-line imaging in the evaluation of febrile UTI is renal ultrasound to detect abnormalities that would warrant further workup.

◆ The spectrum of urachal remnant anomalies, from most common to least common, includes patent urachus, urachal cyst, urachal-umbilical sinus, and vesicourachal diverticulum.

Image Rich 1

■ Case

Match the manifestation of tuberous sclerosis complex (TSC) with the corresponding image.
   A. Subependymal giant cell astrocytoma
   B. Subcortical tubers
   C. Rhabdomyoma
   D. Angiomyolipoma

1.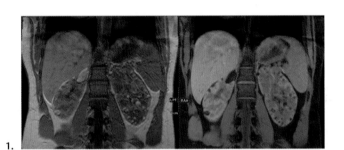

2.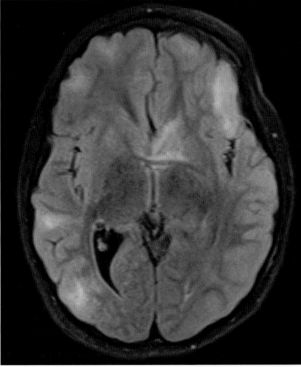

3.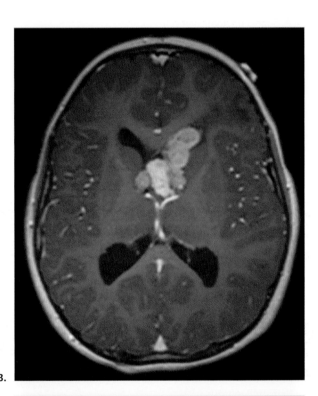

4.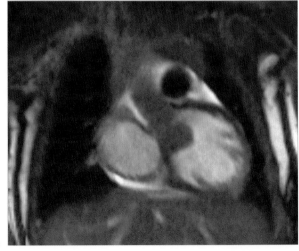

■ Answers and Explanations

1. D. Angiomyolipoma. T1 pre- (*left*) and postcontrast (*right*) with fat saturation images demonstrate multiple fat-suppressing lesions in both kidneys. Some of these lesions demonstrate partial enhancement. They are consistent with renal angiomyolipomas.

2. B. Subcortical tubers. This axial fluid-attenuated inversion recovery image shows multiple hyperintense subcortical lesions representing dysplastic neurons of the tubers. On computed tomography imaging (not shown), 50% of these tubers will calcify.

3. A. Subependymal giant cell astrocytoma. Magnetic resonance imaging T1-weighted image after contrast administration demonstrates a lobular intraventricular enhancing mass. In the setting of TSC, the findings are most consistent with subependymal giant cell astrocytoma. This entity can be differentiated from the precursor, a subependymal nodule, by having a size > 1 cm, contrast enhancement, lack of calcification, predilection for regions near the foramen of Monro, and high choline-to-creatine and low N-acetylaspartate-to-creatine ratios.

4. C. Rhabdomyoma. Noncontrast black-blood magnetic resonance imaging demonstrates an isointense solid mass arising from the intraventricular septum most consistent with an intracardiac rhabdomyoma. These lesions are hamartomatous masses. When they are multiple, this is diagnostic of TSC. When a single lesion is present, approximately 50% of these patients will have TSC.

■ Suggested Readings

Carvalho Neto A de, Gasparetto EL, Bruck I. Subependymal giant cell astrocytoma with high choline/creatine ratio on proton MR spectroscopy. Arquivos de neuro-psiquiatria. 2006;64:877–880

Manoukian SB, Kowal DJ. Comprehensive imaging manifestations of tuberous sclerosis. Am J Roentgenol 2015;204:933–943

Mühler MR, Rake A, Schwabe M, et al. Value of fetal cerebral MRI in sonographically-proven cardiac rhabdomyoma. Ped Radiol 2007;37:467–474

Top Tips

◆ TSC is a hamartomatous disease manifested by skin angiofibromas, subependymal nodules, intracardiac rhabdomyomas, bone islands, renal angiomyolipomas, and lymphangioleiomyomatosis of the lungs.

◆ The presence of multiple intracardiac rhabdomyomas is essentially diagnostic of TSC.

◆ Detection of fat in renal lesions is easily confirmed with fat saturation on magnetic resonance imaging. A fat-containing renal mass is essentially diagnostic of an angiomyolipoma.

Image Rich 2

■ Case

Match the appropriate suprasellar lesion with the provided image.
- A. Langerhans cell histiocytosis
- B. Hypothalamic hamartoma
- C. Craniopharyngioma
- D. Pilocytic astrocytoma

1.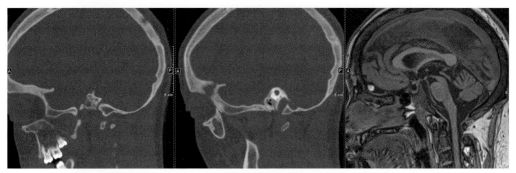

2.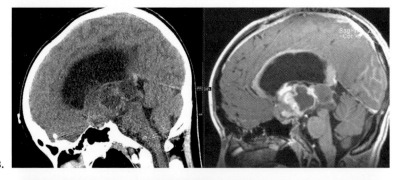

3.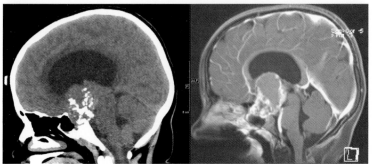

4.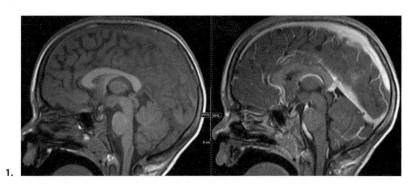

■ Answers and Explanations

1. B. Hypothalamic hamartoma. Sagittal pre- (*left*) and postcontrast (*right*) T1-weighted magnetic resonance imaging (MRI) demonstrates a nonenhancing mass within the hypothalamus near the floor of the third ventricle. This mass has the same signal characteristics as gray matter and represents gray matter heterotopia. These lesions are associated with gelastic seizures (laughing or crying seizures).

2. A. Langerhans cell histiocytosis. Two computed tomography (CT) images in the sagittal plane demonstrate lytic lesions within the parietal bone and the superior orbital rim. The sagittal T1 image in the midline demonstrates absence of the posterior pituitary bright spot. The combination of these findings is diagnostic of Langerhans cell histiocytosis.

3. D. Pilocytic astrocytoma. CT and MRI sagittal plane images in the midline demonstrate an enhancing, partially cystic mass in the suprasellar space without calcification. Pilocytic astrocytomas are the second most common suprasellar mass in children. Many of these tumors (20 to 50%) are associated with neurofibromatosis type 1.

4. C. Craniopharyngioma. CT and MRI sagittal plane images in the midline demonstrate an enhancing, partially cystic mass in the suprasellar space containing coarse calcifications. Of the choices, these findings most closely correlate to a craniopharyngioma, particularly given the associated calcifications. Calcification can be seen in up to 93% of pediatric cases. These are the most common suprasellar masses in children, accounting for 50% of suprasellar tumors. There are two histologic types of craniopharyngioma, but the adamantinomatous type is the most common in children. This type is predominately cystic.

■ Suggested Readings

Kerrigan JF, Ng Y, Chung S, et al. The hypothalamic hamartoma: a model of subcortical epileptogenesis and encephalopathy. Seminars in Ped Neurol 2005;12:119–131

Schroeder JW, Vezina LG. Pediatric sellar and suprasellar lesions. Ped Radiol. 2011;41:287–298

Yildiz AE, Oguz KK, Fitoz S. Suprasellar masses in children: characteristic MR imaging features. J Neuroradiol 2016;43:246–259

Top Tips

◆ A pediatric cystic suprasellar mass containing calcification is likely a craniopharyngioma.

◆ A hypothalamic hamartoma is like any other hamartoma in the body, representing normal tissue in an abnormal location. Because it represents normal tissue (ectopic gray matter), it does not enhance.

◆ Pilocystic astrocytomas are enhancing masses, which can be associated with neurofibromatosis type 1.

Image Rich 3

■ **Case**

Match the appropriate pediatric forearm injury with the provided images.
- A. Greenstick fracture
- B. Monteggia fracture
- C. Galeazzi fracture
- D. Gymnast wrist

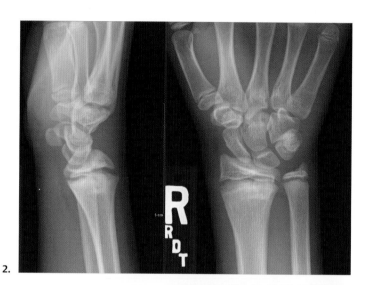

2.

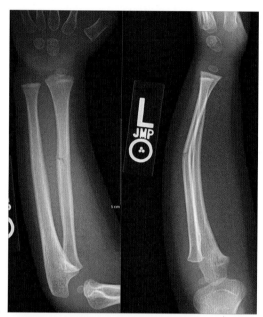

1.

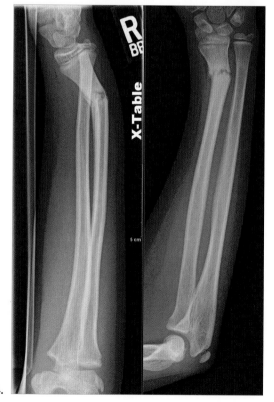

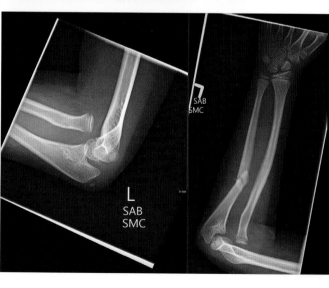

3.

4.

■ Answers and Explanations

1. A. Greenstick fracture. Radiographs demonstrate an incomplete fracture of the radial shaft and bowing deformity of both forearm bones. These findings are consistent with greenstick fractures. The term arises from comparison to fresh tree branches, or greensticks, which tend to bend rather than snap. The plasticity of pediatric bones creates a similar mechanism of injury where the bone bends but does not create a complete fracture. These fractures are fairly common, accounting for up to 50% of all pediatric fractures.

2. D. Gymnast wrist. Radiographs demonstrate distal radial physial widening, irregularity, and mild sclerosis. This injury has been termed "gymnast wrist." These findings are secondary to repetitive trauma to the physis due to abnormal axial loading (hand stands, hand springs, etc.). This injury is classified as a Salter-Harris I fracture.

3. B. Monteggia fracture. Radiographs demonstrate a fracture of the ulna and dislocation of the radial head. Remember that the radiocapitellar joint should be aligned on *every* view of the elbow. To help differentiate this fracture dislocation pattern from the Galeazzi type, the mnemonic "mugger" or MUGR can be used. This memory aid associates the bone that is fractured with the fracture-dislocation type. The *Monteggia* type involves a fracture of the *ulna*, whereas the *Galeazzi* type involves a fracture of the *radius*.

4. C. Galeazzi fracture. Radiographs demonstrate a fracture of the radius and dislocation of the distal radioulnar joint. In addition to frank dislocation of the ulna at the distal radioulnar joint, an avulsion-type fracture at the ulnar epiphysis (Salter-Harris I type) creates a Galeazzi equivalent fracture, even though the distal radioulnar joint may appear intact.

■ Suggested Readings

Little JT, Klionsky NB, Chaturvedi A, Soral A, Chaturvedi A. Pediatric distal forearm and wrist injury: an imaging review. Radiographics 2014;34(2):472–490

Ramski DE, Hennrikus WP, Bae DS, et al. Pediatric monteggia fractures: a multicenter examination of treatment strategy and early clinical and radiographic results. J Ped Orthopaedics 2015;35:115–120

Schmuck T, Altermatt S, Büchler P, et al. Greenstick fractures of the middle third of the forearm. a prospective multi-centre study. Eur J Ped Surg 2010;20:316–320

SECTION X
PEDIATRIC IMAGING

Top Tips

◆ Fracture dislocations of the forearm can be remembered using the mnemonic MUGR, which associates the fractured bone with its eponym. (Monteggia contains a fracture of the ulna, and Galeazzi involves a fracture of the radius.)

◆ The bones of children are more plastic than the bones of adults, and thus, greenstick fractures should be suspected when there is a bowing deformity.

◆ Gymnast wrist is a repetitive Salter-Harris I injury that results in widening of the distal radial physis.

Image Rich 4

■ **Case**

Match the appropriate Todani classification of choledochal cysts with the provided image.
- A. Type 1
- B. Type 3
- C. Type 4
- D. Type 5

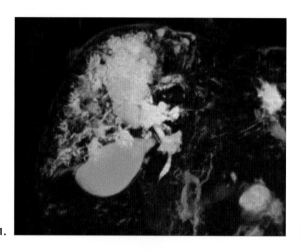

1.

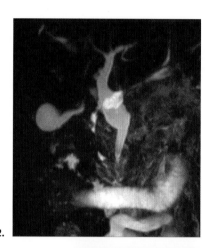

2.

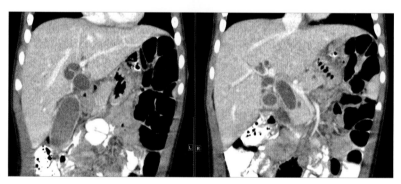

3.

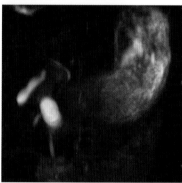

4.

■ Answers and Explanations

1. D. Type 5. This coronal maximum intensity projection (MIP) image of a magnetic resonance cholangiopancreatography (MRCP) exam of the biliary tree demonstrates diffuse multifocal intrahepatic biliary cystic dilation, consistent with Caroli disease. There is no extrahepatic duct involvement. This entity is relatively uncommon, comprising 10% of the Todani classification cases. It can be associated with hepatic fibrosis, autosomal dominant polycystic kidney disease, and medullary sponge kidney.

2. A. Type 1. This coronal MIP image from an MRCP shows fusiform extrahepatic duct dilation. There is no intrahepatic involvement of the biliary tree. This is the most common Todani classification anomaly.

3. C. Type 4. When there is involvement of both the intra- and extrahepatic ducts, the findings are consistent with type 4 choledochal cysts.

4. B. Type 3. This coronal oblique MIP image of the biliary tree demonstrates a focal fluid collection at the level of the duodenum without a discernable neck. The findings are consistent with a choledochocele. This is in contrast to a type 2 cyst (not shown), which will have a small neck (a choledochal diverticulum).

■ Suggested Reading

Lewis VA, Adam SZ, Nikolaidis P, et al. Imaging of choledochal cysts. Abdominal Imaging 2015;40:1567–80

Top Tips

◆ Todani classification of choledochal cyst anomalies increases in number as the lesions become more complex.

◆ Caroli disease (type 5) is associated with hepatic fibrosis and autosomal dominant polycystic disease in children.

◆ Although ultrasound can be used to screen for choledochal cysts, MRCP is the preferred evaluation in children because it is noninvasive, has excellent spatial resolution, and avoids radiation.

SECTION X
PEDIATRIC IMAGING

Image Rich 5

■ **Case**

Match the appropriate entity leading to proximal airway disease with the provided image.
- A. Tracheitis
- B. Epiglottitis
- C. Croup
- D. Retropharyngeal abscess

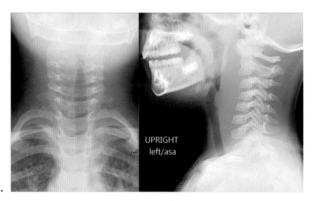

1.

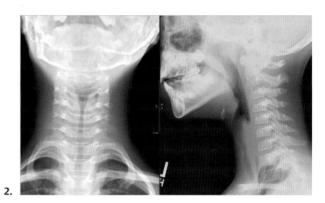

2.

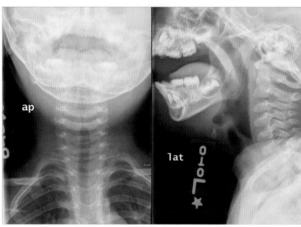

3.

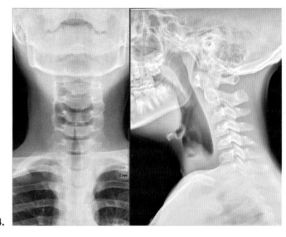

4.

■ Answers and Explanations

1. D. Retropharyngeal abscess. Radiographs demonstrate prevertebral soft tissue swelling with convex margins and reversal of the normal cervical lordosis. Of the choices, retropharyngeal abscess is the only entity with a predominantly prevertebral abnormality. A good rule of thumb is that the prevertebral soft tissues at the C4 level should be less than the anteroposterior width of the C4 cervical vertebral body.

2. A. Bacterial tracheitis. Radiographs show plaque-like irregularities within the subglottic airway at approximately the C7 level. With the appropriate clinical history, the suspicion of bacterial tracheitis should be high. Another sometimes seen finding is visualization of sloughed mucosa in the form of radiopaque bands in the airway.

3. B. Epiglottitis. Thumb-printing at the level of the epiglottis with supraglottic gaseous distention of the airway is consistent with epiglottitis. Additionally, there is swelling of the aryepiglottic folds. Epiglottitis is becoming increasingly rare, and the mean age of presentation has increased. This is due to an effective *Haemophilus* vaccine, the most common causative agent.

4. C. Croup. This frontal view of the neck shows focal narrowing of the subglottic trachea with loss of the normal shouldering, consistent with a steeple sign. These findings are most indicative of croup or laryngotracheobronchitis. These patients present with a classic barking cough. The most common causative agent is parainfluenza.

■ Suggested Reading

Darras KE, Roston AT, Yewchuk LK. Imaging acute airway obstruction in infants and children. Radiographics 2015;35:2064–2079

Top Tips

◆ Normal prevertebral soft tissue thickness should be less than the anteroposterior width of the adjacent vertebral body at the C4 level.

◆ Supraglottic distention should raise your suspicion for an upper airway obstructive process.

◆ Look carefully at the epiglottis for the thumb sign and at the subglottic trachea for the steeple sign, to make the diagnoses of epiglottitis or croup, respectively.

More Challenging 1

■ Case

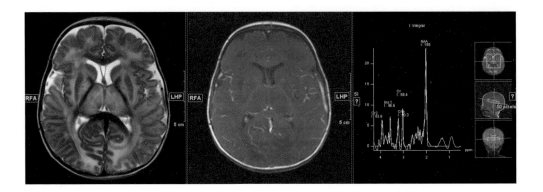

■ Questions

1. Which ONE of the following is an imaging feature of Canavan disease?
   A. Diffuse symmetric involvement of the white matter without extension to the subcortical U-fibers
   B. Involvement of the internal capsule
   C. Increase in the N-acetylaspartate peak
   D. Increase in the choline peak relative to the creatinine peak
   E. Contrast enhancement of the white matter involved

2. Which ONE of the following is a clinical feature of Canavan disease?
   A. Microcephaly
   B. Autosomal dominant inheritance pattern
   C. Lower incidence in the Ashkenazi Jewish population
   D. White matter degeneration is typically not treatable, with very low survival rates
   E. Hypertonia

3. Which ONE of the following leukodystrophies typically presents in a normocephalic infant?
   A. Canavan disease
   B. Alexander disease
   C. X-linked adrenoleukodystrophy
   D. Megalencephalic leukoencephalopathy with cysts

■ Answers and Explanations

Question 1

C. Correct! On single voxel magnetic resonance spectroscopy, Canavan disease demonstrates a dramatic increase in the N-acetylaspartate (NAA) peak. The peak that is typically decreased is the choline peak relative to the creatinine peak. The test case is an example of Canavan disease.

Other choices and discussion

A. The subcortical U-fibers are involved in Canavan disease, which is a progressive white matter disease caused by degeneration of the myelin. As demonstrated in the image, there is diffuse symmetric T2 hyperintense abnormal signal in the white matter extending to the subcortical U-fibers. This white matter involvement demonstrates restricted diffusion but no pathologic contrast enhancement.

B. Canavan disease typically spares the internal capsule. In addition to the internal capsule, the corpus callosum is also spared in this particular white matter disease.

D. With Canavan disease, the choline peak is typically decreased relative to the creatinine peak.

E. With Canavan disease, there is no pathologic enhancement of the white matter.

Question 2

D. Correct! Canavan disease is a devastating white matter degeneration process that does not currently have an effective treatment. Although a juvenile form has been described, afflicted children typically do not survive past 1 year of age.

Other choices and discussion

A. Macrocephaly, not microcephaly, is a helpful clinical feature of infantile white matter disease. Canavan disease is one of the entities that presents with macrocephaly.

B. Canavan disease is caused by a deficiency in aspartoacylase that is inherited in an autosomal recessive, not dominant, pattern. This mutation results in accumulation of NAA in the brain, plasma, and urine.

C. As with a few other conditions, there is a higher, not lower, incidence of Canavan disease in the Ashkenazi Jewish population, as 1 in 40 are carriers of the gene mutation.

E. Canavan disease typically presents as severe hypotonia that is evident by 4 months of age.

Question 3

C. Correct! X-linked adrenoleukodystrophy is not associated with macrocephaly. Magnetic resonance imaging in children most commonly presents with white matter disease that involves the splenium of the corpus callosum and the trigonal regions of the periventricular white matter. This leukodystrophy can also demonstrate contrast enhancement.

Other choices and discussion

A. Canavan disease is associated with macrocephaly. The three leukodystrophies that are most clearly associated with macrocephaly are Canavan disease, Alexander disease, and megalencephalic leukoencephalopathy with cysts (MLC).

B. Alexander disease is associated with macrocephaly. Alexander disease typically has a frontal lobe distribution and is one of the few leukodystrophies that demonstrates contrast enhancement. A decreased NAA peak also helps differentiate this macrocephalic leukodystrophy from Canavan disease.

D. As the name suggests, MLC is associated with macrocephaly. MLC is also known as van der Knaap disease. It manifests as diffuse white matter disease that may involve the cerebellum and corticospinal tracts. The white matter disease does not demonstrate restricted diffusion or contrast enhancement. The associated cysts are subcortical. The NAA peak is normal in MLC.

■ Suggested Readings

Kim JH, Kim HJ. Childhood x-linked adrenoleukodystrophy: clinical-pathologic overview and MR imaging manifestations at initial evaluation and follow-up. Radiographics 2005;25:619–631

van der Knaap MS, Breiter SN, Naidu S, et al. Defining and categorizing leukoencephalopathies of unknown origin: MR imaging approach. Radiology 1999;213:121–133

Top Tips

◆ The leukodystrophies most commonly associated with macrocephaly are Canavan disease, Alexander disease, and MLC.

◆ Canavan disease diffusely involves the white matter, including the subcortical U-fibers, with sparing of the internal capsule. No contrast enhancement should be present. The NAA peak is abnormally elevated.

◆ Alexander disease has a predominant frontal distribution that can demonstrate contrast enhancement.

More Challenging 2

■ Case

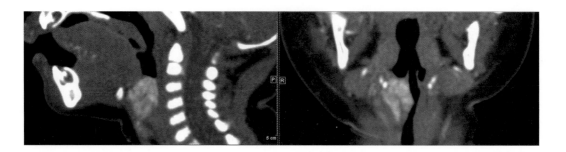

■ Questions

1. In combination with the imaging findings, which ONE of the following histologic or laboratory findings is diagnostic of this lesion?
   A. GLUT-1 positive tissue
   B. Alpha fetoprotein–positive tissue
   C. NMYC amplification
   D. Elevated serum beta-human chorionic gonadotropin

2. Which ONE of the following statements is TRUE regarding congenital hemangiomas?
   A. It is present at birth and does not demonstrate growth.
   B. It is not present at birth and can demonstrate growth.
   C. There are both proliferative and involuting phases of congenital hemangiomas.
   D. It is considered a vascular malformation.
   E. Phleboliths are diagnostic of congenital hemangiomas.

3. The thumb sign on a lateral neck radiograph is most consistent with which ONE of the following?
   A. Croup
   B. Epiglottitis
   C. Tracheitis
   D. Papillomatosis
   E. Retropharyngeal abscess

■ Answers and Explanations

Question 1

A. Correct! This is an infantile hemangioma. The test case shows an intensely enhancing eccentric mass in the subglottic space. GLUT-1 (a glucose transporter 1 protein) positivity is essentially diagnostic for infantile hemangiomas. It is present in 97% of cases. In the subglottic region, infantile hemangiomas are associated with PHACES syndrome (posterior fossa anomalies, hemangioma, arterial lesions, cardiac abnormalities/aortic coarctation, eye abnormalities, and sternal defects). In fact, up to 52% of cases of PHACES syndrome have concurrent subglottic hemangiomas.

Other choices and discussion

B. Alpha fetoprotein is a tumor marker for hepatoblastoma and for certain malignant germ cell tumors such as yolk sac and embryonal carcinomas.

C. NMYC (a proto-oncogene protein) amplification is a marker for neuroblastoma, and its presence portends a worse prognosis.

D. Aside from its use in the diagnosis of pregnancy, an elevated serum beta-human chorionic gonadotropin is a tumor marker for choriocarcinoma and embryonal carcinomas.

Question 2

A. Correct! As opposed to infantile hemangiomas (the presented case), congenital hemangiomas by definition are present at birth and have already developed to their full potential/size. There are two types: rapidly involuting congenital hemangiomas and noninvoluting congenital hemangiomas.

Other choices and discussion

B. Congenital hemangiomas do not continue to grow after birth. However, an infantile hemangioma can demonstrate growth.

C. Infantile hemangiomas, not congenital hemangiomas, demonstrate proliferative, quiescent, and involuting phases.

D. Congenital hemangiomas, as with infantile hemangiomas, should be correctly considered true vascular neoplasms (masses) rather than vascular malformations.

E. Phleboliths are not diagnostic of this entity, and in fact are much more commonly present in venous vascular malformations than in vascular masses.

Question 3

B. Correct! The thumb sign on a radiographic lateral view of the neck is representative of epiglottic swelling and is most consistent with epiglottitis. Epiglottitis is a bacterial infection that is now uncommon due to an effective vaccine.

Other choices and discussion

A. Croup, also known as laryngotracheobronchitis, is a self-limiting viral infection of the upper airway that causes subglottic edema. Classically on the frontal view of the neck, it is characterized by the "steeple" sign, which represents loss of the normal shouldering of the subglottic airway.

C. Tracheitis is typically caused by a bacterial infection. Radiographically, it most commonly presents as tracheal irregularities and linear membranes within the upper airway representing sloughing of the mucosa. When recognized, an urgent call should be made to the referring clinician, and bronchoscopy should be performed.

D. Papillomatosis is caused by maternal transmission to the infant through the birth canal. Most commonly, the entity is characterized by multiple airway nodules. If lung parenchymal involvement is present, it manifests as nodules and cysts.

E. When the prevertebral soft tissues are thickened, retropharyngeal abscess should be suspected. A good rule of thumb for identifying abnormal prevertebral soft tissue thickness in young children is tissue measuring greater than the anteroposterior diameter of the C4 vertebral body.

An adequate lateral view of the soft tissue neck should have the chin away from the neck, and the cervical spine should be extended. If there is a question of adequacy, a repeat examination should be performed.

■ Suggested Readings

Chen TS, Eichenfield LF, Friedlander SF. Infantile hemangiomas: an update on pathogenesis and therapy. Pediatrics 2013;131: 99–108

Huoh KC, Rosbe KW. Infantile hemangiomas of the head and neck. Pediatr Clin North Am 2013;60:937–949

Ngo A-VH, Walker CM, Chung JH, et al. Tumors and tumorlike conditions of the large airways. Am J Roentgenol 2013;201:301–313

Ricafort R. Tumor markers in infancy and childhood. Pediatr Rev 2011;32:306–308

Top Tips

- Both congenital and infantile hemangiomas are vascular masses, not malformations.

- Congenital hemangiomas are present from birth and do not grow, whereas infantile hemangiomas are typically not present at birth and have proliferative, quiescent, and involution phases.

- A good rule of thumb in young children is that prevertebral soft tissue fullness at the C4 level that has an anteroposterior diameter greater than the adjacent C4 vertebral body is concerning for possible retropharyngeal abscess.

More Challenging 3

■ **Case**

An infant presents with history of cyanosis.

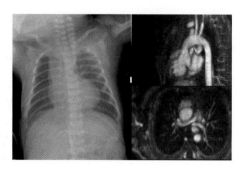

■ **Questions**

1. Which ONE of the following cyanotic heart diseases is typically NOT associated with increased blood flow?
   A. Transposition of the great arteries
   B. Tetralogy of Fallot
   C. Truncus arteriosus
   D. Total anomalous pulmonary venous return
   E. Single ventricle

2. Which ONE of the following cyanotic heart diseases is associated with a narrow superior mediastinum?
   A. Transposition of the great arteries
   B. Tetralogy of Fallot
   C. Truncus arteriosus
   D. Total anomalous pulmonary venous return
   E. Single ventricle

3. Which subtype of total anomalous pulmonary venous return is commonly associated with pulmonary congestion?
   A. Type I (supracardiac)
   B. Type II (cardiac)
   C. Type III (infracardiac)
   D. Type IV (mixed)

■ Answers and Explanations

Question 1

B. Correct! Tetralogy of Fallot (TOF) is not associated with increased blood flow. TOF has four primary features: ventricular septal defect, right ventricular outflow tract obstruction, overriding aorta, and right ventricular hypertrophy. Right ventricular hypertrophy usually develops at birth, secondary to right heart strain both from the ventricular septal defect as well as from the outflow tract obstruction. Outflow tract obstruction can be secondary to a number of causes related to the pulmonary valves (including a bicuspid valve) or a hypoplastic or atretic pulmonary artery. Given the presence of outflow tract obstruction, TOF is often associated with decreased pulmonary blood flow. A concave main pulmonary artery contour can be seen on plain radiographs related to the hypoplasia. The test case is an example of TOF.

Other choices and discussion

A. Transposition of the great arteries (D-TGA) denotes the transposition of the aorta and pulmonary artery relative to the left and right ventricles, respectively. This results in two parallel circuits circulating blood and is not compatible with life without a patent ductus arteriosus. Pulmonary vascularity is normal to increased, given the patent ductus arteriosus.

C. Truncus arteriosus typically presents with increased pulmonary blood flow secondary to admixture of blood through the common vascular trunk.

D. Total anomalous pulmonary venous return (TAPVR) can present with normal to increased pulmonary blood flow depending on if there is obstruction to venous return.

E. Single ventricle morphology can present with normal or increased pulmonary blood flow if there is no associated outflow tract obstruction.

Question 2

A. Correct! D-TGA has been described as having an "egg on a string" appearance on radiographs related to a narrow superior mediastinum. This narrowing is explained both by the orientation of the great vessels with the aorta now positioned anterior to the pulmonary artery, as well as a common association with an atrophic thymus. D-TGA is the most common type of transposition, where the aorta and pulmonary artery are "swapped" in relation to the left and right ventricles. This leads to two parallel circuits of blood flow, with patency of a patent ductus arteriosus needed in order to sustain life until surgical correction.

Other choices and discussion

B. The typical chest radiographic finding in TOF is a "boot-shaped" heart.

C. Truncus arteriosus typically presents with cardiomegaly, increased pulmonary blood flow, and a widened mediastinum. In certain cases, however, a small main pulmonary artery arising from the common trunk will result in a narrow superior mediastinum, mimicking D-TGA.

D. TAPVR has a spectrum of chest radiographic findings; in type I (supracardiac) TAPVR, the classic radiographic finding is the "snowman" sign.

E. Single ventricle morphology can have a variety of chest radiographic findings but is not classically associated with a narrow superior mediastinum.

Question 3

C. Correct! Type III (infracardiac) is the subtype of TAPVR commonly associated with pulmonary congestion. TAPVR describes a condition where all pulmonary veins are connected to systemic venous return rather than to the left atrium. The four different subtypes of TAPVR are listed in the question. Pulmonary venous obstruction can occur in all subtypes secondary to a narrow venous connection or extrinsic compression (e.g., a vertical vein compressed between the left pulmonary artery and left main bronchus in supracardiac TAPVR). Of all these subtypes, infracardiac TAPVR is the most commonly obstructed. In this subtype, the anomalous pulmonary venous drainage can be compressed in multiple ways: the draining vein can be compressed as it courses inferiorly through the diaphragm, there can be impaired drainage at the junction with the portal venous system, or there can be impaired drainage secondary to the venous return being filtered through the portal venous system/hepatic sinusoids before eventually returning to the inferior vena cava.

■ Suggested Readings

Apitz C. Tetralogy of Fallot. Lancet 2009;374:1462–1471

Dillman JR. Imaging of pulmonary venous developmental anomalies. Am J Roentgenol 2009;92:1272–1285

Frank L. Cardiovascular MR imaging of conotruncal anomalies. Radiographics 2010;30:1069–1094

Lapierre C. Segmental approach to imaging of congenital heart disease. Radiographics 2010;30:397–411

Top Tips

♦ The differential diagnosis of cyanotic heart disease can be separated into two broad categories: decreased pulmonary blood flow and normal/increased pulmonary blood flow.

♦ TAPVR has four subtypes; type III is the most likely to cause obstruction to venous return.

♦ The differential for common cyanotic congenital heart diseases can be remembered using the 1-2-3-4-5 mnemonic. Single ventricle and truncus for 1, transposition of the two great vessels for 2, tricuspid atresia for 3, TOF for 4 (can present as either cyanotic or acyanotic), and total anomalous pulmonary venous return for 5.

More Challenging 4

■ Case

A 4-year-old boy presents with hearing loss.

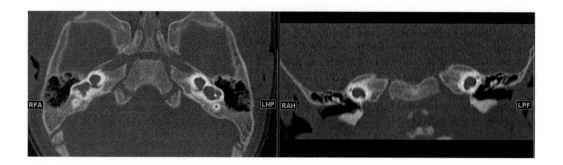

■ Questions

1. Patients with the Mondini anomaly typically present with what type of hearing loss?
   A. Sensorineural
   B. Conductive
   C. Mixed
   D. They do not typically present with hearing loss.

2. All of the following are descriptors of middle and inner ear anomalies EXCEPT:
   A. Baseball cap appearance of the cochlea
   B. Plump apical turn
   C. Blunted scutum
   D. Snail-shaped cochlea
   E. Bulbous endolymphatic sac

3. Bilateral vestibular schwannomas are associated with which ONE of the following conditions?
   A. Neurofibromatosis type 1
   B. Neurofibromatosis type 2
   C. CHARGE syndrome
   D. Fibrous dysplasia

■ Answers and Explanations

Question 1

A. Correct! Patients with the Mondini anomaly typically present with profound sensorineural hearing loss.

Other choices and discussion

B. Conductive hearing loss is a result of the inability to conduct the sound waves. This usually occurs from a malformation with the tympanic membrane or the middle ear ossicles.

C. Mixed hearing loss, a combination of sensorineural and conductive hearing loss, is present in malformations that typically span both the middle and inner ear compartments.

D. Malformations of the middle and inner ear almost always cause hearing loss.

Question 2

D. Correct! A snail shape is the normal appearance of the cochlea and is not associated with any middle or inner ear anomalies. In the axial plane, the normal anatomic appearance of the cochlea is snail-shaped. It should complete 2.5 turns and contain a hyperdense bony center called the modiolus. Absence or distortion of the turns is abnormal and should prompt a closer evaluation of the vestibular aqueduct (completing the Mondini malformation).

Other choices and discussion

A. A baseball cap appearance of the cochlea is used to describe the cochlea when there is absent septation of the apical and middle turns of the cochlea. This is typical of incomplete partition type II. The modiolus may also be absent in this scenario. Incomplete partition type I is characterized by a dysplastic cystic anomaly of the cochlea, and in combination with the vestibule, has been described as a figure 8 or snowman configuration. This is shown in the test case.

B. Plump apical turn is another descriptor used to characterize incomplete septation of the middle and apical turns of the cochlea with incomplete partition type II.

C. Most commonly associated with a cholesteatoma, a blunted scutum is the result of bony erosion from the lesion. The scutum is a sharp bony prominence of the middle ear and creates the lateral margin of Prussak space. Blunting of the scutum can be appreciated on both the axial and coronal planes.

E. A bulbous endolymphatic sac or enlarged vestibular aqueduct is the most common abnormality in sensorineural hearing loss. A vestibular aqueduct that measures > 1.5 mm is abnormal. A good normal internal reference is the width of a normal semicircular canal.

Question 3

B. Correct! Bilateral vestibular schwannomas are associated with neurofibromatosis (NF)-2. NF-2 is also known as MISME syndrome, which stands for multiple inherited schwannomas, meningiomas, and ependymomas. The schwannomas do not necessarily have to be vestibular. In fact, 50% of the cranial nerve schwannomas do not involve cranial nerve VIII. The most common alternative is cranial nerve V.

Other choices and discussion

A. NF-1 is an autosomal dominant condition in which there are multiple plexiform neurofibromas. Some of the lesions may be neurocutaneous, and thus, the condition is categorized as a phakomatosis. Diagnostic criteria includes two or more of the following: six café au lait spots, two or more neurofibromas or one plexiform fibroma, axillary/inguinal freckling, visual pathway glioma, Lisch nodules, distinctive bone lesions such as sphenoid wing dysplasia or thinning of the long bones, or a first-degree relative with NF-1.

C. CHARGE is an acronym that stands for coloboma, heart anomaly, atresia choanae, retardation (mental and somatic development), genital hypoplasia, and ear abnormalities. Although sensorineural hearing loss is associated with CHARGE, it is typically a result of dysplasia or aplasia of the inner ear. Common abnormalities include the Mondini anomaly and semicircular canal aplasia or malformations. Additional clinical clues to the CHARGE syndrome also include external ear abnormalities such as pinna cupping malformation and low set ears.

D. An important clinical complication of fibrous dysplasia that involves the skull base is sensorineural hearing loss. However, this hearing loss is typically due to bony narrowing of the internal auditory canal or other bony neural canals secondary to bony expansion from the fibrous dysplasia.

■ Suggested Readings

Choi JW, Lee JY, Phi JH, et al. Clinical course of vestibular schwannoma in pediatric neurofibromatosis type 2. J Neurosurg Pediatr 2014;13:650–665

DeMarcantonio M, Choo DI. Radiographic evaluation of children with hearing loss. Otolaryngol Clin North Am 2015;48:913–932

Top Tips
- Careful evaluation of the cochlea for 2.5 turns and a bony modiolus is paramount in a patient presenting with neurosensory hearing loss.
- The vestibular aqueduct should present at a level similar to the cochlea in the axial plane and should not be wider than a semicircular canal, or 1.5 mm.
- Other important secondary causes of sensorineural hearing loss include prematurity, infection, hyperbilirubinemia, ototoxins, and tumors such as vestibular schwannomas.

More Challenging 5

■ Case

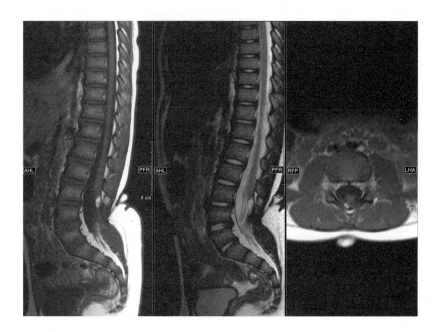

■ Questions

1. Which ONE of the following represents an open neural tube defect?
   A. Diastematomyelia
   B. Myelomeningocele
   C. Meningocele
   D. Myelocystocele
   E. Lipomyelomeningocele

2. After surgical correction of a tethered cord, which ONE of the following imaging findings is diagnostic of retethering?
   A. Decreased motion of the filum on ultrasound
   B. Magnetic resonance imaging contrast enhancement
   C. Intradural calcification on computed tomography
   D. Persistent low-lying conus medullaris
   E. None of the above; this is a clinical diagnosis.

3. The termination of the conus below what level is considered abnormal?
   A. T12
   B. L1
   C. L2
   D. L3

■ Answers and Explanations

Question 1

B. Correct! Myelomeningocele is an open neural tube defect most commonly associated with Chiari 2 malformation. It contains both cord parenchyma and meninges, as the name indicates.

Other choices and discussion

A. Diastematomyelia is a closed neural tube defect in which the spinal canal is longitudinally segmented or split. The split can be asymmetric and fibrous or bony.

C. Meningocele is a skin-covered, closed spinal defect. This is most commonly located in the lumbosacral spine, but can be present in the thoracic or cervical spine.

D. Myelocystocele is a skin-covered, closed spine defect. It contains neural components. It is categorized as nonterminal or terminal, depending on whether it occurs at the end of the thecal sac. The lesion is characterized by protrusion of the central canal spinal canal into a dilated subarachnoid cyst, creating a "cyst in cyst" appearance.

E. Lipomyelomeningocele, as shown in the test case, is a skin-covered spinal defect that contains a fatty mass (the T1 hyperintense signal at L3–L4) with neural tissue, as the components of the name suggests.

Question 2

E. Correct! This is a clinical diagnosis. Although decreased motion of the filum, contrast enhancement, and intradural calcifications can all be seen in retethering syndrome, none are specific imaging findings. The conus often does not move superiorly after a detethering procedure, and thus, position is unreliable. The follow up examination can serve as a new baseline, but correlation with clinical suspicion is required to establish retethering.

Question 3

C. Correct! The conus terminates normally between L1 and L2. In asymptomatic patients, the conus does not terminate below L2. Therefore, when the conus terminates below L2, a tethering mass should be investigated. Most commonly, the cause is a lipoma or thickened filum. The filum terminale should be no thicker than 1 mm.

■ Suggested Readings

Badve CA, Khanna PC, Phillips GS, et al. MRI of closed spinal dysraphisms. Pediatr Radiol 2011;41:1308–1320

Barkovich AJ. Pediatric Neuroimaging. 9th ed. Philadelphia, PA: Lippincott Williams & Wilkins; 2012

Egloff A, Bulas D. Magnetic resonance imaging evaluation of fetal neural tube defects. Semin Ultrasound CT MR 2015;36:487–500

Halevi PD, Udayakumaran S, Ben-Sira L, et al. The value of postoperative MR in tethered cord: a review of 140 cases. Childs Nerv Syst 2011;27:2159–2162

SECTION X
PEDIATRIC IMAGING

Top Tips

◆ Termination of the conus below L2 is abnormal, and the presence of a tethering mass should be investigated.

◆ Myelomeningocele is an open (uncovered) spinal defect that is most commonly associated with Chiari 2 malformation.

◆ The diagnosis of retethering after a detethering procedure is predominately clinical. The postprocedure imaging evaluation can serve as a new baseline.

Essentials 1

■ Case

An asymptomatic 23-year-old foreign exchange student presents with a required health clearance chest radiograph.

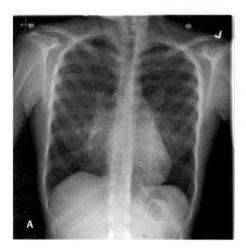
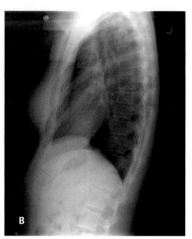

■ Questions

1. What is the next MOST reasonable course of action?
   A. Additional radiographic views
   B. Magnetic resonance imaging of the chest
   C. Treatment with antibiotics
   D. No further action
   E. Computed tomography of the chest

2. What is the MOST likely diagnosis?
   A. Pectus excavatum
   B. Right middle lobe pneumonia
   C. Right lower lobe pneumonia
   D. Right hilar mass
   E. Cardiophrenic angle mass

3. Regarding the diagnosis, which ONE of the following is correct?
   A. A familial occurrence is reported in 70% of cases.
   B. The condition is associated with Down syndrome.
   C. There is a female predominance (female-to-male ratio of 3:1).
   D. Tricuspid regurgitation is reported in 20 to 60% of cases.
   E. Pectus patients may have an abnormal Haller index.

■ Answers and Explanations

Question 1

D. Correct! No further action is needed. The two-view chest confirms a pectus excavatum deformity. In most pectus patients (including the test patient), the abnormality is mild and clinically insignificant. When severe, however, a pectus excavatum deformity can cause pain the chest and back and even impair cardiac and respiratory function. In select symptomatic cases, cross-sectional imaging treatment is sometimes performed.

Other choices and discussion

A. Additional radiographic views are occasionally used to better localize pathology or to differentiate a real finding from overlapping normal tissue. In this case, as the two-view chest successfully excludes a nodule/infiltrate and clearly demonstrates the sternal depression, more views are not required.

B. Additional cross-sectional imaging is not required at this point. The lateral chest radiograph clearly demonstrates the pectus excavatum deformity, and there is no lung or mediastinal abnormality seen on the lateral view.

The most common indications for magnetic resonance imaging of the chest include the assessment of cardiac morphology and function, aortic dissection, pleural and mediastinal masses, and pericardial disease.

C. The patient is asymptomatic and there is no lung consolidation seen on the lateral view, so antibiotic treatment is not indicated.

E. Additional cross-sectional imaging is not required at this point. Computed tomography may be indicated *eventually* in treatment planning for severe cases, but is not needed for the initial diagnosis.

Question 2

A. Correct! The lateral radiograph demonstrates inward displacement of the sternum. This confirms a pectus excavatum deformity, which is a congenital deformity of the anterior thoracic wall in which the sternum has a caved-in or sunken appearance. The depressed sternum replaces aerated lung at the right heart border, and the right heart border appears to be obscured.

Pectus carinatum, also called pigeon chest, is a deformity of the chest characterized by a protrusion of the sternum and ribs.

The other choices are all incorrect. There is no pneumonia, consolidation, or mass, because the lateral view excludes those findings and confirms the pectus deformity.

Question 3

E. Correct! The Haller index is the ratio of the transverse diameter (the horizontal distance of the inside of the ribcage) to the anteroposterior diameter (the shortest distance between the vertebrae and sternum). A normal Haller index is 2.5. A significant pectus excavatum has an index > 3.25.

Other choices and discussion

A. A familial occurrence of pectus deformity is reported in 35% of cases.

B. Pectus deformity can be with Marfan syndrome, Poland syndrome, Noonan syndrome, Ehlers-Danlos syndrome, neurofibromatosis type I, and osteogenesis imperfecta.

C. There is a male predominance (male-to-female ratio of 3:1).

D. Mitral valve prolapse (not tricuspid regurgitation) has been reported in 20 to 60% of cases.

■ Suggested Readings

Dähnert W. Radiology Review Manual. Philadelphia, PA: Lippincott Williams & Wilkins; 2007

Mak SM, Bhaludin BN, Naaseri S, Di Chiara F, Jordan S, Padley S. Imaging of congenital chest wall deformities. Br J Radiol 2016;89(1061):20150595

Restrepo CS, Martinez S, Lemos DF, et al. Imaging appearances of the sternum and sternoclavicular joints. Radiographics 2009;29(3):839–859

Top Tips

- Pectus excavatum is a common developmental anomaly of the anterior chest wall in which the sternum is caved in, creating a sunken appearance of the chest.

- Most patients have a mild and clinically insignificant abnormality. However, severe cases can impair cardiac and respiratory function and cause chest and back pain.

- The diagnosis of pectus excavatum is easily made on frontal and lateral chest radiographs. The right heart border is obscured on the frontal view, whereas the lateral view confirms the pectus deformity and excludes a consolidation.

Essentials 2

■ Case

A 19-year-old man with recurrent pneumonia and hemoptysis.

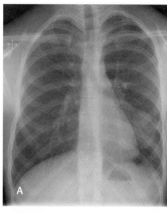

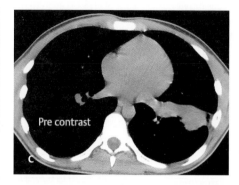

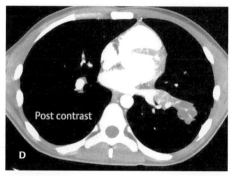

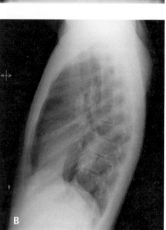

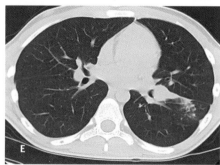

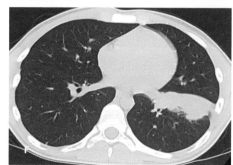

■ Questions

1. What is the MOST likely diagnosis?
   A. Pulmonary sequestration
   B. Lung abscess
   C. Hilar lymphadenopathy
   D. Congenital pulmonary airway malformation
   E. Endobronchial tumor

2. Regarding typical course of this diagnosis, which ONE of the following is correct?
   A. Carcinoid typically demonstrates poor contrast enhancement on CT.
   B. Carcinoid typically demonstrates intense fluorodeoxyglucose (FDG) update on positron emission tomography/CT.
   C. Calcification is seen in approximately 70% of pulmonary carcinoids.

D. A total of 80% of patients with carcinoid tumors are asymptomatic.
E. Pulmonary carcinoid arises from Kulchitsky cells in the bronchial epithelium.

3. Regarding pulmonary neuroendocrine tumors, which ONE of the following is correct?
   A. Small cell lung carcinoma is the most common neuroendocrine lung neoplasm.
   B. Neuroendocrine proliferations such as diffuse idiopathic neuroendocrine cell hyperplasia (DIPNECH) present as large masses.
   C. Large cell neuroendocrine carcinoma (LCNEC) typically presents as a central endobronchial pulmonary mass.
   D. Cushing syndrome is reported in approximately 25% of patients with pulmonary carcinoid.
   E. Carcinoid syndrome is reported in approximately 25% of patients with pulmonary carcinoid.

■ Answers and Explanations

Question 1

E. Correct! This is a pulmonary carcinoid tumor. An enhancing endobronchial lesion typical of a vascular endobronchial pulmonary carcinoid is demonstrated.

Other choices and discussion

A. Pulmonary sequestration refers to the aberrant formation of segmental lung tissue that has no connection to the bronchial tree or pulmonary arteries. Sequestration preferentially affects the lower lobes. A total of 60% of intralobar sequestrations affect the left lower lobe, and 40% of intralobar sequestrations affect the right lower lobe. This entity may present in late childhood or adolescence with recurrent pulmonary infections. Cross-sectional imaging frequently demonstrates the arterial supply originating from the descending aorta and coursing into the lesion (although that is not shown in this case).

B. The chest computed tomography (CT) images demonstrate an enhancing left perihilar endobronchial lesion (note the curvilinear air density posteriorly suggesting an endobronchial location). The low attenuation material within the distal collapsed left lower lobe parenchyma represents accumulated endobronchial secretions. This does not have the appearance of an abscess.

C. The enhancing left endobronchial lesion is suggestive of a vascular tumor, rather than typical hilar lymphadenopathy.

D. CPAM is a multicystic mass comprised of segmental lung tissue with abnormal bronchial proliferation. Five subtypes are currently classified. Type I and II CPAMs demonstrate a multicystic (air-filled) lesion, but in type III, the lesion can present as a nonresolving consolidation. CPAM is typically diagnosed early in life and often in the perinatal period. It usually presents with tachypnea, cyanosis, and respiratory distress. However, rare cases are asymptomatic and undiagnosed until adulthood. There is no associated endobronchial mass in CPAM, as is shown in the test case.

Question 2

E. Correct! Kulchitsky cells are of neuroendocrine origin and are found in the epithelium of the digestive and respiratory tracts. Gastrointestinal tract carcinoids account for 90% of all carcinoids. The lung is the second most common location for a carcinoid tumor.

Other choices and discussion

A. Pulmonary carcinoid tumors typically demonstrate intense enhancement on CT. Postobstructive pneumonitis may be present.

B. FDG positron emission tomography is often negative because of the relatively low metabolism of a typical carcinoid tumor. FDG uptake may be seen in an atypical carcinoid, or one that has undergone dedifferentiation. If a pulmonary carcinoid is diagnosed, a better nuclear medicine test to assess for metastatic disease is an Octreotide scan (somatostatin analogue). This is often successfully used to diagnose and localize occult carcinoid tumors.

C. A total of 30% of pulmonary carcinoids demonstrate calcification on CT (only 5% of cases demonstrate calcification on plain film).

D. A total of 25% of patients with typical lung carcinoid tumors are asymptomatic. In symptomatic patients, the most common presentation is persistent cough, hemoptysis, and recurrent or obstructive pneumonitis. Rarely, paraneoplastic syndromes can be the initial symptoms of either typical or atypical pulmonary carcinoid tumors. Some of the endocrinopathies that can be produced by a pulmonary carcinoid tumor include carcinoid syndrome, hypercortisolism and Cushing syndrome, inappropriate secretion of antidiuretic hormone, increased pigmentation secondary to excess melanocyte-stimulating hormone, and ectopic insulin production resulting in hypoglycemia. Atypical carcinoid sometimes initially presents with metastatic disease. Carcinoid syndrome is most likely to occur when there is metastatic disease to the liver.

Question 3

A. Correct! Small cell lung carcinoma is the most common neuroendocrine lung neoplasm, representing 15 to 20% of invasive lung malignancies. It is also one of the most aggressive cell types of primary lung cancer.

Other choices and discussion

B. DIPNECH is one of the manifestations of neuroendocrine proliferation in the lungs. DIPNECH is seen as multiple pulmonary micronodules, with or without associated mosaic attenuation or air trapping on high-resolution chest CT. Typical symptomatic patients with DIPNECH are females in their fifth to seventh decade with a history of cough and dyspnea. About half of patients with DIPNECH are asymptomatic and diagnosed incidentally on CT.

C. LCNEC typically manifests as a large, peripheral pulmonary mass ranging from 2 to 10 cm. It is a high-grade malignancy with neuroendocrine histologic features. Most patients are males in their fifth or sixth decade with a history of heavy smoking.

D. Pulmonary carcinoid rarely presents with paraneoplastic syndromes. Cushing syndrome is reported in only 2% of bronchial carcinoids. When present, it is characterized by an acute onset high concentration of adrenocorticotropic hormone and hypokalemia.

E. Although carcinoid syndrome is reported in 9% of patients with gastrointestinal carcinoids, it is seen at presentation in only 0.7% of patients with pulmonary carcinoids.

Top Tips

- Carcinoid is a low-grade malignant neuroendocrine neoplasm with metastatic potential.

- Consider pulmonary carcinoid tumor in symptomatic young or middle-aged patients with a well-defined central enhancing mass and an endoluminal component.

- Four major types of neuroendocrine neoplasms are recognized, and these are grouped into three histologic grades. Typical carcinoid is the low-grade malignant neoplasm, atypical carcinoid is the intermediate-grade neoplasm, and LCNEC and small cell lung carcinoma are the high-grade neoplasms.

Essentials 3

■ **Case**

A 26-year-old man with an incidental finding on chest X-ray (CXR).

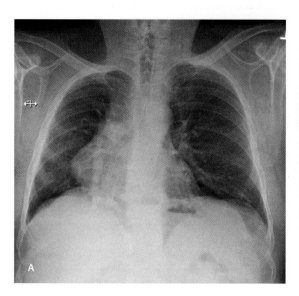
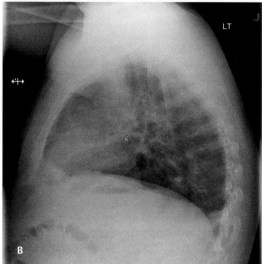

■ **Questions**

1. What is the MOST likely diagnosis?
   A. Fibrosing mediastinitis
   B. Pulmonary sequestration
   C. Swyer-James syndrome
   D. Hypogenetic lung syndrome
   E. Meandering pulmonary vein

2. Which of the following are CORRECT concerning pulmonary venolobar syndrome? (Select ALL that apply.)
   A. Defined as the partial or total anomalous pulmonary venous return of the right lung to the IVC just above or below the diaphragm
   B. Also called Luftsichel syndrome
   C. Associated abnormalities include abnormal right lung lobation and right lung hypoplasia
   D. Scimitar vein is seen in 50% of cases
   E. Majority are right sided

3. Which ONE of the following is correct?
   A. Right PAPVR is associated with high sinus venosus atrial septal defect.
   B. Left PAPVR is associated with high sinus venosus atrial septal defect.
   C. Scimitar syndrome is a type of total anomalous venous drainage.
   D. All cases of scimitar syndrome need surgical correction.
   E. Meandering pulmonary vein is more common on the left side.

■ Answers and Explanations

Question 1

D. Correct! Hypogenetic lung syndrome (aka pulmonary venolobar syndrome or the scimitar syndrome) is a rare congenital disorder that consists of anomalous pulmonary venous drainage of the right lung to the inferior vena cava (IVC; giving rise to the scimitar sign), anomalous systemic arterial supply of the right lower lobe from either the thoracic or abdominal aorta, hypoplasia of the right lung, and resultant cardiac dextroposition and right pulmonary artery hypoplasia.

The curved vertical vein, representing the anomalous venous drainage, is seen paralleling the right heart border and directed toward the IVC, right atrium, or portal vein. CXR findings are that of a small lung with ipsilateral mediastinal shift. In one-third of cases, the anomalous draining vein may be seen as a tubular structure paralleling the right heart border in the shape of a Turkish sword ("scimitar"). There is associated congenital heart disease in 25% of cases.

Other choices and discussion

A. Fibrosing mediastinitis refers to a focal hilar or mediastinal mass that narrows the nearby airways or vessels. Calcification of the mass is common (60 to 90%). There is no mediastinal or hilar mass seen in the test case.

B. Pulmonary sequestration represents nonfunctioning lung tissue that is separated from normal lung and receives its blood supply from a systemic artery that lacks normal communication with the bronchi. On CXR, there is a persistent left-sided (65%) paraspinal mass. There is often a clinical history of recurrent pneumonia. The lung may contain solid, fluid, and cystic components (i.e., some have an air-fluid level). The identification of the systemic artery feeding the abnormal lung on computed tomography or magnetic resonance imaging is diagnostic. These findings are not present in the test case.

C. Swyer-James syndrome is characterized on radiography by a unilateral small lung with hyperlucency and air trapping, but with *normal* pulmonary venous anatomy. There is no vertical vein association with Swyer-James syndrome. This condition typically follows a viral respiratory infection such as adenoviruses or *Mycoplasma pneumoniae* in infancy or childhood.

E. With a meandering pulmonary vein, the scimitar sign is present in the right lung and the anomalous right pulmonary vein drains normally into the left atrium. This may therefore mimic a scimitar syndrome on CXR. However, there is no vascular shunt, and no treatment is required. For this reason, it is important to differentiate this condition from scimitar syndrome. Multidetector computed tomography allows clear depiction of the vascular connections and associated anatomy, and has superseded invasive pulmonary angiography and cardiac catheterization as the investigation of choice for differentiating meandering pulmonary vein from scimitar syndrome.

Question 2

A. Correct! Pulmonary venolobar syndrome is defined as the partial or total anomalous pulmonary venous return of the right lung to the IVC just above or below the diaphragm.

C. Correct! It is associated with abnormal right lung lobation and right lung hypoplasia in nearly all cases.

D. Correct! It has a scimitar (vertical) vein in 50% of patients (70% of pediatric/adult and 10% of infantile).

E. Correct! The majority are right sided.

Other choice and discussion

B. Pulmonary venolobar syndrome is called the "scimitar syndrome," not the "Luftsichel syndrome." The curved vertical vein paralleling the right heart border directed toward the midline is shaped like a "scimitar" (i.e., a Turkish sword).

Question 3

A. Correct! Because this type of atrial septal defect is clinically silent, the associated PAPVR may be the clue leading to the diagnosis of an atrial septal defect.

Other choices and discussion

B. This is incorrect.

C. Scimitar syndrome is a type of partial anomalous venous drainage with an anomalous pulmonary vein that drains into the IVC, the portal vein, or the hepatic veins below the diaphragm, and is associated with right pulmonary hypoplasia.

D. Most frequently, patients with scimitar syndrome are asymptomatic in the absence of associated abnormalities. Surgical correction is recommended for symptomatic patients or asymptomatic patients with a pulmonary to systemic blood flow exceeding 1.5 to 2 (because of their higher likelihood of progression to pulmonary hypertension and right ventricular failure).

E. Meandering pulmonary vein is more common on the right, is not associated with a shunt, and does not require further invasive investigation or management.

**SECTION XI
THORACIC IMAGING**

Top Tips

◆ Scimitar syndrome, also called hypogenetic lung syndrome or congenital pulmonary venolobar syndrome, is a congenital hypoplasia of the right lung and anomalous pulmonary venous drainage, most commonly draining to the IVC.

◆ The vertical vein is a gently curved vein in the right lung directed toward the right costovertebral angle. This vein enlarges as it descends toward the diaphragm. The anomalous vein is shaped like a Turkish sword, hence the name scimitar sign.

◆ The majority are right sided.

Essentials 4

■ Case

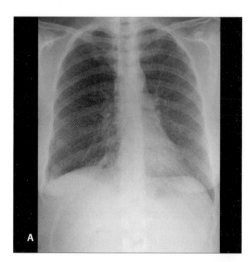

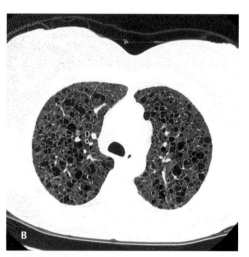

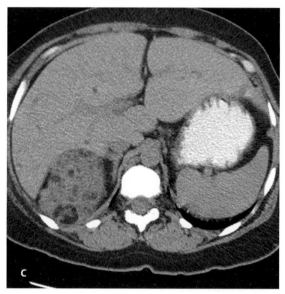

■ Questions

1. Which ONE of the following is the MOST likely diagnosis?
   A. Pulmonary Langerhans cell histiocytosis
   B. Lymphangioleiomyomatosis
   C. Centrilobular emphysema
   D. Cystic fibrosis
   E. Tuberous sclerosis

2. Regarding the diagnosis in the test case, which of the following are correct? (Select ALL that apply.)
   A. The classic triad includes seizures, mental retardation, and adenoma sebaceum.
   B. There are no associated imaging findings in the brain.

C. There is a significantly increased risk of renal cell carcinoma.
D. There is an association with pulmonary arterial hypertension, meconium ileus, pancreatic insufficiency, and cirrhosis.

3. All of the following are appropriate indications for high-resolution chest CT (HRCT) EXCEPT:
   A. Diffuse lung disease
   B. Solitary pulmonary nodule
   C. Restrictive lung disease
   D. Pulmonary hypertension
   E. Obstructive lung disease

■ Answers and Explanations

Question 1

E. Correct! This is tuberous sclerosis (TS). The chest radiograph shows a diffuse reticular pattern. Closer inspection shows innumerable cystic air spaces. Computed tomography (CT) confirms a pattern of diffuse cystic lung disease, with cysts showing well-defined walls. In the abdomen, multiple angiomyolipomas (AMLs) are present in the right kidney. The left kidney is surgically absent.

Other choices and discussion

A. PLCH can be associated with a diffuse bilateral reticulonodular pattern with a predilection for the upper lungs. Later in the course of the disease, the irregular nodules can cavitate, giving the appearance of irregular cysts.

B. LAM can be associated with multiple thin-walled cysts throughout the lungs. Very small cysts can give the appearance of diffuse interstitial markings. Chylous pleural effusion are sometimes present. Associated pneumothorax can be seen with TS, PLCH, and LAM, but the left nephrectomy clips favor TS.

C. Visible walls make emphysema less likely. Lack of associated nodules also argues against emphysema.

D. Cystic fibrosis should show bronchiectasis (tram-tracking).

Question 2

A. Correct! The classic triad of TS includes seizures, mental retardation, and adenoma sebaceum. Less than half of the patients present with the complete triad.

Other choices and discussion

B. Multiple brain imaging findings may be present with TS. These include cortical/subcortical tubers, subependymal hamartomas, subependymal astrocytomas, and various white matter abnormalities.

C. The incidence of renal cell carcinoma in patients with TS is similar to that of the general population, but patients with TS tend to develop them at an earlier age. Angiomyolipoma is the renal mass classically associated with TS and may be multiple, as is demonstrated in the test case. AMLs often occur with aneurysms, which can sometimes be seen with imaging.

D. Pulmonary arterial hypertension, meconium ileus, pancreatic insufficiency and cirrhosis are associated with *cystic fibrosis*.

Question 3

B. Correct! Solitary pulmonary nodule is not typically an appropriate indication for HRCT.

Referring providers often misconstrue the *high-resolution* moniker as an indicator of the best lung evaluation (aka HDTV or 4K TV!). In truth, most centers perform HRCT as a *sampling* of the lung parenchyma with "noncontiguous" series, primarily to assess for patterns of diffuse lung disease, airway disease, or vascular disease. The noncontiguous technique, also referred to as "axial" or "sequential" imaging, is generally used to limit radiation. Thin collimation in HRCT requires more radiation on a per-slice basis to mitigate the extra image noise. Typi-

cal HRCTs include sampling of the lungs with full inspiration at 1-mm slice thickness at 10- to 20-mm intervals (aka 1×10 mm), rendering them inappropriate for initial characterization or follow up of solitary pulmonary nodules. Furthermore, typical HRCT protocols also include separate prone and expiratory imaging, adding additional radiation. These are necessary to assess for early subpleural fibrosis or air-trapping.

Initial workup of solitary pulmonary nodules should include an attempt to characterize three different features of the nodule: size, consistency (i.e., cavitation, calcification, or fat), and margins. Noncontrast standard protocol CT with 2.5- to 5-mm *contiguous* intervals is preferable (aka 2.5×2.5 mm), with contrast added for additional characterization if needed or for mediastinal assessment.

Other choices and discussion

A. HRCT is well suited for characterization of diffuse lung disease, as in the test case. HRCT can identify the predominant pattern and distribution of cystic, interstitial, and fibrotic lung disease. When paired with appropriate clinical inputs, useful differential diagnoses can be generated for guiding further investigations such as medical therapy, biochemical assays (autoimmune workup), or biopsy.

C. When pulmonary function testing indicates restriction or decreased lung volumes, the primary consideration is fibrotic lung disease. Key indicators of fibrotic lung disease on HRCT are honeycombing, traction bronchiectasis, architectural distortion, and decreased lung volume.

D. The majority of pulmonary hypertension is attributable to primary pulmonary arterial hypertension. Two important categories of secondary pulmonary hypertension are lung disease and vascular disease.

E. HRCT can be helpful in detecting both small and large airway obstruction. Small airway disease is typically manifest as air-trapping on expiratory imaging. Large airway disease can be manifest as bronchial wall thickening or large airway collapse involving the trachea or main bronchi on expiratory imaging.

Top Tips

- ◆ Ground glass attenuation on HRCT often suggests an active and potentially reversible process.

- ◆ Pulmonary hypertension is likely in patients older than 50 years of age if the ratio of the diameter of the main pulmonary artery to the ascending aorta (at the same level) is > 1.

- ◆ Typical findings of cystic fibrosis in the lungs include mucous plugging, bronchiectasis, recurrent atelectasis and pneumonitis, and air trapping.

Essentials 5

■ Case

A 42-year-old man undergoes cross-sectional imaging following discovery of an incidental mass on chest X-ray.

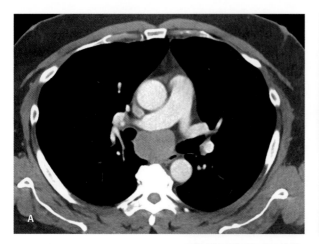

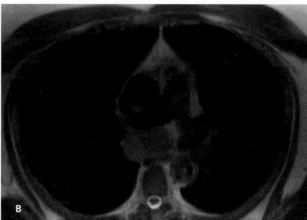

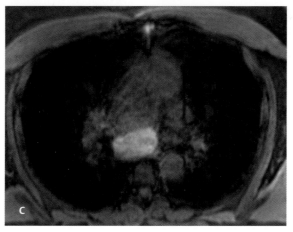

■ Questions

1. What is the MOST likely diagnosis?
   A. Pericardial cyst
   B. Thymic cyst
   C. Castleman disease
   D. Bronchogenic cyst
   E. Intrathoracic pancreatic pseudocyst

2. What is the MOST common location for this lesion?
   A. Subcarinal region
   B. Paratracheal region
   C. Retrocardiac
   D. Intrapulmonary
   E. Pericardium

3. Which are the following is NOT a recognized complication of this lesion?
   A. Fistula
   B. Hemorrhage
   C. Rhabdomyosarcoma
   D. Abscess
   E. Lymphoma

■ Answers and Explanations

Question 1

D. Correct! This is a bronchogenic cyst. The postcontrast computed tomography (CT) demonstrates a soft tissue density subcarinal mass. It demonstrates iso- to mildly hyperintense signal on T2-weighted magnetic resonance imaging (MRI), but it is lower signal intensity than cerebrospinal fluid and is hyperintense on precontrast T1. These imaging features are characteristic of a bronchogenic cyst, a congenital malformation of the bronchial tree. They are the most common type of foregut duplication cyst, accounting for approximately 50% of congenital mediastinal cysts. Bronchogenic cysts can cause symptoms from local compression, but are most often asymptomatic and discovered incidentally. On CT, they may be fluid or soft tissue density, depending on the presence of hemorrhage or proteinaceous contents. This proteinaceous content can cause them to appear iso- to mildly hyperintense signal on T1 MRI, and iso- to mildly hyperintense signal on T2 MRI.

Other choices and discussion

A. Pericardial cysts are typically located at the cardiophrenic angles, most commonly on the right, and are low attenuation on CT.

B. Thymic cysts typically occur in the anterior mediastinum. Congenital thymic cysts tend to be unilocular, with well-defined and frequently imperceptible walls. Multilocular thymic cysts are usually acquired secondary to hemorrhage, infection, or underlying malignancy. On MRI, thymic cysts are typically low signal on T1, high signal on T2, and have no enhancement on postgadolinium T1 imaging.

C. Castleman disease (angiofollicular lymph node hyperplasia or giant lymph node hyperplasia) is characterized by hypervascular lymphoid hyperplasia. This is a B-cell lymphoproliferative condition that commonly presents as a solitary mediastinal mass. It typically contains arborizing calcification on CT and is a solid mass with iso- to low signal intensity on T2-weighted MRI. Multicentric Castleman disease is a rare systemic disease with diffuse lymphadenopathy, anemia, and splenomegaly, and usually occurs in patients with human immunodeficiency virus.

E. Intrathoracic pancreatic pseudocysts are retroperitoneal cystic lesions that extend from the abdomen into the thorax through the aortic or esophageal hiatus. They originate from the pancreas and occur as a complication of pancreatitis.

Question 2

A. Correct! The mediastinum is the most common location for bronchogenic cysts, accounting for 65 to 90% cases, with the subcarinal location accounting for approximately 50% of total cases.

Other choices and discussion

B. Paratracheal location, most commonly on the right, accounts for approximately 20% cases.

C. Retrocardiac is an uncommon location, accounting for <10% of cases.

D. Intrapulmonary is an uncommon location; when present in an intrapulmonary location, they are typically perihilar and found in the lower lobes.

E. Pericardium is an uncommon location. The most common cystic lesion in the pericardium is a pericardial cyst.

Question 3

E. Correct! Lymphomatous transformation is a recognized complication of Castleman disease, but is not described in bronchogenic cysts.

Other choices and discussion

A. Fistula formation with the bronchial tree is a recognized complication of bronchogenic cysts. Instrumentation can lead to fistula formation, and this manifests as an air-fluid level in the cyst.

B. Intralesional hemorrhage is a common complication. It can occur spontaneously or secondary to intervention, manifesting on CT as layered high density material within the cyst.

C. Malignancy transformation is a rare (approximately 0.7%) complication, with reported tumors including rhabdomyosarcoma, leiomyosarcoma, and adenocarcinoma. This manifests on imaging as a new and enhancing solid component within the cyst.

D. Abscess complicates approximately 20% of bronchogenic cysts, usually occurring secondary to fistula formation with the tracheobronchial tree.

■ Suggested Readings

Berrocal T, Madrid C, Novo S, Gutiérrez J, Arjonilla A, Gómez-León N. Congenital anomalies of the tracheobronchial tree, lung, and mediastinum: embryology, radiology, and pathology. Radiographics 2004;24(1)

Ko S-F, Hsieh M-J, Ng S-H, Lin J-W, Wan Y-L, Lee T-Y, et al. Imaging spectrum of Castleman's disease. Am J Roentgenol 2004;3:769–775

Top Tips

◆ Bronchogenic cysts are the most common foregut duplication cyst and are usually found in the subcarinal, paratracheal, or perihilar regions.

◆ On CT, they may be fluid or soft tissue density, depending on the proteinaceous content. They are T2 iso- to mildly hyperintense and do not enhance. Post-contrast subtraction images maybe helpful in lesions with intrinsic precontrast T1 hyperintensity (due to hemorrhage or protein) and also to exclude an enhancing soft tissue component.

◆ Infection is the most common complication, usually occurring secondary to instrumentation of the tracheobronchial tree leading to fistula formation.

Essentials 6

■ Case

A 53-year-old man presents with abdominal distention.

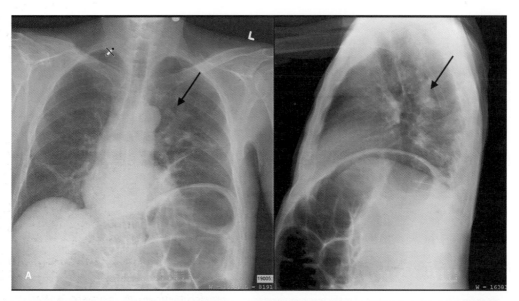
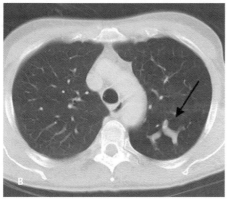
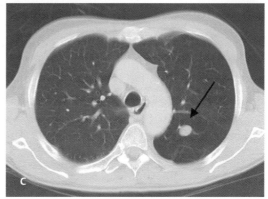

■ Questions

1. What is the MOST common clinical presentation of bronchial atresia?
   A. Asymptomatic patient
   B. Focal wheeze on auscultation
   C. Hemoptysis
   D. Shortness of breath
   E. Recurrent pneumonia

2. What is the MOST common presentation of this diagnosis on chest X-ray?
   A. Hyperinflated lobe
   B. Perihilar nodule
   C. Bronchiectasis
   D. Tubular/branching opacity

3. Where is the MOST common location for bronchial atresia?
   A. Left upper lobe
   B. Right upper lobe
   C. Right middle lobe
   D. Left lower lobe

■ Answers and Explanations

Question 1

A. Correct! Most patients with bronchial atresia are asymptomatic.

Other choices and discussion

This abnormality is usually an incidental finding on chest radiography. However, some patients may present with recurrent pneumonia. Focal wheeze on auscultation, hemoptysis, and shortness of breath are not commonly seen with bronchial atresia.

Question 2

A. Correct! A hyperinflated lobe is the most common radiographic appearance of bronchial atresia.

Other choices and discussion

Typically, chest radiographs of patients with bronchial atresia show an area of lobar hyperlucency (90%) and a hilar nodule or mass (80%). Mucoid-impacted airway may mimic a solitary pulmonary nodule. A hyperlucent lobe may be mistaken for congenital lobar emphysema, obstructing foreign body or, less likely, a Westermark sign (oligemia secondary to pulmonary embolism).

Question 3

A. Correct! The left upper lobe is the most common location for bronchial atresia.

Other choices and discussion

Bronchial atresia is a congenital abnormality thought to arise from a vascular insult in utero, after the fifteenth week of gestation. The result is a short segment obliteration of a lobar segmental or subsegmental bronchus near its origin. It most commonly involves the apical posterior segment of the left upper lobe.

As is seen in this case, computed tomography (CT) imaging typically shows an area of pulmonary hyperlucency secondary to hyperinflation via collateral air drift (pores of Kohn and canals of Lambert) and decreased vascularity (oligemia). The adjacent lung is compressed and displaced. The focal rounded low density lesion represents the mucoid impacted dilated bronchus just distal to the bronchial obliteration. Another common radiographic appearance is tubular and branching densities, representing mucoid impacted airways, distal to the obliterated bronchus. CT is the most sensitive imaging technique for confirmation of the diagnosis.

It is important to make the correct diagnosis, as the main differential diagnosis for bronchial atresia includes endobronchial tumor and foreign body, and bronchoscopy is indicated for those entities. Clinical history that would increase suspicion for foreign body includes aspiration episode and traumatic intubation/recent dental work (i.e., broken tooth). Thin collimation CT is helpful to identify a possible foreign body and to measure the density of the obstructing lesion. A low-density focus (Hounsfield unit <25) is consistent with mucoid impaction if the density is tubular or branching in morphology.

Other less common diagnostic considerations for bronchial atresia include congenital lobar emphysema associated with a patent bronchus, allergic bronchopulmonary aspergillosis, pulmonary varix, arterial venous malformation, and postinfectious bronchial stricture secondary to *Mycobacterium tuberculosis*. Contrast-enhanced CT can better diagnose vascular abnormalities such as pulmonary varix and arterial venous malformation.

■ Suggested Readings

Dillman JR, Yarram SG, Hernandez RJ. Imaging of pulmonary venous developmental anomalies. Am J Roentgenol 2009;192(5):1272–1285

Kinsella D, Sissons G, Williams MP. The radiological imaging of bronchial atresia. Br J Radiol 1992;65(776):681–685

Schuster SR, Harris GB, Williams A, Kirkpatrick J, Reid L. Bronchial atresia: a recognizable entity in the pediatric age group. J Pediatr Surg 1978;13(6D):682–689

Top Tips

◆ Bronchial atresia is usually asymptomatic, but may present with recurrent pneumonia.

◆ The main differential diagnosis for bronchial atresia includes endobronchial tumor and foreign body.

◆ Less common diagnostic considerations for bronchial atresia include congenital lobar emphysema associated with a patent bronchus, allergic bronchopulmonary aspergillosis, pulmonary varix, arterial venous malformation, and postinfectious bronchial stricture secondary to *Mycobacterium tuberculosis*.

Essentials 7

■ Case

A 69-year-old man status post attempted transesophageal echocardiogram; preoperative for atrial flutter ablation.

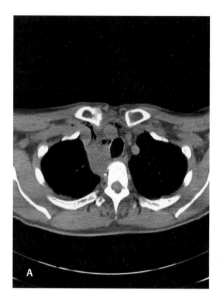

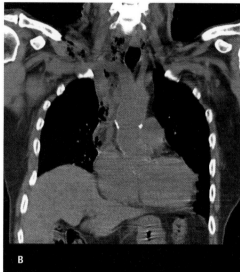

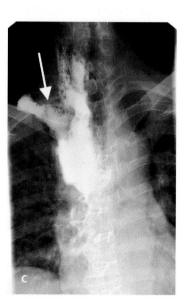

■ Questions

1. What is the MOST likely diagnosis?
   A. Mediastinitis
   B. Esophageal tear
   C. Empyema necessitans
   D. Bronchial rupture

2. Given the location of the defect, what is the MOST common cause?
   A. Boerhaave
   B. Iatrogenic
   C. Caustic ingestion
   D. Perforated ulcer

3. What complication is visualized on the above images?
   A. Esophageal pleural fistula
   B. Esophageal bronchial fistula
   C. Empyema
   D. Mediastinitis

■ Answers and Explanations

Question 1

B. Correct! This is an esophageal tear. Extravasation of contrast on the esophagram is diagnostic.

If an esophageal tear is suspected, the next most appropriate imaging modality is an esophagram with water-soluble contrast. Indirect signs of esophageal perforation on chest radiography include subcutaneous emphysema, widened mediastinum, and left pleural effusion.

The other choices are incorrect.

Question 2

B. Correct! Iatrogenic causes account for the majority of esophageal perforations (56% of cases).

Other choices and discussion

The term Boerhaave syndrome is reserved for esophageal perforations that occur secondary to vomiting (10% of cases). Patients typically present with chest pain that radiates to the back or left shoulder, causing physicians to confuse an esophageal perforation with a myocardial infarction.

While iatrogenic esophageal perforations can occur anywhere, in most cases of Boerhaave syndrome, the tear occurs at the left posterior and lateral aspect of the distal esophagus. The classical presentation is named Mackler triad, which includes chest pain, vomiting, and subcutaneous emphysema.

Other etiologies of perforation include foreign bodies (chicken and fish bones), caustic ingestion, pill esophagitis, Barrett esophagus, and iatrogenic following dilatation for strictures. Of note, a series of esophageal perforations has been reported in the literature as the sequelae of ablation for atrial fibrillation. Ablations occur near the ostia of the pulmonary veins within the left atrium, and the adjacent esophagus traveling along the posterior aspect of the left atrium is sometimes injured.

Question 3

D. Correct! Mediastinitis is demonstrated.

Dreaded complications of esophageal perforation are mediastinitis and sepsis, which can result in high morbidity and mortality. Other complications include abscess, esophageal/bronchial/pleural fistulas, and empyema.

Treatment consists of immediate antibiotic therapy (to prevent mediastinitis and sepsis) and surgical repair of the perforation. In this case, the patient was taken to the operating room to drain the mediastinal collection and to repair the esophageal tear.

■ Suggested Readings

De Lutio di Castelguidone E, Pinto A, Merola S, Stavolo C, Romano L. Role of spiral and multislice computed tomography in the evaluation of traumatic and spontaneous oesophageal perforation. Our experience. Radiol Med 2005;109(3):252–259

Lee S, Mergo PJ, Ros PR. The leaking esophagus: CT patterns of esophageal rupture, perforation, and fistulization. Crit Rev Diagn Imaging 1996;37(6):461–490

Tocino I, Armstrong J. Trauma to the lung. In: Taveras J, ed. Radiology. Philadelphia, PA: Lippincott-Raven; 1996: 1–8

Top Tips

- Fish and chicken bones are best imaged with computed tomography. Fish bones contain less calcium and are less opaque than chicken bones. If plain films are negative and there is a high index of suspicion, either contrast esophagram or computed tomography is indicated.

- Other causes of pneumomediastinum include tracheal injury, excessive coughing, barotrauma (intubated patient with increasing positive end expiratory pressure), rapid rises in altitude (scuba diving), and the use of recreational drugs such as crack cocaine.

- Esophageal perforations have been reported as the sequelae of ablation for atrial fibrillation.

Essentials 8

■ Case

A 53-year-old woman with 20 pack-year smoking history presents with right shoulder pain.

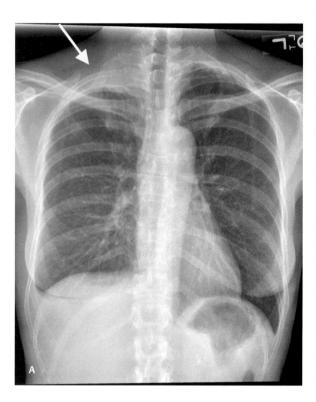

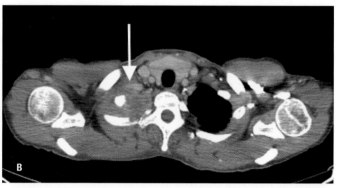

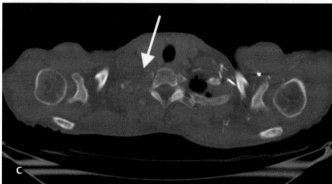

■ Questions

1. What radiographic abnormality is demonstrated?
   A. Neurogenic tumor
   B. Mycobacterial infection (tuberculosis)
   C. Postradiation fibrosis
   D. Lung carcinoma

2. What is the MOST common clinical presentation for this disease entity?
   A. Hemoptysis
   B. Shoulder pain
   C. Horner syndrome
   D. Pleuritic chest pain

3. What is the most common histologic type of this apical abnormality?
   A. Squamous cell
   B. Adenocarcinoma
   C. Neuroendocrine
   D. Sarcomatoid

■ Answers and Explanations

Question 1

D. Correct! This is most likely lung carcinoma.

The differential diagnosis of apical cap/mass includes extrapleural fat, inflammatory disease (tuberculosis), neurogenic tumor, mesothelioma, and radiation fibrosis. Bony destruction of the right apical first rib and a smoking history favor the diagnosis of Pancoast tumor. In this case, both the brachial plexus and subclavian vessels were encased by tumor.

Magnetic resonance imaging with its superior soft tissue contrast permits better evaluation of the brachial plexus, subclavian vessels, and possible chest wall involvement. Positron emission tomography/computed tomography allows assessment of nodal and distant metastasis and is helpful for staging.

The other choices are incorrect.

Question 2

B. Correct! Shoulder pain is the most common clinical presentation. Pancoast (or superior sulcus) tumor is a smoking-related cancer of lung origin. Clinically, patients often present with shoulder pain radiating down the arm due to brachial plexus involvement. (This patient presented with weight loss and shoulder pain.)

Less commonly (25%), patients present with Horner syndrome (ptosis, miosis, and hemifacial anhidrosis) when the stellate plexus is involved. By definition, Pancoast tumors involve the parietal pleura and include periosteal/bony involvement of the upper ribs or apical vertebral bodies. With newer surgical approaches and combined use of chemotherapy and radiation therapy, these tumors may be resectable even with vertebral body or neural foramen involvement.

Question 3

A. Correct! Although Pancoast tumors may be any histologic type, squamous cell is most common.

The other choices are incorrect.

Note that the "pack-year" is a unit for measuring the amount a person has smoked over a long period of time.

Number of pack-years = (number of cigarettes smoked per day/20) × number of years smoked. (One pack has 20 cigarettes.)

For example, if a patient smoked 15 cigarettes per day for 20 years, that amounts to 15 pack-years.

■ Suggested Readings

Heelan RT, Demas BE, Caravelli JF, et al. Superior sulcus tumors: CT and MR imaging. Radiology 1989;170(3 Pt 1):637–641

Pancoast HK. Superior pulmonary sulcus tumor: tumor characterized by pain, Horner's syndrome, destruction of bone and atrophy of hand muscles. JAMA 1932;99:1391–1396

Webb WR, Gatsonis C, Zerhouni EA, et al. CT and MR imaging in staging non-small cell bronchogenic carcinoma: report of the Radiologic Diagnostic Oncology Group. Radiology 1991;178(3):705–713

Top Tips

◆ Number of pack-years = (number of cigarettes smoked per day/20) × number of years smoked.

◆ Musculoskeletal radiologists should keep Pancoast tumor in mind when reviewing dedicated shoulder radiographs for shoulder pain.

◆ Asymmetric pleural thickening has many causes. Benign causes include postinfectious (prior tuberculosis), abscess, radiation fibrosis, idiopathic, and hematoma (posttrauma, aortic injury). Malignant causes include Pancoast tumor, lymphoma, and mesothelioma.

Essentials 9

■ Case

A 53-year-old presents with dyspnea on exertion for past 5 years.

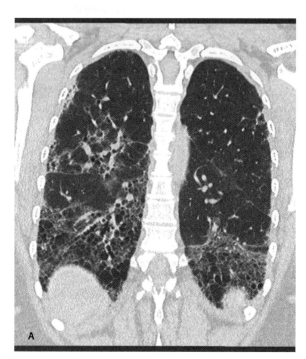

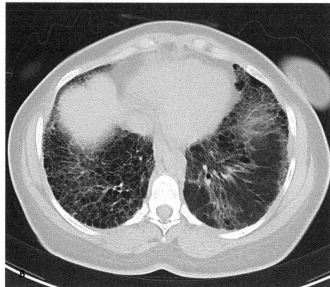

■ Questions

1. The characteristic distribution of usual interstitial pneumonia (UIP) pulmonary fibrosis on chest imaging is
   A. Upper lungs
   B. Diffuse
   C. Peripheral
   D. Basilar

2. Which characteristic feature best differentiates UIP from nonspecific interstitial pneumonia (NSIP)?
   A. Severity
   B. Bronchiectasis
   C. Honeycombing
   D. Ground-glass opacity

3. What is the correct computed tomography categorization of fibrotic lung disease for this patient?
   A. Definite with UIP
   B. Probable UIP
   C. Possible UIP
   D. Inconsistent with UIP

■ Answers and Explanations

Question 1

D. Correct! The UIP pattern of pulmonary fibrosis is most concentrated in the subpleural and basal portions of the lungs.

The other choices are incorrect.

Question 2

C. Correct! Honeycombing (clustered cystic air spaces) is the most specific finding of a UIP pattern on high-resolution computed tomography (HRCT) and is present in the majority of patients with histopathologic UIP.

The differential diagnosis for UIP on HRCT includes other fibrotic diseases, most commonly NSIP and chronic hypersensitivity pneumonitis (HP).

HRCT findings that favor NSIP over UIP include the presence of ground-glass opacity (basal predominant), subpleural sparing, and lack of honeycombing. Chronic HP may be indistinguishable from UIP on HRCT.

Findings suggestive of chronic HP include centrilobular nodules, mosaic attenuation, lobular air-trapping, and mid- to upper lobe predominant fibrosis. In advanced cases, honeycombing may be present.

Question 3

C. Correct! This case is best categorized as probable UIP.

Current guidelines provide three categories of UIP diagnosis by HRCT: definite UIP pattern, possible UIP pattern, and inconsistent with UIP pattern. A *definite UIP* pattern consists of basilar and subpleural fibrosis predominant reticulation, honeycombing with or without traction bronchiectasis, and absence of features suggestive of another diagnosis. A *possible UIP* pattern includes all of the imaging findings of definite UIP pattern except for honeycombing. An *inconsistent with UIP* pattern category occurs if any of the following imaging findings are present: upper or midlung predominance, peribronchovascular predominance, ground-glass opacity more extensive than reticulation, profuse micronodules, discrete cysts, diffuse mosaic attenuation or air-trapping involving three or more lobes (as seen with chronic HP), and consolidation.

Guidelines state that patients with HRCT patterns of possible UIP and inconsistent with UIP require further evaluation and may need a surgical lung biopsy to establish a confident diagnosis. Of the patients with HRCT findings of possible UIP who undergo surgical biopsy, many are indeed found to have a histologic diagnosis of UIP. Given the high morbidity and mortality associated with surgical lung biopsies in this population, avoiding biopsies in the appropriate clinical context is ideal.

The differential for dyspnea on exertion is broad. This patient had hyperlipidemia and a family history of coronary artery disease, and a cardiac origin of the dyspnea was initially suspected. The cardiac workup, which included several missed appointments and waiting for stress test results, delayed making the correct diagnosis. In this patient, a simple chest radiograph would have been helpful in establishing the diagnosis much sooner.

■ Suggested Readings

Monaghan H, Wells AU, Colby TV, du Bois RM, Hansell DM, Nicholson AG. Prognostic implications of histologic patterns in multiple surgical lung biopsies from patients with idiopathic interstitial pneumonias. Chest 2004;125:522–526

Raghu G, Collard HR, Egan JJ, et al. An official ATS/ERS/JRS/ALAT statement: idiopathic pulmonary fibrosis: evidence-based guidelines for diagnosis and management. Am J Respir Crit Care Med 2011;183:788–824

Song JW, Do KH, Kim MY, et al. Pathologic and radiologic differences between idiopathic and collagen vascular disease-related usual interstitial pneumonia. Chest 2009;136:23–30

Top Tips

◆ Surgical lung biopsies carry significant morbidity and mortality in patients with pulmonary fibrosis. Establishing the diagnosis noninvasively, with concordant clinical and radiologic findings, is beneficial to the patient.

◆ One commonly overlooked diagnosis for pulmonary fibrosis is chronic HP. Radiographic findings suggestive of chronic HP include centrilobular nodules, mosaic attenuation, lobular air-trapping, and mid- to upper lobe predominant fibrosis. In advanced cases, honeycombing may be present.

◆ Honeycombing (clustered cystic air spaces) is the most specific finding of a UIP pattern on HRCT.

Essentials 10

■ **Case**

A 68-year-old nonsmoking woman presents with a 3-month history of cough. Temperature and complete blood count are normal. Seven weeks previous, her primary care physician gave her a 7-day course of levofloxacin without improvement.

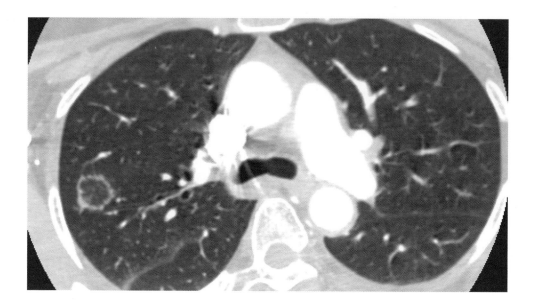

■ **Questions**

1. Which ONE of the following is the MOST likely diagnosis?
   A. Septic embolus
   B. Organizing pneumonia
   C. Adenocarcinoma
   D. Granulomatosis with polyangiitis

2. Which sign is demonstrated on the computed tomography image?
   A. Reverse halo sign
   B. Westermark sign
   C. Flat waist sign
   D. Signet ring sign

3. Histopathology in biopsied areas of the test case would most likely demonstrate _____.
   A. Innumerable neutrophils
   B. Malignant respiratory epithelium
   C. Destruction of alveolar walls
   D. Fibroblast proliferation

■ Answers and Explanations

Question 1

B. Correct! The image demonstrates a focus of minimal central ground glass surrounded by a rim of more consolidated-appearing lung parenchyma in the right lung. This sign has a name, which is discussed in question 2. OP can occur in patients with prior infection that has subsequently organized, or may be the sequela of a drug reaction or an underlying collagen vascular disease.

Other choices and discussion

A. Septic embolus usually presents on imaging with multiple pulmonary nodules, some of which may cavitate. Patients are usually febrile and acutely ill.

C. Adenocarcinoma usually presents as a nodule or a mass. Occasionally, nonnodular forms develop and have the appearance of consolidations, rather than the rim-like appearance shown here.

D. Granulomatosis with polyangiitis (formerly called Wegener granulomatosis) is a multisystem disorder that can affect the lungs, airways, and blood vessels. Cavitating nodules in the lungs are usually found.

Question 2

A. Correct! This is a reverse halo sign. A focus of minimal central ground glass surrounded by a rim of more consolidated-appearing lung parenchyma is termed the reverse halo or "atoll" sign. This is seen in OP in approximately 30% of cases.

The atoll sign name originates from the similar appearance with a coral atoll, which is a ring-shaped coral reef that surrounds a lagoon (peripheral dense coral and central low density water).

Other choices and discussion

B. The Westermark sign refers to unilateral hyperlucency due to oligemia from a large pulmonary embolus.

C. The flat waist sign is associated with left lower lobe collapse.

D. The signet ring sign is associated with bronchiectasis.

Question 3

D. Correct! OP represents the deposition of granulation tissue within the alveolar spaces. This is due to fibroblast proliferation.

Other choices and discussion

A. Innumerable neutrophils would not be found because OP is not an acute infection.

B. Malignant respiratory epithelium would not be found because OP represents the deposition of granulation tissue, not neoplastic tissue, within the alveolar spaces.

C. Destruction of alveolar walls would not be found because the architecture is typically preserved in OP.

■ Suggested Readings

Mueller-Mang C, Grosse C, Schmid K, Stiebellehner L, Bankier AA. What every radiologist should know about idiopathic interstitial pneumonias. Radiographics 2007;27:595–615

Travis WD, Costabel U, Hansell DM, King TE Jr, Lynch DA, Nicholson AG, et al. An official American Thoracic Society/ European Respiratory Society Statement: update of the international multidisciplinary classification of the idiopathic interstitial pneumonias. Am J Respir Crit Care Med 2013;188(6);733–748

Walker CM, Mohammed T-L, Chung JH. Reversed halo sign. J Thor Imaging 2011;26(3):W80

Top Tips

♦ Think of OP in patients with persistent symptoms following treatment of pneumonia. OP can also be seen with drug toxicity, collagen vascular disease, and radiation therapy.

♦ The atoll, or reverse halo sign, is seen in up to 30% of cases of OP.

♦ When a persistent peripheral consolidation is seen, consider both OP and chronic eosinophilic pneumonia in the differential diagnosis.

Details 1

■ Case

A 65-year-old woman undergoes successive computed tomography (CT) examinations, 2 years apart, for chronic cough. She has no other significant past medical history. The referring pulmonologist requests your advice on the best next course of action. Which of the following would you recommend (assuming the CT is otherwise unremarkable)?

A. Follow-up chest X-ray in 1 year
B. Follow-up chest CT in 1 year
C. Serum cytoplasmic antineutrophil cytoplasmic antibody
D. Treat with antibiotics and repeat the CT scan in 6 months
E. Tissue sampling

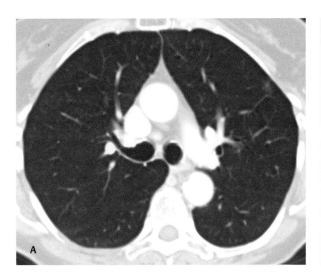
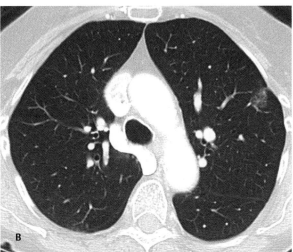

■ The following questions pertain to lung cancer.

1. True or False. The solid component of a part-solid pulmonary nodule should be measured using lung windows on CT.
2. True or False. Adenocarcinoma is the most common type of primary lung malignancy.
3. True or False. Bronchioalveolar carcinoma (BAC) is a distinct subtype of non-small cell lung cancer.
4. True or False. Adenocarcinoma in situ is a typically a uniformly solid nodule on CT.
5. True or False. Minimally invasive adenocarcinoma is commonly indistinguishable from adenocarcinoma in situ on CT.
6. True or False. Lepidic predominant adenocarcinoma often mimics consolidation on CT.
7. True or False. There is a correlation between tumor size and central nervous system metastases in invasive pulmonary adenocarcinoma.
8. True or False. Subsolid nodules are accurately evaluated on chest CT with a slice thickness of ≤ 5 mm.
9. True or False. Clear visualization of pulmonary vessels in an area of consolidation is pathognomonic of pneumonia.

■ Answers and Explanations

E. Correct! Tissue sampling is indicated. The two CT scans demonstrate an approximate doubling in size of the left upper lobe ground glass nodule with a small internal solid component. This is suspicious for a lung adenocarcinoma. The major choice between performing percutaneous CT-guided biopsy or going straight to wedge resection depends on patient and physician preference. This patient with a peripheral subsolid lesion underwent wedge resection, with the pathology demonstrating minimally invasive adenocarcinoma. Positron emission tomography/CT may be helpful if there is a significant solid component, particularly for the evaluation of potential metastatic disease. Positron emission tomography/CT is less sensitive for detecting malignancy in ground glass nodules than in solid nodules.

Other choices and discussion

A. The abnormality is an enlarging ground glass nodule in the left upper lobe. This will not be visible on chest radiography.

B. This ground glass nodule has grown significantly over a 2-year period and is highly concerning for malignancy. Further imaging surveillance at this stage is not appropriate.

C. Serum cytoplasmic antineutrophil cytoplasmic antibody is a useful antibody test for cases of suspected granulomatosis with polyangiitis (previously Wegener granulomatosis) and is positive in > 90% of cases. This is a multisystem disease, characterized by upper respiratory tract, pulmonary, and renal involvement. Pulmonary involvement manifests on CT as multiple pulmonary nodules, which cavitate in 50% of cases.

D. This ground glass nodule has been present for 2 years and is unlikely to be related to infection. Current Fleischner society guidelines do not recommend a course of antibiotics in the management of ground glass nodules.

Question 1

False. When assessing a part-solid pulmonary nodule, the total size, including the solid and nonsolid (ground glass) components, should be measured. In addition, the solid component by itself should also be measured. For consistency, the solid component should be measured on mediastinal windows and the ground glass component measured on lung windows.

Question 2

True. Lung cancer is the most common cause of cancer mortality worldwide. It is broadly divided into non-small cell (80%) and small cell carcinoma (20%). Adenocarcinoma is now the most common type of lung cancer overall (35%) and is the most common type in nonsmokers. Squamous cell carcinoma (30%) is strongly associated with smoking and is the most common primary lung cancer subtype to cavitate. Large cell carcinoma (15%) is the least common type of non-small cell carcinoma; these lesions tend to be peripherally located and can grow to a large size before diagnosis.

Question 3

False. Since the 2011 updated classification of lung adenocarcinoma, BAC is no longer considered a distinct type of non-small cell lung cancer. It has been incorporated into the spectrum of lung adenocarcinoma. The histopathologic term lepidic (growth along alveolar walls) has replaced BAC.

Question 4

False. Adenocarcinoma in situ refers to a purely lepidic (growth along alveolar walls) and noninvasive adenocarcinoma of 3 cm or smaller. When resected, it is associated with excellent survival, with reported 5-year survival rates of close to 100%. The classical CT appearance is a non-solid ground glass nodule of < 3 cm, which may have a part solid or bubble-like appearance.

Question 5

True. There is significant overlap in the imaging appearances of the preinvasive lesions of adenocarcinoma and of minimally invasive adenocarcinoma. Minimally invasive adenocarcinoma refers to a 3 cm or smaller lepidic predominant adenocarcinoma with an invasive component of 5 mm or smaller.

Question 6

False. Invasive mucinous adenocarcinoma commonly mimics consolidation on CT, with air bronchograms in a peribronchovascular distribution. It may be multifocal and multicentric, often with lower lobe predominance, and was formerly called mucinous/multifocal BAC. Lepidic predominant adenocarcinoma is a form of nonmucinous invasive adenocarcinoma with a predominant lepidic growth pattern. Its characteristic appearance on CT is a part-solid, part-nonsolid lesion, with an occasional bubble-like appearance.

Question 7

True. There is a correlation between tumor size and the risk of central nervous system metastasis in invasive pulmonary adenocarcinoma. For example, a 6-cm primary adenocarcinoma has a 65% probability of central nervous system metastases, versus 15% for a 2-cm primary tumor.

Question 8

False. Subsolid nodules are best evaluated on thin section CT with a slice thickness of ≤ 3 mm to accurately assess for the presence of an internal solid component.

Question 9

False. Invasive mucinous adenocarcinoma often mimics pneumonia on CT. The clear visualization of pulmonary vessels in areas of consolidation, the so-called CT-angiogram sign, has been described in relation to invasive mucinous adenocarcinoma.

Top Tips

◆ Consider lung adenocarcinoma for persisting or enlarging ground glass nodules on CT, especially those with a new or enlarging solid component.

◆ The size of the solid component in lepidic lung adenocarcinoma corresponds with the likelihood of invasion.

◆ Mucinous invasive adenocarcinoma may mimic consolidation on chest radiographs and CT.

Details 2

■ Case

A 32-year-old female smoker with progressive shortness of breath undergoes a chest CT. What is the MOST likely diagnosis based on the CT appearance?

A. Centrilobular emphysema
B. Sporadic lymphangioleiomyomatosis (LAM)
C. Pulmonary Langerhans cell histiocytosis (LCH)
D. Lymphocytic interstitial pneumonia (LIP)
E. Desquamative interstitial pneumonia (DIP)

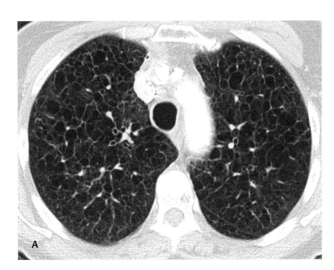

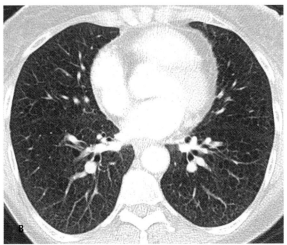

■ The following questions pertain to cystic lung disease.

1. True or False. In patients with cystic lung disease, pneumothorax is pathognomonic of LAM.
2. Which of the following cystic lung diseases is associated with renal cell carcinoma?
   A. Pulmonary LCH
   B. LIP
   C. Birt-Hogg-Dube (BHD)
   D. Erdheim-Chester disease
   E. Sporadic LAM

3. True or False. Regarding cystic lung disease, patients with pulmonary LCH have an increased incidence of meningiomas.
4. True or False. Regarding pulmonary LCH, smoking cessation is uniformly effective as a therapeutic intervention.

■ Answers and Explanations

C. Correct! This is pulmonary Langerhans cell histiocytosis (LCH). LCH is a single or multisystem disease caused by proliferation or organ infiltration by Langerhans cells, a type of dendritic cell. CT appearances vary according to the stage of disease; centrilobular and bronchocentric nodules predominate in the early stage (corresponding with Langerhans cell granulomas). These may cavitate, leading to thick-walled cysts ("Cheerio" sign). Thin-walled cysts may be seen much later in the course of disease. As demonstrated in this case, cysts in pulmonary LCH are typically bizarre shaped and unequal in size and occur predominately in the upper lobes, with relative sparing of the lung bases, medial middle lobe and lingula.

Other choices and discussion

A. The predominant abnormality is the presence of multiple pulmonary cysts of varying sizes. Pulmonary cysts are parenchymal lucencies containing air with a thin, perceptible wall (2- to 3-mm thick). In contrast to pulmonary cysts, areas of centrilobular emphysema are typically not surrounded by a wall. The presence of a central core centrilobular artery in the low attenuation cystic air space is classic for centrilobular emphysema.

B. Sporadic LAM is a multisystem cystic lung disease characterized by infiltration of immature smooth muscle cells in the airways and along the chest lymphatics. It is almost exclusive to women of childbearing age and commonly presents with recurrent pneumothoraces. On CT, the typical pattern is multiple diffusely distributed pulmonary cysts. Unlike LCH, these cysts may involve the juxtaphrenic recesses, and tend to spare the lung apices.

D. LIP is a rare, benign, lymphoproliferative disorder caused by diffuse lymphocytic infiltrate and is often associated with collagen vascular disorders, especially Sjogren syndrome. Ground glass opacities and nodules are universal features on CT. Cysts occur in approximately two-thirds of patients. Lung cysts are usually small (< 3 cm), thin-walled, and randomly distributed. Lung biopsy is required to exclude low-grade lymphoma.

E. Desquamative interstitial pneumonia is an uncommon smoking-related interstitial lung disease caused by macrophage accumulation within alveoli. Diffuse ground glass opacification in the lower lung zones is the dominant finding on CT; small cysts are interspersed in the ground glass in one-third of patients.

Question 1

False. Pneumothorax is common in LAM, but is not pathognomonic. It can occur in any cystic lung disease. Pulmonary LCH is complicated by pneumothorax due to rupture of a subpleural cyst in 25% of cases, and pneumothorax is a common presentation of other cystic lung diseases, such as Birt-Hogg-Dube (BHD).

Question 2

C. Correct! BHD is associated with renal cell carcinoma. BHD is a rare multisystem disease caused by a mutation on the FLCN gene on chromosome 17. It is characterized by multiple lung cysts, spontaneous pneumothoraces, cutaneous angiofibromas, and multiple bilateral renal tumors, particularly chromophobe renal cell cancer and oncocytoma.

Other choices and discussion

A. Patients with pulmonary LCH are usually smokers and thus have an increased risk of lung malignancy. Pulmonary LCH is also associated with an increased risk of lymphoma. However, there is no known association with renal malignancy.

B. LIP is a benign lymphoproliferative disorder often associated with connective tissue disease. It sometimes requires lung biopsy to distinguish it from low-grade pulmonary lymphoma. It is unclear whether LIP confers an increased risk of lymphoma.

D. Erdheim-Chester disease is a rare systemic non-LCH histiocytic disorder. It affects middle-aged adults and is characterized by xanthomatous infiltrates of foamy histiocytes. Skeletal manifestations are common, with bone pain often the major presenting feature; bilateral symmetrical sclerosis of the long bones is a characteristic radiographic feature.

E. Sporadic LAM is not associated with renal malignancy. Patients with tuberous sclerosis (TS) may have LAM-like pulmonary involvement, and these patients do have an increased risk of renal malignancy. Renal angiomyolipomas can occur in sporadic LAM, as well as in TS-LAM complex.

Question 3

False. Patients with sporadic LAM, not pulmonary LCH, are at increased risk for meningiomas. Because meningiomas are progesterone-sensitive tumors, brain magnetic resonance imaging is recommended prior to commencement of progesterone therapy for patients with sporadic LAM. Approximately 10% of patients with TS develop subependymal giant cell tumors.

Question 4

False. Although smoking cessation is the most effective therapeutic intervention in pulmonary LCH, up to a quarter of patients with PLCH will still progress. Poor prognostic features include multiorgan involvement, extensive pulmonary cysts on imaging, recurrent pneumothoraces, reduced diffusion capacity, and pulmonary hypertension.

Top Tips

- Pulmonary cysts on CT are parenchymal lucencies containing air with a thin, perceptible wall (2- to 3-mm thick).

- Centrilobular emphysema is characterized by parenchymal lucencies that are not typically surrounded by a wall. The presence of a central core centrilobular artery in the low attenuation cystic air space is characteristic.

- Pulmonary LCH is characterized by multiple bizarre pulmonary cysts and centrilobular nodules in a young smoker.

Details 3

■ Case

A patient presents with shortness of breath. Which ONE of the following is the MOST likely diagnosis?
- A. Sarcoidosis
- B. Subacute hypersensitivity pneumonitis
- C. Alveolar proteinosis
- D. Pulmonary edema

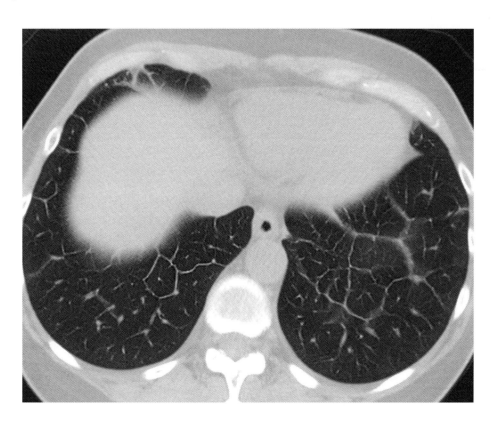

■ The following questions pertain to the secondary pulmonary lobule.

1. What structure(s) comprise the central "dot" seen in the secondary pulmonary lobule?
2. What structure(s) comprise the "walls" of the lobules?
3. Interlobular septal thickening with superimposed ground glass opacities is known as a _____ pattern.
4. Nodular interlobular septal thickening and peribronchovascular studding is known as which kind of micronodular pattern?
5. Unilateral interlobular septal thickening can be seen with _____.

6. On chest radiography, short and thickened septal lines in the periphery perpendicular to the pleural surface are known as _____.
7. Diffuse ground glass nodules, which are located within the middle of the lobules in a nonsmoker, are most often associated with _____.
8. An _____ is the portion of each lobule supplied by a terminal bronchiole.
9. Centrilobular bronchial impaction from mucus or infection that branches along the anatomy of the airway is termed _____.

■ Answers and Explanations

D. Correct! This is most likely pulmonary edema. The image demonstrates bilateral, smooth, interlobular septal thickening. This finding can also be accompanied by peribronchial interstitial thickening and subpleural interstitial thickening, as the interstitium in these anatomic locations is contiguous with the interlobular septa.

Other choices and discussion

A. Sarcoid is an upper lobe predominant process, often demonstrating micronodules. Chronic sarcoid can cause upper lobe fibrosis.

B. Subacute hypersensitivity pneumonitis shows ill-defined centrilobular ground glass nodules.

C. Pulmonary alveolar proteinosis usually has a crazy paving pattern (ground glass opacity with superimposed interlobular septal thickening).

Question 1

The airway, artery, and lymphatics comprise the central "dot" seen in the secondary pulmonary lobule.

Question 2

The veins and lymphatics comprise the "walls" of the lobules.

Question 3

Interlobular septal thickening with superimposed ground glass opacities is known as a crazy paving pattern.

Question 4

Nodular interlobular septal thickening and peribronchovascular studding is known as a perilymphatic pattern.

Question 5

Unilateral interlobular septal thickening can be seen with lymphangitic spread of malignancy.

Question 6

On chest radiography, short and thickened septal lines in the periphery perpendicular to the pleural surface are known as Kerley B lines.

Question 7

Diffuse ground glass nodules, which are located within the middle of the lobules in a nonsmoker, are most often associated with hypersensitivity pneumonitis.

Question 8

An acinus is the portion of each lobule supplied by a terminal bronchiole.

Question 9

Centrilobular bronchial impaction from mucus or infection that branches along the anatomy of the airway is termed tree-in-bud.

High-resolution computed tomography of the chest requires a slice thickness of at most _____ mm.

High-resolution computed tomography of the chest requires a slice thickness of at most 1.5 mm.

■ Suggested Reading

Webb R. Thin-section CT of the secondary pulmonary lobule: anatomy and the image—the 2004 Fleischner lecture. Radiology 2006;239(2):322–338

Top Tips

◆ The interlobular septa contain pulmonary veins and lymphatics.

◆ Septal thickening may be smooth, nodular, or be part of another pattern such as crazy paving.

◆ Tree-in-bud nodularity is indicative of bronchiolitis and is most commonly seen in infection.

Details 4

■ Case

An asymptomatic 40-year-old African-American man undergoes a chest CT. There is no history of flushing, nausea, or oc-cupation exposure. Blood cell counts are normal. What is the MOST likely diagnosis based upon the information given and these CT findings?

A. Untreated lymphoma
B. Silicosis
C. Sarcoidosis
D. Carcinoid
E. Pneumoconiosis

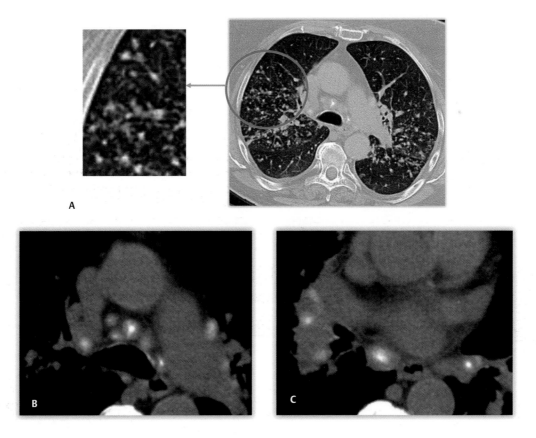

A

B

C

■ The following questions pertain to thoracic infection.

1. The 1-2-3 sign on chest radiography refers to _____.
2. Regarding the images presented for this case, what is the stage of the disease?
3. True or False. The calcification pattern for lymph nodes related to silicosis is typically central.
4. A chest CT shows a large mediastinal mass with many associated chunky calcifications. Subsequent tissue sampling demonstrates Congo Red stains that are apple-green birefringent under polarized light. What is the likely final diagnosis?
5. What is the usual cause of broncholithiasis?
6. Why do benign calcified mediastinal/hilar nodes on fluorodeoxyglucose positron emission tomography/CT sometimes have falsely elevated uptake?

7. Within the context of pulmonary tuberculosis, the combination of a Ghon lesion and a calcified node is called _____.
8. A patient presents with hoarseness, elevated calcito-nin, a painless thyroid nodule, and superior mediasti-nal lymph nodes containing fine calcifications. What is the likely diagnosis?
9. What is the typical appearance of a calcified lymph node on magnetic resonance imaging?
10. What is one cause of lymph node visualization on bone scan?

■ Answers and Explanations

C. Correct! This is sarcoidosis. The lung findings are in a peri-lymphatic distribution, meaning that the nodules seen are along the location of the pulmonary lymphatics. This, in combination with the enlarged symmetrical hilar and right paratracheal nodes, is a classic pattern for sarcoid involvement of the chest. After several years, the nodes sometimes calcify. The pattern of calcification is variable but most commonly focal. Pulmonary sarcoidosis is a noncaseating granulomatous process and is most common among females, African-Americans, and those between 20 and 40 years of age. Approximately 50% of patients with sarcoidosis are asymptomatic.

Other choices and discussion

The differential for the perilymphatic lung findings would also include lymphatic carcinomatosis, silicosis, and pneumoconiosis.

A. With lymphoma, abnormal blood counts may be seen, and *treated* rather than untreated lymphoma would have calcified lymph nodes.

B. Silicosis would require inhalational occupational exposure.

D. The symptom of flushing would direct one toward carcinoid. The lymph nodes of carcinoid calcify in 30% of cases and are typically avidly enhancing. Pulmonary manifestations of carcinoid include well-defined lung nodules, rather than the pattern seen here.

E. Pneumoconiosis would require inhalational occupational exposure.

Question 1

The 1-2-3 sign on chest radiography refers to the pattern of enlarged nodes in the mediastinum/hilar regions for sarcoid—bilateral hilar and right paratracheal nodes. This is also referred to as the Garland triad or the pawnbroker sign. The nodes themselves are sometimes called potato nodes.

Question 2

This patient has stage II disease, which means nodal and parenchymal involvement. Stage 0 = normal, Stage I = nodal only, Stage II = nodal and parenchymal involvement, Stage III = parenchymal only, and Stage IV = end-stage pulmonary fibrosis. This staging system was originally based upon chest radiography, but CT is more sensitive for detecting enlarged nodes and subtle parenchymal involvement.

Question 3

False. The nodal calcification pattern for silicosis is typically an eggshell appearance, with the calcification either diffuse or at the periphery of the nodes (in 2% of patients).

Question 4

This patient has a mediastinal amyloidoma. Congo Red is the most useful stain for diagnosing amyloid. Amyloid proteins appear apple-green under polarized light. Amyloid nodal involvement can, in fact, have a variable associated calcification appearance.

Question 5

Broncholithiasis is endobronchial calcified material. It is usually caused by adjacent calcified lymph node erosion.

Question 6

Calcification within a node is of higher density than a noncalcified node. Therefore, there is overcorrection from the CT-based attenuation correction protocol. This can also occur with other dense materials, such as metal.

Question 7

Within the context of pulmonary tuberculosis, the combination of a Ghon lesion and an ipsilateral calcified node is called a Ranke complex. A Ghon lesion is a tuberculoma (caseating granuloma) and is the sequelae of primary pulmonary tuberculosis.

Question 8

This patient likely has medullary thyroid carcinoma.

Question 9

On magnetic resonance imaging, calcified lymph nodes are dark on all sequences.

Question 10

One cause of lymph node visualization on bone scan is calcium deposition in the node(s).

■ Suggested Readings

Fraser R, Müller NL, Colman N. Inhalation of inorganic dust (pneumoconiosis). In: Fraser R, Müller N, Colman N, eds. Diagnosis of Diseases of the Chest. 4th ed. Philadelphia, PA: Saunders; 1999: 2386–2484

Pickford HA, Swensen SJ, Utz JP. Thoracic cross-sectional imaging of amyloidosis. Am J Roentgenol 1997;168:351–355

Wells A. High resolution computed tomography in sarcoidosis: a clinical perspective. Sarcoidosis Vasc Diffuse Lung Dis 1998;15(2):140–146

SECTION XI
THORACIC IMAGING

Top Tips

◆ Most causes of calcified nodes in the chest are benign.

◆ Treated lymph nodes often calcify.

◆ Granulomatous disease is the most common cause of thoracic calcified lymph nodes.

Details 5

■ Case

A patient presents with chest pain and fever. Which ONE of the following is the most likely diagnosis?
- A. Empyema
- B. Pneumatocele
- C. Aspergilloma
- D. Abscess
- E. Round pneumonia

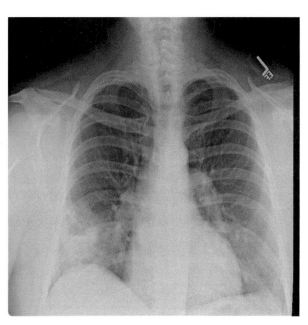 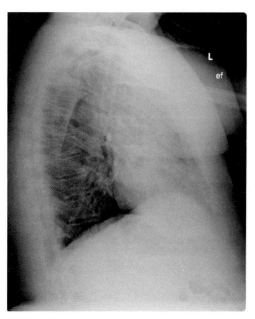

Posteroanterior and lateral

■ The following questions pertain to infection on plain film.

1. The "claw" sign on chest radiography refers to a(n) _____.
2. True or False. Round pneumonia is most commonly seen in the upper lobes.
3. Another term to describe an intracavitary mycetoma (as with aspergilloma) surrounded by a crescent of air is _____.
4. In a patient with pneumonia, a silhouette sign along the interface of the lung and left heart border indicates infection localization to which lung lobe?
5. A patient has a history of viral respiratory infection. Chest X-ray shows a unilateral small hyperlucent lung. What is the name of this syndrome?
6. Lemierre syndrome develops as a complication from a bacterial oropharyngeal infection. Besides thrombophlebitis, what can be seen in the lungs?
7. What are some chest X-ray manifestations of bronchitis?
8. A "shaggy" appearance of the heart on chest X-ray is representative of this type of pneumonia.
9. Which lobes are most commonly affected by acute aspiration pneumonia?
10. The differential diagnosis for calcified mediastinal and hilar nodes as related to infection/inflammation includes _____.

■ Answers and Explanations

D. Correct! This is an abscess. A pulmonary abscess is round in shape on both posteroanterior and lateral projections and contains an air-fluid level. Typically, all margins are seen, unless obscured by adjacent opacities/consolidation, and an acute angle is formed with the chest wall/costal surface.

Other choices and discussion

A. An empyema is lentiform in shape with an obtuse angle. This is consistent with pleural-based pathology.

B. A pneumatocele is also in the differential, but the walls are usually thinner and smoother, and the opacity contains little to no fluid. With an abscess, the walls are typically more irregular.

C. An aspergilloma is surrounded by crescent-shaped air.

D. Round pneumonia is a well-defined area of consolidation usually found in pediatric patients.

Question 1

The "claw" sign on chest radiography refers to an abscess with an acute angle.

Question 2

False. Round pneumonia is most commonly seen in the superior segments of the lower lobes.

Question 3

Another term to describe an intracavitary mycetoma (as with aspergilloma) surrounded by a crescent of air is the "Monad" sign.

Question 4

A silhouette sign along the interface of the lung and left heart border indicates infection localization to the lingula/left upper lobe.

Question 5

A unilateral small hyperlucent lung that develops after a viral respiratory infection is termed Swyer-James syndrome. This condition typically follows adenovirus or *Mycoplasma pneumoniae* lung infection in infancy or childhood.

Question 6

Septic emboli can be seen in the lungs of a patient with Lemierre syndrome. The most common bacterial cause is *Fusobacterium necrophorum*.

Question 7

Chest X-ray manifestations of bronchitis include peribronchial cuffing or thickening, "dirty" hilum, and hyperinflation.

Question 8

A shaggy appearance of the heart on chest X-ray is associated with *Bordetella pertussis* pneumonia. There is classically an associated whooping cough.

Question 9

Acute aspiration pneumonia in the erect patient is most commonly seen in the right middle lobe, lingula, and the bilateral basal segments. Aspiration pneumonia in the recumbent patient is most commonly seen in the posterior segment upper lobes and superior segment lower lobes.

Question 10

The differential diagnosis for calcified mediastinal and hilar nodes as related to infection/inflammation includes old granulomatous disease (histoplasmosis, tuberculosis, sarcoidosis), pulmonary coccidioidomycosis, silicosis, and *Pneumocystis carinii* pneumonia.

■ Suggested Readings

Bramson RT, Griscom NT, Cleveland RH. Interpretation of chest radiographs in infants with cough and fever. Radiology 2005;236(1):22–29

Jeung MY, Gangi A, Gasser B, et al. Imaging of chest wall disorders. Radiographics 1999;19(3):617–637

SECTION XI THORACIC IMAGING

Top Tips

◆ Consider aspiration pneumonia in patients with central nervous system disorders, swallowing disorders, and head and neck surgery.

◆ Septic emboli at-risk patients include alcoholics, intravenous drug abusers, immunodeficiency, concomitant infection such as peritonsillar abscess or infected thrombophlebitis, and infected lines.

◆ Classic patterns of pneumonia: pneumatocele: *Staphylococcus*; perihilar interstitial: pneumocystis/viral; lobar: *Streptococcus*; bulging fissure: *Klebsiella*.

Image Rich 1

■ Case

Match the appropriate description to the provided image.
- A. A condition seen in smokers characterized by small, well-defined or poorly defined areas of low attenuation surrounded by normal lung.
- B. An idiopathic syndrome of progressive lung disease described in association with cigarette smoking, marijuana, sarcoidosis, alpha-1-anti-trypsin deficiency, Marfan syndrome, and tuberculosis.
- C. A pattern of emphysema that involves destruction of the entire acinus distal to the respiratory bronchioles and has a predilection for the lower lobes.
- D. An emphysematous condition not associated with any significant symptoms or physiologic impairment.

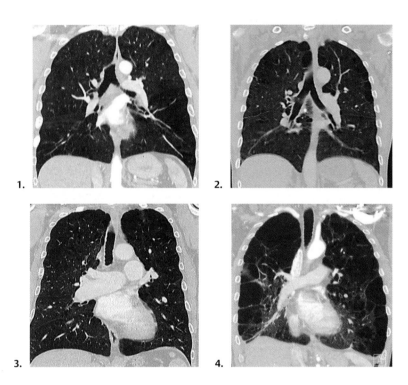

1.

2.

3.

4.

■ Answers and Explanations

1. C. A pattern of emphysema that involves destruction of the entire acinus distal to the respiratory bronchioles and has a predilection for the lower lobes.

Pan lobular emphysema refers to diffuse emphysematous destruction of the entire acinus, in contrast to the centrilobular distribution found in smokers. Pan lobular emphysema affects the lower lobes more severely. This pattern of emphysema is associated with alpha-1-antitrypsin deficiency, which is a hereditary metabolic disorder that results in the unopposed action of neutrophil elastase, with subsequent severe basal emphysema and respiratory symptoms. Pan lobular emphysema may also be seen with the intravenous drug use of methylphenidate, also known as Ritalin lung.

2. D. An emphysematous condition not associated with any significant symptoms or physiologic impairment.

Paraseptal emphysema refers to emphysema caused by selective destruction of the distal acinus. It has a predilection for peripheral subpleural lobules along the peripheral pleura and fissures, and is usually most marked in the middle and upper lungs and along the mediastinum. The patient is usually asymptomatic, although spontaneous pneumothorax can occur. On computed tomography (CT), small focal lucencies up to 10 mm in size are seen in the subpleural space. When these are > 10 mm, they are referred to as subpleural blebs or bullae.

3. A. A condition seen in smokers characterized by small, well-defined or poorly defined areas of low attenuation surrounded by normal lung.

Centrilobular emphysema affects the proximal respiratory bronchioles, particularly of the upper zones. It is strongly associated with smoking in a dose-dependent fashion. The pathologic process of centrilobular emphysema begins near the center of the secondary pulmonary lobule in the region of the proximal respiratory bronchiole. Early centrilobular emphysematous lesions are seen as small low attenuating holes with ill-defined borders, located in the central portion of the secondary pulmonary nodule around the centrilobular artery. As the condition progresses, the low-attenuation areas become confluent, and the surrounding normal lung parenchyma becomes compressed. On CT, poorly defined areas of low attenuation surrounded by normal lung are seen. The pulmonary vessels in areas of severe emphysema are small, with shunting of blood flow to lung parenchyma that can better exchange air and maintain matched ventilation and perfusion.

4. B. An idiopathic syndrome of progressive lung disease described in association with cigarette smoking, marijuana, sarcoidosis, alpha-1-anti-trypsin deficiency, Marfan syndrome, and tuberculosis.

Idiopathic giant bullous emphysema (or vanishing lung syndrome) is a progressive condition characterized by giant emphysematous bullae, which commonly develop in the upper lobes and occupy at least one-third of a hemithorax. It affects mainly young male smokers. This condition has been described in association with cigarette smoking, marijuana, sarcoidosis, alpha-1-anti-trypsin deficiency, Marfan syndrome, and Ehler-Danlos syndrome. High-resolution CT is the most accurate means of diagnosing the condition and determining the extent of disease. CT features include extensive paraseptal emphysema coalescing into giant bullae, often compressing the normal lung parenchyma.

■ Suggested Readings

Litmanovich D, Boiselle PM, Bankier AA. CT of pulmonary emphysema - current status, challenges, and future directions. Eur Radiol 2008;19(3):537–551

Lynch DA, Austin JHM, Hogg JC, et al. CT-Definable subtypes of chronic obstructive pulmonary disease: a statement of the Fleischner Society. Radiology 2015;277(1):192–205

Top Tips

Pulmonary emphysema can be classified into three major subtypes based on the disease distribution within secondary pulmonary lobules.

◆ Centrilobular emphysema is most common and is strongly associated with smoking in a dose-dependent fashion. It is upper zone predominant.

◆ Pan lobular emphysema is associated with alpha-1-antitrypsin deficiency (exacerbated by smoking) and the intravenous injection of methylphenidate. It is lower lobe predominant.

◆ Paraseptal emphysema is associated with subpleural cyst-like lucenies/bullae, involving more than the lung apices, and may cause spontaneous pneumothorax. It is middle and upper lungs and paramediastinal predominant.

Image Rich 2

■ Case

Match the appropriate description to the provided image.

    C. A 42-year-old woman with wheezing and hemoptysis

    E. A 57-year-old man with hemoptysis and weight loss

    D. A 28-year-old man with asthma and peripheral eosinophilia

    B. A 47-year-old man with recurrent pneumonia

    A. A 36-year-old woman with recurrent pneumonia and pancreatic insufficiency

    F. A 78-year-old woman with cough and night sweats

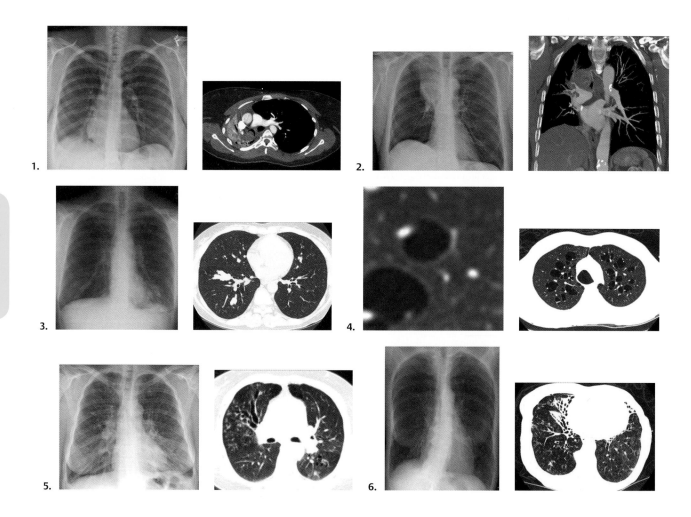

■ Answers and Explanations

1. C. A 42-year-old woman with wheezing and hemoptysis. This is an endobronchial carcinoid. With symptoms of cough and hemoptysis in a younger patient (typically fourth decade), endobronchial carcinoid is the best match. Chest X-ray (CXR) shows a subtle right main bronchial filling defect expanding the lumen. The tumor is better seen on the follow-up computed tomography (CT), with postobstructive atelectasis. Note that while avid enhancement and calcifications are helpful in diagnosing carcinoid, not all carcinoids exhibit these features, including this case.

2. E. A 57-year-old man with hemoptysis and weight loss. This is bronchogenic carcinoma. In a middle-aged or older patient with cough and hemoptysis, bronchogenic carcinoma is the best match. CXR shows the "Golden S" sign of a right hilar mass with postobstructive right upper lobe collapse. Note the elevated right hemidiaphragm and the hyperlucent, overexpanded right lower lobe. CT shows the obliterated right upper lobe bronchus.

3. D. A 28-year-old man with asthma, peripheral eosinophilia. This is allergic bronchopulmonary aspergillosis (ABPA). In a younger patient with a history of asthma and imaging findings that include the "finger in glove" sign of branching, mucoid impaction, and a bronchiectatic airway, ABPA is the best match.

4. B. A 47-year-old man with recurrent pneumonia. This is Mournier-Kuhn syndrome (primary tracheobronchomegaly). The CT first impression may be of cystic lung disease. However, closer inspection shows the "signet ring" sign of bronchiectasis along with the markedly dilated trachea. This makes Mournier-Kuhn syndrome the best match.

5. A. A 36-year-old woman with recurrent pneumonia and pancreatic insufficiency. This is cystic fibrosis. In a younger patient with pancreatic insufficiency and recurrent pneumonia, cystic fibrosis is the best match. CXR shows the typical "tram track" appearance of bronchiectasis and bronchial wall thickening, shown better on the accompanying CT. Note scattered tree-in-bud nodules, indicating distal bronchiolar mucoid impaction, and associated lucencies of air-trapping.

6. F. A 78-year-old woman with cough and night sweats. This is *Mycobacterium avium* complex infection or Lady Windermere syndrome. In an elderly patient with fever and night sweats, mycobacterial infection is the best fit. CT shows bronchiectasis and volume loss (aka middle lobe syndrome), compatible with chronic endobrachial infection found in atypical mycobacteria or *Mycobacterium avium* complex (rather than *M. tuberculosis*).

■ Suggested Readings

Albelda SM, Kern JA, Marinelli DL, Miller WT. Expanding spectrum of pulmonary disease caused by nontuberculous mycobacteria. Radiology 1985;157:289–296

Dunne MG, Reiner B. CT features of tracheobronchomegaly. J Comput Assist Tomogr 1988;12(3):388–391

Jeung MY, Gasser B, Gangi A, et al. Bronchial carcinoid tumors of the thorax: spectrum of radiologic findings. Radiographics 2002;22(2):351–365

SECTION XI THORACIC IMAGING

Top Tips

◆ The Mounier-Kuhn syndrome of tracheobronchomegaly predisposes to recurrent infection. One method of diagnosis is measuring the anteroposterior diameter of the trachea 2 cm above the aortic arch. An anteroposterior measurement of 3 cm or greater is consistent with the diagnosis.

◆ Finger-in-glove sign: Found in obstructive conditions (bronchial carcinoid, bronchogenic carcinoma and bronchial atresia), and nonobstructive conditions (asthma, ABPA, and cystic fibrosis)

◆ Mycobacterium avium infection is often seen in patients with preexisting pulmonary conditions, but may also be seen in healthy elderly woman who intentionally suppress the cough reflex (Lady Windermere syndrome).

Image Rich 3

■ Case

Match the appropriate description to the provided image.
- B. A 35-year-old woman with dysphagia and restrictive lung function
- A. A 54-year-old man with progressive dyspnea and weight loss over 1 month
- D. A 67-year-old man with progressive dyspnea and dry cough over 2 years
- C. A 41-year-old female smoker with 5-month history of cough and low-grade fever

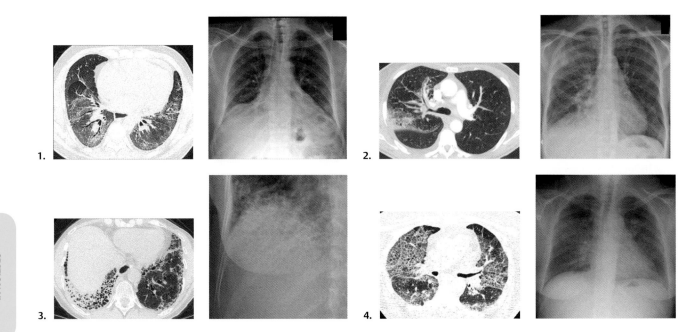

1.

2.

3.

4.

■ Answers and Explanations

1. B. 35-year-old woman with dysphagia and restrictive lung function. This is scleroderma. Computed tomography (CT) shows ground glass opacities and intralobular interstitial thickening (without interlobular septal thickening). Note the patulous esophagus. Traction bronchiectasis indicates underlying fibrosis. This suggests the fibrotic subtype of nonspecific interstitial pneumonia, in contrast to the cellular subtype comprised of isolated ground glass. Chest X-ray (CXR) shows a basilar predominant interstitial pattern, with hazy obscuration of the diaphragm. There is also a positive "spine" sign on the lateral projection; normally, the lung become progressively more lucent toward the base on the lateral projection. That lucency is not present in this case.

2. A. A 54-year-old man with progressive dyspnea and weight loss over 1 month. This is lymphangitic carcinomatosis. CT shows extensive peribronchovascular interstitial thickening. Note the unilateral involvement, with thickening of the right upper lobe bronchi compared to the left upper lobe, pleural thickening, and pleural effusion. CXR shows similar findings.

3. D. A 67-year-old man with progressive dyspnea and dry cough over 2 years. This is idiopathic pulmonary fibrosis. CT shows multiple rows of lung cysts, or honeycombing, indicating end-stage fibrotic change. Coned down posteroanterior and lateral radiograph shows similar findings.

4. C. A 41-year-old female smoker with 5-month history of cough and low-grade fever. This is alveolar proteinosis. CT shows "crazy paving" pattern of ground glass opacities with both interlobular septal thickening (between secondary pulmonary lobules) and intralobular interstitial thickening (within the lobules themselves). On CXR, it is difficult to compartmentalize the opacities as either alveolar or interstitial, owing to involvement of both.

■ Suggested Readings

Al-Jahdali H, Rajiah P, Allen C, Koteyar SS, Khan AN. Pictorial review of intrathoracic manifestations of progressive systemic sclerosis. Ann Thorac Med 2014;9(4):193–202

Ikezoe J, Godwin JD, Hunt KJ, et al. Pulmonary lymphangitic carcinomatosis: chronicity of radiographic findings in long-term survivors. Am J Roentgenol 1995;165(1):49–52

Rossi SE, Erasmus JJ, Volpacchio M, et al. "Crazy-paving" pattern at thin-section CT of the lungs: radiologic-pathologic overview. Radiographics 2003;23(6):1509–1519

Top Tips

◆ Pulmonary alveolar proteinosis is rare, but when present, often shows crazy paving.

◆ Common causes of crazy paving: bacterial pneumonia, acute respiratory distress syndrome, acute interstitial pneumonia.

◆ Up to 50% of patients with histologic evidence of lymphangitic carcinomatosis are occult on CXR.

Image Rich 4

■ Case

Match the appropriate description to the provided image.

    F. A 53-year-old asymptomatic man

    D. A 28-year-old woman with human immunodeficiency virus and fever

    B. A 65-year-old woman with abnormal bone scan

    A. A 44-year-old man with abnormal echocardiogram

    C. A 35-year-old woman with renal transplant and cough

    E. A 47-year-old man with renal failure and recurrent hemoptysis

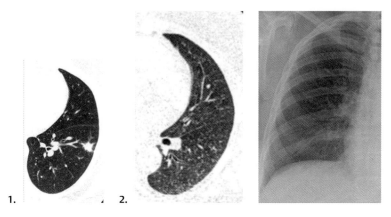

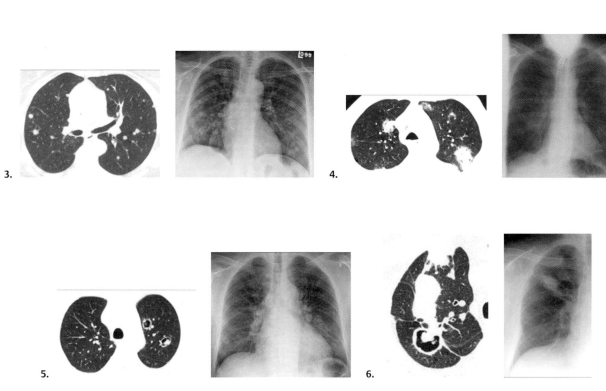

■ Answers and Explanations

1. F. A 53-year-old asymptomatic man. This is organizing pneumonia (OP). Computed tomography (CT) shows a spiculated, solitary pulmonary nodule in the left lower lobe. Differential diagnosis includes early malignancy (non-small cell lung cancer) and unusual infection (e.g., fungal). The lesion showed minimal hypermetabolic activity on positron emission tomography, and a transthoracic needle biopsy suggested OP. Because OP can occur locally in response to malignancy, the nodule was excised with thoracoscopy, confirming OP and excluding adjacent malignancy. OP is a diagnosis of exclusion, and it should only be suggested when a lesion has proven stable after months of follow up.

2. D. A 28-year-old woman with human immunodeficiency virus and fever. This is miliary tuberculosis. CT shows diffuse 2- to 3-mm miliary nodules. Coned radiographic views of the right lung and anterior chest show a diffuse nodular pattern. Note that, in general, diffuse processes involving the upper lobes are often best appreciated in the retrosternal clear space on chest X-ray (CXR).

3. B. A 65-year-old woman with abnormal bone scan. This is metastatic breast cancer. CT and corresponding CXR show multiple well-circumscribed nodules. These are typical of intrathoracic metastatic disease, as the mass effect tends to "push" normal lung parenchyma aside. This in contrast to infectious or inflammatory nodules that tend to have more poorly defined or "infiltrative" appearing margins.

4. A. A 44-year-old man with abnormal echocardiogram. These are septic emboli. CT and CXR show multiple poorly defined nodules. These nodules demonstrate an infiltrative appearance of the margins, suggesting a locally aggressive process typical of active infection or, less commonly, perilesional hemorrhage. On CXR, the margins are barely perceptible. On CT, the internal noncavitary lucencies represent traversing airway or islands of spared airspaces typical of nodular consolidation (rather than mass). Primary consideration is multifocal pneumonia, and this case represented septic emboli in a patient with aortic vegetations.

5. C. A 35-year-old woman with renal transplant and cough. This is mucormycosis infection. CT and CXR show multiple thin-walled cavitary nodules. The largest in the left upper lobe shows an internal mycetoma. Smooth, thin-walled cavitary nodules favor infection, whereas thick- or irregular-walled cavitary nodules favor tumor.

6. E. A 47-year-old man with renal failure and recurrent hemoptysis. This is Wegener granulomatosis. CT and CXR show coalescent irregular thick-walled cavitary nodules in the right upper lobe. The cavitation is new from 2 years prior. The primary differential diagnosis is cavitary neoplasm. Cavitary infection is less likely, given the large solid components, thick walls, and lack of surrounding inflammatory change. Nodules and masses are commonly seen at initial presentation of Wegener (up to 70%), and may either involute to form discoid scarring or progress to cavitation.

■ Suggested Readings

Aberle DR, Gamsu G, Lynch D. Thoracic manifestations of Wegener granulomatosis: diagnosis and course. Radiology 1990;174(3 Pt 1):703–709

Argiriadi PA, Mendelson DS. High resolution computed tomography in idiopathic interstitial pneumonias. Mt Sinai J Med 2009;76(1):37–52

Koutsopoulos AV, Mitrouska I, Dambaki KI, et al. Is a miliary chest pattern always indicative of tuberculosis or malignancy? Respiration 2006;73(3):379–381

Top Tips

◆ Miliary nodules are 1 to 4 mm in size and have a broad differential diagnosis in addition to tuberculosis, including other infections, neoplasm, noninfectious inflammatory conditions, and pneumoconiosis. For classification purposes, it is useful to begin with febrile versus nonfebrile causes.

◆ The most common thoracic radiographic findings with Wegener granulomatosis are nodules (which may cavitate) and mass-like opacities (which sometimes contain hemorrhage).

◆ About half of benign lung nodules are not calcified. Fat is a reliable indicator of a benign pulmonary hamartoma and is found in 50% of hamartomas.

Image Rich 5

■ Case

Four patients present for initial staging of non-small cell lung cancer. Match the image findings with the appropriate lung cancer stage. Images provided are the only pertinent findings (i.e., all positive lung nodules and/or lymph nodes are shown for each case unless otherwise noted).

A. Stage I
B. Stage II
C. Stage III
D. Stage IV
E. Stage not listed

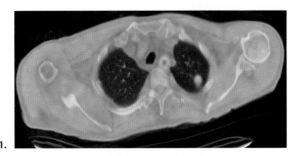

1.

Lung nodule = 1.5 cm

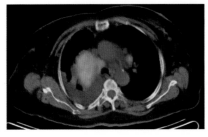 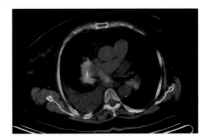

2.

Lung mass = 7.5 cm

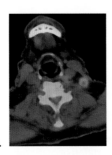 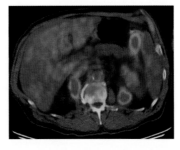

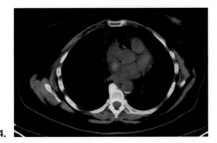 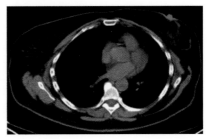

3.

Not shown is a positive 4-cm left lung mass (surrounded by lung and not invading adjacent structures).

4.

Axial images: fludeoxyglucose positron emission tomography/computed tomography and computed tomography selected slices through the chest.

■ Answers and Explanations

1. C. Stage III. This is T1, N2, M0. The staging for lung cancer is based upon the TNM system, with the seventh edition the most current. Tumor size < 3 cm (such as this one) is considered T1 (this is broken down further, but not discussed here). This image shows a positive ipsilateral high paratracheal node which is an N2 category node. N1 = ipsilateral hilar; N2 = ipsilateral paratracheal, prevascular, paraesophageal, subcarinal; N3 = any contralateral, any enlarged supraclavicular

2. C. Stage III. This is T4, N3, M0. Any lung mass > 7 cm in size is classified as T3. Other T3 categories include lung nodules in the same lobe as the primary nodule, endobronchial lesions < 2 cm distal to the carina, and invasion of the chest wall, diaphragm, mediastinal pleura, or parietal pericardium. However, this case is actually classified as T4, as the lung mass also invades the mediastinum and not just the mediastinal pleura. A T4 lung tumor can be of any size if there is mediastinal, tracheal, esophageal, great vessels, or adjacent vertebral body invasion. T4 also includes separate tumor nodules in lobes other than the site of the primary and malignant pleural effusions. As described previously, any contralateral lymph node involvement is classified as N3. In this case, there are ipsilateral and contralateral hilar nodes involved as well as a positive subcarinal node.

3. D. Stage IV. This is T2, N3, M1. By the "T" size criteria, this is a T2 tumor, as these are > 3 to ≤ 7 cm in size. The "N" category for this case is N3, as there is a positive supraclavicular node. The images also show bilateral adrenal gland metastases, which automatically classifies this patient as Stage IV, regardless of the primary lung tumor size, nodal locations, etc.

4. E. Stage not listed. This activity is not related to lung cancer or lymph nodes. If you look closely, you can see that the focal fludeoxyglucose uptake localizes to interatrial fat, a common location for physiologic brown fat uptake.

■ Suggested Readings

De Wever W, Ceyssens S, Mortelmans L, et al. Additional value of PET-CT in the staging of lung cancer: comparison with CT alone, PET alone and visual correlation of PET and CT. Eur Radiol 2007;17:23–32

Goldstraw P, Crowley J, Chansky K, et al. The IASLC Lung Cancer Staging Project: proposals for the revision of the TNM stage groupings in the forthcoming (seventh) edition of the TNM classification of malignant tumours. J Thorac Oncol 2007;2: 706–714

Lardinois D, Weder W, Hany TF, et al. Staging of non-small-cell lung cancer with integrated positron-emission tomography and computed tomography. N Engl J Med 2003;348:2500–2507

Top Tips

◆ Distinguishing between stages IIIA and IIIB is critical, as IIIB+ stages are surgically unresectable.

◆ Any distant metastases is Stage IV.

◆ Fludeoxyglucose positron emission tomography/ computed tomography is very useful in identifying positive nodes.

More Challenging 1

■ Case

A patient status post placement of transvenous pacer. Chest X-ray and computed tomography images are presented.

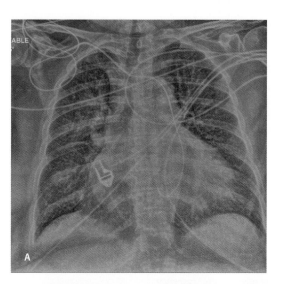

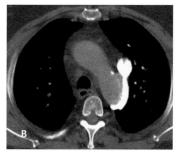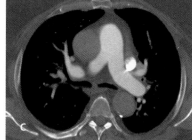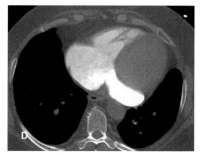

■ Questions

1. What is the MOST likely diagnosis?
   A. Enlarged left superior intercostal vein
   B. Hemiazygos continuation of the inferior vena cava
   C. Partial anomalous pulmonary venous return (PAPVR)
   D. Persistent left superior vena cava (PLSVC)
   E. Left internal thoracic vein

2. Which ONE of the following is true for PLSVC?
   A. The vast majority of cases of this congenital venous anomaly are symptomatic.
   B. The most commonly associated congenital heart abnormalities include atrial septal defect and ventricular septal defect.
   C. The right SVC is absent.
   D. The coronary sinus is usually normal.

3. Which ONE of the following statements is true for PAPVR?
   A. Approximately 80% of patients with right-sided PAPVR have an atrial septal defect (ASD).
   B. PAPVR is a cyanotic left-to-right shunt.
   C. The anomalous pulmonary vein drains into the right-sided circulation.
   D. Surgical correction is always the treatment of choice.
   E. Scimitar syndrome is the type of PAPVR most often associated with ASD.

■ Answers and Explanations

Question 1

D. Correct! This is a PLSVC. Pathognomonic findings (which are present in this case) include a dilated vessel opacified with contrast that drains inferiorly across the left hilar region and into the coronary sinus. This is typically associated with a dilated coronary sinus. A PLSVC is the most common congenital thoracic venous anomaly, with an incidence of 0.3 to 0.5% in the general population. If isolated, no treatment is necessary. Surgical correction is indicated if there is a significant shunt. The right superior vena cava (SVC) may be normal, small, or absent. The left brachiocephalic (bridging) vein is frequently absent (65%).

Other choices and discussion

A. When a central venous catheter is abnormally located to the left of the mediastinum, the differential diagnosis includes a left-sided SVC, left internal thoracic vein, left superior intercostal vein, and left pericardiophrenic vein.

Normally, the left superior intercostal vein drains the second through fourth intercostal spaces and courses anteriorly into the left innominate vein. A catheter in the superior intercostal vein would be expected to follow the aortic knob. However, in the test case, the left superior intercostal vein drains into a large venous structure that courses in a caudal direction to the coronary sinus and further drains into the right atrium.

B. The hemiazygos vein is located on the left side of the lower thoracic spine, curving to the right to drain into the azygous vein. These findings are not present in the test case.

C. PAPVR is a congenital pulmonary venous anomaly involving drainage of some (between one and three, but not all four) pulmonary veins into the systemic venous circulation or the right atrium. This creates an extracardiac left-to-right shunt. However, the shunt is usually hemodynamically insignificant. PAPVR is most commonly seen in the left upper lobe (47%) and in the right upper lobe (38%).

The best diagnostic clue to this diagnosis is visualization of the direct drainage of a pulmonary vein into the systemic circulation (e.g., SVC, inferior vena cava, right atrium, left brachiocephalic vein). In left upper lobe PAPVR, a vertical vein drains from the medial aspect of the left upper lobe into the left brachiocephalic vein. This may be confused with a persistent left SVC. However, no connection to the coronary sinus will be seen, and the left superior intercostal vein will not connect to the vertical vein associated with left upper lobe PAPVR.

E. Malposition of central venous catheters is usually limited to the larger tributaries of the SVC. On a frontal chest radiograph, a catheter within the internal thoracic vein would be located more laterally, and on a lateral radiograph, the catheter would overlie the anterior mediastinum.

Question 2

B. Correct! The congenital heart abnormalities most commonly associated with PLSVC include atrial septal defect and ventricular septal defect, followed by aortic coarctation, transposition of the great vessels, tetralogy of Fallot, and anomalous connections of the pulmonary vein.

Other choices and discussion

A. The vast majority of cases of PLSVC are asymptomatic. The abnormality is usually detected incidentally.

C. The right SVC may be normal, small, or absent.

D. The coronary sinus is enlarged in the majority of cases. If an enlarged coronary sinus is seen on echocardiography or on cross-sectional imaging, PLSVC must be suspected.

Question 3

C. Correct! The anomalous pulmonary vein drains into the right-sided circulation (SVC, azygos, brachiocephalic, inferior vena cava, coronary sinus, right atrium).

Other choices and discussion

A. In approximately 40% of patients with right-sided PAPVR, an ASD is seen.

B. PAPVR is usually an acyanotic left-to-right shunt. Most patients are asymptomatic and the finding is detected incidentally on imaging. It is symptomatic only if the shunt is large or associated with other cardiopulmonary anomalies.

D. Surgical correction is only recommended if the pulmonary-to-systemic flow ratio is > 1.5 (to avoid progression to pulmonary hypertension and right ventricular failure).

E. In some cases, an anomalous vein that drains into the inferior vena cava is seen as a crescentic shadow of vascular opacity along the right cardiac border. This is called scimitar syndrome. In these patients, pulmonary sequestration and anomalous arterial supply to the affected lobe of the lung are encountered, rather than an ASD.

■ Suggested Readings

Goyal SK, Punnam SR, Verma G, Ruberg FL. Persistent left superior vena cava: A case report and review of literature. Cardiovasc Ultrasound 2008;6(1):50

Kazerooni EA, Gross BH. Cardiopulmonary Imaging. Philadelphia, PA: Lippincott Williams & Wilkins; 2004

Sonavane SK, Milner DM, Singh SP, Abdel Aal AK, Shahir KS, Chaturvedi A. Comprehensive imaging review of the superior Vena Cava. Radiographics 2015;35(7):1873–1892

Top Tips

- PLSVC is the most common anatomic variation of the thoracic central veins.
- With PLSVC, the right SVC may be normal, small, or absent.
- PLSVC is of potential clinical relevance when pacemaker wires are deployed or central venous catheters are placed.

More Challenging 2

■ Case

A 58-year-old man with no significant past medical history undergoes investigation for progressive dyspnea.

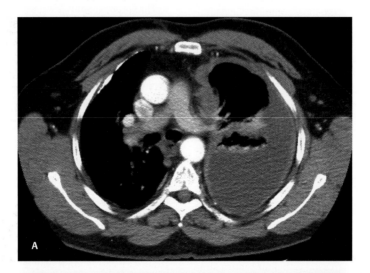

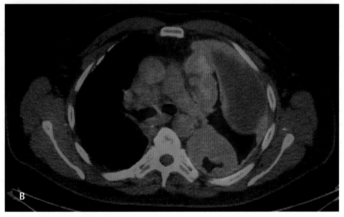

■ Questions

1. What is the MOST likely diagnosis?
    A. Metastatic thymoma
    B. Benign pleural thickening
    C. Solitary fibrous tumor
    D. Benign asbestos related pleural disease
    E. Malignant mesothelioma

2. The thoracic surgeon wants an assessment of local chest wall or diaphragmatic invasion. What test would you recommend?
    A. 18-FDG PET/CT
    B. Magnetic resonance imaging (MRI) with gadolinium
    C. Percutaneous biopsy
    D. Chest CT
    E. Ultrasound

3. Which ONE of the following is NOT a recognized primary site of malignant mesothelioma?
    A. Pleura
    B. Peritoneum
    C. Pericardium
    D. Meninges
    E. Tunica vaginalis

■ Answers and Explanations

Question 1

E. Correct! This is a case of malignant mesothelioma. The computed tomography (CT) demonstrates a rind of circumferential nodular pleural thickening in the left hemithorax with a loculated pleural effusion, and there is corresponding intense fludeoxyglucose (FDG) uptake on 18-FDG positron emission tomography (PET)/CT. These features are consistent with a diagnosis of malignant mesothelioma, an aggressive malignant tumor of the pleura. Mesothelioma is strongly associated with asbestos exposure (especially crocidolite fibers). The typical appearance on CT is a pleural-based soft tissue density nodular mass that spreads along the pleural surfaces and into the fissures, creating a pleural rind. Calcification is seen in 20% of cases, usually due to engulfed calcified pleural plaques rather than true tumoral calcification. Malignant mesothelioma is FDG avid on 18-FDG PET/CT, which can be useful to distinguish between benign and malignant pleural thickening. There are three histologic subtypes of malignant mesothelioma: epithelial (60%), sarcomatoid (15%), and mixed (25%), which are often hard to distinguish on imaging. The sarcomatoid variants may demonstrate calcification due to osteo- or chondrosarcomatoid de-differentiation.

Other choices and discussion

A. Metastatic thymoma is in the differential diagnosis for an FDG-avid pleural mass. However, thymoma is frequently associated with solid pleural implants in the lower hemithorax and costophrenic sulci (drop metastases) ipsilateral to the site of the mediastinal mass. Presence of effusions is rare, and "dry pleural disease" is frequently noted in these patients. The lack of a mediastinal mass and presence of a pleural effusion makes metastatic thymoma unlikely.

B. The presence of pleural thickening along the mediastinal border anterior to the vertebral bodies is a key feature of malignant pleural disease. Circumferential pleural thickening and a thickness of > 1 cm are other features that can help to distinguish malignant from benign pleural disease.

C. Solitary fibrous tumor is a pleural-based mass that typically presents as a solitary pleural based soft tissue attenuation mass. It can be associated with a small pleural effusion and is typically not FDG-avid on 18-FDG PET/CT.

D. Benign asbestos-related pleural disease is a spectrum of pleural disease comprising pleural effusions and pleural thickening. The pleural thickening is usually focal, discontinuous, and calcified, but diffuse pleural thickening may occur. In the test case, calcified pleural plaques are seen in the right hemithorax consistent with previous asbestos exposure, but the extent of nodular pleural thickening and FDG-avidity in the left hemithorax is consistent with malignant mesothelioma.

Question 2

B. Correct! Chest MRI with gadolinium is the most sensitive imaging modality for chest wall and diaphragmatic invasion due to its superior soft tissue resolution. The pleural thickening is typically iso- to hyperintense to skeletal muscle on T1 images and enhances on postcontrast imaging.

Other choices and discussion

A. Malignant mesothelioma is FDG-avid on PET/CT in the regions of pleural thickening, but is suboptimal in delineating local extension due to its low spatial resolution. PET/CT is useful in assessing for local and distal metastases and also has a role in treatment response.

C. Percutaneous biopsy should be avoided in cases of suspected mesothelioma due to the risk of seeding the biopsy tract.

D. Chest CT is often the initial modality used to investigate cases of suspected mesothelioma and is excellent at depicting the extent of tumor and presence of local metastases. However, CT is inferior to MRI in the assessment of local chest wall, pericardial, and diaphragmatic invasion owing to its inferior soft tissue resolution.

E. Chest ultrasound can be useful to distinguish pleural fluid from thickening, but it is not a sensitive modality to assess chest wall or diaphragmatic invasion.

Question 3

D. Correct! Meningeal metastases are described in mesothelioma, but not as a primary location.

Other choices and discussion

A. The pleura is the most common site of primary mesothelioma.

B. Approximately 20 to 30% of all mesotheliomas arise from the peritoneal serosal lining. There is a strong association between peritoneal mesothelioma and asbestos exposure. Typical CT appearances are solid, enhancing, peritoneal masses with ascites. Concurrent pleural involvement is common.

C. Pericardial primary site is rare, accounting for < 1% of cases, presenting as either diffuse pericardial thickening or a focal mass with a coexistent pericardial effusion.

E. Mesothelioma arising from the tunica vaginalis testis is an extremely rare, but recognized, entity. Asbestos exposure is present in < 50% of cases. It can present as single or multiple paratesticular masses, or papillary excrescences on the inner surface of a hydrocele.

Top Tips

- Circumferential pleural thickening, thickening extending along the mediastinal border, and a pleural thickness of > 1 cm are key features of malignant pleural disease on CT.

- Malignant mesothelioma is FDG-avid on 18F-FDG PET/CT.

- MRI with gadolinium is the best imaging modality for the assessment of local chest wall, diaphragmatic, and pericardial invasion in malignant pleural mesothelioma.

More Challenging 3

■ Case

A 50-year-old woman with a cough undergoes chest computed tomography (CT) after discovery of a mass on chest X-ray.

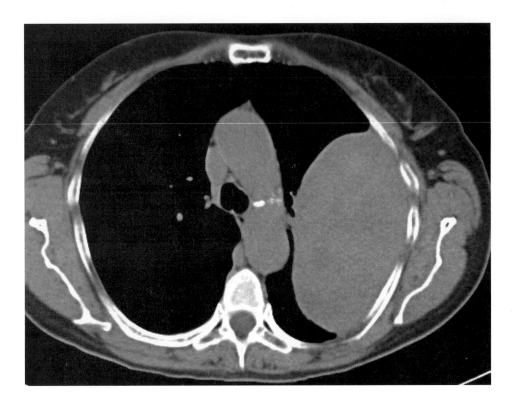

■ Questions

1. What is the most likely diagnosis?
   A. Lung cancer
   B. Mesothelioma
   C. Solitary fibrous tumor
   D. Pleural lipoma
   E. Metastases

2. Which ONE of the following is NOT associated with this diagnosis?
   A. Hyperglycemia
   B. Wrist pain
   C. Chest wall invasion
   D. Pleural effusion
   E. Diaphragmatic invasion

3. Which ONE of the following is associated with malignancy in this lesion?
   A. Sessile morphology
   B. Pedunculated morphology
   C. Unifocality
   D. Prior tobacco use
   E. Previous asbestos exposure

■ Answers and Explanations

Question 1

C. Correct! Solitary fibrous tumors (SFTs) account for approximately 5% of primary pleural tumors, arising from the visceral pleura in 80% cases. The pleural-based origin is best demonstrated on CT, with an obtuse or right angle to the adjacent pleura. These masses are usually well-marginated and isodense compared to adjacent muscle on noncontrast CT, as is demonstrated in this case. They generally enhance avidly on postcontrast imaging.

Other choices and discussion

A. The test case is a pleural-based mass, forming an obtuse angle with the pleural surface, making primary lung cancer unlikely.

B. Mesothelioma is in the differential diagnosis for pleural-based masses, but typically presents as circumferential pleural thickening.

D. Pleural lipomas are usually fat attenuation on CT, rather than soft tissue density.

E. Metastases are included in the differential for a solitary pleural mass, but pleural metastases are generally multifocal and smaller in size than SFTs.

Question 2:

A. Correct! Hypoglycemia, not hyperglycemia, is a rare complication in approximately 2 to 4% of cases, due to production of insulin-like growth factor 2 by the tumor. This is known as Doege-Potter syndrome.

Other choices and discussion

B. Hypertrophic pulmonary osteoarthropathy is associated with SFT in approximately 20% of cases.

C. Malignant change can be seen in up to 40% of cases of SFT. These often manifest on imaging as chest wall or diaphragmatic invasion.

D. Pleural effusions are associated with SFT in approximately 25% of cases.

E. Malignant change can be seen in up to 40% of cases of SFT. These often manifest on imaging as chest wall or diaphragmatic invasion.

Question 3:

A. Correct! Factors predicting malignancy include large tumor size at presentation, symptomatic patients, sessile morphology, and multifocality. Owing to the risk of malignancy in SFT, further investigation is appropriate. Magnetic resonance imaging with gadolinium can be used to define the tumor border more accurately than on CT, and can be used to assess for chest wall and diaphragmatic invasion. 18-fludeoxyglucose (FDG) positron emission tomography/CT has a role in differentiating benign SFT from other malignant pleural neoplasms: benign SFTs are generally not FDG-avid, whereas those with increased FDG uptake are more likely to be malignant. Intense FDG uptake in the mass suggests an alternate diagnosis, such as lymphoma, mesothelioma, or metastatic disease. Most centers pursue a confirmatory biopsy, which can be performed percutaneously under CT guidance. No known association with asbestos or tobacco exposure is reported.

The other choices are incorrect.

■ Suggested Readings

Cardillo G, Carbone L, Carleo F, Masala N, Graziano P, Bray A, et al. Solitary fibrous tumors of the pleura: an analysis of 110 patients treated in a single institution. Ann Thorac Surg 2009;88(5):1632–1637

Keraliya AR, Tirumani SH, Shinagare AB, Zaheer A, Ramaiya NH. Solitary fibrous tumors: 2016 imaging update. Radiol Clin North Am 2016;3:565–579

Top Tips

- SFT is a primary pleural tumor of varying malignant potential. These can be sessile or pedunculated. The presence of a pedicle can be inferred if the mass demonstrates mobility on serial imaging.

- Known associations include hypoglycemia and hypertrophic pulmonary osteoarthropathy.

- Factors predicting malignancy include large tumor size, symptomatic patients, sessile morphology, and multifocality.

More Challenging 4

■ Case

A 58-year-old with a history of asthma.

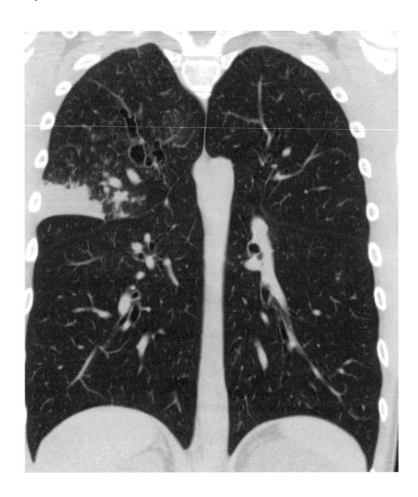

■ Questions

1. Which ONE of the following is the MOST likely diagnosis?
   A. Aspiration pneumonia
   B. Cystic fibrosis
   C. Bronchial atresia
   D. Allergic bronchopulmonary aspergillosis (ABPA)

2. Which ONE of the following statements is true?
   A. The "air crescent" sign develops in invasive aspergillosis as the host immunity recovers.
   B. A mycetoma occurs in immunocompromised patients.
   C. Bronchiolectasis is the most prominent finding in ABPA.
   D. Traction bronchiectasis results from an intrinsic defect within the airway wall.

3. Which ONE of the following is a MAJOR criterion for diagnosis of the test case?
   A. Elevated serum immunoglobulin E levels
   B. Aspergillus in the sputum
   C. Expectoration of mucus plugs
   D. Delayed hypersensitivity reaction with intradermal injection

■ Answers and Explanations

Question 1

D. Correct! ABPA develops in patients with a history of asthma. Imaging features include central bronchiectasis and mucoid impaction (both seen in this case). The contents of the impacted mucus often have high attenuation (not shown).

Other choices and discussion

A. The image demonstrates central bronchiectasis in the right upper lobe along with several impacted bronchi and a peripheral consolidation. Bronchiectasis would not be found with aspiration. In addition, aspiration is more commonly seen in the lower lobes (in the erect patient).

B. Cystic fibrosis results in diffuse central and upper lobe bronchiectasis, which is not seen in the test case.

C. Bronchial atresia is a congenital disorder of a focal bronchial branch with resultant impaction of the distal airway and associated distributional hyperinflation. No parenchymal lucency is seen here to suggest this diagnosis.

Question 2

A. Correct! The "air crescent" sign develops in invasive aspergillosis as the host immunity recovers. Invasive aspergillus infection most commonly presents as a pulmonary nodule in immunocompromised patients. As host immunity improves, a small crescent of air forms around the nodule. This is not to be confused with the air surrounding a mycetoma, which occurs when a fungus ball inhabits a preexisting cavity.

Other choices and discussion

B. Mycetomas occur in immunocompetent patients. They form within cavities created by old granulomatous disease.

C. APBA causes central airway dilation. Bronchioles are anatomically peripheral and are not seen with APBA.

D. Potential causes of bronchiectasis include infection (most common), congenital disorders (e.g., cystic fibrosis), obstruction, and iatrogenic (e.g., radiation). The traction type of bronchiectasis results from the adjacent fibrotic lung parenchyma "pulling" on the bronchus and causing it to enlarge. Traction bronchiectasis does not result from an intrinsic defect within the airway wall.

Question 3

A. Correct! Elevated serum immunoglobulin E levels is a major criterion for this diagnosis. Patients with ABPA have a hypersensitivity reaction to endobronchial *Aspergillus* proliferation. Typical features of an allergic response (such as an elevated immunoglobulin E and positive skin tests) aid in confirming the diagnosis of ABPA.

Other choices and discussion

B. Aspergillus in the sputum is a minor criterion for ABPA.

C. Expectoration of mucus plugs is a minor criterion for ABPA.

D. Delayed hypersensitivity reaction with intradermal injection is a minor criterion for ABPA. (Major criteria include elevated immunoglobulin E levels and immediate type I positive skin test.)

■ Suggested Readings

Abramson S. Signs in imaging—the air crescent sign. Radiology 2001;218(1):230–232

Agarwal R. Allergic bronchopulmonary aspergillosis. Chest 2009;135(3):805–826

Gipson MG, Cummings KW, Hurth KM. Bronchial atresia. Radiographics 2009;29:1531–1535

Silva CI, Colby TV, Muller NL. Asthma and associated conditions: high-resolution CT and pathologic findings. Am J Roentgenol 2004;183(3):817–824

Thompson BH, Stanford W, Galvin JR, Kurihara Y. Varied radiologic appearances of pulmonary aspergillosis. Radiographics 1995;15:1273–1284

**SECTION XI
THORACIC IMAGING**

Top Tips

◆ Think of APBA if you see central bronchiectasis, particularly in a patient with a history of asthma or cystic fibrosis.

◆ *Aspergillus* can manifest in the lungs in four major ways: mycetoma within a preformed cavity (normal hosts), semi-invasive form, invasive form (immunocompromised patients), and ABPA (hypersensitivity reaction in asthmatics).

◆ The "air crescent" sign is seen in invasive aspergillosis as host immunity improves.

More Challenging 5

■ Case

A severely immunocompromised leukemia patient presents with fever that is unresponsive to antibiotics.

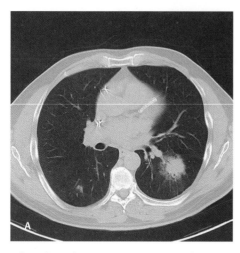 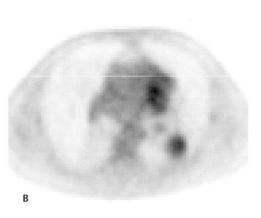

Left: High-resolution noncontrast computed tomography. Right: Corresponding fludeoxyglucose positron emission tomography.

■ Questions

1. What is the MOST likely diagnosis for this patient?
   A. Pulmonary Kaposi sarcoma
   B. Adenocarcinoma in situ
   C. Vasculitis
   D. Invasive aspergillosis
   E. Angiosarcoma

2. What is the MOST likely primary cause of the perilesional ground glass attenuation surrounding this lung abnormality?
   A. Lepidic spread of tumor cells
   B. Spread of an inflammatory infiltrate from the nodule
   C. Peripheral alveolar or pulmonary hemorrhage
   D. Postradiation change around a treated lung carcinoma

3. In a different scenario, you notice several pulmonary nodules with halo signs and enlarged bilateral hilar nodes on a noncontrast chest computed tomography. You also notice that the patient has an elevated angiotensin-converting enzyme level. Which entity does this patient MOST likely have?
   A. Granulomatosis with polyangiitis
   B. Churg-Strauss syndrome
   C. Pulmonary Kaposi sarcoma
   D. Invasive aspergillosis
   E. Sarcoidosis

■ Answers and Explanations

Question 1

D. Correct! This is invasive aspergillosis. A "halo" sign is present in this case. Angioinvasive aspergillosis is the most common cause of the halo sign in the chest in an immunocompromised patient. Other fungal infections can also demonstrate this appearance, although are less common. These include *Mucor* infection, pulmonary candidiasis, and coccidioidomycosis.

Other choices and discussion

A. Although the pulmonary nodules of Kaposi sarcoma can have perilesional ground glass attenuation, those nodules are typically more flamed-shaped than are shown in the test case. Also, the clinical history provided favors infection over neoplasm.

B. Adenocarcinoma in situ was previously referred to as bronchoalveolar carcinoma. This entity can demonstrate nodules with a halo sign.

C. Various inflammatory and/or vasculitis etiologies can cause this appearance (pulmonary hemorrhage and hemorrhagic lung nodules), including Wegener granulomatosis, eosinophilic pneumonia, organizing pneumonia, and even endometriosis. However, the clinical information given for the test case does not match these causes.

E. Based on imaging alone, metastatic disease cannot be excluded, as metastatic disease can also demonstrate a halo sign. This can be seen, for example, with angiosarcoma, osteosarcoma, or choriocarcinoma, and is likely due to fragility of the neovascular tissue with resultant perilesional alveolar hemorrhage. The clinical scenario favors an infection over a neoplasm.

Not shown here, there is also a "reverse halo" sign, aka the "atoll" sign. With this sign, the central portion of the nodule demonstrates ground glass density while the peripheral consolidation is more dense. The ground glass area corresponds to alveolar inflammation, and the peripheral area is typically due to granulomatous tissue.

Question 2

C. Correct! The ground glass density is most likely the result of peripheral alveolar or pulmonary hemorrhage. This ground glass density is best seen on the lung window setting. Most cases represent peripheral alveolar or pulmonary hemorrhage (i.e., a hemorrhagic nodule).

The computed tomography halo sign is often seen in neutropenic patients who have undergone bone marrow or organ transplantation. As mentioned above, the most common cause in this patient population is angioinvasive aspergillosis. The fungus invades the pulmonary vasculature, resulting in peripheral ground glass areas of thrombosis, infarction, and hemorrhage.

Other choices and discussion

A. Lepidic spread refers to tumor that spreads along an alveolar structure. However, the given history of an immunocompromised patient favors infection over tumor.

B. Spread of inflammatory infiltrate from the nodule is the mechanism for an inflammatory and/or vasculitis etiology. However, this is less likely than peripheral hemorrhage.

D. There was no history given that the patient had prior lung cancer and radiation treatment. In addition, radiation-induced change in the lungs would tend to follow a more linear pattern of infiltrate along the zone of radiation.

Question 3

E. Correct! This patient most likely has sarcoid. Angiotensin-converting enzyme levels are typically elevated in patients with sarcoidosis. Bilateral enlarged paratracheal and hilar nodes are common (sometimes called "potato nodes").

Other choices and discussion

The computed tomography halo sign can also be seen with all of the following.

A. Granulomatosis with polyangiitis is the newer terminology for Wegener granulomatosis. This is an autoimmune disease with necrotizing granulomatous inflammation and vasculitis. The most common pulmonary findings are single or multiple nodules/masses, which may cavitate. Cytoplasmic antineutrophil cytoplasmic antibodies are associated with this entity.

B. Churg-Strauss syndrome is also known as eosinophilic granulomatosis with polyangiitis. This is an autoimmune disease with associated vasculitis in an individual with a history of airway allergic hypersensitivity. Perinuclear antineutrophil cytoplasmic antibodies are associated with this entity.

C. A human herpesvirus-8 viral load is seen in immunocompromised patients with pulmonary Kaposi sarcoma.

D. The diagnosis of invasive aspergillosis could include a positive galactomannan assay.

■ Suggested Readings

Franquet T, Muller NL, Gimenez A, Guembe P, de La TJ, Bague S. Spectrum of pulmonary aspergillosis: histologic, clinical, and radiologic findings. Radiographics 2001;21:825–837

Gaeta M, Blandino A, Scribano E, Minutoli F, Volta S, Pandolfo I. Computed tomography halo sign in pulmonary nodules: frequency and diagnostic value. J Thorac Imaging 1999;14:109–113

Kumazoe H, Matsunaga K, Nagata N, et al. "Reversed halo sign" of high-resolution computed tomography in pulmonary sarcoidosis. J Thorac Imaging 2009;24:66–68

Top Tips

◆ The computed tomography halo sign may the first indication of a fungal infection.

◆ The reverse halo sign was initially thought to be fairly specific for cryptogenic organizing pneumonia, but a variety of pathologies, including opportunistic fungal infection, sarcoid, and tuberculosis, can have this appearance.

◆ The fludeoxyglucose positron emission tomography image shown demonstrates increased uptake in this infectious hemorrhagic lung nodule. Lung infection can show increased fludeoxyglucose uptake similar in intensity to malignancy. Therefore, the clinical scenario is of utmost importance in making the correct diagnosis.

Essentials 1

■ Case

A patient has intense tenderness when the sonographer presses the transducer probe over the right upper quadrant of the abdomen. Grayscale longitudinal image of the right upper quadrant (a) and longitudinal image of the right upper quadrant with Doppler (b) are shown.

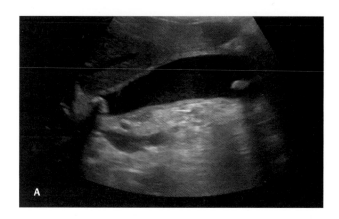

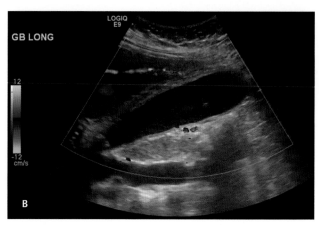

■ Questions

1. Which ONE of the following is the most likely diagnosis?
   A. Acute acalculous cholecystitis
   B. Acute calculous cholecystitis
   C. Adenomyomatosis
   D. Gallbladder carcinoma
   E. Emphysematous cholecystitis

2. Which ONE of the following is the most sensitive sign for this condition?
   A. Air within the gallbladder lumen
   B. Sonographic Murphy sign
   C. Presence of gallstones
   D. Decreased vascular flow to the gallbladder wall on Doppler
   E. Gallbladder distention

3. Which ONE of the following is a feature of emphysematous cholecystitis?
   A. More common in women than men
   B. Gallstones are present in 85% of cases
   C. Gallstones are almost never present
   D. Isolated condition not usually associated with systemic metabolic disorders
   E. Surgical emergency due to risk of perforation

■ Answers and Explanations

Question 1

B. Correct! This is acute calculous cholecystitis. This has the classic appearance of an obstructing stone in the gallbladder neck, with wall thickening, and wall hyperemia on Doppler. (As noted in the history, there was a reported positive sonographic Murphy sign as well.)

Other choices and discussion

A. Gallstones are present, excluding acalculous cholecystitis. Acute inflammation of the gallbladder in the absence of stones is termed acalculous cholecystitis.

C. The classic "comet-tail" artifact of adenomyomatosis is not present in this case.

D. No mass lesion or mass-like wall thickening is present to suggest neoplasm.

E. No air or "dirty shadowing" is present to suggest emphysematous cholecystitis.

Question 2

B. Correct! The sonographic Murphy sign is the most sensitive sign for this diagnosis. A sonographic Murphy sign refers to pain from transducer palpation over the gallbladder with inspiration. A sonographic Murphy sign is associated with 90% of cases of acute cholecystitis. Typically, the gallbladder is visualized, and the patient is instructed to take a deep breath while the sonographer increases transducer pressure.

Other choices and discussion

A. Air within the gallbladder *lumen* is a very uncommon finding. In the setting of emphysematous cholecystitis, air is present within the *wall* of the gallbladder.

C. The presence of gallstones (cholelithiasis) is common, but not the most sensitive finding. In addition, gallstones are often seen in the absence of acute inflammation. Gallstones may be clinically asymptomatic or result in intermittent biliary colic.

D. Vascular flow is typically increased in the setting of acute cholecystitis, although this is not the most sensitive finding. Pronounced flow in the cystic artery is occasionally seen with Doppler.

E. Gallbladder distention commonly occurs with fasting in normal patients.

Question 3

E. Correct! Emphysematous cholecystitis is a surgical emergency. Emphysematous cholecystitis refers to acute inflammation of the gallbladder due to gas-forming bacteria. It carries an increased risk of gallbladder perforation, peritonitis, sepsis, and death. Therefore, emergent cholecystectomy is indicated.

Other choices and discussion

A. Emphysematous cholecystitis is seven times more common in males than in females.

B. Up to half of the patients with emphysematous cholecystitis do not have gallstones.

C. Up to half of the patients with emphysematous cholecystitis do not have gallstones.

D. The prevalence of emphysematous cholecystitis is increased in patients with metabolic disorders. Up to one-half of the patients with emphysematous cholecystitis have diabetes mellitus.

■ Suggested Readings

Cooperberg PL, Burhenne HJ. Real-time ultrasonography. Diagnostic technique of choice in calculous gallbladder disease. N Engl J Med 1980;302:1277–1279

Konno K, Ishida H, Naganuma H, et al. Emphysematous cholecystitis: sonographic findings. Abdom Imaging 2002;27:191–195

Singer AJ, McCracken G, Henry MC, Thode HC Jr, Cabahug CJ. Correlation among clinical, laboratory, and hepatobiliary scanning findings in patients with suspected acute cholecystitis. Ann Emerg Med 1996;28:267–272

SECTION XII
US/REPRODUCTIVE/
ENDOCRINOLOGY IMAGING

Top Tips

◆ The patient should fast for at least 4 hours prior to an ultrasound examination for possible acute cholecystitis. (The gallbladder should be distended during the ultrasound examination for optimal assessment.)

◆ The hallmark of gallbladder carcinoma is a discrete immobile mass with vascular flow. Conversely, gallstones and sludge will move to the dependent portion of the gallbladder and are avascular vascularity. Use mobility and vascularity to differentiate these two entities.

◆ Be careful when concluding that there is a positive sonographic Murphy sign. Many people use the term loosely to describe pain on transducer palpation anywhere in the right upper quadrant. A true positive sign refers to pain directly over the visualized gallbladder with transducer pressure and patient inspiration.

Essentials 2

■ Case

The patient is currently asymptomatic. Grayscale longitudinal image of the right upper quadrant (a) and grayscale longitudinal decubitus image of the right upper quadrant (b) are shown.

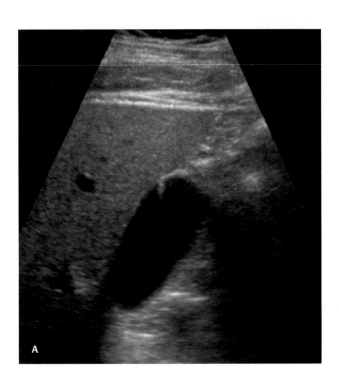

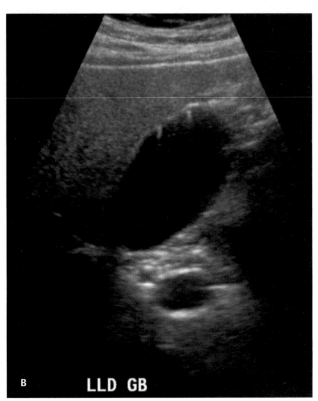

■ Questions

1. Which ONE of the following the most likely diagnosis?
   A. Acute acalculous cholecystitis
   B. Acute calculous cholecystitis
   C. Adenomyomatosis
   D. Gallbladder carcinoma
   E. Emphysematous cholecystitis

2. What is the malignant potential of this condition?
   A. No malignant potential
   B. Premalignant condition that develops into gallbladder carcinoma in 20% of cases
   C. If untreated, nearly always leads to cholangiocarcinoma
   D. Questionable association with carcinoma, but incidentally found on nearly all specimens of resected gallbladder cancer
   E. Associated with sarcomatous transformation

3. What is the etiology of this condition?
   A. Small gallstones adherent to the gallbladder wall
   B. Intramural gas within the gallbladder wall
   C. Prominent Rokitansky-Aschoff sinuses
   D. Intraluminal calculi
   E. Inflammatory polyps

■ Answers and Explanations

Question 1

C. Correct! This is adenomyomatosis. Pictured is the classic "comet-tail" artifact, which occurs secondary to ultrasound wave reflections off cholesterol crystals within sinuses of the gallbladder wall.

Other choices and discussion

A. No sonographic signs are seen to suggest cholecystitis, such as gallbladder wall thickening or pericholecystic fluid. In addition, the patient is reportedly asymptomatic.

B. No gallstones are seen.

D. No mass lesion or mass-like wall thickening is seen.

E. Air would result in more pronounced shadowing in the gallbladder wall than is seen in the test case, and the patient would likely be symptomatic with emphysematous cholecystitis.

Question 2

A. Correct! Adenomyomatosis has no malignant potential. While adenomyomatosis has been identified in some resected gallbladder carcinoma specimens, no direct relationship between the two conditions has been definitively established.

Discussion

The other options are incorrect. Surgical treatment of isolated adenomyomatosis is not indicated in the absence of symptoms.

Question 3

C. Correct! The hallmark of adenomyomatosis is prominent epithelial sinuses (Rokitansky-Aschoff sinuses), which herniate into the gallbladder wall. Cholesterol crystals may deposit in these sinuses, giving a characteristic comet-tail artifact.

Other choices and discussion

A. This is not due to adherent gallstones.

B. This is not due to intramural gas. Intramural gas is seen in the setting of emphysematous cholecystitis and is a surgical emergency, due to the risk of gallbladder perforation. It does not progress to adenomyomatosis.

D. Patients with adenomyomatosis may also have cholecystitis. However, this condition does not lead to the formation of adenomyomatosis.

E. Inflammatory polyps are a less common form of gallbladder polyposis. They are usually associated with longstanding cholelithiasis.

■ Suggested Readings

Nishimura A, Shirai Y, Hatakeyama K. Segmental adenomyomatosis of the gallbladder predisposes to cholecystolithiasis. J Hepatobiliary Pancreat Surg 2004;11:342–347

Raghavendra BN, Subramanyam BR, Balthazar EJ. Sonography of adenomyomatosis of the gallbladder: radiologic-pathologic correlation. Radiology 1983;146:747–752

Top Tips

- Adenomyomatosis is commonly asymptomatic and can be an incidental finding on gallbladder ultrasound.

- Adenomyomatosis should not be confused with "adenomyosis," which is a condition affecting the uterine endometrium and myometrium. (Clue: adenomyomatosis has a "T" in it, and is located at the "top" of the abdomen.)

- Cholecystectomy is often recommended for gallbladder polyps that are > 1 cm, increasing in size, or symptomatic.

Essentials 3

■ Case

Ultrasound of the right upper quadrant was obtained in a 20-year-old patient with intermittent abdominal pain. Grayscale longitudinal images of the liver with (a) and without (b) Doppler are shown.

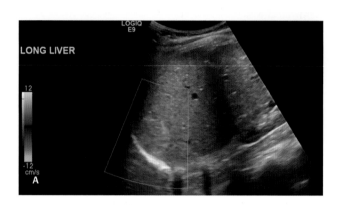

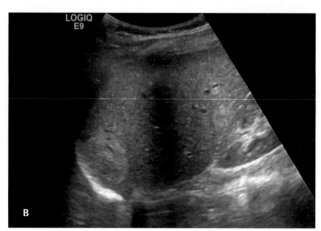

■ Questions

1. Which ONE of the following is the most likely diagnosis?
   A. Hemangioma
   B. Fibrolamellar hepatocellular carcinoma
   C. Abscess
   D. Cirrhosis
   E. Postbiopsy pseudoaneurysm

2. What is the MOST common presentation of this disorder?
   A. Incidental finding on imaging
   B. Acute intrahepatic hemorrhage
   C. Elevated transaminases
   D. Thrombocytopenia
   E. Metastasis

3. Which ONE of the following is a common imaging characteristic of this disorder on ultrasound?
   A. Size > 6 cm
   B. Intense vascular flow on Doppler
   C. Heterogeneous appearance with internal necrosis
   D. Anechoic signal
   E. Homogeneous hyperechoic mass

■ Answers and Explanations

Question 1

A. Correct! This is a hemangioma. Hepatic hemangiomas typically present as well-defined hyperechoic masses with no flow on Doppler. They are common incidental findings on imaging of the liver, with some studies reporting them in up to 20% of the population.

Other choices and discussion

B. Fibrolamellar hepatocellular carcinoma is a hepatic mass that typically presents in 20- to 40-year-olds. Although it is less aggressive than hepatocellular carcinoma, it does not produce symptoms until later in the disease, so it often presents as a large mass, unlike the test case.

C. Abscess would present as a complex fluid collection.

D. This patient does not have the nodular liver contour or heterogeneous echotexture seen in cirrhosis.

E. Pseudoaneurysm is a highly vascular lesion. It is usually the result of trauma or prior intervention.

Question 2

A. Correct! Cavernous hemangiomas are frequently found incidentally on ultrasound, computed tomography, and magnetic resonance imaging examinations. They are the most common benign liver lesion.

Other choices and discussion

B. While large hemangiomas (> 5 cm) can hemorrhage, most cavernous hemangiomas are smaller and do not bleed.

C. Most hemangiomas are asymptomatic and do not affect liver enzyme levels.

D. Consumptive coagulopathy can occur in the setting of Kasabach-Merritt syndrome in infants, but the vast majority of hemangiomas are asymptomatic.

E. This is a benign lesion, so it would not present with metastatic disease.

Question 3

E. Correct! A homogeneous hyperechoic mass is the most common sonographic appearance of a hepatic cavernous hemangioma.

Other choices and discussion

A. Giant and symptomatic hemangiomas can occur, although the majority of cavernous hemangiomas are small (< 5 cm).

B. While some hemangiomas can have flow, that flow is typically slow and may not be visualized on Doppler. In fact, most hemangiomas have no flow on Doppler.

C. Necrosis is not a typical feature of cavernous hemangiomas.

D. Hepatic hemangiomas can have a varied appearance on ultrasound, but most are hyperechoic.

■ Suggested Readings

McArdle CR. Ultrasonic appearances of a hepatic hemangioma. J Clin Ultrasound 1978;6:124

Mungovan JA, Cronan JJ, Vacarro J. Hepatic cavernous hemangiomas: lack of enlargement over time. Radiology 1994;191:111–113

Perkins AB, Imam K, Smith WJ, Cronan JJ. Color and power Doppler sonography of liver hemangiomas: a dream unfulfilled? J Clin Ultrasound 2000;28:159–165

Tait N, Richardson AJ, Muguti G, Little JM. Hepatic cavernous haemangioma: a 10 year review. Aust N Z J Surg 1992;62:521–524

SECTION XII
US/REPRODUCTIVE/
ENDOCRINOLOGY IMAGING

Top Tips

◆ Computed tomographic (CT) features of hemangioma include peripheral, nodular, discontinuous enhancement. Areas of discontinuous enhancement will later fill in and become more homogeneous on delayed phases. Larger hemangiomas sometimes do not completely fill in centrally.

◆ Some hemangiomas may show fast homogenous enhancement, termed "flash filling." These are usually smaller.

◆ A typical hemangioma matches the blood pool on all phases of contrast.

Essentials 4

■ Case

Transverse images of the liver with (a) and without (b) Doppler are shown.

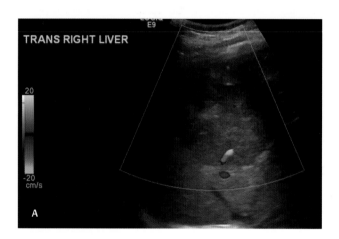

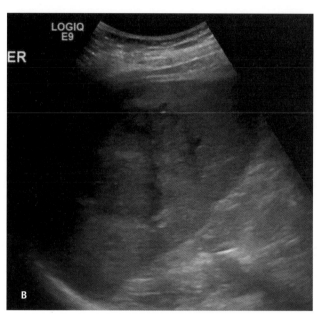

■ Questions

1. Which ONE of the following is the most likely diagnosis?
   A. Hepatocellular carcinoma
   B. Acute hepatitis
   C. Abscess
   D. Hemangioma
   E. Biliary obstruction

2. Which ONE of the following is NOT a predisposing factor for developing this disorder?
   A. Hepatitis B
   B. Hepatitis C
   C. Hepatitis E
   D. Alcohol abuse
   E. Aflatoxins

3. Which ONE of the following is a characteristic of fibrolamellar hepatocellular carcinoma?
   A. Found in elderly patients
   B. Small tumor size
   C. Multifocal distribution
   D. Contains calcification
   E. Associated decreased serum alpha-fetoprotein level

■ Answers and Explanations

Question 1

A. Correct! A large solid mass is present in the right lobe of the liver. Doppler demonstrates vascular flow within the lesion.

Other choices and discussion

B. Acute hepatitis can present as an enlarged liver with a somewhat hypoechoic hepatic parenchyma. The portal triads remain echogenic, giving the "starry sky" appearance.

C. Abscess presents as a complex fluid collection.

D. Hemangiomas typically present as well-defined hyperechoic masses with no flow on Doppler.

E. Biliary obstruction would cause biliary dilation, which is not seen in this case.

Question 2

C. Correct! Hepatitis E causes acute viral hepatitis and is commonly a co-infection with other viral types. However, it *does not* predispose to the development of hepatocellular carcinoma (HCC).

Discussion

The other options are incorrect—that is, they are all risk factors for developing HCC. This includes chronic hepatitis B and C, chronic alcohol use, and aflatoxins (fungal toxins used in grains).

Question 3

D. Correct! Fibrolamellar HCC commonly demonstrates internal calcification, which is a distinguishing feature.

Other choices and discussion

A. Fibrolamellar HCC typically presents in patients before the fourth decade of life, and it may occur in adolescents.

B. Fibrolamellar HCC typically presents as a large circumscribed mass lesion and has been reported at > 20 cm in size at the time of diagnosis.

C. Fibrolamellar HCC typically presents as a large solitary mass lesion and is rarely multifocal.

E. Alpha-fetoprotein levels are usually normal in patients with fibrolamellar HCC. Less than 10% of cases have increased levels.

■ Suggested Readings

El-Serag HB, Davila JA. Is fibrolamellar carcinoma different from hepatocellular carcinoma? A US population-based study. Hepatology 2004;39:798–803

El-Serag HB, Kanwal F. Epidemiology of hepatocellular carcinoma in the United States: where are we? Where do we go? Hepatology 2014;60:1767–1775

Jemal A, Bray F, Center MM, et al. Global cancer statistics. CA Cancer J Clin 2011;61:69–90

Kuniholm MH, Purcell RH, McQuillan GM, et al. Epidemiology of hepatitis E virus in the United States: results from the Third National Health and Nutrition Examination Survey, 1988-1994. J Infect Dis 2009;200:48–56

SECTION XII
US/REPRODUCTIVE/
ENDOCRINOLOGY IMAGING

Top Tips

- Patients at high risk for developing HCC should be screened with imaging every 6 months.

- Abnormal findings on ultrasound should prompt further workup with computed tomography and/or magnetic resonance imaging.

- Fibrolamellar carcinoma is a rare form of HCC seen most commonly in young patients. It is less aggressive than typical HCC, although the stage at presentation is often advanced, as symptoms usually present late.

Essentials 5

■ Case

Grayscale transverse image of the left kidney (a) and longitudinal image of the left kidney with Doppler (b) are shown.

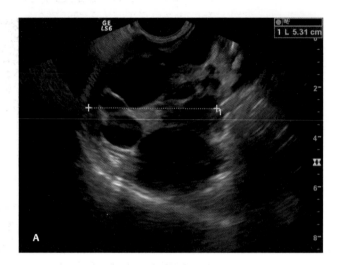

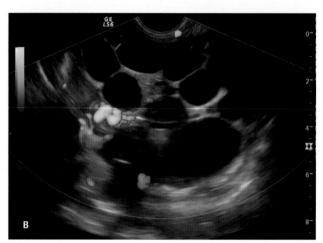

■ Questions

1. Which of the following is(are) in the differential diagnosis? Select ALL that apply.
   A. Multicystic dysplastic kidney
   B. Acquired renal cystic disease
   C. Autosomal dominant polycystic kidney disease
   D. Lithium nephrotoxicity
   E. Renal lymphoma

2. Which ONE of the following is a feature of this condition?
   A. Common cause of cystic renal disease in utero and in infancy
   B. Usually progresses to fulminant renal failure
   C. Multiple cysts communicate with one another and with the collecting system
   D. Commonly bilateral

3. Which ONE of the following is included in the management of multicystic dysplastic kidney?
   A. Screening the contralateral kidney for reversible abnormalities
   B. Percutaneous nephrostomy
   C. Retrograde ureteral stent placement
   D. Biopsy at diagnosis to exclude superimposed neoplasm
   E. Surgical resection of the affected kidney

■ Answers and Explanations

Question 1

A. Correct! Multicystic dysplastic kidney (MCDK) is characterized by multiple, large, noncommunicating cysts that distort the normal renal parenchyma.

B. Correct! Acquired renal cystic disease arises in patients who have undergone chronic dialysis therapy. It is characterized by multiple cysts of varying sizes. The intervening renal parenchyma is shrunken and echogenic.

C. Correct! Autosomal dominant polycystic kidney disease is characterized by numerous cysts. Patients may also have cystic involvement of the liver and pancreas.

Other choices and discussion

D. Lithium toxicity is a cause of cystic renal disease. However, the kidney develops microcysts, which are much smaller than the ones shown in the test case.

E. Renal lymphoma is an infiltrative process presenting as renal enlargement and solid masses that are usually hypoechoic. Cysts are not typical.

Question 2

A. Correct! MCDK is the most common cause of cystic renal disease early in life.

Other choices and discussion

B. Most cases are unilateral with preservation of contralateral renal function.

C. MCDK is characterized by multiple, noncommunicating cysts with a markedly distorted renal parenchyma. The cysts do not communicate with the collecting system, which differentiates this condition from ureteropelvic junction (UPJ) obstruction.

D. MCDK is commonly unilateral. If both kidneys are involved, it can be lethal.

E. Contralateral abnormalities, including vesicoureteral reflux and UPJ obstruction, have been reported in over 25% of patients with MCDK. These contralateral conditions require prompt diagnosis and correction to prevent the progression to renal failure.

Question 3

A. Correct! Screening of the contralateral kidney is indicated. Contralateral abnormalities, including vesicoureteral reflux and UPJ obstruction, have been reported in over 25% of patients with MCDK. These contralateral conditions may impair renal function, and cause hypertension.

Other choices and discussion

B. Because the affected kidney is nonfunctional, percutaneous nephrostomy is not indicated.

C. The collecting system of the nonfunctional kidney often cannot be visualized. Ureteral stent placement would not affect patient outcome.

D. MCDK is typically self-limiting. The cysts and the kidney tend to decrease in size with time.

E. Resection is rarely necessary, usually when when the kidney is massively enlarged.

■ Suggested Readings

Eckoldt F, Woderich R, Smith RD, Heling KS. Antenatal diagnostic aspects of unilateral multicystic kidney dysplasia—sensitivity, specificity, predictive values, differential diagnoses, associated malformations and consequences. Fetal Diagn Ther 2004;19:163–169

Onal B, Kogan BA. Natural history of patients with multicystic dysplastic kidney-what followup is needed? J Urol 2006;176:1607–1611

Stuck KJ, Koff SA, Silver TM. Ultrasonic features of multicystic dysplastic kidney: expanded diagnostic criteria. Radiology 1982;143:217–221

Top Tips

- In patients with MCDK, imaging of the contralateral kidney is necessary to screen for UPJ obstruction and reflux. These must be corrected in order to preserve renal function.

- Real-time cine imaging is helpful in differentiating multiple noncommunicating cysts from hydronephrosis.

- When evaluating for hydronephrosis, always check postvoid to make sure that it persists, and always use Doppler to exclude vessels that can mimic hydronephrosis.

Essentials 6

■ Case

History of recent endoscopic retrograde cholangiopancreatography to remove a retained distal bile duct stone after chole-cystectomy. Grayscale transverse images of the liver are shown.

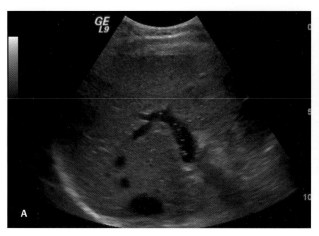
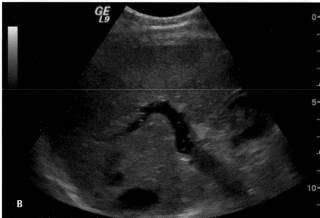

■ Questions

1. Which ONE of the following is the most likely diagnosis?
    A. Acute uncomplicated cholecystitis
    B. Cholangiocarcinoma
    C. Pneumobilia
    D. Hepatic granulomatous disease
    E. Biliary polyps

2. Select ALL of the following conditions that may result in this disorder.
    A. Emphysematous cholecystitis
    B. Biliary-enteric fistula
    C. Mesenteric ischemia
    D. Sphincterotomy at the sphincter of Oddi
    E. Acute cholangitis

3. Which ONE of the following is the recommended treatment for emphysematous cholecystitis?
    A. Follow up ultrasound in 8 hours after confirming fasting status
    B. Repeat ultrasound in 1 week
    C. No follow up is necessary
    D. Long-term therapy with broad-spectrum antibiotics
    E. Emergent cholecystectomy

■ Answers and Explanations

Question 1

C. Correct! This is pneumobilia. Punctate echogenic foci within the biliary system are seen, consistent with air.

Other choices and discussion

A. Air would not be present within the biliary system in uncomplicated acute cholecystitis. This patient is status post cholecystectomy.

B. Cholangiocarcinoma would demonstrate biliary wall thickening and/or a mass lesion, not air.

D. Hepatic granulomatous disease would present as echogenic foci within the hepatic parenchyma, not within the biliary tree.

E. Polyps are discrete masses, not intraluminal mobile foci.

Question 2

A. Correct! With emphysematous cholecystitis, air collects in the gallbladder wall and may enter the biliary system. Emphysematous cholecystitis is a life-threatening condition and occurs more frequently in diabetics.

B. Correct! Biliary-enteric fistulae are commonly created surgically or can arise spontaneously in the setting of a gallstone ileus. Such fistulae allow air in the bowel to communicate with the biliary tree.

D. Correct! A sphincterotomy is sometimes performed during endoscopy to remove obstructing stones and to image the common bile duct. As a result, air may pass retrograde from the duodenum through the sphincter of Oddi and into the biliary tree.

E. Correct! Acute cholangitis classically presents with the Charcot triad: fever, jaundice, and right upper quadrant pain. Progression of this condition can sometimes lead to pneumobilia. Parasitic infections such as *Clonorchis* may be responsible. Ultrasound often demonstrates biliary sludge or air. Emergent treatment is necessary to decompress the biliary system.

Discussion

The other choice is incorrect. Mesenteric ischemia is a life-threatening condition seen with necrotic bowel. Air dissects from the necrotic bowel wall into the portal venous system, not the biliary tree. Portal venous gas usually has a more peripheral location on imaging than does biliary air, which is typically located centrally.

Question 3

E. Correct! Immediate surgical intervention is indicated for emphysematous cholecystitis.

The other choices are incorrect.

■ Suggested Readings

Bennett GL, Balthazar EJ. Ultrasound and CT evaluation of emergent gallbladder pathology. Radiol Clin N Am 2003;41:1203–1216

Sherman SC, Tran H. Pneumobilia: benign or life-threatening. J Emer Med 2006;30:147–153

Top Tips

◆ Biliary air presents as echogenic intraluminal foci within the biliary tree. Real-time imaging demonstrates that the air predominates centrally, mimicking the flow of bile.

◆ Portal venous air occurs within the vessels and implies mesenteric ischemia, which can be life-threatening.

◆ Portal venous air has a more peripheral distribution than does biliary air.

Essentials 7

■ Case

This patient presents for routine screening ultrasound of the abdomen. Grayscale longitudinal image of the right upper quadrant (a) and grayscale longitudinal image of the spleen (b) are shown.

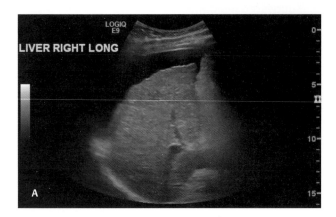

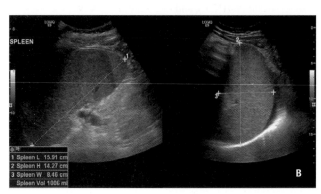

■ Questions

1. Which ONE of the following is the most likely diagnosis?
   A. Portal hypertension
   B. Hepatocellular carcinoma
   C. Acute hepatitis
   D. Ascending cholangitis
   E. Hepatic metastatic disease

2. What is the MOST common malignancy associated with cirrhosis?
   A. Hepatocellular carcinoma
   B. Fibrolamellar carcinoma
   C. Angiosarcoma
   D. Hepatic hemangioma
   E. Focal nodular hyperplasia

3. Which ONE of the following is a feature of chronic portal venous occlusion?
   A. Antegrade flow in the portal vein
   B. Expansion of the main portal vein diameter
   C. Malignant thrombosis
   D. Collateral vessels converging to flow into the portal system
   E. Cavernous transformation of the portal vein

■ Answers and Explanations

Question 1

A. Correct! Findings in this case include a nodular, undulating contour of the liver, consistent with cirrhosis. There is also ascites, and the spleen is enlarged.

Other choices and discussion

B. Patients with cirrhosis are at an increased risk for hepatocellular carcinoma (HCC), and thus commonly have screening examinations. However, no mass lesion is present in this case.

C. Acute hepatitis may present as an enlarged liver with diffusely hypoechoic echotexture. The portal triads remain echogenic, giving the "starry sky" appearance.

D. Patients with cholangitis may present with signs of biliary obstruction, including ductal dilation, thickening, and biliary sludge.

E. No masses are seen on this exam.

Question 2

A. Correct! HCC is the most common hepatic malignancy associated with cirrhosis. In the western hemisphere, HCC is commonly associated with chronic hepatitis B and C infections, alcohol use, and cirrhosis.

Other choices and discussion

B. Fibrolamellar carcinoma is a distinct hepatic malignancy that is less common than HCC. It usually occurs in young adults in the second and third decades of life.

C. Angiosarcoma is a rare malignancy that is sometimes associated with toxic agents such as Thorotrast and polyvinyl chloride.

D. Cavernous hemangiomas are the most common benign hepatic neoplasm. The incidence is high, with some studies reporting hemangiomas in up to 20% of the population. These commonly present on ultrasound as small hyperechoic lesions with increased through transmission. They have no malignant potential.

E. Focal nodular hyperplasia is a benign hepatic mass and is more common in females than males. Imaging characteristics often include a central scar on computed tomography and magnetic resonance imaging, early arterial phase enhancement, and delayed uptake on hepatocyte-specific contrast magnetic resonance imaging.

Question 3

E. Correct! Cavernous transformation usually occurs in the setting of longstanding portal venous thrombosis. The characteristic appearance of this condition is the presence of numerous small vessels at the porta hepatis due to collateral circulation.

Other choices and discussion

A. In the setting of portal hypertension or venous occlusion, portal vein flow is away from the liver. This is referred to as retrograde or hepatofugal flow.

B. The main portal vein does not expand with longstanding thrombosis.

C. Malignant thrombosis can be seen in the setting of HCC. However, isolated chronic venous thrombosis does not itself lead to malignancy. Doppler ultrasound can be used to differentiate malignant thrombus (which may have flow) from bland thrombus (which does not have flow).

D. Multiple collateral vessels arise in the setting of longstanding venous occlusion. However, these vessels divert flow *away from*, not toward, the portal system.

■ Suggested Readings

Amitrano L, Guardascione MA, Brancaccio V, et al. Risk factors and clinical presentation of portal vein thrombosis in patients with liver cirrhosis. J Hepatol 2004;40:736–741

Guichelaar MM, Benson JT, Malinchoc M, et al. Risk factors for and clinical course of non-anastomotic biliary strictures after liver transplantation. Am J Transplant 2003;3:885–890

Trichopoulos D, Bamia C, Lagiou P, et al. Hepatocellular carcinoma risk factors and disease burden in a European cohort: a nested case-control study. J Natl Cancer Inst 2011;103:1686–1695

Van Gansbeke D, Avni EF, Delcour C, et al. Sonographic features of portal vein thrombosis. Am J Roentgenol 1985;144:749–752

Top Tips

♦ Findings of portal hypertension include cirrhosis, splenomegaly, and ascites.

♦ Patients with cirrhosis have an increased risk for developing HCC and are typically routinely screened with ultrasound.

♦ Malignant thrombus may demonstrate vascular flow on Doppler.

Essentials 8

■ Case

A 70-year-old man with pulsatile groin mass following cardiac catheterization. Longitudinal image of the right femoral artery with Doppler (a) and spectral Doppler image of the right femoral vessels (b) are shown.

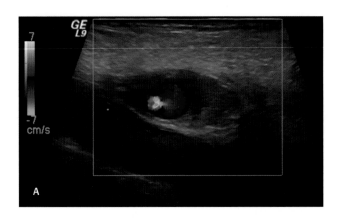

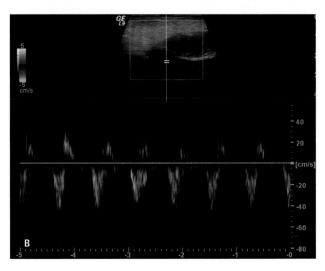

■ Questions

1. Which ONE of the following is the most likely diagnosis?
   A. Femoral artery stenosis
   B. Femoral artery occlusion
   C. Normal waveform
   D. Pseudoaneurysm
   E. True aneurysm

2. Which of the following choices is (are) reasonable INITIAL steps in the management of this disorder, assuming a clinically stable patient? (Select ALL that apply.)
   A. Ultrasound-guided compression
   B. Ultrasound-guided thrombin injection
   C. Covered stent placement
   D. Surgical excision and re-anastomosis
   E. Balloon angioplasty

3. Which ONE of the following is a common Doppler imaging finding of a pseudoaneurysm sac?
   A. Low systolic velocity
   B. Constant unidirectional flow
   C. "Yin-yang" appearance
   D. *Parvus et tardus* waveform
   E. Low resistance waveform

■ Answers and Explanations

Question 1

D. Correct! This is a pseudoaneurysm. Spectral Doppler performed over the neck of the aneurysm demonstrates flow both above and below the baseline on the Doppler spectrum.

Femoral pseudoaneurysms are commonly iatrogenic and secondary to arterial catheterization.

Other options and discussion

A. No stenosis is seen.

B. Flow is present.

C. A normal peripheral arterial waveform has a rapid upstroke with systole and a lower velocity with diastole. Flow is not normally reversed (unlike the test case, which shows diastolic signal below baseline).

E. A true aneurysm is a dilatation involving all three vascular layers and would not have the waveform shown here.

Question 2

A. Correct! Direct manual compression performed using the ultrasound transducer is a reasonable first-line treatment. It should be performed for approximately 30 minutes.

B. Correct! Ultrasound-guided injection of 1000 units of thrombin into the pseudoaneurysm sac is a reasonable first-line treatment.

Other choices and discussion

C. Covered stent placement is not routinely performed as initial therapy.

D. Surgical re-anastomosis is not routinely performed as initial therapy.

E. Angioplasty is not indicated.

Question 3

C. Correct! The "yin-yang" appearance is typical of a pseudoaneurysm. This appearance results from bidirectional flow in the aneurysm sac with swirling of contents.

Other choices and discussion

A. Velocities are elevated within the pseudoaneurysm.

B. Flow is typically bidirectional with to-and-fro flow through the neck of the pseudoaneurysm.

C. *Parvus et tardus* waveform is seen in the setting of arterial stenosis, not pseudoaneurysm.

D. Low resistance waveforms are seen with arteriovenous fistulas. These can result from puncture of artery and vein.

■ Suggested Readings

Foshager MC, Finlay DE, Longley DG, et al. Duplex and color Doppler sonography of complications after percutaneous interventional vascular procedures. Radiographics 1994;14:239–253

Kreuger K, Zaehringer M, Strohe D, et al. Postcatheterization pseudoaneurysm; results of US-guided thrombin percutaneous injection in 240 patients. Radiology 2005;236:1104–1110

SECTION XII US/REPRODUCTIVE/ ENDOCRINOLOGY IMAGING

Top Tips

◆ A "yin-yang" appearance is seen in a pseudoaneurysm sac due to swirling turbid flow.

◆ Waveform analysis over the neck of a pseudoaneurysm shows bidirectional flow, indicated by signal both above and below the baseline.

◆ Pseudoaneurysms that are symptomatic and/or are > 2 cm are frequently treated.

Essentials 9

■ **Case**

A 65-year-old man with microscopic hematuria. Longitudinal image of the right kidney with Doppler (a) and grayscale longitudinal image of the right kidney (b) are shown.

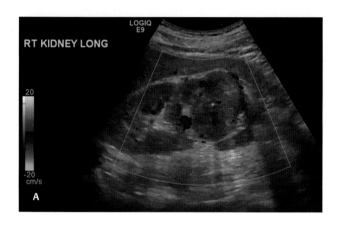

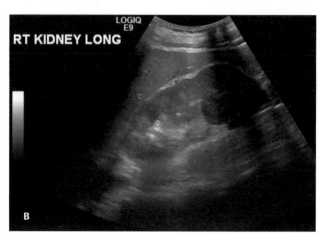

■ **Questions**

1. Which ONE of the following is the most likely diagnosis?
   A. Dromedary hump
   B. Nephrolithiasis
   C. Renal cell carcinoma
   D. Hydronephrosis
   E. Angiomyolipoma

2. What is the most common subtype of renal cell carcinoma?
   A. Clear cell
   B. Papillary
   C. Chromophobe
   D. Collecting duct
   E. Medullary

3. In the absence of distant metastatic disease, what is the stage of disease for renal cell carcinoma once the tumor has invaded the inferior vena cava?
   A. Carcinoma in situ
   B. Stage I
   C. Stage II
   D. Stage III
   E. Stage IV

■ Answers and Explanations

Question 1

C. Correct! A solid hypoechoic mass is seen arising from the lower pole cortex. Doppler confirms vascularity in the lesion. This finding on ultrasound should prompt further workup with computed tomography and/or magnetic resonance imaging, and by imaging this is renal cell carcinoma until proven otherwise.

Other choices and discussion

A. A dromedary hump is a contour variant of the renal cortex, which may mimic a mass lesion. The images shown in the test case demonstrate a discrete renal mass. For problem cases, a nuclear medicine renal scan can sometimes be used to confirm normal renal tissue within a dromedary hump.

B. No calculi are visualized. Renal calculi are highly echogenic and often demonstrate posterior acoustic shadowing. When Doppler is applied over a calculus, there is a characteristic "twinkle" artifact.

D. The collecting system is not dilated.

E. An angiomyolipoma is typically a hyperechoic mass on ultrasound.

Question 2

A. Correct! Clear cell is the most common subtype of renal cell carcinoma, accounting for over 70% of cases. Incidence rates of RCC are increased in patients with von Hippel-Lindau syndrome and in the setting of acquired renal cystic disease (seen in patients who have received long-term dialysis).

Other choices and discussion

B. Papillary carcinoma is the second most common subtype and accounts for approximately 10% of RCC. This subtype is typically slower growing and has a more favorable prognosis than clear cell RCC.

C. On computed tomography and magnetic resonance imaging evaluation, chromophobe carcinomas demonstrate less enhancement and have a more favorable prognosis than clear cell RCC.

D. Collecting duct RCC is a rare and aggressive subtype, accounting for < 1% of RCC.

E. Medullary carcinoma is a rare and aggressive subtype, most commonly found in African-American males with sickle cell disease.

Question 3

D. Correct! This is stage III. Renal vein and inferior vena cava invasion are classified as T3. In the absence of distant metastasis, this renders a stage III classification.

Other choices and discussion

There is no in situ classification of RCC. Staging is as follows:

- Stage I: T1 lesion ($\leq$ 7 cm, limited to the kidney) without nodal or distant metastases
- Stage II: T2 lesion ($\leq$ 10 cm, limited to the kidney) without nodal or distant metastases
- Stage III: T3 lesion without nodal or distant metastases
- Stage IV: T4 lesion (spread beyond Gerota fascia and/or invasion of the ipsilateral adrenal gland), or the presence of distant metastatic disease with any primary lesion

■ Suggested Readings

American Joint Committee on Cancer. Kidney. In: American Joint Committee on Cancer Staging Manual. New York: Springer; 2009: 447

Coogan CL, McKiel CF Jr, Flanagan MJ, et al. Renal medullary carcinoma in patients with sickle cell trait. Urology 1998;51:1049–1050

Patard JJ, Leray E, Rioux-Leclercq N, et al. Prognostic value of histologic subtypes in renal cell carcinoma: a multicenter experience. J Clin Oncol 2005;23:2763–2771

SECTION XII
US/REPRODUCTIVE/
ENDOCRINOLOGY IMAGING

Top Tips

- Clear cell is the most common subtype of RCC.
- Chromophobe RCC demonstrates less enhancement and has a more favorable prognosis than clear cell RCC.
- Invasion of the inferior vena cava is classified as a T3 lesion. Extension into the ipsilateral adrenal gland is classified as a T4 lesion.

Essentials 10

■ Case

A 45-year-old man presents with palpable mass in the scrotum. Grayscale longitudinal image of the left testicle (a) and transverse image of the left testicle with Doppler (b) are shown.

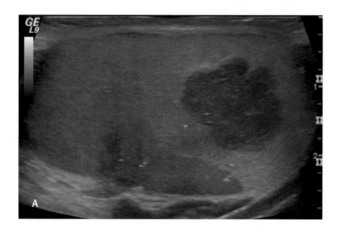

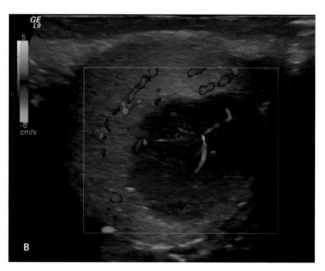

■ Questions

1. Which ONE of the following is the most likely diagnosis?
   A. Testicular carcinoma
   B. Testicular torsion
   C. Orchitis
   D. Tubular ectasia of the rete testis
   E. Abscess

2. What is the most common subtype of testicular carcinoma?
   A. Seminoma
   B. Mixed germ cell tumor
   C. Embryonal cell carcinoma
   D. Teratoma
   E. Choriocarcinoma

3. Which ONE of the following is a common feature of testicular seminoma?
   A. Bilateral masses
   B. Childhood presentation
   C. Late stage presentation
   D. Elevated alpha-fetoprotein
   E. Radiosensitive metastases

■ Answers and Explanations

Question 1

A. Correct! Ultrasound demonstrates a hypoechoic solid intratesticular mass with vascularity.

Other choices and discussion

B. Doppler confirms flow to the testicle, excluding torsion.

C. Orchitis presents with intense hypervascularity on Doppler evaluation of the affected testicle. Note that these patients are very sensitive to testicular manipulation and to pressure from the ultrasound transducer during scanning. If orchitis is detected, look carefully for abscess.

D. Tubular ectasia is a benign condition characterized by tiny anechoic tubular foci seen arising from the mediastinum testis. The incidence of ectasia is higher in patients after vasectomy.

E. There is no fluid collection to suggest abscess. Abscess may form after longstanding orchitis. In this patient, the images show vascularity to this solid lesion.

Question 2

A. Correct! Seminoma is the most common subtype of testicular carcinoma. Approximately 95% of testicular carcinomas are germ cell tumors, of which seminoma accounts for 50%. The most common age of incidence is between 35 and 50 years. Treatment is orchiectomy.

Other choices and discussion

B. Mixed germ cell tumors are classified as nonseminomatous germ cell tumors. They are the second most common subtype of testicular carcinoma. This subtype is typically more aggressive than seminoma, with a higher rate of metastasis at presentation. Laboratory examination may reveal elevated serum alpha-fetoprotein (AFP) levels.

C. Embryonal carcinomas account for 2 to 3% of testicular neoplasms. These tumors are classified as nonseminomatous germ cell tumors and typically present in patients between the ages of 25 and 35 years.

D. Teratomas of the testicle typically present in childhood. On ultrasound, they are characterized with varying echogenicity due to the presence of different cellular types and densities (e.g., calcium, fat, soft tissue).

E. Choriocarcinoma is a rare, aggressive type of testicular carcinoma. When this tumor is present, laboratory values typically include an elevated serum beta-human chorionic gonadotropin (β-HCG).

Question 3

E. Correct! Seminomas have a more favorable prognosis, in part, due to the radiosensitivity of their nodal metastases.

Other choices and discussion

A. Seminomas typically present as a unifocal, unilateral testicular mass.

B. Most patients present between the ages of 35 and 50 years.

C. Seminoma is the least aggressive subtype of testicular carcinoma.

D. Patients with seminoma typically present with normal AFP levels. Elevated AFP levels occur in patients with nonseminomatous germ cell tumors.

■ Suggested Readings

Einhorn LH. Treatment of testicular cancer: a new and improved model. J Clin Oncol 1990;8:1777–1781

Gilligan TD, Seidenfeld J, Basch EM, et al. American Society of Clinical Oncology Clinical Practice Guideline on uses of serum tumor markers in adult males with germ cell tumors. J Clin Oncol 2010;28:3388–3404

Marth D, Scheidegger J, Studer UE. Ultrasonography of testicular tumors. Urol Int 1990;45:237–240

SECTION XII
US/REPRODUCTIVE/
ENDOCRINOLOGY IMAGING

Top Tips

◆ With scrotal masses, it is critical to determine if the mass is intratesticular (highly suspicious for malignancy) or extratesticular (much less commonly malignant).

◆ Treatment of seminoma, the most common type of testicular carcinoma, includes orchiectomy and radiotherapy to nodal metastases.

◆ Choriocarcinoma is an aggressive subtype of testicular neoplasm and may be associated with elevated serum beta-human chorionic gonadotropin levels.

Details 1

■ Case

A 28-year-old G4P0 woman presents to the emergency room at 20 weeks' gestation with vague lower abdominal pain but no vaginal bleeding. Transabdominal and transvaginal images are presented. Which ONE of the following is the mostly likely diagnosis?

    A. Incompetent cervix
    B. Abortion in progress
    C. Placenta previa
    D. Normal pregnancy in labor

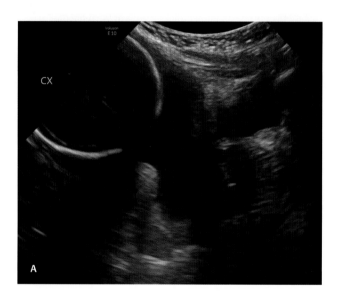 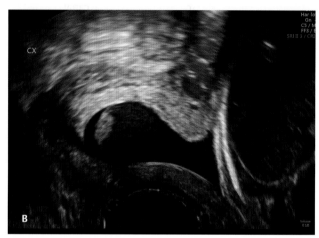

■ The following questions pertain to ultrasound of the cervix.

1. True or False. A cervical length of < 2.5 cm increases the risk for preterm labor.
2. True or False. Transvaginal sonography is contraindicated in pregnant women beyond the first trimester.
3. True or False. A marginal placenta previa extends to the internal os without crossing the endocervical canal.
4. True or False. Fluid in the vaginal canal in early pregnancy is a sure sign of fetal loss.
5. True or False. Hourglass membranes are seen with abortion in progress.
6. True or False. Recurrent pregnancy loss is highly suggestive of cervical incompetence.
7. True or False. Cervical cerclage may be done emergently in spite of the presence of hourglass membranes.
8. True or False. In the absence of active labor, cervical cerclage may be performed after 30 weeks.
9. True or False. Cervical length is most accurately measured with ultrasound by using the transvaginal approach.
10. True or False. The cervical length should be measured on two or more examinations before intervention.

■ Answers and Explanations

A. Correct! This is an incompetent cervix. The longitudinal image of the lower uterine segment and cervix shows a wide-open cervix that contains debris (which is best seen on the transvaginal image). In a patient who is not in labor, cervical dilation is indicative of cervical incompetence.

Other choices and discussion

B. These images could be compatible with an abortion in progress in a patient who is experiencing contractions and has passed amniotic fluid and/or products of conception. However, the absence of these findings in the patient's history makes this diagnosis unlikely.

C. With the cervical canal wide open, the posterior lip of the cervix may be mistaken for placenta previa. However, careful analysis of the transabdominal image instead reveals an intact amniotic sac herniated into the dilated cervical canal.

D. Cervical dilation is the first sign of active labor after the onset of uterine contractions. Although premature labor can happen at 20 weeks, the absence of active contractions makes this diagnosis unlikely.

Question 1

True. Although a cervical length of 3 cm is often used as the normal standard, 2.5 cm is the lower limit of normal and is a better predictor of premature labor.

Question 2

False. Transvaginal ultrasound (TVUS) may be performed at any time during pregnancy, without any absolute contraindications. TVUS is recommended for the definitive diagnosis of placenta previa when the urinary bladder cannot be filled optimally to visualize the cervix. Although historically there have been concerns about performing TVUS in pregnant women with vaginal bleeding or ruptured membranes, there has been no evidence to support these concerns.

Question 3

True. The previa location in marginal placenta previa usually resolves as the uterus grows and the inferior edge of the placenta moves to a more superior position. This change results from lengthening of the lower uterine segment and trophotropism, which allows for the unidirectional growth of the placenta toward the fundus. Although these factors contribute to the tendency of marginal placenta previa to resolve; those that persist after 32 weeks remain a previa in more than 70% of cases.

Question 4

False. If there is suspicion of amniotic fluid extending into the vagina due to cervical incompetence, cerclage may be performed to prevent premature labor.

Question 5

True. Intact amniotic membranes prolapsing into the vagina ("hourglass membranes") can be a sign of early labor in term gestation or an abortion in progress in early pregnancy.

Question 6

True. A history of recurrent pregnancy loss is often an indication to perform a cerclage.

Question 7

False. The prolapsed membrane must be replaced into the uterine cavity prior to cerclage to avoid membrane rupture. Cerclage is contraindicated in clinical scenarios where the procedure is unlikely to reduce the risk of preterm delivery or improve the fetal outcome. Such scenarios include fetal anomaly incompatible with life, intrauterine infection, active bleeding, active preterm labor, preterm premature rupture of membranes, and fetal demise.

Question 8

False. At this stage in gestation (30 weeks or later), the fetus can survive even if premature delivery occurs. In addition, it is technically difficult to perform an adequate cerclage at this time.

Question 9

True. Visualizing the internal os and cervical canal is best done through a transvaginal approach. In situations where transvaginal exam cannot be performed, a translabial approach can be attempted, although is often met with limited success.

Question 10

True. Measurement of cervical length on two or more examinations is good practice to confirm the findings before intervention. Transient shortening of the cervix has been reported.

■ Suggested Readings

Iams JD, Goldenberg RL, Meis PJ, et al. The length of the cervix and the risk of spontaneous premature delivery. N Engl J Med 1996;334:567–572

McGahan JP, Phillips HE, Bowen MS. Prolapse of the amniotic sac: ultrasound appearance. Radiology 1981;140(2):463–466

Scheerer LJ, Lam F, Bartolucci L, Katz M. A new technique for reduction of prolapsed fetal membranes for emergency cervical cerclage. Obstet Gynecol 1989;74:408–412

SECTION XII US/REPRODUCTIVE/ ENDOCRINOLOGY IMAGING

Top Tips

♦ Visualization and measurement of cervical length should be performed in any obstetric ultrasound examination, even when there is no clinical suspicion of cervical incompetence. This assessment may be performed transabdominally through a full bladder or transvaginally with an empty bladder.

♦ Active labor may be misinterpreted as cervical incompetence and should always remain in the differential diagnosis.

♦ Cervical cerclage is recommended to prevent premature delivery until the early second trimester.

Details 2

■ Case

A primigravida female was referred for dating of pregnancy due to poor menstrual history. Which ONE of the following is the most likely diagnosis?

A. Dichorionic diamniotic twins
B. Monochorionic diamniotic twins
C. Monochorionic monoamniotic twins
D. Conjoined twins

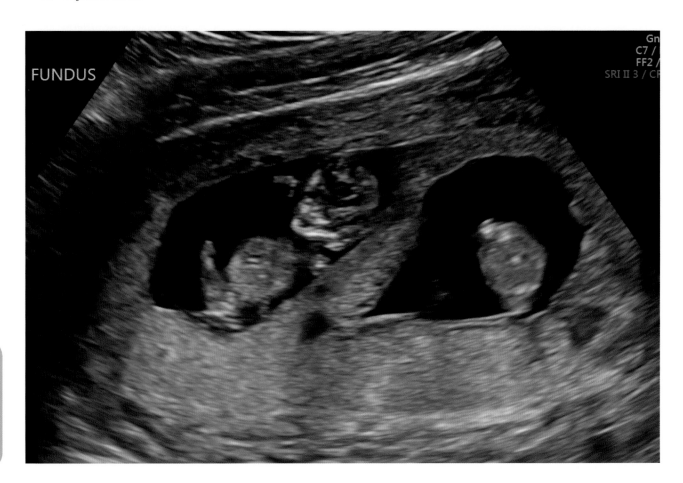

■ The following questions pertain to twins.

1. True or False. Dizygotic twins are always dichorionic.
2. True or False. Dichorionic twins can be either dizygotic or monozygotic.
3. True or False. Determination of chorionicity is achieved most accurately in the first trimester of pregnancy.
4. True or False. In monozygotic twins, dichorionic pregnancies are secondary to the division of the fertilized egg 5 days after fertilization.
5. True or False. Dizygotic twins are more common than monozygotic twins.
6. True or False. Twin transfusion syndrome has a higher incidence in monochorionic twins.
7. True or False. Monochorionic twins demonstrate the lambda or chorionic peak sign in the second or third trimester.
8. True or False. The most reliable sign of chorionicity in the third trimester is discordant fetal sexes.
9. True or False. There is a high mortality rate in diamniotic gestations due to entanglement of fetal parts.
10. True or False. Conjoined twins can occur in dichorionic gestations.

■ Answers and Explanations

A. Correct! This is dichorionic diamniotic twins. There are two fetuses in two separate gestational sacs. The examination was performed in the first trimester when the number of sacs signifies the number of placentas/chorions. This type of twinning represents one-third of all monozygotic twins and all dizygotic twins. In monozygotic twins, division of the fertilized egg happens within 4 days after fertilization.

Determination of amnionicity and chorionicity in the second and third trimesters is based on the following findings, in order of decreasing accuracy:

- Discrepant sexes
- Two separate placentas
- Chorionic peak sign (lambda sign or twin peak sign)
- Thickness of separating membrane

Other choices and discussion

B. Monochorionic diamniotic twins possess one placenta but two amniotic sacs. This type of twinning represents approximately two-thirds of monozygotic twins. Division of the fertilized egg into two embryos occurs at 4 to 8 days post fertilization. Before 10 weeks, there is only one gestational sac. The amniotic sacs will not be defined until around 8 menstrual weeks, but the number of amniotic sacs can be predicted by demonstrating two yolk sacs earlier in pregnancy.

C. Monochorionic monoamniotic twins represent 1 to 3% of monozygotic twins. The fertilized egg does not divide until 8 to 12 days after fertilization. There is only one placenta and one amniotic sac, thus creating a high-risk environment where fetal demise of one or both twins can occur in up to 50% of cases. This type of twinning is suspected when only one yolk sac is seen but two fetuses are visible. No intervening membrane is found.

D. In conjoined twins, the fertilized egg does not divide until 13 days or later after fertilization, resulting in fusion of certain body parts of the twins with one another.

Question 1

True. Two fertilized eggs will have individual placentas.

Question 2

True. A monozygotic pregnancy can result in dichorionic twins if the division of the fertilized egg occurs in the first 3 days after fertilization.

Question 3

True. In the first trimester, visualization of two separate sacs indicates two separate placentas, and is therefore dichorionic.

Question 4

False. The chorion differentiates before 4 days and division of the fertilized egg after 4 days from fertilization results in monochorionic twins.

Question 5

True. The incidence is about 70% for dizygotic and 30% for monozygotic twins in the absence of assisted reproduction techniques.

Question 6

True. The existence of intertwin vascular communication is much higher in twins who share one placenta.

Question 7

False. The lambda sign or chorionic peak sign is found in dichorionic twins where two contiguous placentas produce a triangular placental peak at the point of contact.

Question 8

True. In late pregnancy, it may be difficult to distinguish separate placentas using other criteria. Discordant sexes confirm the dizygotic nature of the pregnancy.

Question 9

False. The presence of a dividing amniotic membrane prevents fetal entanglement. This problem is more common in monoamniotic gestation.

Question 10

False. Conjoined twins can only occur in monochorionic monoamniotic gestations where the fertilized egg divided 13 days or more post fertilization.

■ Suggested Readings

Lee YM, Cleary-Goldman J, Thaker HM, et al. Antenatal sonographic prediction of twin chorionicity. Am J Obstet Gynecol 2006;195:863–868

Shetty A, Smith AP. The sonographic diagnosis of chorionicity. Prenat Diagn 2005;25:735–740

Wood SL, St Onge R, Connors G, et al. Evaluation of the twin peak or lambda sign in determining chorionicity in multiple pregnancy. Obstet Gynecol 1996;88:6–12

Top Tips

- Determination of chorionicity and amnionicity is most accurate in the first trimester. Surveillance, prognosis, and subsequent management of the pregnancy depend upon the accuracy of these findings.

- Closer surveillance of monochorionic pregnancies is warranted due to the higher incidence of fetal complications (compared to the incidence with dichorionic pregnancies).

- The identification of discordant sexes is the most definitive proof of dizygosity and, therefore, dichorionicity.

Details 3

■ Case

A 22-year-old woman with vague abdominal pain and vaginal spotting. Transverse and transvaginal images of the uterus are provided. Which ONE of the following is the most likely diagnosis?
   A. Early normal pregnancy
   B. Ovarian mature follicle
   C. Corpus luteum cyst
   D. Tubal ectopic pregnancy

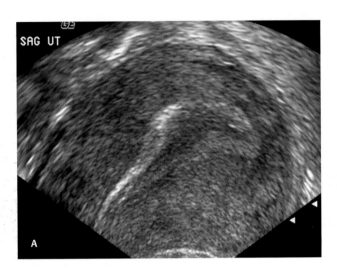
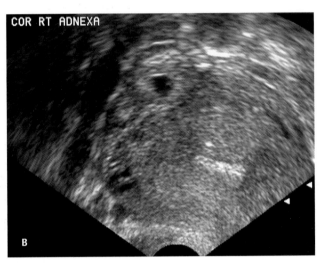

■ The following questions pertain to ectopic pregnancy.

1. What is the discriminatory serum beta-human chorionic gonadotropin (hCG) level at which an intrauterine gestational sac is expected?
2. The MOST appropriate treatment for patients with an ectopic pregnancy who are hemodynamically stable is _____.
3. A fluid collection in the uterus that is associated with an ectopic pregnancy is referred to as what?
4. Vascularity around a suspected ectopic pregnancy is referred to as _____.
5. In a normal pregnancy, serum levels of beta-hCG typically double with what frequency?

6. The MOST common location for an ectopic pregnancy is _____.
7. An ectopic pregnancy that implants in the first 1 to 2 cm of the Fallopian tube is referred to as _____.
8. Which type of ectopic pregnancy can be confused with an abortion in progress?
9. An ectopic pregnancy implanted within the peritoneal cavity is referred to as _____.
10. An ectopic pregnancy that is associated with a concomitant intrauterine pregnancy is referred to as _____.

■ Answers and Explanations

D. Correct! This patient has a tubal ectopic pregnancy. No gestational sac is seen in the endometrial cavity, and the endometrium itself is thickened. The intact gestational sac is extrauterine in location and demonstrates a typical echogenic chorionic ring.

Other choices and discussion

A. While the findings in the uterus may be seen in a very early intrauterine gestation prior to the appearance of a gestational sac, the adnexal findings favor a tubal ectopic pregnancy.

B. The diagnosis of a mature ovarian follicle is made in the setting of a negative pregnancy test. Additionally, the adnexal mass in this case has a thick rind of echogenic chorionic ring, which would not be seen in a mature follicle.

C. A corpus luteum cyst can be seen in both pregnant and nonpregnant patients. However, the echogenic ring seen here is more consistent with an ectopic pregnancy. Note also that the cystic structure that could represent the corpus luteum cyst is not within the ovary.

Question 1

The value recently suggested by the Society of Radiologists in Ultrasound consensus panel as the discriminatory level at which an intrauterine gestation is expected is 3000 mIU/mL.

Question 2

Methotrexate is given to hemodynamically stable patients with ectopic pregnancies who are willing and able to comply with post-treatment follow up and who have hCG level < 5000 mIU/mL, no embryo with cardiac activity, and an ectopic mass size < 3 to 4 cm (hCG and size criteria may vary from institution to institution).

Question 3

A fluid collection in the uterus that is associated with an ectopic pregnancy is referred to as a pseudo-gestational sac. This is differentiated from a normal intrauterine pregnancy by its central location in the endometrial cavity. Recall that a true gestational sac is eccentric relative to endometrial canal.

Question 4

Vascularity around an ectopic pregnancy is often referred to as a "ring of fire." In ectopic gestations, this finding on color Doppler indicates chorionic vascularity. However, studies have shown that this sign is more commonly seen around corpus luteum cysts than ectopic gestations. Thus, the "ring of fire" is not pathognomonic for an ectopic gestation and, in addition, may be absent in a ruptured ectopic.

Question 5

In a normal pregnancy, serum levels of beta-hCG typically double every 48 hours. The doubling time for serum β-hCG is typically slower for ectopic pregnancies than normal gestations and cannot be used reliably to exclude this diagnosis.

Question 6

Ectopic gestations are most frequently located in the fallopian tubes, with tubal ectopics accounting for about 98% of all ectopic pregnancies. Among all tubal ectopics, implantation in the ampullary portion of the tube is particularly common, with ectopic gestations found in this region 75 to 80% of the time.

Question 7

An ectopic pregnancy that implants within the first 1 to 2 cm of the fallopian tube is referred to as an interstitial pregnancy. The old term "cornual pregnancy" is no longer used for ectopic pregnancies located within the first 1 to 2 cm of the tube, and has been more recently reserved for pregnancies occurring in a bicornuate uterus. Bicornuate uteri can be diagnosed with ultrasound by documenting a uterine fundus with two separate uterine horns and uterine cavities. In cases where the images of the uterine fundus are not optimal, magnetic resonance imaging can be confirmatory.

Question 8

The "cervical ectopic" type of ectopic pregnancy can be confused with an abortion in progress. An ectopic pregnancy that is implanted in the wall of the cervix can be distinguished from an abortion in progress by demonstrating the cervical canal, which is intact in a cervical pregnancy but not in an abortion.

Question 9

An ectopic pregnancy implanted within the peritoneal cavity is referred to as an "abdominal pregnancy." Abdominal pregnancies can result either from rupture of a tubal ectopic or from retrograde progression of the fertilized egg. These ectopics are implanted in the peritoneal cavity. They are sometimes asymptomatic and can be carried into the third trimester.

Question 10

A heterotopic pregnancy is a rare type of ectopic pregnancy resulting from two simultaneous pregnancies with different implantation sites. The most common combination is tubal and intrauterine, but dual tubal pregnancies can occur. Heterotopic pregnancy has increased in incidence from 1:30,000 to 1:3,900 due to the popularity of assisted reproduction techniques, which carry a higher risk of extrauterine pregnancy.

■ Suggested Readings

Doubilet PM, Benson CB, Bourne T, Blaivas M. Diagnostic criteria for nonviable pregnancy early in the first trimester. N Engl J Med 2013;369:1443–1451

Top Tips

◆ Ectopic pregnancy should be suspected when the serum beta-hCG is 3000 mIU/mL or more and no intrauterine gestation is seen.

◆ Although a transabdominal ultrasound may not be absolutely necessary in cases where the transvaginal exam adequately documents a normal pregnancy, it is nevertheless still recommended to exclude unexpected adnexal masses or ectopic pregnancies that may be outside of the standard transvaginal field of view.

◆ Ectopic pregnancy occurs most commonly in the fallopian tube (98%), particularly in the ampulla or isthmus.

Details 4

■ Case

A 30-year-old G2P1 asymptomatic patient presents at 18 weeks' gestational age by last menstrual period. She is referred for routine dating ultrasound exam. Presented are two images of the fundus of the uterus, obtained 13 minutes apart. Which ONE of the following is the most likely diagnosis?

  A. Uterine myoma
  B. Focal myometrial contraction (FMC)
  C. Succenturiate placenta
  D. Chorioangioma
  E. Placental hemorrhage

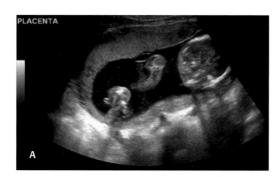
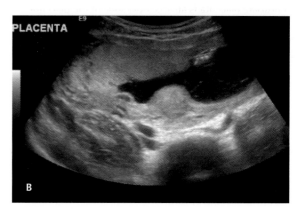

■ The following questions pertain to FMC and mimics.

1. True or False. The most reliable differentiating point between an FMC and a myoma is the transient nature of a FMC.
2. True or False. FMC is asymptomatic.
3. True or False. FMC is also known as a Braxton-Hicks contraction.
4. True or False. Uterine myomas grow during pregnancy due to the influence of beta-human chorionic gonadotropin.
5. True or False. FMC can result in an incorrect cervical length measurement.
6. True or False. FMC is more commonly demonstrated by transvaginal scanning than by transabdominal scanning.
7. True or False. Large myomas can degenerate during pregnancy and cause symptoms of an acute abdomen.
8. True or False. FMC can result in an abortion.
9. True or False. Submucosal myomas can result in placental insufficiency.
10. True or False. Chorioangiomas are avascular.

■ Answers and Explanations

B. Correct! The mass-like structure in the posterior uterine wall is a transient muscular contraction that is asymptomatic and only discovered incidentally during scanning. It distorts only the endometrial surface, not the serosal surface of the uterus. It resolves usually within 30 to 60 minutes. The other choices are incorrect and will not resolve within minutes.

Other choices and discussion

A. Uterine myoma is a tumor arising from the myometrium that can be subserosal, submucosal, or intramural. When subserosal, myomas usually create a distortion of the serosal surface of the uterus but not of the endometrium.

C. Succenturiate placenta is an accessory lobe of the placenta that is usually not attached to the main placenta. It persists until delivery and may be retained if not diagnosed prenatally.

D. Chorioangioma is a benign tumor of the placenta that is not clinically significant unless it becomes enlarged to > 5 cm, in which case it carries a risk for high output failure in the fetus due to arteriovenous shunting.

E. Placental hemorrhage usually occurs within the placental substance, not separate from the main bulk of the placenta as in this case.

Question 1

True. Although FMC may resolve in a few minutes, some can persist for as long as a few hours.

Question 2

True. FMC is typically asymptomatic and discovered incidentally on routine ultrasound.

Question 3

True. FMC and Braxton-Hicks are both sporadic uterine contractions that may be present in the first trimester, but are often not felt until the late second or third trimester.

Question 4

False. Estrogen is the main stimulus for growth of myomas, which occurs in about 20 to 30% of cases of pregnancy, although other factors such as progesterone, human chorionic gonadotropin, and vascular supply may also influence growth. The majority of myomas (50 to 60%) remain stable or show < 10% growth during pregnancy. The radiologist should report the location of myomas, particularly if present in the lower uterine segment, as enlargement of these myomas could complicate vaginal delivery. Additionally, the presence of multiple myomas at the site of placental implantation can cause placental insufficiency and result in intrauterine growth restriction.

Question 5

True. The inaccurate cervical length measurement can occur when FMC or myomas are located near the internal os.

Question 6

False. The large field of view of the transabdominal scan increases the chances of FMC detection.

Question 7

True. Large myomas frequently outstrip their blood supply and undergo what is sometimes painful degeneration.

Question 8

False. FMCs are mild and not forceful enough to result in an abortion.

Question 9

True. Placental insufficiency can occur with submucosal myomas, especially when multiple subplacental myomas are present.

Question 10

False. Chorioangiomas are malformations involving the angioblastic tissues of the placenta. This primary tumor of the placenta is usually echogenic, with evidence of internal vascularity, and is located within the placental substance.

■ Suggested Readings

Tadmor OP, Rabinowitz R, Diamant YZ. Ultrasonic demonstration of local myometerial thickening in early intrauterine pregnancy. Ultrasound Obstet Gynecol 1995;5:44–46

Togashi K, Kawakami S, Kimura I, et al. Sustained uterine contractions: a cause of hypointense myometrial bulging. Radiology 1993;187:707–710

Wilson RL, Worthen NJ. Ultrasonic demonstration of myometrial contractions in intrauterine pregnancy. Am J Roentgenol 1979;132:243–247

Top Tips

◆ FMC is commonly encountered in routine evaluation of early pregnancy. It is always best to reimage the area of suspected FMC at the end of the exam to prove its transient nature. If persistent, follow up study in a few days may be necessary.

◆ Comparing the echogenicity of the contraction to the adjacent myometrium is a simple and accurate way of making the diagnosis. Focal myometrial contraction will have the same echogenicity as the adjacent myometrium, whereas a small or uncomplicated myoma will be relatively hypoechoic.

◆ Although Doppler evaluation has limited value in the assessment of uterine masses, it may be helpful in showing the hypervascularity of a chorioangioma, the relative hypovascularity of a myoma, and the avascular nature of a placental hemorrhage. Occasionally, magnetic resonance imaging is needed to more accurately assess the size or degree of degeneration of a large myoma.

Details 5

■ Case

A 30-year-old G3P3 woman reports to the emergency room complaining of intermittent vaginal bleeding since a normal vaginal delivery 2 weeks prior. Which ONE of the following is the most likely diagnosis?

A. Polyp
B. Endometrial cancer
C. Retained products of conception (RPOC)
D. Uterine myoma

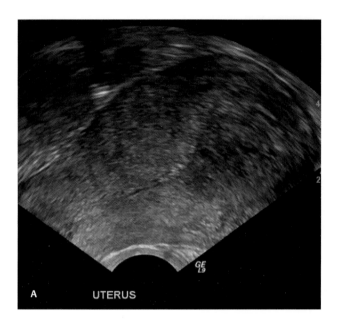
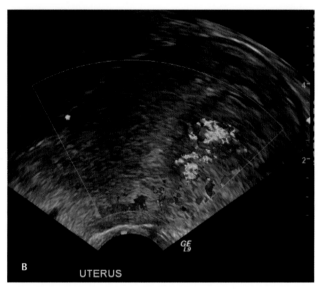

■ The following questions pertain to bleeding after vaginal delivery.

1. True or False. Polyps typically display one central feeding artery.
2. True or False. Myomas have vascularity randomly scattered throughout the mass.
3. True or False. RPOC can manifest as avascular debris in the uterus.
4. True or False. Endometrial cancer is the second most common gynecologic cancer in developed countries.
5. True or False. Hysteroscopy is not as effective as sonohysterography in the diagnostic workup of intrauterine masses.

6. True or False. Routine evaluation for RPOC is recommended after termination of pregnancy.
7. True or False. Asherman syndrome is a known complication of instrumentation of the postabortal uterus.
8. True or False. Measurement of the endometrial thickness is not a good predictor for the presence of RPOC.
9. True or False. Doppler evaluation of intrauterine masses is important in differentiating the nature of the pathology.
10. True or False. Postpartum endometritis should be suspected in the presence of air within the uterine cavity.

■ Answers and Explanations

C. Correct! The presence of a vascularized soft tissue mass within the endometrial cavity in the postpartum period is pathognomonic for RPOC. Without the postpartum history and based only on the ultrasound appearance, all of the other choices are possible differential diagnostic considerations. Biopsy is needed to prove the diagnosis. When interpreting findings in suspected cases of RPOC, only a thin endometrium should be reported as having "no evidence of RPOC."

Other choices and discussion

B. The patient history is not consistent with a polyp. Also, the vascularity of a polyp is usually central and classically has a single feeding vessel.

C. Although endometrial cancer may be seen in premenopausal patients, it is more commonly found in the older and postmenopausal patient.

D. A very vascular uterine myoma that is intracavitary in location could mimic this finding. However, the postpartum history makes this option less likely.

Question 1

True. Although not always present, the presence of a central feeding artery is the classic finding that can differentiate a polyp from the other choices.

Question 2

True. Unlike polyps, myomas are vascularized from the periphery with vessels that are randomly scattered throughout the mass.

Question 3

True. When RPOC is no longer attached to the vascular supply of the uterus, it can mimic blood clots, necrotic tissue, and infected material.

Question 4

True. Endometrial cancer is the most common gynecologic cancer in developed countries but second to cervical cancer in underdeveloped countries.

Question 5

True. Hysteroscopy is very good at defining focal irregularities in the uterine cavity and can distinguish a free-floating echogenic mass from a mass adherent to the uterine wall. It also has the potential to both diagnose and treat during a single procedure. However, saline infusion sonohysterography allows complete visualization of the endometrial cavity and can demonstrate pathology that may be missed on hysteroscopy.

Question 6

False. Routine evaluation for RPOC is likely to result in false positive diagnoses and unnecessary interventions, as RPOC do not always lead to morbidity. Evaluation should be reserved for patients with bleeding that is heavy or prolonged, and for patients with fever, uterine tenderness, or abdominopelvic pain. Complete evacuation of products of conception should demonstrate an empty uterine cavity with ultrasound.

Question 7

True. Uterine synechiae, also known as Asherman syndrome, are due to scarring within the uterine cavity. They range from inconsequential filmy adhesions to very thick scars that obliterate the endometrium, leading to amenorrhea or hypomenorrhea and infertility. To visualize the band of Asherman syndrome, the uterine cavity should be distended with fluid during saline infusion sonohysterography. Without fluid distension, this can only be suspected but not confirmed.

Question 8

True. Measurement of endometrial thickness following miscarriage or pregnancy termination should not be used as a test for RPOC or as a predictor of the need for surgical intervention. Sonographic findings correlate poorly with clinical symptoms and histologic results, as the appearance of necrotic decidua and blood clots can mimic RPOC.

Question 9

True. Doppler can be helpful in determining if viable tissue is present in the uterus and can also help decide if surgical intervention is necessary. However, Doppler characteristics are nonspecific for the various vascular masses and are not helpful in masses where no flow is demonstrated.

Question 10

True. Although the diagnosis of postpartum endometritis is usually made clinically, the diagnosis can be suggested if the ultrasound findings include intrauterine debris mixed with echogenic air trapped in the endometrial cavity.

Top Tips

♦ RPOC refers to placental and/or fetal tissue that remains in the uterus after spontaneous pregnancy loss, planned pregnancy termination, or delivery. This tissue may spontaneously pass or need evacuation by dilation and curettage, when persistent or complicated by bleeding or infection.

♦ The presence of a focal echogenic abnormality in the endometrium, particularly with evidence of blood flow by Doppler imaging, is the best predictor of RPOC. However, the decision to intervene should be based on clinical need rather than on an isolated ultrasound finding.

♦ The goal of the ultrasound evaluation is to determine whether RPOC is the probable source of the woman's symptoms or whether another diagnosis is more likely. Other possible diagnoses include unsuspected uterine vascular malformations, polyps, or myomas (that may have been undiagnosed prenatally).

Image Rich 1

■ Case

Match the appropriate diagnosis to the provided first trimester ultrasound image.

A. Perigestational hemorrhage
B. Chorionic bump
C. Intradecidual sign
D. Open rhombencephalon

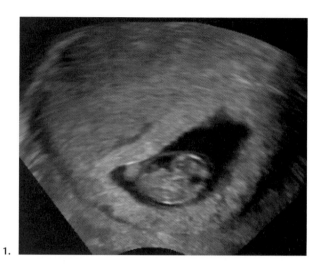

1.

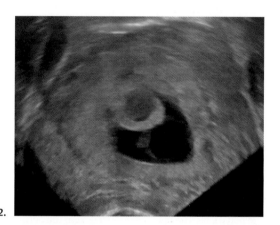

2.

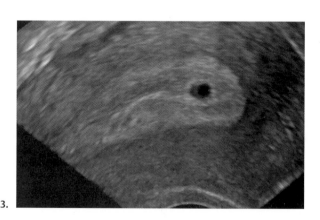

3.

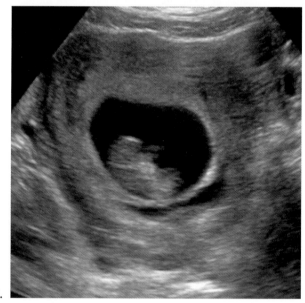

4.

■ Answers and Explanations

1. D. Open rhombencephalon. The open rhombencephalon is a small cystic structure (3 to 4 mm) in the posterior aspect of the cranium, which corresponds to the rhomboid fossa or hindbrain. The open rhombencephalon is a normal first trimester finding in all fetuses, and may be seen starting at the 8th to 10th menstrual weeks. It develops into the normally proportioned fourth ventricle after the 11th menstrual week when the vermis and cerebellar hemispheres form the posterior roof of the fourth ventricle. Until that time, the rhombencephalon remains open. The rhombencephalon disappears late in the first trimester. No follow up of this finding is necessary, unless a perfect midsagittal view cannot be obtained on the initial exam. In that instance, a confirmatory test is indicated later in the first trimester.

2. B. Chorionic bump. The chorionic bump is a relatively uncommon (incidence 0.7%), irregular, convex bulge from the choriodecidual surface into the first trimester gestational sac. On serial sonograms, most bumps become hypoechoic and smaller over time with no untoward pregnancy outcome. However, the chorionic bump is associated with a guarded prognosis in early pregnancy due to its potential correlation with nonviability. Thus, this finding should be followed until a normal live embryo is documented in the first trimester.

Although the etiology of the chorionic bump is unknown, it is reasonable to assume that it represents a hematoma or small area of hemorrhage that resolves with time. On the other hand, the bump may represent a blighted second pregnancy undergoing resorption, and has been observed in some infertility treatment patients.

3. C. Intradecidual sign. The intradecidual sign is produced by the implantation of the blastocyst on one side of the decidua in early intrauterine pregnancy, resulting in an eccentric position of the gestational sac relative to the endometrial canal. When present, this sign signifies that an intrauterine fluid collection is due to pregnancy even before definite visualization of a yolk sac or embryo. The development of an early pregnancy should be confirmed by the eventual development of a yolk sac and embryo.

The intradecidual sign is usually seen at five to six menstrual weeks, but may be absent in 35% of normal gestational sacs. Its eccentric location within the endometrial cavity helps to distinguish it from the pseudogestational sac of ectopic pregnancy, which is centrally located within the endometrial cavity.

4. A. PGH. PGH will appear on ultrasound as a fluid collection in the intrauterine cavity that separates the decidua capsularis from the chorion laeve. PGH is synonymous with subchorionic hemorrhage and includes the suspected peri-implantation hemorrhage that may be seen in the uterine cavity in a minority of first trimester gestations. PGH is the most common cause of first trimester bleeding and occurs in 18% of pregnancies. The vast majority of PGH resolves spontaneously, but if the hemorrhage occupies more than two-thirds of the chorionic sac diameter, there is a nearly 20% rate of spontaneous abortion.

PGH should be differentiated from the chorioamniotic separation that may be seen as a normal developmental variation up to 17 to 18 weeks' gestational age. This latter finding usually subsequently resolves when fusion of membranes occurs. PGH may be difficult to differentiate from twin fetal demise, unless a prior ultrasound exam had documented a yolk sac/embryo in the fluid collection.

Follow up in 1 to 2 weeks is recommended to document progression or resolution of hemorrhage.

■ Suggested Readings

Bronshtein M, Zimmer EZ, Blazer S. Isolated large fourth ventricle in early pregnancy—a possible benign transient phenomenon. Prenat Diagn 1998;18:997–1000

Doubilet PM, Benson CB, Bourne T, et al. Diagnostic criteria for nonviable pregnancy early in the first trimester. N Engl J Med 2013;369:1443–1451

Harris RD, Couto C, Karpovsky C, Blanchette Porter MM, Ouhilal S. The chorionic bump: a first-trimester pregnancy sonographic finding associated with a guarded prognosis. J Ultrasound Med 2006;25:757–763

SECTION XII US/REPRODUCTIVE/ ENDOCRINOLOGY IMAGING

Top Tips

- A gestational sac should be present in the uterine cavity when serum beta-human chorionic gonadotropin levels reach 3000 mIU/mL. A yolk sac is usually detectable once the mean sac diameter measurement reaches 10 mm, and an embryo should be present at a mean sac diameter measurement of 25 mm or more.

- Cardiac activity should be detected in an embryo with a crown–rump length of 7 mm or more.

- Although signs of normal pregnancy development can be seen prior to the detection of a yolk sac or live embryo, follow up ultrasound examination should be performed until these benchmarks are demonstrated.

Image Rich 2

■ Case

Match the appropriate diagnosis to the provided image of an adnexal mass in a nonpregnant patient.

A. Hydrosalpinx
B. Ovarian hyperstimulation syndrome
C. Hemorrhagic cyst
D. Teratoma

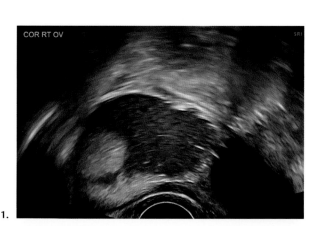

1.

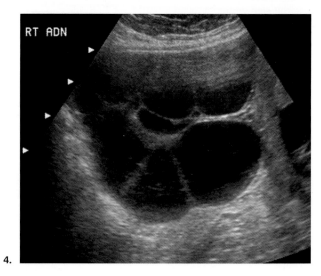

2.

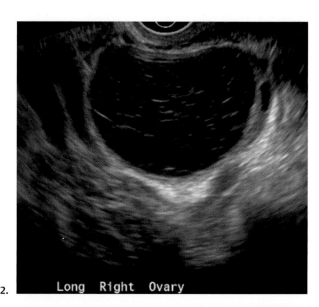

3.

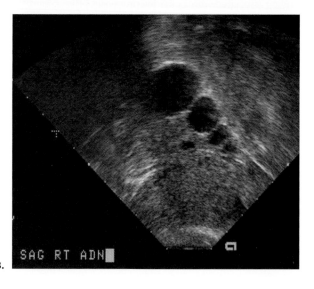

4.

■ Answers and Explanations

1. D. Teratoma. The "teratoma" is the most common type of germ cell tumor, and refers to a neoplasm that differentiates toward somatic-type cell populations—ectoderm, endoderm and mesoderm—that can be typical of either adult or embryonic development. Teratomas, composed of tissues that range from immature to well-differentiated, are foreign to the anatomic site in which they are found. Most, but not all, teratomas are benign. In addition, most are cystic and composed of mature differentiated elements; these are better known as dermoid cysts.

Dermoid cysts account for > 95% of all ovarian teratomas and are the most common ovarian tumor in the second and third decades of life. They are bilateral in about 15% of cases. Most women with dermoid cysts are asymptomatic. Larger dermoids are more likely to be symptomatic, and torsion may occur. Dermoid cysts have a characteristic ultrasound appearance, which allows for reasonably accurate noninvasive diagnosis in most cases.

2. C. Hemorrhagic cyst. The majority of hemorrhagic ovarian cysts are physiologic and result during the normal formation of a corpus luteum following ovulation. These cysts can reach 5 to 12 cm in diameter. The sonographic appearance of a hemorrhagic cyst is highly dependent upon the timing of detection. In the acute phase of hemorrhage, the cyst is uniformly echogenic. With involution, there are typically increased internal echoes and septations within the cyst, secondary to debris and resolving clot.

In the absence of pain or intraperitoneal bleeding, observation for a period of 2 weeks to 3 months is appropriate. Most hemorrhagic cysts will involute during this observation period. If the hemorrhagic cyst persists, consider endometrioma as a diagnostic possibility.

3. A. Hydrosalpinx. A hydrosalpinx is most often tubular in shape. However, depending on the plane of imaging, it may instead appear as a series of cysts of decreasing caliber—known as the "string of pearls" sign. The visualized nodules are due to thickened endosalpingeal folds and may raise concern for ovarian malignancy, if one does not recognize the extraovarian location of the mass.

In addition, the hydrosalpinx may have septations or nodules in its wall. These "septations" are not true septations, but actually represent the wall of the tube folded in on itself. Typically, the septations will appear to be incomplete. Hydrosalpinx should always be included in the differential diagnosis when incomplete or partial septations are identified.

On gross examination, a hydrosalpinx is frequently filled with clear fluid that is sometimes the chronic sequela of infection or hemorrhage. However, when filled with debris in the acute phase of pelvic inflammatory disease, it may be difficult to differentiate hydrosalpinx from pyosalpinx or hematosalpinx with ultrasound. Acute pelvic pain may resolve after conservative management of the acute infection, but the hydrosalpinx may persist on ultrasound (often remaining asymptomatic.)

4. B. OHSS. OHSS is an exaggerated ovarian response to ovulation induction, frequently performed in the setting of planned in vitro fertilization. However, OHSS may be seen occasionally during normal pregnancy in women with a low threshold for human chorionic gonadotropin stimulation.

OHSS is characterized by bilateral ovarian enlargement with multiple follicular and corpus luteum cysts, abdominal distention and discomfort, mild nausea, and, less frequently, vomiting and diarrhea. In severe cases, ascites and pleural effusions may develop. When associated with normal pregnancy, patients are often asymptomatic.

Resolution typically occurs after withdrawal of the human chorionic gonadotropin source, which may be > 6 weeks postpartum.

■ Suggested Readings

Ayhan A, Bukulmez O, Genc C, Karamursel BS, Mature cystic teratomas of the ovary: case series from one institution over 34 years. Eur J Obstet Gynecol Reprod Biol 2000;88:153–157

Patel MD, Acord DL, Young SW. Likelihood ratio of sonographic findings in discriminating hydrosalpinx from other adnexal masses. Am J Roentgenol 2006;186:1033–1038

Valentin L, Ameye L, Jurkovic D, et al. Which extrauterine pelvic masses are difficult to correctly classify as benign or malignant on the basis of ultrasound findings and is there a way of making a correct diagnosis? Ultrasound Obstet Gynecol 2006;27:438–444

SECTION XII
US/REPRODUCTIVE/
ENDOCRINOLOGY IMAGING

Top Tips

◆ The adnexa contains the ovary and fallopian tube, as well as associated vessels, ligaments, and connective tissue. In addition to these structures, pathology in this area may arise from the uterus, bowel, retroperitoneum, or as metastasis from another site—typically the breast or stomach.

◆ Adnexal masses may be found in females of all ages. The overall risk of malignancy within an adnexal mass increases with age after menarche and is reportedly 6 to 11% in premenopausal women and 29 to 35% in postmenopausal women.

◆ Past medical history and clinical findings can provide important predictive information in the diagnosis of adnexal masses. For example, while ascites identified on physical exam can be associated with both benign and malignant processes, it is more common with malignancy.

Image Rich 3

■ Case

Match the appropriate diagnosis to the provided fetal head image.

    A. Schizencephaly
    B. Dandy-Walker malformation
    C. Trisomy 21
    D. Alobar holoprosencephaly

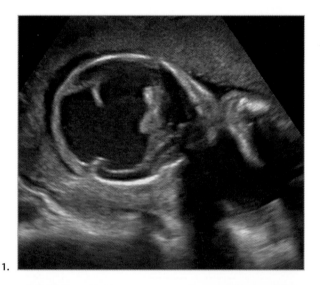

1.

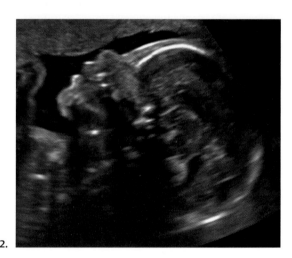

2.

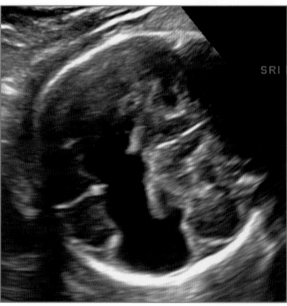

3.

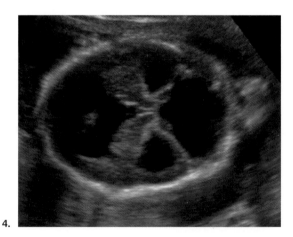

4.

■ Answers and Explanations

1. D. Alobar holoprosencephaly. The holoprosencephaly sequence develops from failure of the prosencephalon (forebrain) to differentiate into two cerebral hemispheres and lateral ventricles between the fourth and eighth postmenstrual weeks. This failure results in partial to complete fusion of the cerebral hemispheres, in addition to lateral ventricles that partially or fully communicate across the midline. The three main types of holoprosencephaly are, in decreasing order of severity: alobar, semilobar, and lobar. Variable degrees of facial dysmorphism may also be present, with alobar holoprosencephaly associated with the most severe facial dysmorphism.

Alobar holoprosencephaly is a lethal anomaly characterized by complete failure of cleavage of the prosencephalon. The cerebral hemispheres are fused, there is a single large midline fluid collection (ventricle), and there is absence of the corpus callosum and falx cerebri. The cerebrum is smaller than normal, and the thalami are usually completely fused.

Alobar holoprosencephaly has been diagnosed as early as menstrual week 10 and has been associated with trisomy of chromosome 18.

2. C. Trisomy 21 (Down syndrome). Down syndrome is the most common autosomal trisomy among live births, with an incidence of 1 in every 700 live births. Trisomy 21 is associated with advanced maternal age—35% of infants with trisomy 21 are born to mothers > 35 years of age. Mean survival is 20 years. Cardiac defects are common, affecting 40% of infants with Down syndrome, and severe cardiac anomalies are associated with the poorest survival.

Approximately one-third of fetuses with trisomy 21 have one or more sonographically detectable structural malformations in the following systems: cardiovascular, central nervous system, gastrointestinal, and craniofacial structures. In particular, nonvisualization of the nasal bone (shown in the test case) at around 13 weeks' gestation is a specific finding in fetuses with Down syndrome. Also, by 15 to 20 weeks' gestation, 40 to 50% of fetuses with Down syndrome will have a thickened nuchal fold of ≥ 6 mm. These imaging findings are useful adjuncts to screening, especially when other studies such as the quad screen show a borderline or high risk of Down syndrome.

3. A. Schizencephaly. Schizencephaly is a rare disorder of neuronal migration in which one or more fluid-filled clefts in the cerebral hemisphere communicate with the lateral ventricle. It can be unilateral or bilateral, and frequently is seen in association with microcephaly and other brain anomalies.

Two types of schizencephaly have been described. Type 1 is characterized by small symmetrical clefts, with the edges of the clefts fused within a pia-ependymal seam that is continuous with the ependyma of the lateral ventricle. Type 2 is characterized by extensive clefts extending from the ventricle to the surface of the brain and subarachnoid space, with the edges of the clefts not fused.

The degree of functional impairment in patients with schizencephaly depends on the location of the cleft, whether it is unilateral or bilateral, whether it is type 1 or 2, and whether there are associated malformations.

4. B. DWM. DWM refers to a complex developmental anomaly of the fourth ventricle that occurs at the sixth to seventh postmenstrual week; thus, it is perhaps easy to predict many of the concurrent anomalies. The incidence of DWM is 1 in 30,000 births.

Sonographic findings of DWM include dilation of the fourth ventricle, a large posterior fossa cyst extending from the cisterna magna to the fourth ventricle (Dandy-Walker cyst), hypoplasia or complete agenesis of the cerebellar vermis, an elevated tentorium, and, frequently, dilation of the third and lateral ventricles. Hydrocephaly is present in three-quarters of cases of DWM, and DWM is present in up to 12% of cases of congenital hydrocephaly. In the syndromic form of DWM, malformations of the heart, face, limbs, and/or gastrointestinal or genitourinary system may be present.

■ Suggested Readings

Bethune M. Literature review and suggested protocol for managing ultrasound soft markers for Down syndrome: thickened nuchal fold, echogenic bowel, shortened femur, shortened humerus, pyelectasis and absent or hypoplastic nasal bone. Australas Radiol 2007;51:218–222

Guibaud L, Larroque A, Ville D, et al. Prenatal diagnosis of "isolated" Dandy-Walker malformation: imaging findings and prenatal counselling. Prenat Diagn 2012;32:185–193

International Society of Ultrasound in Obstetrics & Gynecology Education Committee. Sonographic examination of the fetal central nervous system: guidelines for performing the "basic examination" and the "fetal neurosonogram." Ultrasound Obstet Gynecol 2007;29:109–116

Kutuk MS, Gorkem SB, Bayram A, Doganay S, Canpolat M, Basbug M. Prenatal diagnosis and postnatal outcome of schizencephaly. J Child Neurol 2015;30:1388–1394

Top Tips

♦ In the fetal brain, it is recommended that three structures are routinely documented and commented upon in the ultrasound imaging report:

♦ Ventricular atria—should be no more than 10 mm in transverse diameter; any measurements > 10 mm should be reported as ventriculomegaly

♦ Cavum septi pellucidi—should always be present in the fetus; no measurements are needed

♦ Cisterna magna—should always be present in a normal fetus and should be no more than 10 mm in depth at midline

♦ "Soft markers" refer to ultrasound findings typically associated with normal fetuses, have no clinical sequelae, and are transient. Examples of soft markers include slightly shortened humerus/femur, echogenic intracardiac foci, echogenic bowel, and urinary tract dilation. Isolated soft markers are identified in 11 to 17% of normal fetuses. The prevalence is higher in aneuploid fetuses, and the likelihood of aneuploidy is significantly increased when more than one marker is present.

♦ Fetuses with sonographic evidence of a structural anomaly are at increased risk of having a chromosomal abnormality, with the magnitude of risk highly dependent upon the specific malformation.

Image Rich 4

■ **Case**

Match the appropriate diagnosis to the provided phase of the normal endometrium

    A. Secretory
    B. Late follicular
    C. Periovulatory
    D. Early follicular

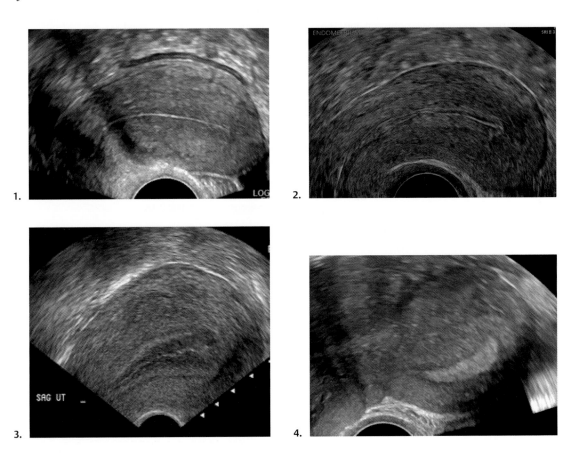

1.   2.

3.   4.

■ Answers and Explanations

1. D. Early follicular. After menses, the endometrium appears as a thin hyperechoic line as a result of shedding of the functional layer. Proliferation from the basal layer begins soon thereafter and continues throughout the follicular phase under the influence of increasing estradiol secretion.

The early follicular phase is the ideal time for performance of transvaginal sonography, as pathology that might increase the thickness of the endometrium can be easily distinguished from the normally thin endometrium. Measurements are usually not necessary, as the thin endometrial stripe is characteristic. If workflow issues make early follicular phase examination impractical, the ultrasound study may be done at any time as long as the option for follow up in the follicular phase is offered, if needed. The demonstration of the dynamic changes of the endometrium is sufficient to exclude pathology.

2. B. Late follicular. Increasing proliferation of the basal layer results in a "triple-line" appearance on ultrasonography. The functional layer becomes hypoechoic in contrast to the thin echogenic basal layers. By the end of the follicular phase, the endometrium measures between 8 and 12 mm.

3. C. Periovulatory. The "triple" line is at its thickest just before ovulation. The thin echogenic basal layer remains the same, but the hypoechoic functional layer increases in thickness. Measurements should be made that include the echogenic basal layer.

4. A. Secretory. After ovulation, the "triple-line" disappears and is replaced by a hyperechoic stripe of 10 to 14 mm in thickness. The brightness of this stripe appears to be related to increasing length and tortuosity of endometrial glands with mucin and glycogen storage within the functionalis layer.

■ Suggested Readings

Bakos O, Lundkvist O, Bergh T. Transvaginal sonographic evaluation of endometrial growth and texture in spontaneous ovulatory cycles—a descriptive study. Hum Reprod 1993;8:799–806

Fleischer AC, Kalemeris GC, Entman SS. Sonographic depiction of the endometrium during normal cycles. Ultrasound Med Biol 1986;12:271–277

Randall JM, Fisk NM, McTavish A, Templeton AA. Transvaginal ultrasonic assessment of endometrial growth in spontaneous and hyperstimulated menstrual cycles. Br J Obstet Gynaecol 1989;96:954–959

Top Tips

◆ In a premenopausal woman, the endometrial stripe is thinnest during the follicular phase (5 mm) and thickest in the midsecretory phase when it can measure up to 13 mm. Absolute measurements are not as important as the demonstration of the dynamic changes of the endometrium throughout the menstrual cycle. In postmenopausal women, 5 mm is usually the upper limit of normal for endometrial thickness, although it may be up to 8 mm when the patient is on hormonal replacement. Beyond this limit, further evaluation with magnetic resonance imaging or endometrial biopsy is recommended.

◆ A "triple line" indicates thickening of the endometrium due to the increase in the functionalis layer as it approaches ovulation. The basal echogenic layer remains stable.

◆ The early proliferative phase is the ideal time to perform endovaginal sonography, when the endometrium is at its thinnest.

Image Rich 5

■ Case

Match the appropriate diagnosis to the provided ultrasound image of the nongravid uterus.

- A. Endometrial polyp
- B. Fibroid
- C. Adenomyosis
- D. Endometrial cancer

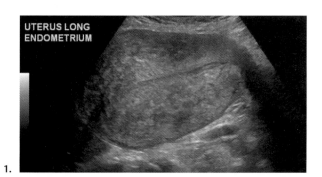

1.

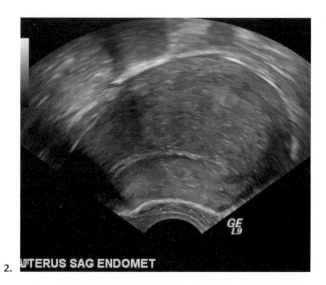

2.

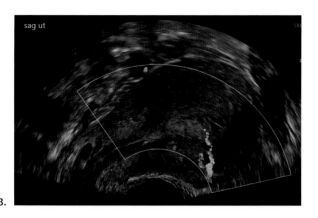

3.

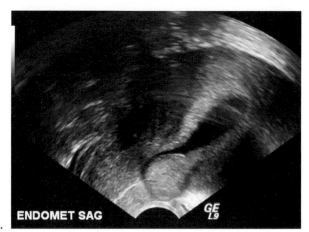

4.

■ Answers and Explanations

1. C. Adenomyosis. Adenomyosis is a disorder in which endometrial glands and stroma are present within the uterine musculature. The ectopic endometrial tissue appears to induce hypertrophy and hyperplasia of the surrounding myometrium, which results in a diffusely enlarged uterus. The uterus only rarely exceeds the size of a pregnant uterus at 12 weeks of gestation.

Adenomyosis is more common in parous than nulliparous women. It typically presents as heavy menstrual bleeding and painful menstruation, occurring in approximately 60% and 25% of women, respectively. Chronic pelvic pain may occur. Symptoms typically develop between the ages of 40 and 50 years. Both transvaginal ultrasound and magnetic resonance imaging are increasingly used for clinical decision making. With both modalities, evidence of adenomyosis includes asymmetric thickening of the myometrium (with the posterior myometrium typically thicker), myometrial cysts, linear striations radiating from the endometrium, loss of a clear endomyometrial border, and increased myometrial heterogeneity.

Ultrasound diagnosis is predicated upon the presenting symptoms outlined above. When clinical symptoms are suggestive, the contour of the uterus is usually the first clue, followed by other signs. Myometrial cysts are highly suggestive.

2. D. Endometrial cancer. This is uterine cancer. Uterine cancer is the most common gynecologic malignancy in developed countries and is the second most common gynecologic cancer in developing countries (cervical cancer is more common). Adenocarcinoma of the endometrium is the most common histologic type of uterine cancer. Endometrial carcinoma is most common in women who are postmenopausal and with increasing age in premenopausal women.

Endometrial carcinoma typically presents with abnormal uterine bleeding. In postmenopausal women, transvaginal ultrasound evaluation of the endometrial thickness (normally ≤ 5 mm) may be used as an initial study to evaluate for endometrial neoplasia in selected women. In premenopausal women with suspected endometrial neoplasia, sonographic measurement of endometrial thickness cannot be used as an alternative to endometrial sampling. Differentiating endometrial hyperplasia from carcinoma relies upon the identification of smooth, homogeneous thickening of the endometrium in hyperplasia, in contrast to the irregular, heterogeneous thickening present in carcinoma. Sonohysterography can help with this distinction.

3. A. Endometrial polyp. Endometrial polyps are one of the most common etiologies of abnormal vaginal bleeding in both premenopausal and postmenopausal women. Polyps consist of localized hyperplastic overgrowth of endometrial glands and stroma around a vascular core that form a sessile or pedunculated projection from the surface of the endometrium. They can develop anywhere in the uterine cavity.

Polyps develop in 2 to 36% of postmenopausal women treated with tamoxifen. Approximately 95% of endometrial polyps are benign. However, malignant transformation of an endometrial polyp is more frequent in women on tamoxifen. Premalignant or malignant histology has also been associated with polyps > 1.5 cm in diameter.

4. B. Fibroid. This is a uterine leiomyoma. Uterine leiomyomas (fibroids or myomas) are the most common pelvic tumor in women. Leiomyomas are benign monoclonal tumors arising from the smooth muscle cells of the myometrium. They arise in reproductive-aged women and typically present with symptoms of heavy or prolonged menstrual bleeding or pelvic pain and pressure. Uterine fibroids may also have reproductive effects (e.g., infertility and adverse pregnancy outcomes).

Fibroids are often described according to their location in the uterus, although many fibroids have more than one location designation. An International Federation of Gynecology and Obstetrics (FIGO) staging scheme for fibroid location has been proposed:

- Submucosal myoma (FIGO type 0, 1, 2)—These leiomyomas derive from myometrial cells just below the endometrium and protrude into the uterine cavity. A type 0 fibroid is completely intracavitary, a type I has < 50% of its volume in the uterine wall, and a type II has 50% or more of its volume in the uterine wall. Types 0 and I are hysteroscopically resectable.
- Intramural myoma (FIGO type 3, 4, 5)—These leiomyomas develop from within the uterine wall and may enlarge sufficiently to distort the uterine cavity or serosal surface. Some fibroids can be transmural and extend from the serosal to the mucosal surface.
- Subserosal myoma (FIGO type 6, 7)—These leiomyomas originate from the myometrium at the serosal surface of the uterus. They can have a broad or pedunculated base and may be intraligamentary (i.e., extending between the folds of the broad ligament).
- Cervical myoma (FIGO type 8)—These leiomyomas are located in the cervix, rather than the uterine corpus.

Transvaginal ultrasound has high sensitivity (95 to 100%) for detecting myomas in uteri < 10 weeks' size, and is the most widely used modality due to its broad availability and cost-effectiveness.

Top Tips

- Polyp, fibroid, adenomyosis, and cancer can all manifest as vaginal bleeding involving the nongravid uterus.
- Ultrasound can help in narrowing this differential diagnosis. Rapid growth, increased vascularity, pain, and bleeding in a "fibroid" raises suspicion for leiomyosarcoma, which is typically large and demonstrates a high degree of necrosis.
- If ultrasound findings are equivocal, sonohysterography or magnetic resonance imaging should be performed for further evaluation. For small submucosal myomas, sonohysterography can outline the endometrial encroachment of the mass. Magnetic resonance imaging is more accurate in defining the borders of the myoma prior to resection, especially in women who desire to preserve fertility.

More Challenging 1

■ Case

Grayscale transverse images of the right upper quadrant (a) and Doppler transverse images of the right upper quadrant (b) are shown.

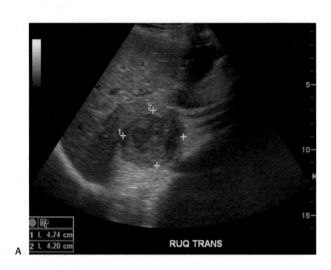

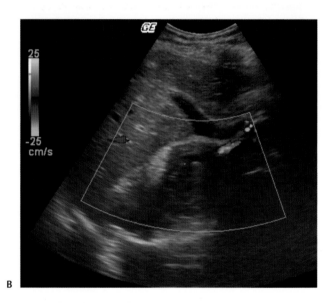

■ Questions

1. Which of the following is(are) included in the differential diagnosis of the mass pictured in the test case? (Select ALL that apply.)
   A. Renal cell carcinoma
   B. Adrenal adenoma
   C. Hepatocellular carcinoma
   D. Malignant thrombus
   E. Myelolipoma

2. Which ONE of the following is the most common adrenal mass detected incidentally on sonography?
   A. Pheochromocytoma
   B. Adrenal cortical carcinoma
   C. Myelolipoma
   D. Adenoma
   E. Metastasis

3. What is the most common location and what is the most common mechanism for adrenal hemorrhage?
   A. Left-sided predominance due to direct arterial supply from the aorta
   B. Left-sided predominance due to splenic compression
   C. Right-sided predominance due to circuitous venous outflow into the right renal vein
   D. Right-sided predominance due to direct compression from the liver
   E. No lateral predilection exists with adrenal hemorrhage

■ Answers and Explanations

Question 1

A. Correct! Renal cell carcinoma is possible. The right kidney is included in the evaluation of the right upper quadrant with ultrasound. In particular, lesions arising from the upper pole may be in close proximity to the liver and the adrenal gland.

B. Correct! Adrenal adenoma is possible. It is difficult to visualize the adrenal gland routinely on ultrasound. However, a sufficiently large mass can be seen sonographically. Most adrenal masses have nonspecific sonographic appearances, and further characterization with computed tomography (CT) and/or magnetic resonance imaging (MRI) should be performed upon discovery.

C. Correct! Hepatocellular carcinoma is possible. Careful attention should be given as to whether a lesion is an exophytic mass arising from the liver or an extrinsic mass arising adjacent to the liver.

D. Correct! Malignant thrombus is possible. When the inferior vena cava is distended with malignant thrombus, that thrombus may be seen on ultrasound. Malignant thrombus sometimes occurs in the setting of metastatic renal cell carcinoma. When it does, the thrombus often demonstrates internal flow on Doppler. This flow differentiates it from bland thrombus.

E. Correct! Myelolipoma is possible. Myelolipomas are benign masses that contain fat and hematopoietic elements resembling bone marrow. This often results in a predominantly hyperechoic, but heterogeneous, mass.

Question 2

D. Correct! Adenomas are the most common adrenal masses and are typically incidental findings on abdominal imaging. Commonly, the ultrasound appearance is that of a homogeneously hypoechoic mass. Due to the varied and nonspecific appearance of an adenoma, however, further imaging with adrenal protocol CT and/or adrenal MRI may be necessary for complete characterization.

Other choices and discussion

A. Pheochromocytomas are rare tumors that often present as large masses and may be symptomatic due to catecholamine release.

B. Adrenal cortical carcinoma is a rare condition. When it does occur, the mass is often hyperfunctioning and symptomatic.

C. Myelolipomas are less common than adrenal adenomas. They are typically discovered incidentally. The sonographic appearance reflects that of macroscopic fat, with elements of hyperechoic tissue.

E. The adrenal glands are the fourth most common site in the body for metastatic involvement. However, even in patients with a history of carcinoma, adenomas statistically remain the most likely adrenal masses.

Question 3

D. Correct! Adrenal hemorrhage is more commonly right-sided. This right-sided predominance is thought to result from hepatic compression between the liver and the spine.

The other choices are incorrect. The adrenal veins drain directly into the inferior vena cava, not the renal vein.

■ Suggested Readings

Dunnick NR, Korobkin M, Francis I. Adrenal radiology: distinguishing benign from malignant adrenal masses. Am J Roentgenol 1996;167:861–867

Murphy BJ, Casillas J, Yrizarry JM. Traumatic adrenal hemorrhage: radiologic findings. Radiology 1998;169:701–703

Top Tips

◆ Adrenal masses are difficult to visualize on ultrasound but may be seen when large. The most common adrenal mass is an adenoma.

◆ Complete adrenal characterization with ultrasound alone is difficult. Most masses should have further characterization with CT and/or MRI.

◆ Adrenal hemorrhage is more commonly right-sided due to hepatic compression.

More Challenging 2

■ Case

Grayscale longitudinal images (a) of the left internal carotid artery and spectral Doppler images (b) of the left internal carotid artery are shown.

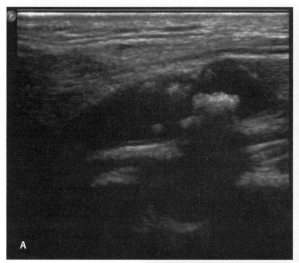
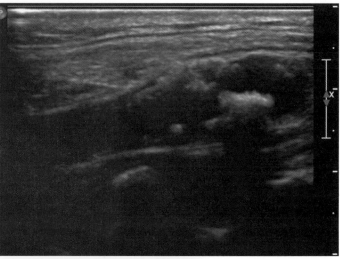

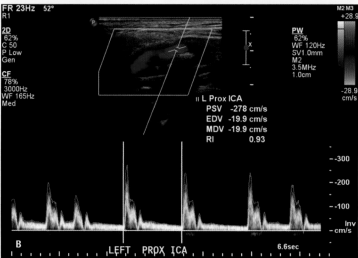

■ Questions

1. What is the most likely diagnosis?
   A. Normal
   B. < 50% stenosis
   C. 50 to 69% stenosis
   D. ≥70% stenosis
   E. Total occlusion

2. Which is the recommended angle of the transducer when imaging the carotid to maximize Doppler shift?
   A. Zero degrees
   B. 1 to 60 degrees
   C. 61 to 89 degrees
   D. 90 degrees
   E. The angle has no effect on velocity measurement.

3. Which criteria is seen with an internal carotid artery stenosis of > 70% without complete occlusion?
   A. PSV < 125 cm/sec
   B. PSV = 125 to 230 cm/sec
   C. Internal carotid artery/common carotid artery peak systolic velocity ratio 2.0 to 4.0
   D. Internal carotid artery/common carotid artery PSV ratio > 4.0
   E. Internal carotid artery end-diastolic volume < 40

■ Answers and Explanations

Question 1

D. Correct! There is ≥70% stenosis. This patient's peak systolic velocity (PSV) is 278 cm/sec. In general, PSV > 230 cm/sec is consistent with ≥70% stenosis (without occlusion). In addition, this patient has a large degree of visible shadowing calcific plaque. Plaque estimate for this category of stenosis is ≥50%.

Other choices and discussion

A. A normal carotid artery has a peak systolic velocity < 125 cm/sec, with little or no visible plaque.

B. PSV for < 50% stenosis is < 125 cm/sec with estimated visible plaque < 50%.

C. PSV for 50 to 69% stenosis is 125 to 230 cm/sec.

E. Doppler confirms flow and velocities are detectable, excluding complete occlusion.

Question 2

B. Correct! A Doppler shift of < 60 degrees (nonzero) is recommended. Doppler shift is calculated as the difference between frequencies transmitted and frequencies reflected back to the transducer. This is a function of the angle transmitted into the material, and this is used to calculate velocity. Doppler shift is maximized when patients are imaged with an angle of 30 to 60 degrees.

Other choices and discussion

A. While a zero-degree angle would maximize the Doppler shift for the velocity equation, an angle of zero is rarely attainable when imaging a vessel.

C. Angles > 60 degrees will lessen the Doppler shift, which results in possible errant velocity measurement.

D. The velocity equation is dependent on the cosine of the Doppler angle. As Cos(90) = 0, velocity cannot be measured at 90 degrees.

E. The velocity equation is dependent on the cosine of the Doppler angle.

Question 3

D. Correct! An internal carotid artery (ICA)/common carotid artery (CCA) ratio of > 4.0 is seen with an ICA stenosis of > 70% without complete occlusion. Additional diagnostic criteria include PSV > 230 cm/sec and end-diastolic volume > 100 cm/sec.

The other options are incorrect.

■ Suggested Readings

Bushberg JT, Seibert JA, Leidholdt EM, Boone JM. The Essential Physics of Medical Imaging. 2nd ed. Philadelphia: Lippincott Williams and Wilkins; 2002: 531–533

Grant EG, Benson CB, Moneta GL, et al. Carotid artery stenosis: gray-scale and Doppler US diagnosis - Society of Radiologists in Ultrasound consensus conference. Radiology 2003;229:340–346

Grant EG, Duerinckx AJ, El Saden SM, et al. Ability to use duplex ultrasound to quantify internal carotid arterial stenoses: fact or fiction? Radiology 2000;214:247–252

Top Tips

♦ Velocity measurements are dependent on the Doppler angle, which is maximized between 30 to 60 degrees. Velocity cannot be measured with the transducer positioned at 90 degrees to the direction of flow.

♦ Velocities cannot be reliably measured in patients with total or near-total occlusion of a vessel. Differentiating occlusion from severe stenosis is critical and often requires further imaging beyond ultrasound.

♦ Several parameters to know:

Normal: (primary) ICA PSV < 125 cm/sec, no visible plaque; (secondary) ICA/CCA ratio < 2.0; ICA EDV < 40 cm/sec

Less than 50% stenosis: (primary) ICA PSV < 125 cm/sec, < 50% visible plaque; (secondary) ICA/CCA ratio < 2.0; ICA EDV < 40 cm/sec

50 to 69% stenosis: (primary) ICA PSV 125 to 230 cm/sec, > 50% visible plaque; (secondary) ICA/CCA ratio 2.0 to 4.0; ICA EDV 40 to 100 cm/sec

≥ 70% stenosis but less than near occlusion: ICA PSV > 230 msec; ICA/CCA ratio > 4.0; ICA EDV > 100 cm/sec

More Challenging 3

■ Case

A male patient presents with groin pain. Grayscale transverse image of the left inguinal canal (a) and grayscale transverse image of the left inguinal canal with Doppler (b) are shown.

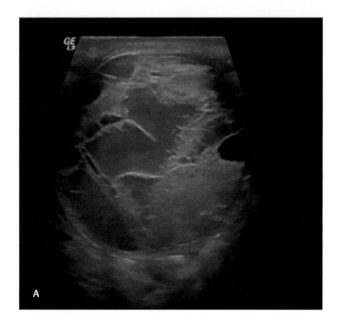

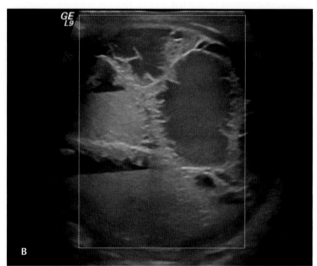

■ Questions

1. Which of the following is (are) in the differential diagnosis? (Select ALL that apply.)
   A. Inguinal hernia
   B. Inguinal hematoma
   C. Testicular carcinoma
   D. Hydrocele
   E. Abscess

2. Which ONE of the following is a characteristic of an indirect inguinal hernia?
   A. Occurs lateral to the inferior epigastric artery
   B. Acquired rather than congenital
   C. Presents as a pulsatile groin mass
   D. Occurs medial to the femoral vein
   E. Rarely requires surgery

3. Which ONE of the following aids in the sonographic diagnosis of herniated bowel?
   A. Vascular flow on Doppler
   B. Increased posterior acoustic transmission
   C. Reverberation artifact
   D. Presence of hydrocele
   E. Real-time visualization of peristalsis

■ Answers and Explanations

Question 1

A. Correct! Inguinal hernia is in the differential diagnosis. Bowel may enter the inguinal canal in an indirect hernia. On real-time cine imaging, this would present as an inguinal mass exhibiting peristalsis.

B. Correct! Inguinal hematoma is in the differential diagnosis and, in fact, is the correct diagnosis. This patient is postoperative day 5 following inguinal hernia repair. Increasing swelling and pain were reported by the patient. Ultrasound demonstrates a heterogeneous mass with no Doppler flow and no peristalsis. Surgical consultation was obtained, and the findings resolved after 1 month of observation.

C. Correct! Testicular carcinoma is in the differential diagnosis. Undescended testes (cryptorchidism) may reside in the inguinal canal. These undescended testicles are at an increased risk to develop into malignancy. Careful surveillance must be performed in all patients with cryptorchidism, and the undescended testicle may require removal due to this heightened risk of neoplasm.

Other choices and discussion

D. Hydrocele is characterized by simple anechoic fluid, which sometimes tracks into the inguinal canal. This is not demonstrated in this case.

E. Abscess may arise postoperatively or in the setting of untreated epididymoorchitis. An abscess is usually heterogeneous. However, it usually contains a component of fluid and has peripheral hyperemic tissue, neither of which are present in this case.

Question 2

A. Correct! Indirect inguinal hernias occur lateral to the inferior epigastric artery within the inguinal canal.

Other choices and discussion

B. Indirect hernias are usually congenital, due to a patent processus vaginalis.

C. The presence of pulsatility would raise suspicion for a vascular etiology, such as a femoral pseudoaneurysm.

D. Occurrence medial to the femoral vein is characteristic of an acquired femoral hernia.

E. Surgical correction is necessary for some indirect hernias (those exhibiting incarceration or strangulation).

Question 3

E. Correct! A mass exhibiting peristalsis on imaging is characteristic of bowel. This is often better captured with cine images through the groin.

Other choices and discussion

A. Vascularity can be observed within herniated bowel, solid masses, and vascular masses.

B. Increased posterior acoustic transmission is not a characteristic feature of herniated bowel.

C. Reverberation artifact is not a characteristic feature of herniated bowel.

D. Fluid can be seen in the setting of a hernia, but this is a nonspecific finding.

■ Suggested Readings

Bradley M, Morgan D, Pentlow B, Roe A. The groin hernia – an ultrasound diagnosis? Ann R Coll Surg Engl 2003;85:178–180

Robinson A, Light D, Nice C. Meta-analysis of sonography in the diagnosis of inguinal hernias. J Ultrasound Med 2013;32:339–346

Shadbolt CL, Heinze SBJ, Dietrich RB. Imaging of groin masses: inguinal anatomy and pathologic conditions revisited. Radiographics 2001;21:S261–S271

SECTION XII US/REPRODUCTIVE/ENDOCRINOLOGY IMAGING

Top Tips

◆ Indirect inguinal hernias are more commonly congenital, whereas direct inguinal hernias are more commonly acquired. Direct hernias typically occur in elderly males and are associated with weakened abdominal musculature.

◆ Real-time visualization of peristalsis on ultrasound is a highly specific finding of inguinal hernia.

◆ Ultrasound is highly accurate for diagnosing the presence of an inguinal hernia and for differentiating between indirect inguinal, direct inguinal, and femoral hernias.

More Challenging 4

■ Case

A patient status post liver transplant. Spectral Doppler image of the hepatic artery (a), grayscale transverse image of the right upper quadrant (b), and transverse ultrasound image of the right upper quadrant with Doppler (c) are shown.

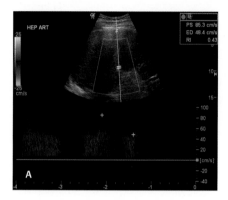
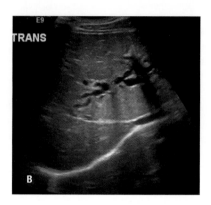
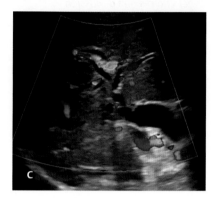

■ Questions

1. Which ONE of the following is the most likely diagnosis?
   A. Biliary sludge
   B. Portal vein thrombosis
   C. Hepatic artery pseudoaneurysm
   D. Complete hepatic artery occlusion
   E. Hepatic artery stenosis

2. Which ONE of the following is a characteristic ultrasound finding of this disorder?
   A. Increased resistive indices
   B. Decreased resistive indices
   C. Diffuse biliary sclerosis
   D. Acute hepatic necrosis
   E. Rapid systolic arterial upstroke on spectral Doppler of the intraparenchymal arterial vessels

3. When the test case diagnosis is suggested on ultrasound, which of the following is/are included in its management? (Select ALL that apply.)
   A. Doppler evaluation of the entire hepatic artery
   B. Computed tomography angiography
   C. Catheter angiography and angioplasty
   D. Biliary stenting
   E. Surgical re-anastomosis

■ Answers and Explanations

Question 1

E. Correct! Hepatic artery stenosis is the most likely diagnosis. The spectral Doppler demonstrates a *parvus et tardus* waveform distal to the occlusion. This waveform shows a diminished and slowed systolic upstroke with depressed velocities.

Other choices and discussion

A. Sludge would present as echogenic material within the bile duct lumen.

B. The main portal vein is not imaged on this study.

C. Spectral Doppler over a pseudoaneurysm classically demonstrates a bidirectional "to-and-fro" waveform, which is not present in this case.

D. No aneurysm is seen on these images.

Question 2

B. Correct! Decreased resistive indices is a characteristic finding of hepatic artery stenosis. Resistive indices in the hepatic artery are decreased to < 0.5. This occurs because of diminished flow in the vessel distal to the site of stenosis.

Other choices and discussion

A. Resistive indices in the hepatic artery are decreased (not increased) due to diminished flow in the vessel distal to the site of stenosis.

C. The intrahepatic bile ducts and proximal common bile duct receive blood flow from the hepatic artery. Stenosis may lead to biliary ischemia and necrosis, which can present as diffuse or segmental biliary dilation, with occasional biloma formation.

D. While hepatic artery stenosis can ultimately lead to graft failure, acute liver necrosis does not occur. The liver receives a dual blood supply from both the hepatic artery and the portal vein. Note, however, that *biliary* necrosis can occur, as these structures receive blood solely from the hepatic artery.

E. Elevated peak systolic velocity occurs at the site of narrowing, usually at or adjacent to the surgical anastomosis. The intrahepatic arterial system will have delayed arterial upstroke on spectral Doppler, leading to a *parvus et tardus* waveform.

Question 3

B. Correct! Computed tomography angiography (CTA) is indicated. The area of hepatic artery stenosis is rarely visualized by ultrasound. Secondary signs of hepatic artery stenosis are more commonly found on ultrasound. These secondary signs include decreased resistive indices (< 0.5) in the intrahepatic arterial vessels and *parvus et tardus* waveform on Doppler. If stenosis is suspected on ultrasound, further imaging with angiography or computed tomography angiography is recommended.

C. Correct! Catheter angiography and angioplasty are indicated. In patients with hepatic artery stenosis, catheterization and angioplasty can restore blood flow to the graft. Such therapy results in lower rates of graft failure and longer life of the graft.

D. Correct! Biliary stenting is indicated. Longstanding hepatic artery stenosis is a cause of biliary ischemia. This sometimes results in nonanastomotic biliary strictures, which can lead to focal and segmental intrahepatic biliary dilatation. When symptomatic, these strictures can be treated with percutaneous or retrograde biliary intervention with stenting to decompress the biliary system.

E. Correct! Surgical re-anastomosis is indicated. Most cases of hepatic artery stenosis occur near the site of arterial re-anastomosis. Surgical re-anastomosis may correct blood flow around this region. Additionally, patients who undergo repeated catheter angiography are at a higher risk for developing arterial dissection, and surgical intervention may be necessary to treat this condition.

The other choice is incorrect. Further Doppler evaluation is unlikely to help. Direct visualization of the entire hepatic artery is difficult, and the site of thrombosis is rarely seen by ultrasound. More commonly, secondary signs are seen.

■ Suggested Readings

Hamby BA, Ramirez DE, Loss GE. Endovascular treatment of hepatic artery stenosis after liver transplantation. J Vasc Surg 2013;57:1067–1072

Koegan MT, McDermott VG, Price SK, et al. The role of imaging in the diagnosis and management of biliary complications after liver transplantation. Am J Roentgenol 1999;173:215–219

Verdonk RC, Buis CI, Porte RJ, et al. Anastomotic biliary strictures after liver transplantation: Causes and consequences. Liver Transpl 2006;12:726–735

Top Tips

♦ Spectral Doppler within a vessel distal to a hepatic arterial stenosis has a characteristic *parvus et tardus* waveform.

♦ The liver has a dual supply of oxygenated blood: the hepatic arterial tree and the portal vein.

♦ Vascular supply to the biliary tree is via the hepatic artery.

More Challenging 5

■ Case

A 61-year-old woman with hypothyroidism. Grayscale image of the thyroid is shown.

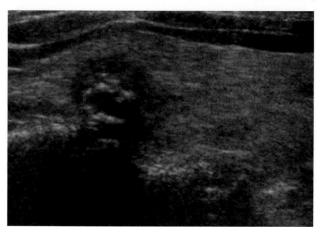 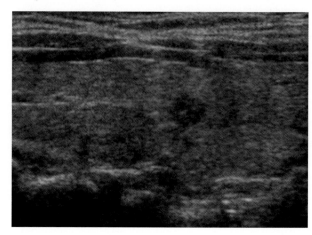

■ Questions

1. Which ONE of the following is the most appropriate next step in management of this nodule?
   A. Do not report this nodule, as it is < 2 cm in size.
   B. Mention this nodule in the report, but no further follow up is necessary.
   C. Follow up this nodule in 6 months, then yearly to confirm stability.
   D. Recommend fine needle aspiration of this nodule.
   E. Recommend thyroidectomy.

2. Which ONE of the following is a feature of papillary thyroid carcinoma?
   A. Most common in the second decade of life
   B. Affects men more often than women
   C. Rarely spreads into cervical lymph nodes
   D. Often presents as a mass with microcalcifications
   E. High mortality at diagnosis

3. For which ONE of the following conditions is fine needle aspiration indicated?
   A. Solitary thyroid nodule 1 cm in size with microcalcifications
   B. Entirely cystic thyroid nodule
   C. Solitary thyroid nodule 1 cm in size with coarse calcifications
   D. Cystic thyroid nodule stable in size and appearance for 5 years by ultrasound
   E. Spongiform nodule 1.3 cm in size

■ Answers and Explanations

Question 1

D. Correct! Tissue sampling with fine needle aspiration (FNA) is indicated for this nodule. The suspicious characteristics on imaging in this case include a nodule that is solid, hypoechoic, has mildly ill-defined margins peripherally, and has internal calcifications. Several of these calcifications are coarse, but a few are smaller. At FNA, this was confirmed to represent papillary carcinoma. A smaller 5 mm nodule (see image below) in the same patient was also biopsied. Even though it was small, it was hypoechoic, had slightly ill-defined margins, and had minimal internal calcification. This was also confirmed papillary carcinoma at FNA.

The other options are incorrect. This nodule has suspicious features, which warrant tissue diagnosis. FNA is the next best step (rather than thyroidectomy).

Question 2

D. Correct! On ultrasound, papillary thyroid carcinoma typically presents as a solid thyroid nodule with internal microcalcifications. Often, tiny microcalcifications do not demonstrate the typical shadowing of larger calcifications. Differentiating microcalcifications from colloid is an important distinction, as microcalcifications are suspicious and colloid is benign. Colloid has comet-tail artifact due to internal reverberation.

Other choices and discussion

A. Papillary thyroid carcinoma is usually diagnosed in the fourth to sixth decades of life.

B. Papillary thyroid carcinoma more frequently affects females.

C. Papillary thyroid carcinoma often presents with microscopic involvement of cervical lymph nodes. The prognosis for patients with such micrometastases remains good.

E. Papillary thyroid carcinoma typically has a favorable prognosis, with cancer-related mortality between 4 to 8% at two decades from diagnosis.

Question 3

A. Correct! Size of ≥1 cm with microcalcifications is a highly specific finding of thyroid carcinoma.

Other choices and discussion

B. FNA is usually unnecessary for predominately cystic nodules.

C. FNA should be performed for nodules ≥1.5 cm in size with coarse calcifications.

D. FNA is usually unnecessary for nodules demonstrating stability by imaging, if the lesions do not exhibit suspicious imaging features (e.g., microcalcifications or a solid and markedly hypoechoic component). Such lesions should, however, be sampled if there is significant interval growth. Nodules should be measured using the largest diameter of the lesion.

E. Spongiform nodules are considered a very low suspicion pattern.

■ Suggested Readings

Davies L, Welch HG. Current thyroid cancer trends in the United States. JAMA Otolaryngol Head Neck Surg 2014;140:317–322

Frates MC, Benson CB, Charboneau JW, et al. Management of thyroid nodules detected at US: Society of Radiologists in Ultrasound consensus conference statement. Radiology 2005;237:794–800

Haugen BR, Alexander EK, Bible KC, Doherty GM, Mandel SJ, Nikiforov YE, et al. 2015 American Thyroid Association Management Guidelines for Adult Patients with Thyroid Nodules and Differentiated Thyroid Cancer. Thyroid 2016;261–133

Hay ID, McConahey WM, Goellner JR. Managing patients with papillary thyroid carcinoma: insights gained from the Mayo Clinic's experience of treating 2,512 consecutive patients during 1940 through 2000. Trans Am Clin Climatol Assoc 2002;113:241–260

SECTION XII US/REPRODUCTIVE/ ENDOCRINOLOGY IMAGING

Top Tips

According to the American Thyroid Association guidelines from 2015, thyroid FNA is recommended for:

◆ Thyroid nodules > 1 cm in greatest dimension with a high suspicion or intermediate suspicion sonographic pattern and for thyroid nodules > 1.5 cm with a low suspicion sonographic pattern.

◆ High suspicion sonographic patterns include microcalcifications, hypoechoic nodule, irregular margin, taller than wide, and interrupted rim calcification with soft tissue extrusion.

◆ Low suspicion sonographic patterns include hyperechoic or isoechoic solid, regular margin, and partially cystic with irregular solid areas.

Essentials 1

■ Case

A 35-year-old woman with multiple uterine fibroids presents for pre-embolization workup. Shown here is the maximum intensity projection magnetic resonance angiography (MRA) image of the pelvis.

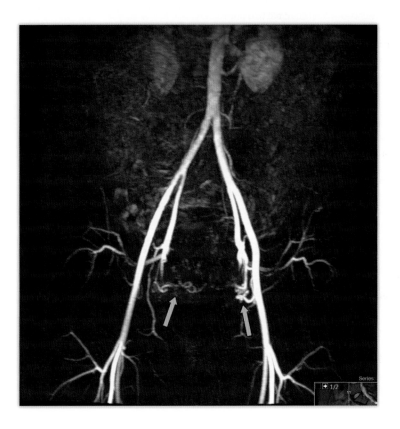

■ Questions

1. What vessels are demonstrated (*arrows*)?
   A. Uterine branch of the ovarian artery
   B. Helicine branches of the uterine artery
   C. Inferior gluteal artery
   D. Vaginal artery
   E. Internal pudendal artery

2. Magnetic resonance imaging with magnetic resonance angiography is a time-consuming and expensive examination for evaluation of uterine leiomyomas. What are the specific indications for this study? (Select ALL that apply.)
   A. Localization and characterization of fibroids
   B. Determination of uterine vascular (arterial) anatomy
   C. Measurement of vascular dimensions
   D. Assessment of effectiveness of treatment (embolization)
   E. Evaluation for presence of an arteriovenous shunt

3. True or False. Magnetic resonance angiography cannot be performed without gadolinium administration.

■ Answers and Explanations

Question 1

B. Correct! The arrows point to the helicine branches of the uterine artery. The uterine artery is a branch of the anterior division of the internal iliac artery. It courses lateral to medial in the base of the broad ligament and ascends along the lateral aspect of the body of the uterus. Helicine arteries (supply the uterus), ovarian branch (anastomoses with the ovarian artery), vaginal branch (anastomoses with the vaginal artery), and tubal branch (supplies the fallopian tubes) are the branches of the uterine artery. Helicine branches, which supply the uterus, have a characteristic corkscrew configuration, and this helps in identification.

Other choices and discussion

A. The ovarian artery arises anterolaterally from the abdominal aorta immediately below the level of the renal arteries. It courses in the retroperitoneum with the gonadal vein and ureter. In the pelvis, it courses through the ovarian suspensory ligament to supply the ovary. It anastomoses with the ovarian branch of the uterine artery but does not have a uterine branch.

C. The inferior gluteal artery is also a branch of the anterior division of the internal iliac artery. It traverses in the lateral pelvis and exits through the greater sciatic foramen to supply the gluteal region and thigh.

D. The vaginal artery arises from the anterior division of the internal iliac artery. It anastomoses with the vaginal branch of the uterine artery.

E. The internal pudendal artery is a branch of the anterior division of the internal iliac artery and arises anterior to the inferior gluteal artery. It exits the pelvis through the greater sciatic foramen and re-enters through the lesser sciatic foramen to supply the perineum.

Question 2

A. Correct! Although pelvic ultrasound is the initial imaging study for the evaluation of fibroids, magnetic resonance imaging (MRI) adds value, especially in cases of multiple fibroids for better demonstration of features such as size, location, and presence or absence of degeneration.

B. Correct! Determination of uterine vascular (arterial) anatomy is an essential step prior to embolization. Presence of an ovarian arterial supply results in unsuccessful embolization.

D. Correct! MRI can be performed after embolization to assess the degree of fibroid degeneration/necrosis and, therefore, the ultimate effectiveness of treatment.

E. Correct! Evaluating for the presence of an arteriovenous shunt is indispensable before embolization. There is a risk of shunting of the beads into the pulmonary arterial system in the presence of an arteriovenous shunt.

The other choice is incorrect. Measurement of the dimensions of the vessels is not required.

Question 3

False. Magnetic resonance angiography (MRA) can be performed even without the administration of intravenous contrast. This is extremely helpful in nephrotoxic patients, pregnant women, and in patients with contrast allergy. The three techniques to perform MRA without contrast include time-of-flight angiography, phase contrast imaging, and three-dimensional electrocardiograph-triggered half Fourier fast spin echo. Generally, these techniques take longer to acquire compared to post-contrast angiography.

■ Suggested Readings

Bulman JC, Ascher SM, Spies JB. Current concepts in uterine fibroid embolization. Radiographics 2012;32(6):1735–1750

Stepansky F, Hecht EM, Rivera R, et al. Dynamic MR angiography of upper extremity vascular disease: pictorial review. Radiographics 2008;28:e28

Top Tips

- ◆ Helicine branches of the uterine artery provide blood supply to the uterus. They have a typical corkscrew appearance.

- ◆ MRI and MRA of the pelvis is the imaging tool of choice for potential uterine fibroid embolization candidates. MRI performed before and after uterine fibroid embolization is critical for demonstrating and localizing leiomyomas, identifying red flags regarding vascular supply, assessing the likelihood of symptom relief after therapy on the basis of imaging characteristics, and monitoring the response of leiomyomas to therapy.

- ◆ MRA can be performed without the use of intravenous contrast.

Essentials 2

■ Case

A 64-year-old man had a follow up computed tomography angiography 6 months after aortic stent graft placement for aneurysm.

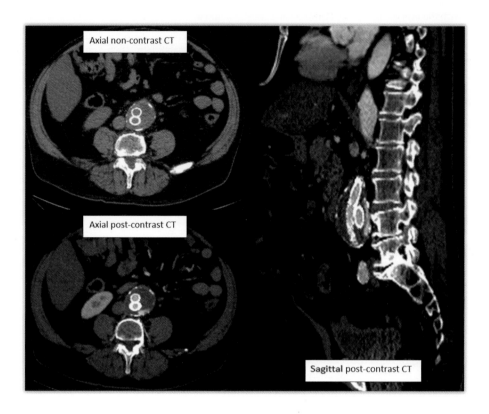

■ Questions

1. What is the diagnosis?
   A. Type I endoleak
   B. Type II endoleak
   C. Type III endoleak
   D. Type IV endoleak
   E. Type V endoleak

2. What is the overall most common type of endoleak?
   A. Type I endoleak
   B. Type II endoleak
   C. Type III endoleak
   D. Type IV endoleak
   E. Type V endoleak

3. Which type(s) of endoleak requires immediate intervention? (Select ALL that apply.)
   A. Type I endoleak
   B. Type II endoleak
   C. Type III endoleak
   D. Type IV endoleak
   E. Type V endoleak

■ Answers and Explanations

Question 1

B. Correct! Type II endoleak occurs due to retrograde flow of blood into the aneurysmal sac from branches (inferior mesenteric artery, lumbar arteries) of the aorta. It is most commonly encountered in abdominal aortic aneurysms. Contrast located in the periphery of the aneurysmal sac without communication with the stent is indicative of a type II endoleak. If located anteriorly, the inferior mesenteric artery is the culprit, whereas those located posterolaterally arise from the lumbar arteries. Another diagnostic clue is tubular configuration of the contrast abutting the aortic wall on coronal or sagittal reformatted images.

Other choices and discussion

A. Type I endoleak occurs due to inadequate apposition between the stent graft and the aneurysm sac. On computed tomography angiography, the diagnosis of type I endoleak is made when contrast is identified in the aneurysmal sac in communication with the proximal or distal attachment sites.

C. Type III endoleak is due to defective components of the endograft, such as stent graft fractures or rupture/tear of the graft material. The underlying cause is proposed to be repetitive stress on the graft from arterial pulsations. Contrast pooling around the stent graft with peripheral sparing is suggestive of type III endoleak.

D. Type IV endoleak is a diagnosis of exclusion and is due to stent-graft porosity. These occur at the time of implantation and are self-limited once the coagulation profile is normalized.

E. Type V endoleak, also called endotension, is defined as an increase in size of the aneurysmal sac without imaging evidence of endoleak.

Question 2

B. Correct! Type II endoleak is the overall most common type of endoleak encountered in clinical practice (40%). Of note, type I endoleak is the most common type of endoleak that occurs in *thoracic* aortic aneurysms.

The other choices are incorrect.

Question 3

A. Correct! Type I endoleak represents direct communication between the systemic arterial system and the aneurysmal sac, and is therefore at greater risk of rupture of the sac. They are usually treated by securing the attachment sites with balloons, stents, or stent graft extensions.

C. Correct! Type III endoleak also represents direct communication between the high-pressure arteries and the native aneurysmal sac and therefore requires immediate intervention. The defect is usually covered with stent graft extension.

Other choices and discussion

B. A total of 40% of type II endoleaks spontaneously thrombose. They are repaired if the patient is symptomatic or if the sac increases in size over time.

D. Type IV endoleak occurs at the time of implantation and autocorrects after normalization of the coagulation profile. Therefore, no treatment is necessary.

E. Once endotension (type V endoleak) is confirmed, open surgical repair is required. However, it is not an emergency.

■ Suggested Readings

Bashire MA, Ferral H, Jacobs C, et al. Endoleaks after endovascular abdominal aortic aneurysm repair: management strategies according to CT findings. Am J Roentgenol 2009;193:W178–186

Stavropoulos SW, Charagundla SR. Imaging techniques for detection and management of endoleaks after endovascular aortic aneurysm repair. Radiographics 2007;243:641–655

Top Tips

◆ Type II endoleak is the most common type of endoleak.

◆ Type I and III endoleaks require emergent treatment.

◆ Type IV endoleak is self-limited and does not require treatment. Type II and V leaks can be managed conservatively with close follow up. Treatment is necessary if the patient has symptoms or if the aneurysmal sac continues to increase in size.

Essentials 3

■ Case

A 45-year-old woman presents with a 5-day history of progressive left lower extremity swelling. Computed tomography of the abdomen and pelvis with contrast was performed. Venous phase images are shown.

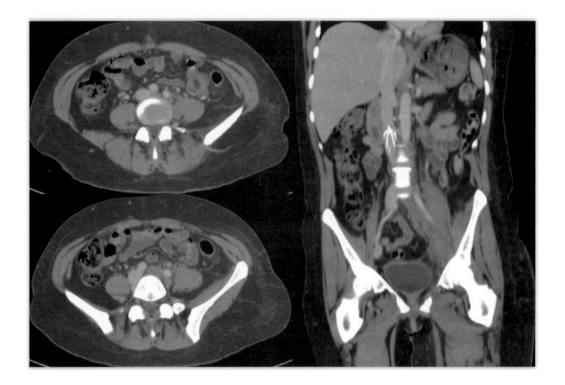

■ Questions

1. Where is the abnormality?
   A. Inferior vena cava
   B. Left common iliac artery
   C. Left common iliac vein
   D. Right common iliac vein

2. What is the diagnosis?
   A. Paget-Schroetter syndrome
   B. Lemierre syndrome
   C. May-Thurner syndrome
   D. Budd-Chiari syndrome

3. What is the appropriate management of May-Thurner syndrome?
   A. Systemic anticoagulation
   B. Catheter-directed thrombolysis and endovascular stent placement
   C. Catheter-directed thrombolysis alone
   D. Nothing

■ Answers and Explanations

Question 1

C. Correct! There is a large occlusive thrombus in the left common iliac vein.

The other choices are incorrect.

Question 2

C. Correct! May-Thurner syndrome is alternatively called Cockett syndrome. It is characterized by compression of the left common iliac vein by the right common iliac artery against the vertebral body. This in turn results in left lower extremity swelling with or without thrombosis of the left common iliac vein. It generally affects young and middle-aged adults and predominantly women. The presence of a pelvic mass must be excluded as the cause of thrombosis before making this diagnosis.

Other choices and discussion

A. Paget-Schroetter syndrome is a thoracic outlet syndrome characterized by subclavian vein thrombosis between the first rib and the clavicle. It is also referred to as effort thrombosis and is typically seen in young athletic males. It is thought to be due to vigorous overhead arm physical activity.

B. Lemierre syndrome, also called postanginal sepsis, is characterized by thrombophlebitis of the internal jugular vein secondary to adjacent oropharyngeal infection. The critical feature is the spread of infection into the chest that manifests as pulmonary septic emboli.

D. The key imaging findings in Budd-Chiari syndrome are thrombosis of the hepatic veins and/or inferior vena cava.

Question 3

B. Correct! Catheter-directed thrombolysis followed by endovascular stent placement has evolved as an alternate to surgery and is now the preferred management technique. It has a high success rate of 95% and excellent 1-year patency rates of 90 to 100% (mean 96%).

Other choices and discussion

A. Systemic anticoagulation was the first line of treatment prior to thrombolysis. It is no longer used due to a very low patency rate. Oral anticoagulants are used after stent placement to prevent recurrence of thrombosis.

C. Catheter-directed thrombolysis alone is effective and has a higher patency rate at 6 months than oral anticoagulation alone. However, a recurrence rate of 73% has been reported when the primary cause of obstruction has not been addressed.

D. May-Thurner syndrome can lead to dreadful complications such as pulmonary embolism and acute limb ischemia. Therefore, treatment is necessary.

■ Suggested Readings

Eliahou R, Sosna J, Bloom AI. Between a rock and a hard place: clinical and imaging features of vascular compression syndromes. Radiographics 2012;32:E33–49

Lamba R, Tanner DT, Sekhon S, et al. Multidetector CT of vascular compression syndromes in the abdomen and pelvis. Radiographics 2014;34:93–115

Top Tips

◆ Compression with or without thrombosis of the left common iliac vein by the right common iliac artery is defined as May-Thurner syndrome.

◆ Catheter-directed thrombolysis with endovascular stent placement has emerged as the treatment of choice.

◆ Pulmonary embolism and acute limb ischemia (phlegmasia cerulea dolens) are the two potential complications.

Essentials 4

■ Case

A 35-year-old man is status post a high-speed motor vehicle accident. Images are from chest computed tomography with contrast.

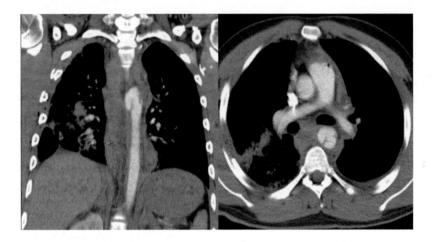

■ Questions

1. What is the diagnosis?
   A. Aortic dissection
   B. Intimal tear
   C. Normal ductus diverticulum
   D. Aortic transection with pseudoaneurysm

2. What is the MOST common location for this entity?
   A. Diaphragmatic hiatus
   B. Aortic root
   C. Aortic isthmus
   D. Ascending aorta

3. What is the treatment for aortic transection with pseudoaneurysm?
   A. Observation
   B. Open surgical repair
   C. Angioplasty
   D. Endovascular stent graft placement

■ Answers and Explanations

Question 1

D. Correct! This is a classic case of aortic transaction with pseudoaneurysm formation. The direct signs of abnormal contour and outpouching of the aorta representing the pseudoaneurysm are noted. In addition, the indirect sign of the presence of periaortic hematoma without a fat plane between the hematoma and the aorta is also seen.

Other choices and discussion

A. Aortic dissection is an extremely rare sequelae of trauma. It is characterized by intimal tear with resultant accumulation of blood between the intima and the adventitia, and the formation of a second false lumen. On imaging, an intimal flap and two lumens are the clues for diagnosis.

B. Intimal tear in the trauma setting is categorized under minimal aortic injury (MAI). It is characterized by intimal flap or intraluminal aortic thrombus. Intramural hematoma also falls under the same category. The diagnosis of MAI has increased since the advent of thin-slice computed tomography.

C. Although this is the typical location for a ductus diverticulum, the presence of periaortic hematoma precludes that diagnosis. Other clues of a ductus diverticulum include a smooth contour and obtuse margins of the diverticulum with the aortic wall.

Question 2

C. Correct! Aortic transaction occurs more commonly (90%) at the isthmus because of the relative immobility of this region due to tethering by the ligamentum arteriosum. This results in shearing injury during high-speed motor vehicle collisions.

Other choices and discussion

A. A total of 5% of acute traumatic aortic injuries occur in the region of the diaphragmatic hiatus.

B. The aortic root is not a typical location for an acute traumatic injury.

D. A total of 5% of acute traumatic aortic injuries occur in the ascending aorta.

Question 3

D. Correct! Endovascular stent graft placement has recently emerged as the treatment of choice. The advantages of this method over open repair include the avoidance of single lung ventilation, aortic cross-clamping, cardiopulmonary bypass, and systemic anticoagulation. In addition, with endovascular stent graft placement, there is reduced blood loss and reduced surgical time.

Other choices and discussion

A. Conservative management is reserved for patients with MAI or patients with other critical comorbid injuries.

B. Open surgical repair has been the treatment of choice for decades. However, its use is fading due to the associated risks of anesthesia and the surgery itself.

C. Angioplasty is not an appropriate treatment for aortic injury.

■ Suggested Readings

Cullen EL, Lantz EJ, Johnson M, et al. Traumatic aortic injury: CT findings, mimics, and therapeutic options. Cardiovasc Diagn Ther 2014;4:238–244

Morgan TA, Steenburg SD, Siegel EL, et al. Acute traumatic aortic injuries: posttherapy multidetector CT findings. Radiographics 2010;44:158–163

Steenburg SD, Ravenel JG, Ikonomidis JS, et al. Acute traumatic aortic injury: imaging evaluation and management. Radiology 2008;248:748–762

Top Tips

◆ Acute traumatic aortic injury occurs most commonly at the aortic isthmus.

◆ Endovascular therapy is now the treatment of choice.

◆ Pretherapy multidetector computed tomography should document the following: caliber of the aorta proximal and distal to the injury, distance from the left subclavian artery to the injury, length of the vascular injury, and presence of any anatomic variants.

Essentials 5

■ Case

A 61-year-old man presents to the emergency room with severe acute chest pain. Computed tomography of the chest was performed.

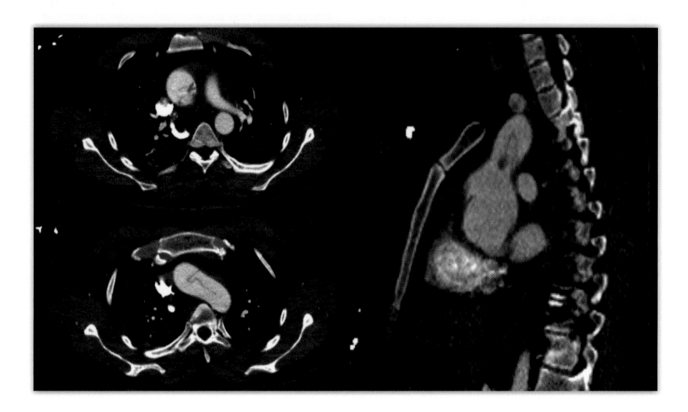

■ Questions

1. What is the diagnosis?
   A. Stanford type A dissection
   B. Stanford type B dissection
   C. DeBakey type III dissection
   D. Stanford type C dissection

2. True or False. All dissections of the type presented in this case are typically treated surgically.

3. What are the primary indications for repair of type B dissection? (Select ALL that apply.)
   A. All type B dissections
   B. Ruptured aorta or descending aortic diameter > 6 cm
   C. Renal or visceral vascular compromise
   D. Uncontrolled hypertension

■ Answers and Explanations

Question 1

A. Correct! Two classifications exist for aortic dissection: Stanford and DeBakey. Aortic dissections involving the ascending aorta regardless of the distal extent are referred to as Stanford type A dissections. Sixty percent of dissections are type A. Acute aortic dissections are those diagnosed within 14 days of the onset of symptoms, whereas chronic dissections are older than 14 days. Hypertension is the most common risk factor for aortic dissection. Other contributing factors include pregnancy, aortic stenosis, or the presence of connective tissue disorders such as Marfan syndrome, cystic medial necrosis, Ehlers-Danlos syndrome, and Turner syndrome.

Other choices and discussion

B. Aortic dissection distal to the origin of the left subclavian artery with sparing of the ascending aorta is termed a Stanford type B dissection.

C. DeBakey type III dissection also involves the descending thoracic aorta distal to the origin of the left subclavian artery (this is similar to a Stanford type B). DeBakey type I involves both ascending and descending aorta, whereas type II involves only the ascending aorta (both come under Stanford type A).

D. Stanford type C dissection does not exist.

Question 2

True. All type A dissections require immediate intervention. The dreaded complications of type A dissection include rupture of the dissection into the pericardium with progressive pericardial tamponade, occlusion of the supra-aortic vessels, extension of the dissection into the coronary arteries resulting in ischemia, and severe aortic insufficiency with acute heart failure.

Question 3

B. Correct! Irregularity of the aortic wall, extravasation of contrast, hemothorax, hemopericardium, and hyperattenuating mediastinal fluid collections are indicative of aortic rupture, when immediate intervention is required. A descending aortic diameter of > 6 cm is at great risk for rupture, and therefore, necessitates emergent intervention.

C. Correct! Extension of the intimal flap into the branches of the aorta (renal, celiac, superior and inferior mesenteric arteries) can cause end-organ ischemia. This is considered a surgical emergency.

D. Correct! Most type B dissections are managed conservatively by controlling the blood pressure. However, in patients with hypertension refractory to medical therapy, surgical management is necessary to prevent rupture.

The other choice is incorrect. Approximately 40% of the dissections are type B in nature. Most of these can be treated conservatively.

■ Suggested Reading

Sebastia C, Pallisa E, Quiroga S, et al. Aortic Dissection: diagnosis and follow-up with helical CT. Radiographics 1999;19:45–60

Top Tips

- Aortic dissections have two classifications: Stanford and DeBakey. Stanford is the most commonly used classification.

- Stanford type A dissections require immediate intervention.

- Stanford type B dissections are treated conservatively, unless there is uncontrolled hypertension, end-organ ischemia, ruptured aorta, or aortic diameter > 6 cm.

Essentials 6

■ Case

A 66-year-old man presents for evaluation of left flank pain. He is status-post renal biopsy one day earlier. Computed tomography of the abdomen and pelvis with contrast was performed.

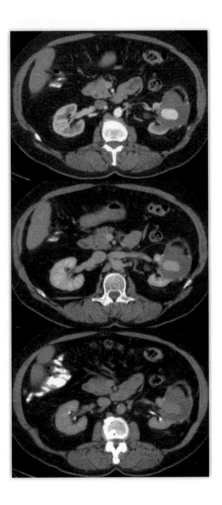

■ Questions

1. What is the diagnosis?
   A. Active extravasation of contrast
   B. Subcapsular hematoma
   C. Pseudoaneurysm
   D. True aneurysm

2. What is the MOST common nontraumatic abdominal visceral arterial aneurysm?
   A. Hepatic artery
   B. Celiac artery
   C. Superior mesenteric artery
   D. Splenic artery

3. Which of these visceral arterial aneurysms requires intervention regardless of size in otherwise normal patients?
   A. Hepatic artery
   B. Renal artery
   C. Superior mesenteric artery
   D. Splenic artery

■ Answers and Explanations

Question 1

C. Correct! This patient has a pseudoaneurysm. Pseudoaneurysm is an entity seen secondary to trauma, infection, or iatrogenic causes such as percutaneous biopsy or drainage. It is the result of partial or complete disruption of the aortic wall with resultant formation of a sac contained by media, adventitia, or connective tissue, or simply by soft tissue structures surrounding the vessel wall. On computed tomography, it appears as a smooth, well-circumscribed round or oval-shaped focus of contrast that does not enlarge or increase in attenuation on the more delayed images. Pseudoaneurysms have a greater risk of rupture due to the deficient arterial wall. Therefore, immediate intervention is warranted.

Other choices and discussion

A. Active extravasation of contrast is depicted as an irregularly shaped pooling of contrast with ill-defined edges on the arterial phase that increases in size on the venous and delayed phases. An adjacent hematoma with various stages of blood products is usually associated with active extravasation. Treatment includes angiographic embolization.

B. Subcapsular hematoma is a well-known complication of renal biopsy. It is represented as a curvilinear high-density hematoma surrounding the kidney. Because of the subcapsular location of the hematoma, there is compression of the renal parenchyma, which can result in a Page kidney. Page kidney is defined as the phenomenon of developing hypertension due to compression of the renal parenchyma and vasculature with resultant activation of the renin-angiotensin system.

D. True aneurysms are typically seen with atherosclerotic disease. They have all three layers of the vessel wall intact. They are usually fusiform in shape, whereas pseudoaneurysms are saccular. Visceral arterial aneurysms are less common than visceral pseudoaneurysms, especially with a history of trauma or surgical intervention.

Question 2

D. Correct! Splenic artery aneurysm is the most common type of abdominal visceral arterial aneurysm and accounts for 60 to 80% of cases. It has a male-to-female ratio of 1:4. Predisposing conditions include pregnancy, multiparity, portal hypertension, systemic hypertension, medial fibroplasia, and alpha-1 antitrypsin deficiency. Rupture is seen in 3 to 10% of cases. The mortality rate in nonpregnant patients is 10 to 25%, but that rate increases to approximately 70% during pregnancy.

Other choices and discussion

A. True aneurysms involving the common hepatic artery, hepatic artery proper, or intrahepatic arterial branches account for 20% of the cases. They are the second most common type of abdominal visceral arterial true aneurysm.

B. Celiac artery aneurysm is the fourth most common type of visceral arterial true aneurysm. They can be associated with abdominal aortic aneurysms in up to 18% of cases and with other visceral arterial aneurysms in about 50% cases. Therefore, presence of one aneurysm necessitates a search for another.

C. Superior mesenteric artery aneurysm is the third most common type of nontraumatic visceral arterial aneurysm. Unlike other visceral artery aneurysms, 70 to 90% of these aneurysms are symptomatic and associated with a high incidence of ischemic bowel complications.

Question 3

C. Correct! Unlike other visceral artery aneurysms, 70 to 90% of superior mesenteric artery aneurysms are symptomatic and associated with a high incidence of ischemic bowel complications. The risk of rupture is estimated to be 50%, and the surgical mortality rate in the setting of a ruptured aneurysm is 38%. On the other hand, no deaths have been reported in cases with elective intervention. The success rates for treatment of these aneurysms vary from 75 to 100%. Considering all of these factors, superior mesenteric artery aneurysms are treated irrespective of the size.

Other choices and discussion

A. Hepatic arterial true aneurysms are treated if the patient is symptomatic or when the size exceeds 2 cm. However, in patients with polyarteritis nodosa or fibromuscular dysplasia, treatment is recommended regardless of the size. The mortality rate associated with rupture is 21%.

B. Intervention is required in renal arterial aneurysms if the size is > 2 cm or if the patient is symptomatic. However, treatment is deemed necessary in pregnant women regardless of the size.

D. Symptomatic patients and splenic artery aneurysms > 2 cm require intervention in otherwise normal patients. However, with pregnancy, portal hypertension, connective tissue disorders, and alpha-1 antitrypsin deficiency, treatment is initiated regardless of the size.

■ Suggested Readings

Jesinger RA, Thoreson AA Lamba R, et al. Abdominal and pelvic aneurysms and pseudoaneurysms: imaging review with clinical, radiologic, and treatment correlation. Radiographics 2013;33:E71–96

Saad EA, Saad WEA, Davies MG, et al. Pseudoaneurysms and the role of minimally invasive techniques in their management. Radiographics 2005;25(Suppl 1):S173–189

Top Tips

- ◆ Pseudoaneurysms are more common than true aneurysms in the setting of trauma, infection, or iatrogenic etiologies. Pseudoaneurysms require emergent intervention due to high risk of rupture.

- ◆ Splenic artery aneurysm is the most common type of visceral arterial true aneurysm.

- ◆ All superior mesenteric arterial true aneurysms require elective intervention.

Essentials 7

■ Case

A 77-year-old man with chronic history of abdominal pain had a computed tomography angiogram of the abdomen and pelvis with contrast performed. Pre- and postcontrast axial computed tomography images are shown.

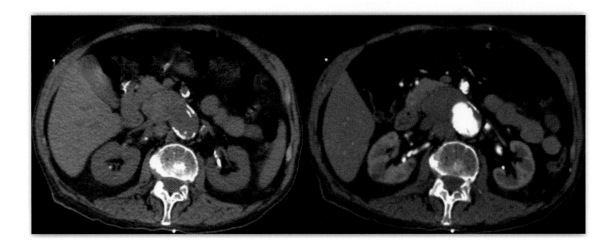

■ Questions

1. What is the most complete diagnosis?
   A. Abdominal aortic aneurysm
   B. Abdominal aortic aneurysm with impending rupture
   C. Abdominal aortic aneurysm with contained rupture
   D. Aortoenteric fistula

2. At what size are abdominal aortic aneurysms typically treated?
   A. 3 cm
   B. 4 cm
   C. 5 cm
   D. 6 cm

3. What is the MOST common complication after endo-vascular stent-graft placement for abdominal aortic aneurysm?
   A. Endoleak
   B. Graft thrombosis
   C. Shower embolism
   D. Graft infection

■ Answers and Explanations

Question 1

C. Correct! This patient has an abdominal aortic aneurysm with a contained rupture.

The computed tomography (CT) features of chronic contained rupture include discontinuity of the wall or rim calcification of the aneurysm, well-defined soft tissue density adjacent to the aorta (as seen here), displaced viscera, and no contrast material in the hematoma. Draping of the posterior aspect of the aorta over the adjacent vertebral body is suggestive of a contained rupture of the posterior wall of the aorta and is termed the "draped aorta" sign. Frank and acute ruptures demonstrate significant retroperitoneal hemorrhage with or without contrast extravasation.

Other choices and discussion

A. There is abnormal dilatation of the abdominal aorta, consistent with an aneurysm. However, there is more here than just a simple aneurysm.

B. A well-defined peripheral crescent of increased attenuation within the thrombus of a large abdominal aortic aneurysm on a noncontrast study is a CT sign of acute or impending rupture. It is the earliest and most specific imaging manifestation of impending rupture, but is not seen here.

D. In the presence of a patent fistula, CT with contrast would demonstrate extravasation of contrast into the adjacent bowel. In this case, the duodenum is displaced, but there is no contrast material in the lumen.

Question 2

C. Correct! Abdominal aortic aneurysms ≥ 5 cm in size are associated with a greater risk of rupture and thus are often treated at this size. The other criterion is > 10 mm increase in size of the aneurysm per year. With this criterion, aneurysms < 5 cm are also treated.

The other choices are incorrect.

Question 3

A. Correct! Endoleak is the most common complication. Leakage into the aneurysm status post stent graft placement is referred to as an endoleak. This is the most common complication after endovascular repair of abdominal aortic aneurysm, with rates ranging from 2.4 to 45.5%. Five types of endoleak have been described. Types I and III require immediate intervention. Type II endoleak is the most common type of endoleak.

Other choices and discussion

B. The rate of graft thrombosis ranges from 3 to 19%. The thrombosis can be parietal, circular, or semicircular within the stent-graft. Short-term follow up studies are performed to determine the prognosis.

C. Shower embolism is one of the most serious complications of abdominal aortic aneurysm repair and is seen more commonly with endovascular repair than with conventional surgery. This condition is associated with high perioperative mortality.

D. Graft infection with pseudoaneurysm formation is also a rare complication associated with high morbidity and mortality rates.

■ Suggested Readings

Mita T, Arita T, Matsunaga N, et al. Complications of endovascular repair for thoracic and abdominal aortic aneurysm: an imaging spectrum. Radiographics 2000;20:1263–1278

Rakita D, Newatia A, Hines JJ, et al. Spectrum of CT findings in rupture and impending rupture of abdominal aortic aneurysms. Radiographics 2007;27:497–507

SECTION XIII
VASCULAR IMAGING

Top Tips

◆ A high attenuation crescent sign is indicative of impending rupture of an abdominal aortic aneurysm.

◆ The draped aorta sign is suggestive of a contained rupture of an aortic aneurysm.

◆ Endoleak is the most common complication after abdominal aortic aneurysm repair.

Essentials 8

■ Case

A 45-year-old man had a computed tomographic angiography performed. Coronal and sagittal reformatted images are shown.

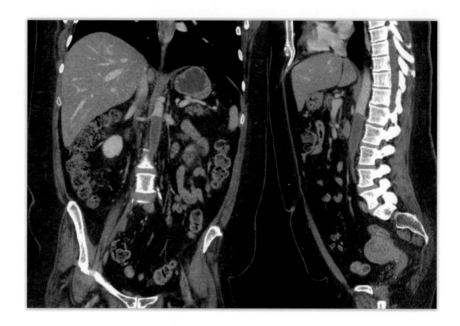

■ Questions

1. What is the classic clinical triad of symptoms that patients with this diagnosis present with?
   A. Paraplegia, pain, and paresthesia
   B. Thigh, hip, or buttock claudication, absent/diminished femoral pulse, and impotence
   C. Thigh, hip, or buttock claudication, absent/diminished femoral pulse, and quadriplegia
   D. Abdominal pain, back pain, and impotence

2. Which of the following best describes midaortic dysplastic syndrome?
   A. Aneurysmal dilatation of the abdominal aorta and its branches
   B. Thrombotic occlusion of the abdominal aorta and its branches
   C. Narrowing of the abdominal aorta and its branches
   D. Dissection of the abdominal aorta extending into its branches

3. What is the BEST diagnostic study for evaluation of abdominal aortic stenotic/occlusive disease?
   A. Computed tomographic angiography
   B. Ultrasound with Doppler
   C. Magnetic resonance angiography
   D. Digital subtraction angiography

■ Answers and Explanations

Question 1

B. Correct! These images demonstrate thrombotic occlusion of the infrarenal abdominal aorta, which is consistent with Leriche syndrome. The classic clinical triad of Leriche syndrome includes thigh, hip, or buttock claudication; absent/diminished femoral pulse; and impotence. Three main subtypes have been described based on the location of the thrombus: juxtarenal or within 5 mm of the lower renal arterial origin; infrarenal or cephalic to the origin of the inferior mesenteric artery; and inframesenteric, which is caudal to the origin of the inferior mesenteric artery. The etiology of Leriche syndrome is atherosclerotic disease.

The other choices are incorrect.

Question 2

C. Correct! Midaortic dysplastic syndrome (also called abdominal aortic coarctation) is characterized by narrowing of the abdominal aorta and its branches. It is an uncommon condition typically affecting children and young adults. Refractory hypertension and a weakened or absent femoral pulse are the presenting features of this entity. These patients die by age 35 to 40 due to progressive hypertension, if not treated. Aortic reconstruction with prosthetic or autologous venous grafts is a treatment option.

The other choices are incorrect.

Question 3

A. Correct! Computed tomographic angiography (CTA) is best diagnostic modality for evaluation of arterial (aortic) pathology because of the great spatial resolution, fast acquisition time (requiring less time), and ability to reconstruct and reformat the images. Radiation is the precluding factor for CTA in pregnant women and children. The contraindications for CTA include contrast allergy and renal failure.

Other choices and discussion

B. Ultrasound with Doppler is good for evaluation of the peripheral arteries and the superficial and deep venous structures. Deeper structures such as the aorta may be difficult to visualize due to overlying bowel gas. Therefore, ultrasound is not a reliable modality for accurate evaluation of the abdominal aorta.

C. Magnetic resonance angiography (MRA) has good contrast resolution but has lower spatial resolution than CTA. The major disadvantages of MRA include long acquisition time, resultant motion artifacts, and greater cost. Contraindications for MRA are contrast allergy, pregnancy, and renal failure. MRA without contrast (time-of-flight or phase contrast angiography) can be performed in nephrotoxic patients. Generally, scan time is longer with these techniques compared to postcontrast MRA.

D. Digital subtraction angiography is a gold standard for arterial pathology. However, it is invasive and is not generally used for diagnostic purposes since the advent of CTA.

■ Suggested Readings

Bhatti AM, Mansoor J, Younis U, Siddique K, Chatta S. Mid aortic syndrome: a rare vascular disorder. J Pak Med Assoc 2011;61:1018–1020

Sebastia C, Quiroga S, Boye R, et al. Aortic stenosis: spectrum of diseases depicted at multisection CT. Radiographics 2003;23:S79–S91

> ## Top Tips
>
> - Leriche syndrome is atherosclerotic occlusion of the infrarenal abdominal aorta with a classic clinical triad of thigh, hip, or buttock claudication; absent/diminished femoral pulse; and impotence.
>
> - Midaortic dysplastic syndrome (also called coarctation of the abdominal aorta) is characterized by narrowing of the abdominal aorta and its branches. Children and young adults present with uncontrolled hypertension.
>
> - CTA is the diagnostic modality of choice for abdominal aortic pathology.

SECTION XIII
VASCULAR IMAGING

Essentials 9

■ Case

Postcontrast magnetic resonance images of a 51-year-old woman are shown.

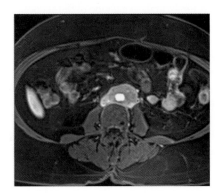

Axial postcontrast T1 fat-saturated image in arterial phase

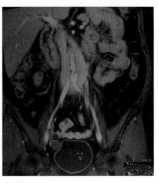

Coronal postcontrast T1 fat-saturated image in delayed phase

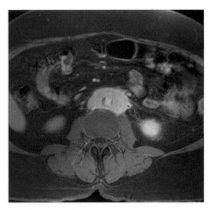

A   Axial postcontrast T1 fat-saturated image in delayed phase

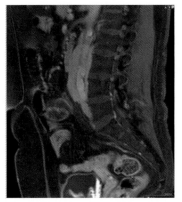

B   Sagittal postcontrast T1 fat-saturated image in delayed phase

■ Questions

1. What is the diagnosis?
   A. Retroperitoneal hematoma
   B. Infectious aortitis
   C. Perianeurysmal fibrosis
   D. Retroperitoneal fibrosis

2. What is the classic feature suggestive of this disorder on intravenous pyelography and retrograde pyelography?
   A. Lateral bowing of the ureters
   B. Medial deviation of the ureters
   C. Delayed excretion of contrast by the ureters
   D. Hydronephrosis

3. True or False. A catheter can be easily passed through the narrowed area of the ureter in retroperitoneal fibrosis, unlike in the presence of intrinsic or extrinsic obstructive ureteral lesions.

■ Answers and Explanations

Question 1

D. Correct! This patient has retroperitoneal fibrosis (RPF; aka Ormond disease). RPF is characterized by proliferation of fibroinflammatory tissue typically surrounding the infrarenal abdominal aorta, inferior vena cava, and iliac vessels. It can extend to neighboring structures, especially the ureters, and ultimately lead to renal failure. Two subtypes of RPF have been described: idiopathic and secondary. Idiopathic RPF is an autoimmune condition and can lead to obstructive uropathy in 56 to 100% of patients, deep vein thrombosis (due to entrapment of retroperitoneal lymphatics), and varicocele (secondary to gonadal vein involvement) formation. The secondary form can be benign (from ingestion of drugs) or malignant. Malignant RPF is a described as a desmoplastic response to retroperitoneal primary tumors (lymphoma or sarcoma) or metastatic disease (breast, colon, stomach, lung, thyroid, carcinoid, and genitourinary tract).

Owing to the poor prognosis of malignant RPF, it is important to differentiate benign from malignant RPF. Anterior displacement of the aorta from the spine is usually seen with malignant RPF; however, there are exceptions (as in this case). In idiopathic RPF, the mass envelopes the retroperitoneal structures rather than exerting mass effect, as in malignant RPF. A retroperitoneal mass that has low signal intensity on T2-weighted images is highly suggestive of benign RPF in the late inactive stage. On the other hand, high T2 signal intensity is seen in both malignant and early stage idiopathic RPF, and this appearance is therefore nonspecific. Ultimately, histopathologic examination is often mandatory to establish the definitive diagnosis in suspicious cases with a possibility of malignancy. The mainstay of treatment for idiopathic RPF is steroid administration.

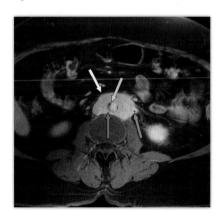

This postcontrast T1 fat-saturated image in delayed phase demonstrates an enhancing soft tissue mass (*white arrow*) encasing the infrarenal abdominal aorta (*yellow arrow*) and the left ureter (*blue arrow*). There is elevation of the posterior wall of the aorta from the vertebral body (*green arrow*), which is unsual for idiopathic retroperitoneal fibrosis.

Other choices and discussion

A. Retroperitoneal hematoma is usually seen with aortic aneurysm rupture or trauma-related aortic injury.

B. Infectious aortitis is characterized by aortic wall thickening, fluid or stranding in the periaortic soft tissues with rapidly progressing saccular aneurysm or pseudoaneurysm, and rarely, air in the aortic wall. The most common inciting organisms include *Staphylococcus aureus* and *Salmonella*.

C. Perianeurysmal fibrosis can have morphologic features similar to RPF. However, the encased aorta should also be aneurysmally dilated.

Question 2

B. Correct! Although not pathognomonic, medial deviation of the middle third of both ureters at the level of the lower lumbar spine or upper sacrum on fluoroscopy is a classic feature of RPF.

Other choices and discussion

A. RPF typically does not cause mass effect on the neighboring structures. Therefore, the ureters are not laterally bowed or displaced.

C. Delayed excretion of contrast is seen with RPF but is also seen with several other conditions, especially intrinsic or extrinsic obstructive lesions.

D. Hydronephrosis is seen with RPF, but is more commonly found with other intrinsic or extrinsic obstructive lesions.

Question 3

True! The narrowed portion of the ureter in RPF can be traversed easily by a catheter, because the cause of obstruction in RPF is impairment of the normal ureteral peristalsis due to encasement by the fibroinflammatory tissue, rather than mechanical compression or invasion. This technique is especially helpful in performing retrograde pyelography for nephrotoxic patients who cannot receive intravenous contrast.

■ Suggested Readings

Caiafa RO, Vinuesa AS, Izguierdo RS, et al. Retroperitoneal fibrosis: role of imaging in diagnosis and follow-up. Radiographics 2013;33:535–552

Cronin CG, Lohan DG, Blake MA, Roche C, McCarthy P, Murphy JM. Retroperitoneal fibrosis: a review of clinical features and imaging findings. Am J Roentgenol 2008;191:423–431

Top Tips

- ◆ RPF is described as a fibrotic reaction typically intimately bordering the infrarenal abdominal aorta, extending to involve the inferior vena cava and bilateral ureters, and leading to renal failure.

- ◆ Although the soft tissue mass in RPF does not typically extend posterior to the aorta, a few cases with "lifting" of the aorta from the spine have been reported.

- ◆ A very classic, but not pathognomic, feature of RPF on fluoroscopy is medial deviation of the middle third of the ureters.

Essentials 10

■ Case

A patient has lower extremity pain and swelling. This grayscale ultrasound image demonstrates a patent common femoral vein (*white arrow*), which compresses completely (*yellow arrow*).

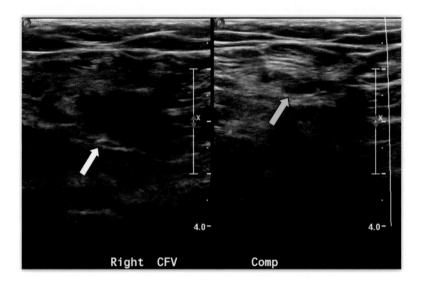

■ Questions

1. What is the MOST accurate study for the diagnosis of deep venous thrombosis?
   A. Computed tomography venography
   B. Magnetic resonance venography
   C. Ultrasound
   D. Catheter venography

2. Which of the following is the principal feature used to diagnose deep venous thrombosis with venous Doppler?
   A. Echogenic thrombus in the lumen
   B. Absence of augmentation
   C. Expansion of the vein
   D. Inability to compress the vein on transverse view

3. A 46-year-old woman with new onset of left lower extremity edema presents for evaluation. Lower extremity venous Doppler demonstrates a normally compressible and patent common femoral vein with absence of respiratory phasicity. What is the suspected diagnosis?
   A. Popliteal venous thrombosis
   B. Iliac venous thrombosis
   C. Saphenous vein thrombosis
   D. Superficial femoral vein thrombosis

■ Answers and Explanations

Question 1

C. Correct! Ultrasound (US) is recognized as the most accurate first-line tool for the diagnosis of deep venous thrombosis (DVT). The sensitivity and specificity of compression US alone are 95% and 98%, respectively. The major advantages of this modality include its portability, lack of ionizing radiation, no requirement for intravenous contrast, low cost, and faster acquisition time without complications. Limitations include difficult visualization of deeper structures, especially in patients with a large body habitus.

Other choices and discussion

A. Computed tomography venography is an emerging modality for the diagnosis of DVT. Despite accurate timing of the contrast, an undesired mixing effect can be seen in some cases. Another major hurdle is its ionizing radiation, especially if multiple phases are performed. In addition, contrast cannot be administered in patients with renal failure. Computed tomography venography may be advantageous in the evaluation of obese patients and for deeper structures, such as the iliac veins.

B. Magnetic resonance venography is not used for routine evaluation of DVT owing to its longer acquisition time, high cost, and the presence of artifacts. Contrast allergy and nephrotoxicity are contraindications for magnetic resonance venography.

D. Catheter venography is not used as a diagnostic tool, unless therapeutic intervention is planned concurrently. The invasive nature with potential complications, presence of ionizing radiation, and longer imaging times preclude the usage of catheter venography as a diagnostic modality for DVT.

Question 2

D. Correct! Absence of compressibility of a vein is the most sensitive and specific diagnostic feature for DVT on venous Doppler US. All of the other answer choices suggest the presence of DVT; however, lack of venous compression is required to confirm the diagnosis.

Other choices and discussion

A. Identification of an echogenic thrombus within the lumen of a vein leads to the diagnosis of DVT. However, in cases of acute thrombosis, the clot is not hyperechoic and it can sometimes be hard to differentiate from a normal vein. Therefore, echogenic thrombus is not present in all cases of DVT.

B. Compression below the site of examination to determine patency below the site of examination is termed augmentation. Absence of augmentation suggests distal thrombosis. However, this is a less sensitive feature for the diagnosis of DVT.

C. Expansion of the vein is a feature of acute venous thrombosis and is not typically seen with chronic DVT.

Question 3

B. Correct! The iliac vein is located proximal to the common femoral vein. Thrombosis/occlusion of the iliac vein leads to failure of transmission of the right atrial/inferior vena cava pressure changes into the distal veins, thus leading to a lack of respiratory phasicity of the venous waveform. This technique is extremely important, as the iliac veins are deeper structures, not well visualized, and can only be secondarily evaluated by interrogating the common femoral veins.

Other choices and discussion

A. The popliteal vein is located distal to the common femoral vein. Thrombosis of the popliteal vein, therefore, will lead to absence of augmentation, not respiratory phasicity.

C. The saphenous vein is a superficial vein and is not diagnosed by lack of respiratory phasicity.

D. The superficial femoral vein is also located distal to the common femoral vein. Thrombosis of this vein, therefore, will lead to absence of augmentation, not respiratory phasicity.

■ Suggested Readings

Divittorio R, Bluth EI, Sullivan MA. Deep vein thrombosis: diagnosis of a common clinical problem. Ochsner J 2002;4:4–17

Fraser JD, Anderson DR. Deep venous thrombosis: recent advances and optimal investigation with US. Radiology 1999;211:9–24

SECTION XIII VASCULAR IMAGING

Top Tips

◆ Venous Doppler is the modality of choice for the diagnosis of DVT.

◆ Compressibility is the most reliable feature to diagnose DVT using venous Doppler.

◆ Lack of augmentation suggests the presence of DVT distal to the examination site, whereas lack of respiratory phasicity suggests thrombosis proximal to the examination site.

Essentials 11

■ Case

Precontrast and computed tomography angiographic images of a 65-year-old white man who presented to the emergency department with acute onset of chest pain are shown.

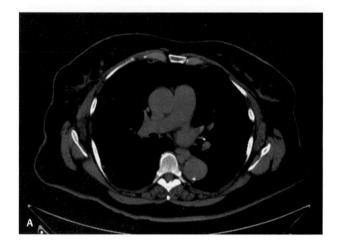

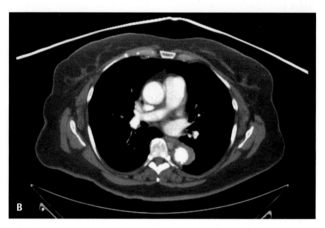

■ Questions

1. What is the diagnosis?
   A. Aortic dissection
   B. Aortic transection
   C. Penetrating aortic ulcer
   D. Intramural hematoma

2. What is the pathogenesis of the condition presented here?
   A. Intimal tear
   B. Spontaneous rupture of the vasa vasorum
   C. Thrombosis of the false lumen in aortic dissection
   D. Mural thrombus in aortic aneurysm

3. What is the next step after the diagnosis of a Stanford type B aortic intramural hematoma?
   A. Emergent surgery
   B. Endovascular graft placement
   C. Conservative management with antihypertensives
   D. Do nothing

■ Answers and Explanations

Question 1

D. Correct! This patient has an intramural hematoma. Intramural hematoma is one of the three entities that constitute acute aortic syndrome. The other two are aortic dissection and penetrating aortic ulcer. Intramural hematoma is also termed atypical dissection, as the clinical presentation is similar to aortic dissection. It is commonly seen in hypertensive patients and rarely as a result of trauma.

Other choices and discussion

A. Aortic dissection is characterized by an intimal tear with resultant accumulation of blood between the intima and the adventitia and the formation of a second false lumen. On imaging, an intimal flap and two lumens are demonstrated.

B. Aortic transection is defined as laceration of all three layers of the aortic wall, also known as aortic rupture. The rupture can be contained by hematoma or a thin layer of adventitia forming a pseudoaneurysm, which is depicted as an irregular outpouching from the aortic wall. Aortic transection is usually posttraumatic in origin, rather than spontaneous.

C. Penetrating aortic ulcer is described as an atherosclerotic ulcer that penetrates the intima and further progresses into the aortic wall. This can resolve or remain stable. However, it can also penetrate the wall and lead to grave consequences such as aortic rupture or aneurysm formation. On computed tomography angiography, it appears as a contrast-filled pouch extending into the thickened aortic wall with no intimal flap or false lumen.

Question 2

B. Correct! Acute intramural hematoma is characterized by spontaneous rupture of the vasa vasorum with resultant hemorrhage into the media and ultimately weakening of the aortic wall. This may further progress into the adventitia resulting in aortic rupture or into the intima leading to aortic dissection. Hypertension is the most common predisposing factor. The Stanford classification used for aortic dissection is applicable for intramural hematoma as well. Type A involves the ascending aorta, whereas type B involves the aorta distal to the origin of the left subclavian artery.

Other choices and discussion

A. Intimal tear/flap is a feature of aortic dissection and is depicted as a curvilinear flap in the aorta with resultant formation of true and false lumens.

C. Thrombosis of the false lumen in aortic dissection is also subintimal in location and similar to intramural hematoma. Identification of an intimal flap helps in differentiating between the two.

D. Mural thrombus in an aortic aneurysm usually lies superficial to the intima (which can show calcifications), whereas intramural hematoma is subintimal.

Question 3

C. Correct! Intramural hematoma of the aorta distal to the origin of the left subclavian artery can be managed conservatively with antihypertensives and close follow up. The indicators for emergent intervention of type B intramural hematoma include rapidly increasing size of the intramural hematoma, extensive degree of luminal compromise, and aortic size > 5 cm.

Other choices and discussion

A. Acute intramural hematoma of the ascending aorta is typically treated emergently because of the increased risk of aortic rupture or dissection.

B. Endovascular graft placement is not usually performed for an intramural hematoma.

D. Aortic rupture and aortic dissection are the grave consequences of aortic dissection. Therefore, conservative management is necessary to monitor and prevent progression.

■ Suggested Readings

Chao CP, Walker TG, Kalva SP. Natural history and CT appearances of aortic intramural hematoma. Radiographics 2009;29:791–804

Macura KJ, Corl FM, Fishman EK, et al. Pathogenesis in acute aortic syndromes: aortic dissection, intramural hematoma, and penetrating atherosclerotic aortic ulcer. Am J Roentgenol 2003;181:309–316

Top Tips

- Intramural hematoma is one of the three entities that constitute acute aortic syndrome and is commonly secondary to hypertension, and rarely, due to trauma.
- A curvilinear hyperdensity on noncontrast computed tomography is characteristic of intramural hematoma.
- Management of intramural hematoma is similar to that of aortic dissection. Type A intramural hematomas require surgery, whereas type B are managed conservatively.

Essentials 12

■ Case

Computed tomography angiographic images through the chest are shown.

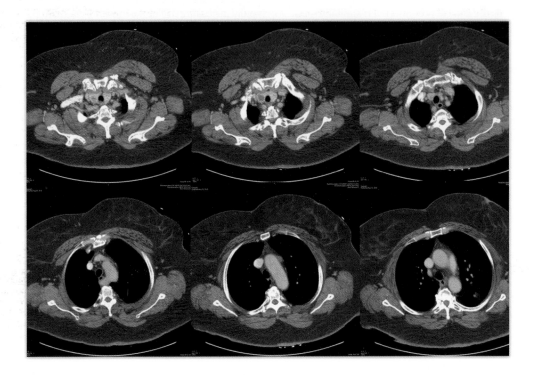

■ Questions

1. What is the diagnosis?
   A. Direct origin of the left vertebral artery from the aortic arch
   B. Left aortic arch with aberrant right subclavian artery
   C. Right aortic arch with aberrant left subclavian artery
   D. Normal

2. Which of the following vascular anomalies causes posterior indentation on the trachea and anterior indentation on the esophagus on esophagram?
   A. Double aortic arch
   B. Right aortic arch with aberrant left subclavian artery
   C. Left aortic arch with aberrant right subclavian artery
   D. Anomalous origin of the left pulmonary artery

3. What is a bovine aortic arch?
   A. Common origin of innominate artery and left common carotid artery
   B. Common origin of left common carotid and subclavian arteries
   C. Common origin of innominate artery and left subclavian artery
   D. Common origin of right and left common carotid arteries

■ Answers and Explanations

Question 1

B. Correct! This patient has a left aortic arch with an aberrant right subclavian artery. The right subclavian artery is typically the first branch off of the aortic arch (left aortic arch in this case). It arises as a fourth branch in 1% of cases, in which it is called an aberrant right subclavian artery or arteria lusoria. It courses posterior to the esophagus 80% of the time, between the trachea and esophagus in 15% of cases, and anterior to the trachea or main stem bronchus in 5%. Anomalous course of the aberrant right subclavian artery posterior to the esophagus can result in dysphagia, which is referred to as "dysphagia lusoria." Aneurysmal dilatation of the origin of the aberrant right subclavian artery results in a pouch, which is termed "diverticulum of Kommerell."

Other choices and discussion

A. The left vertebral artery typically originates from the left subclavian artery. Direct origin of the left vertebral artery from the aortic arch is seen in approximately 3% of the cases.

C. Right aortic arch with an aberrant left subclavian artery is the mirror image of left aortic arch with an aberrant right subclavian artery. This condition is seen in 39.5% of right-sided aortic arch cases.

D. Normal branches of the left aortic arch include the right brachiocephalic trunk, also called the innominate artery, left common carotid artery, and left subclavian artery.

Question 2

D. Correct! The only vascular anomaly to cause both posterior indentation on the trachea and anterior indentation on the esophagus on an esophagram is an anomalous (aberrant) left pulmonary artery, also called a pulmonary artery sling. In this case, the left pulmonary artery arises from the right pulmonary artery instead of the main pulmonary trunk. After originating from the right pulmonary artery, the left pulmonary courses between the trachea (or bronchus intermedius) and the esophagus, thus causing posterior indentation on the trachea and anterior indentation on the esophagus. This can lead to stridor or even lung collapse. Associations with this anomaly include tracheomalacia and bronchus suis (right upper lobe bronchus originating from the trachea). The three most important anatomic variant causes of stridor are double aortic arch, right arch with aberrant right subclavian artery, and pulmonary artery sling. Of these, pulmonary artery sling is the only vascular anomaly to cause stridor in a patient with a normal (left) aortic arch.

Other choices and discussion

A. Double aortic arch is the most common symptomatic aortic arch anomaly. Both left- and right-sided aortic arches are existent and encircle the trachea and esophagus, thus causing anterior indentation on the trachea and posterior indentation on the esophagus. Right dominant arch is seen in 75 to 80% of double aortic arches, left dominant arch is seen in 25%, and codominant arch is present in 5%.

B. Right aortic arch with aberrant left subclavian artery is the mirror image of a left aortic arch with aberrant right subclavian artery. This condition is seen in 39.5% of right-sided aortic arch cases and is typically asymptomatic.

C. Left aortic arch with aberrant right subclavian artery, also called arteria lusoria, courses posterior to the esophagus 80% of the time, between the trachea and esophagus in 15% of cases, and anterior to the trachea or main stem bronchus in 5%.

Question 3

A. Correct! Bovine aortic arch is defined as a common origin of the innominate artery and left common carotid artery. This is the most common aortic arch variant. This condition is seen in 15% of the population and is more common in people of African descent. A slight variation of this anomaly includes origin of the left common carotid artery from the innominate artery, where the left common artery arises distally rather than having a common trunk. The term "bovine arch" is a misnomer as in cattle, only one artery arises from the aortic arch which further branches into a bicarotid trunk and bilateral subclavian arteries.

The other choices are incorrect.

■ Suggested Readings

Berdon WE. Rings, slings, and other things: vascular compression of the infant trachea updated from the midcentury to the millennium—the legacy of Robert E. Gross, MD, and Edward B. D. Neuhauser, MD. Radiology 2000;216:624–632

Kau T, Sinzig M, Gasser J, et al. Aortic development and anomalies. Semin Intervent Radiol 2007;24:141–152

Top Tips

◆ Left aortic arch with aberrant right subclavian artery can cause posterior compression on the esophagus and lead to dysphagia (dysphagia lusoria).

◆ The only vascular anomaly to cause both posterior indentation on the trachea and anterior indentation on the esophagus on esophagram is an anomalous (aberrant) left pulmonary artery, also called a pulmonary artery sling.

◆ The three most important anatomic variant causes of stridor are double aortic arch, right arch with aberrant right subclavian artery, and pulmonary artery sling. Of these, pulmonary artery sling is the only vascular anomaly that causes stridor in a patient with a normal (left) aortic arch.

Essentials 13

■ Case

Selected computed tomography angiographic images of the heart are shown.

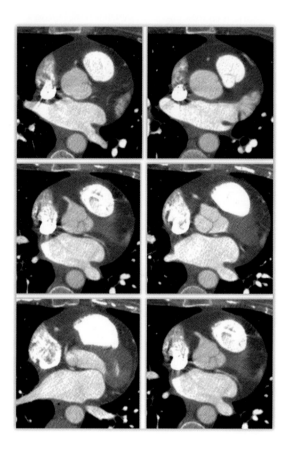

■ Questions

1. What is the BEST explanation for the findings in these images?
   A. Right coronary artery arising from the left coronary sinus
   B. Left anterior descending artery arising from the left coronary sinus
   C. Common origin of the right coronary artery, left anterior descending artery, and left circumflex arteries from the right coronary sinus
   D. Left coronary artery arising from the left coronary sinus

2. Which of the following coronary artery courses is considered malignant?
   A. Retroaortic
   B. Prepulmonic
   C. High origin of the coronary artery
   D. Interarterial

3. What is Bland-White-Garland syndrome?
   A. Anomalous origin of left coronary artery from pulmonary artery
   B. Myocardial bridging
   C. Right coronary artery arising from the left coronary sinus
   D. Left coronary artery arising from the right coronary sinus

■ Answers and Explanations

Question 1

C. Correct! Three coronary sinuses and three coronary arteries are seen on these limited images. The right coronary artery (RCA), left anterior descending (LAD) artery, and left circumflex (LCx) arteries arise from the right coronary sinus, which is located anteriorly. The coronary sinus is situated on the left posteriorly. The noncoronary sinus is seen on the right posteriorly and does not typically give rise to any coronary artery. The four recognized patterns of anomalous origin of a coronary artery from the opposite or noncoronary sinus are (1) RCA arising from the left coronary sinus, (2) left coronary artery (LCA) arising from the right coronary sinus, (3) LCx or LAD arteries arising from the right coronary sinus, and (4) LCA or RCA (or a branch of either artery) arising from the noncoronary sinus.

The other choices are incorrect.

Question 2

D. Correct! Interarterial is considered a malignant course. A coronary artery arising from the opposite or noncoronary sinus has one of these four anomalous courses: (1) retroaortic, (2) prepulmonic, (3) septal, or (4) interarterial. If the artery courses between the ascending aorta and pulmonary artery, this is referred to as an "interarterial course." This course is considered malignant as pulsations of the aorta and/or pulmonary artery, especially during exertion, can result in compression of the coronary artery and ultimately lead to sudden cardiac death. Immediate surgical bypass grafting is recommended for interarterial course of the LCA. Surgical intervention for interarterial course of the RCA is controversial and is typically recommended in symptomatic patients.

Other choices and discussion

A. A retroaortic artery courses posteriorly between the aorta and the interatrial septum. This anomalous course is considered benign.

B. In a prepulmonic course, the anomalous artery travels anterior to the pulmonary artery. This anomalous course is considered benign.

C. High coronary artery origin is defined as origin of a coronary artery > 1 cm above the sinotubular junction. This anomalous origin is considered benign.

Question 3

A. Correct! ALCAPA is also termed Bland-White-Garland syndrome. This is a very rare but very serious coronary artery anomaly. ALCAPA has been recognized to constitute 0.25 to 0.5% of cases of congenital heart disease. Most affected patients are infants with a 90% mortality rate in the first year, if left untreated. Treatment is surgical with either direct implantation of the anomalous coronary artery (in children) or ligation of the anomalous vessel in conjunction with bypass grafting (in adults).

Other choices and discussion

B. The coronary arteries normally course epicardially throughout their length. Myocardial bridging is described as a band of myocardium overlying a portion of the coronary artery. This entity commonly involves the middle segment of the LAD. This is also called the "tunneled artery." Although this is a congenital anomaly, patients do not typically become symptomatic until the third decade of life. The standard of reference for diagnosing myocardial bridging is coronary angiography in which a typical "milking" effect and a "step down–step up" phenomenon induced by systolic compression of the tunneled segment may be seen. Treatment is not indicated for asymptomatic patients. In symptomatic cases, conservative medical management is the first-line treatment. In unresponsive cases, stent implantation, surgical myotomy, or coronary bypass grafting can be performed.

C and **D** are incorrect.

■ Suggested Readings

Kim SY, Seo JB, Do KH, et al. Coronary artery anomalies: classification and ECG-gated multi–detector row CT findings with angiographic correlation. Radiographics 2006;26:317–333

Shriki JE, Shinbane JS, Rashid MA, et al. Identifying, characterizing, and classifying congenital anomalies of the coronary arteries. Radiographics 2012;32:453–468

Top Tips

- The four recognized patterns of anomalous origin of a coronary artery from the opposite or noncoronary sinus are (1) RCA arising from the left coronary sinus, (2) LCA arising from the right coronary sinus, (3) LCx or LAD arteries arising from the right coronary sinus, and (4) LCA or RCA (or a branch of either artery) arising from the noncoronary sinus.

- A coronary artery arising from the opposite or noncoronary sinus has one of these four anomalous courses: (1) retroaortic, (2) prepulmonic, (3) septal, and (4) interarterial. An interarterial course is considered malignant.

- ALCAPA is also termed Bland-White-Garland syndrome, a very rare but very serious coronary artery anomaly. Treatment is surgical.

Essentials 14

■ Case

A 52-year-old man presents with shortness of breath and lower extremity edema.

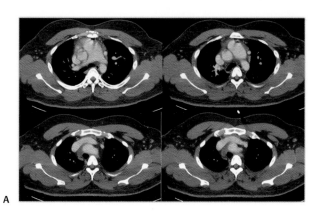

A

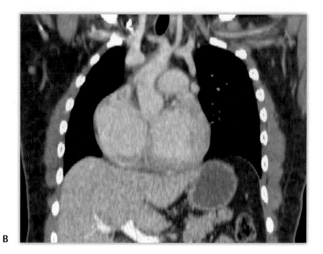

B

■ Questions

1. What is the salient finding?
   A. Saddle pulmonary embolus
   B. Aortic dissection
   C. Left superior vena cava
   D. Partial anomalous pulmonary venous return

2. What is an associated finding with the condition illustrated by this case?
   A. Atrial septal defect
   B. Small right atrium and ventricle
   C. Snowman sign on chest X-ray
   D. Pulmonary edema

3. Which of the following is associated with scimitar syndrome? (Choose ALL that apply.)
   A. Partial anomalous pulmonary venous return
   B. Hypoplasia of the right lung
   C. Dextroversion of the heart
   D. Turkish sword

■ Answers and Explanations

Question 1

D. Correct! Following the images from left to right, one notices a vascular structure coursing alongside the left side of the mediastinum. The vessel is seen emptying into the left innominate vein, which is best appreciated on the coronal image. The vessel is a vertical vein, which is formed by the coalescence of the left upper lobe pulmonary veins.

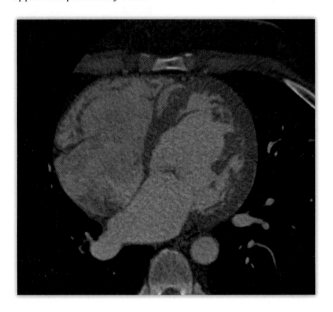

Other choices and discussion

A. The main pulmonary artery as well as its bifurcation are demonstrated on the first image. There are no filling defects visualized.

B. While the aorta is not seen throughout its entirety, the visualized portion of the aorta shows no convincing evidence for a dissection flap. There is motion along the ascending aorta near the aortic arch.

C. A left superior vena cava (SVC) is indeed a consideration. However, a left SVC typically drains into the right coronary sinus.

Question 2

A. Correct! When a partial anomalous pulmonary venous return (PAPVR) connection to the SVC or right atrium exists, an atrial septal defect is also present in 90% of patients, whereas when the anomalous vein connects to the inferior vena cava, only 15% have an atrial septal defect.

Other choices and discussion

B. When an entire lung is drained by an anomalous vein or the shunt is > 2:1, there can be enlargement of the right atrium and ventricle.

C. The snowman sign is typically seen with total anomalous pulmonary venous return.

D. PAPVR is usually an incidental finding with most patients having no clinical symptoms, unless the shunt is > 2:1.

Question 3

A, **B**, **C**, and **D**. **Correct!** Scimitar syndrome is a form of PAPVR in which the anomalous vein drains any or all of the right lung. The anomalous vein can be seen draining below the diaphragm into the inferior vena cava and occasionally into the portal vein, hepatic vein, or right atrium. The vein resembles a Turkish sword (scimitar). Other findings include a small right lung with dextroposition of the heart.

■ Suggested Readings

Ferguson EC, Krishnamurthy R, Oldham S. Classic imaging signs of congenital cardiovascular abnormalities. Radiographics 2007;5:1323–1334

Miller SW. Cardiac Imaging: The Requisites. 2nd ed. Philadelphia, PA: Elsevier Mosby; 2005

SECTION XIII
VASCULAR IMAGING

Top Tips

- ◆ If an anomalous vein associated with PAPVR is seen on the left, it is typically vertical and empties into the left innominate vein.

- ◆ Scimitar syndrome is a form of PAPVR where an anomalous vein can be seen on imaging draining from the chest to below the diaphragm.

Essentials 15

■ Case

A 63-year-old man status post angioplasty 1 day ago now presents with slowly progressive groin swelling. There is no fever or leukocytosis. Computed tomographic angiography was performed.

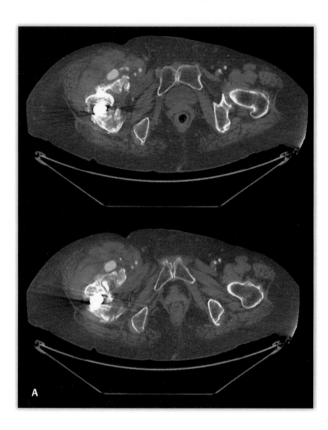

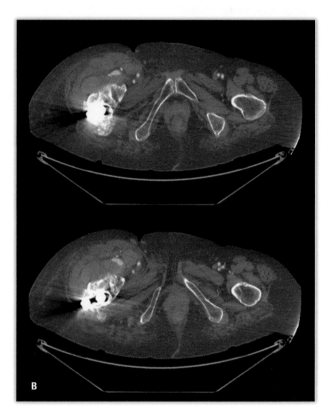

■ Questions

1. What is the pertinent finding?
   A. Groin abscess
   B. Common femoral artery pseudoaneurysm
   C. Aneurysm of the common femoral artery
   D. Dissection of the common femoral artery

2. What is the diagnostic sign of this entity on ultrasound?
   A. Tardus parvus
   B. Posterior acoustic enhancement
   C. Posterior acoustic shadowing
   D. Yin-yang sign

3. What is the initial treatment of choice for a postcatheterization pseudoaneurysm > 1 cm?
   A. Ultrasound-guided percutaneous thrombin injection
   B. Surgery
   C. Ultrasound-guided compression
   D. Observation

■ Answers and Explanations

Question 1

B. Correct! This patient has a pseudoaneurysm (PSA). PSA is described as a contained rupture of an artery with disruption of all three layers of the wall. Postcatheterization PSA is one of the most common vascular complications of cardiac and peripheral angiographic procedures. The incidence of PSA after diagnostic catheterization ranges from 0.05 to 2%. The most common presentation of a PSA is groin pain and/or swelling after catheterization. Any patient who experiences pain that is disproportionate to that expected after a percutaneous procedure should undergo an ultrasound examination to exclude the presence of a PSA (regardless of the presence of a bruit or not).

Other choices and discussion

A. Groin abscess or infection does not occur in the immediate postprocedural period. Also, this patient does not have any signs or symptoms to suggest infection.

C. Aneurysm of an artery is most commonly secondary to atherosclerotic disease, and this does not occur after angiography.

D. No intimal flap is identified to suggest dissection.

Question 2

D. Correct! The "yin-yang" sign is diagnostic of PSA. US with color and spectral Doppler is the initial imaging study of choice in suspected cases of PSA. Grayscale imaging demonstrates an anechoic outpouching, which is connected to a vessel. A swirling, turbulent flow pattern is identified in the chamber on color Doppler. On spectral Doppler, a "to and fro" signal is identified, which suggests bidirectional flow. This is alternatively termed the "yin-yang" sign. This feature is indicative of a PSA. The sensitivity of duplex ultrasound to identify a PSA is 94% with a specificity of 97%.

Other choices and discussion

A. Tardus parvus waveform is typically observed with arterial stenosis. It is characterized by a longer systolic rise time with a blunted arterial upstroke and low peak systolic velocity.

B. Posterior acoustic enhancement, also called increased through-transmission, refers to hyperechogenicity deep to a fluid-filled structure. This feature is diagnostic of simple cysts, the gallbladder, and the urinary bladder. Fluid attenuates sound less than the surrounding structures and, therefore, deeper tissues are hyperechoic.

C. Posterior acoustic shadowing is typically found with calculi. Calculi attenuate almost all of the incident sound beam and, therefore, no signal is seen beyond them.

Question 3

A. Correct! Ultrasound (US)-guided percutaneous thrombin injection has emerged as the treatment of choice for postcatheterization PSA. The principle behind thrombin injection into the PSA is based on the fact that thrombin facilitates the conversion of fibrinogen to fibrin. Thus, a clot is formed almost instantaneously (despite the presence of antiplatelet therapy or anticoagulation therapy) with US-guided thrombin injection, whereas it may

take up to several hours with US-guided compression. Successful treatment ranges from 91 to 100%. The most dreaded complication with this treatment is deep venous thrombosis. This is due to inadvertent injection of thrombin into the neighboring vein and can, in turn, lead to pulmonary embolism. Arterial thrombosis can also occur if the thrombin is injected into the tract of the PSA or the artery itself. Thrombin injection is indicated for postcatheterization PSA only and not for mycotic PSAs. Additionally, a PSA that occurs at the anastomosis of a synthetic graft and native artery should be treated surgically.

Other choices and discussion

B. Surgical management is reserved for specific conditions such as (1) PSA occurring at the site of anastomosis, (2) mycotic aneurysms, and (3) large postcatheterization PSAs (due to the risk of skin necrosis). The complications of surgery include bleeding, infection, neuralgia, prolonged hospital stay, perioperative myocardial infarction and, rarely, death.

C. US-guided compression is a safe and noninvasive method for treatment of postcatheterization PSAs, with a success rate of 75 to 98%. However, the success rate decreases to about 30 to 73% in patients who are on anticoagulation. The main limiting factors include longer compressive times (10 to 120 minutes), treatment failure and recurrence, significant pain associated with the procedure, and technical difficulty in maintaining pressure in the correct position for prolonged periods of time. Rare reported complications include vasovagal reactions, PSA rupture, skin necrosis, and deep venous thrombosis.

D. PSAs do not have a true wall and, therefore, are at an increased risk of rupture compared to true aneurysms. Observation is not ideal in such situations.

■ Suggested Readings

Demirbas O, Batyraliev T, Eksi Z, Pershukov I. Femoral pseudoaneurysm due to diagnostic or interventional angiographic procedures. Angiology 2005;56:553–556

Webber GW, Jang J, Gustavson S, Olin JW Contemporary management of postcatheterization pseudoaneurysms. Circulation 2007;115:2666–2674

Top Tips

- Any patient with pain disproportionate to that expected after a percutaneous procedure should undergo an US examination to exclude the presence of a PSA.
- Yin-yang sign = to and fro (bidirectional) flow into the aneurysmal sac. This is diagnostic of a PSA.
- US-guided percutaneous thrombin injection has emerged as the treatment of choice for postcatheterization PSAs.

Essentials 16

■ Case

A 45-year-old woman with chest pain underwent this contrast-enhanced chest computed tomography.

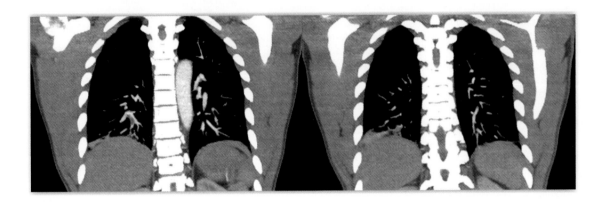

■ Questions

1. What is the most complete diagnosis?
   A. Pulmonary artery thrombosis
   B. Pulmonary vein thrombosis
   C. Pulmonary artery thrombosis with pulmonary infarct
   D. Normal

2. What is an important radiologic feature that suggests acute right ventricular failure?
   A. Enlarged right atrium with or without reflux of contrast into the hepatic veins
   B. Hypertrophic right atrium
   C. Enlarged right ventricle with or without reflux of contrast into the hepatic veins
   D. Hypertrophic right ventricle

3. What is the potential complication of longstanding pulmonary embolus?
   A. Pulmonary arterial hypertension, which further leads to cor pulmonale
   B. Pulmonary venous hypertension
   C. Left heart failure
   D. Aortic enlargement

■ Answers and Explanations

Question 1

C. Correct! The test case images demonstrate a filling defect in a right lower lobe pulmonary arterial branch consistent with pulmonary embolus (PE). In addition, consolidative air space opacification is present in the right lung base representing an infarct. The CT angiogram diagnostic criteria for an acute PE includes (1) filling defect with enlargement of the vessel, (2) partial filling defect surrounded by contrast material producing the "polo mint" sign on axial images and "railway track" sign on coronal images, and (3) a peripheral intraluminal filling defect that forms an acute angle with the arterial wall.

Other choices and discussion

A. There is thrombosis in a right lower lobe branch of the pulmonary artery. Additionally, consolidation is seen in the right lung base representing an infarct.

B. Pulmonary vein thrombosis is difficult to diagnose on a computed tomography performed for pulmonary embolus, as there is typically inadequate opacification of the pulmonary venous system.

D. The study is not normal. See answer C.

Question 2

C. Correct! RV failure can occur with acute PE. Computed tomography features that suggest the presence of right ventriclular failure include (1) RV dilatation (in which the right ventricle is wider than the left ventricle in short axis), with or without contrast material reflux into the hepatic veins, (2) deviation of the interventricular septum toward the left ventricle, and/or (3) a PE index > 60%.

Other choices and discussion

A. The right atrium alone typically does not enlarge in the case of acute PE.

B. The atrial wall is thick and hypertrophied in patients with tricuspid stenosis.

D. The RV demonstrates hypertrophy in cases of pulmonary stenosis or pulmonary arterial hypertension.

Question 3

A. Correct! Pulmonary arterial hypertension resulting in cor pulmonale is the most common complication of chronic PE. Pulmonary arterial trunk diameter > 33 mm is suggestive of this diagnosis. The diagnostic criteria for chronic PE include (1) filling defect in a vessel that is typically smaller in caliber compared to the adjacent patent vessels; (2) a peripheral, crescent-shaped intraluminal defect that forms obtuse angles with the vessel wall; and (3) secondary signs, including extensive bronchial or other systemic collateral vessels, an accompanying mosaic perfusion pattern, or calcification within eccentric vessel thickening.

The other choices are incorrect.

■ Suggested Readings

Wittram C, Kalra MK, Maher MM, et al. Acute and chronic pulmonary emboli: angiography–CT correlation. Am J Roentgenol 2006;186:S421–S429

Wittram C, Maher MM, Yoo AJ, et al. CT angiography of pulmonary embolism: diagnostic criteria and causes of misdiagnosis. Radiographics 2004;24:1219–1238

Top Tips

◆ A partial filling defect of an acute PE can be eccentric but forms acute angles with the vessel wall. Moreover, the caliber of the vessel is enlarged.

◆ A partial filling defect of a chronic PE can be eccentric but forms obtuse angles with the vessel wall. The important differentiating feature is that the involved vessel has a smaller diameter compared to the adjacent normal vessels.

◆ RV failure can occur with acute PE. Pulmonary arterial hypertension resulting in cor pulmonale can occur with chronic PE.

Essentials 17

■ Case

Coronal and axial magnetic resonance images of the abdomen in the portal venous phase are shown.

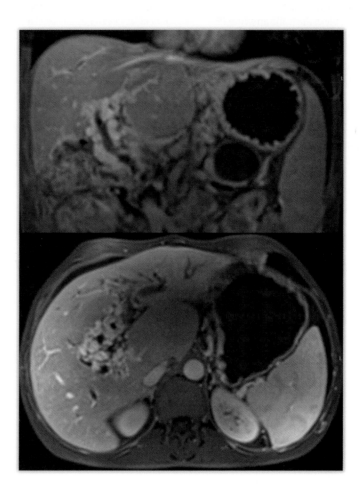

■ Questions

1. What is the diagnosis?
   A. Portahepatic collaterals due to cirrhosis
   B. Portal cavernoma
   C. Portahepatic collaterals due to hepatic artery occlusion
   D. Portahepatic collaterals due to hepatic venous occlusion

2. What is a potential complication that can occur with the condition presented in this test case?
   A. Portal venous thrombosis
   B. Hepatic arterial thrombosis
   C. Malignant transformation
   D. Portal biliopathy

3. What is the MOST common cause of portal vein thrombosis?
   A. Hepatocellular carcinoma
   B. Hypercoagulable state
   C. Cirrhosis
   D. Cholangiocarcinoma

■ Answers and Explanations

Question 1

B. Correct! This patient has a portal cavernoma. Portal cavernoma (also called cavernous transformation of the portal vein [PV]) is characterized by chronic thrombosis of the extrahepatic PV and resultant multiple collateral formation in the porta hepatis. These vessels drain variably into the left and right PV or more distally into the liver. The diagnosis can be made on ultrasound with Doppler, computed tomography with contrast, or magnetic resonance imaging with contrast and magnetic resonance cholangiopancreatography.

Other choices and discussion

A. Collateral vessels from portal hypertension in cirrhosis are typically seen around the esophagus, gastric fundus, and splenic hilum. A recanalized paraumbilical vein may be visualized. Also, the main portal demonstrates normal contrast opacification and can be larger in caliber owing to the portal hypertension.

C. Collateral vessels secondary to hepatic arterial occlusion are not present in the porta hepatic region. When present, they opacify in the arterial phase and not the portal venous phase as in this case.

D. Hepatic venous occlusion results in Budd-Chiari syndrome. Collateral vessels secondary to hepatic arterial occlusion are not present in the porta hepatic region.

Question 2

D. Correct! Portal biliopathy (also referred to as portal cavernoma cholangiopathy) is defined as biliary ductal changes manifested in patients with cavernous transformation of the PV. It has been reported in 70 to 100% of patients with extrahepatic PV obstruction. The proposed mechanisms include (1) narrowing of the biliary duct due to extrinsic compression by large collateral vessels and (2) fibrosis and stricture of the biliary duct secondary to ischemia from venous thrombosis. The disease can progress from asymptomatic elevation of liver function tests to secondary biliary cirrhosis. Magnetic resonance cholangiopancreatography imaging demonstrates narrowing (stricture) of the extrahepatic biliary duct with upstream dilatation.

Other choices and discussion

A. Portal venous thrombosis is the cause, not the effect, of portal cavernoma.

B and **C** are incorrect.

Question 3

C. Correct! Cirrhosis is the most common cause of PV thrombosis. It remains unclear whether this is a consequence of severe liver disease, a factor aggravating underlying liver disease, or both. In patients with cirrhosis, the thrombus is bland, whereas in patients with hepatocellular carcinoma, the thrombus can represent tumor thrombus.

The other choices are incorrect.

■ Suggested Readings

Kalra N, Shankar S, Khandelwal N. Imaging of portal cavernoma cholangiopathy. J Clin Exp Hepatol 2013;4:S44–52

Shin SM, Kim S, Lee KW, et al. Biliary abnormalities associated with portal biliopathy: evaluation on MR cholangiography. AM J Roentgenol 2007;188:W341–347

Vilgrain V, Condat B, Bureau C, et al. Atrophy-hypertrophy complex in patients with cavernous transformation of the portal vein: CT evaluation. Radiology 2006;241:149–155

Top Tips

◆ Portal cavernoma (cavernous transformation of the PV) is characterized by chronic thrombosis of the extrahepatic PV with resultant multiple collateral vessel formation in the porta hepatis.

◆ Portal biliopathy (portal cavernoma cholangiopathy) is defined as biliary ductal changes in patients with cavernous transformation of the PV.

◆ Cirrhosis is the most common cause of PV thrombosis.

Essentials 18

■ Case

The patient is a 48-year-old woman who presents with acute onset of pain in the left lower extremity. She has a history of peripheral vascular disease, but reports no related symptoms since prior intervention until this current episode.

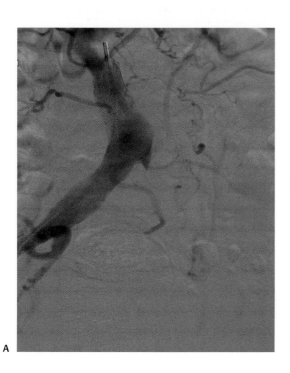

A

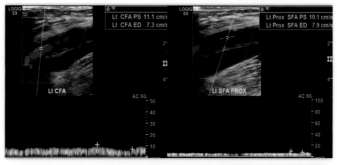

B

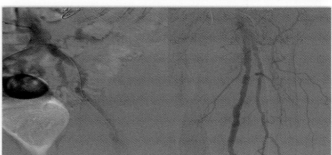

C

■ Questions

1. What is the salient finding?
   A. Dissection of the common iliac artery
   B. Stenosis of the common iliac artery
   C. Contrast extravasation
   D. Occlusion of the common iliac artery

2. What would be the expected findings of the left lower extremity on arterial duplex ultrasound?
   A. Low velocity, monophasic waveform
   B. High velocity, spectral broadening
   C. No flow
   D. To and fro flow outside of the vessel lumen

3. Which are treatment options for acute lower extremity arterial occlusion? (Select ALL that apply.)
   A. Surgical thrombectomy
   B. Percutaneous thrombolysis
   C. Antiplatelet therapy
   D. Surgical thrombectomy + percutaneous thrombolysis
   E. Surgical thrombectomy + percutaneous thrombolysis + antiplatelet therapy

■ Answers and Explanations

Question 1

D. Correct! There is lack of opacification of the left common iliac artery consistent with occlusion of this vessel. This angiographic image of the pelvis was obtained with the catheter near the aortic bifurcation.

Other choices and discussion

A. Typically, a dissection is characterized by a linear flap representing the division between the true lumen of the vessel and the false lumen. However, a dissection can lead to complete thrombosis of a vessel. Most commonly, dissections occur in the setting of some form of trauma.

B. No clinically significant stenosis is seen in the patent vessels.

C. All of the visualized contrast is contained within the blood vessels.

Question 2

A. Correct! There is typically reconstitution of flow around occlusions via collaterals. This provides for limited flow, which can be seen on ultrasound as low velocity and with "flat" waveforms. The normal triphasic waveform will not be present.

Other choices and discussion

B. High velocity, spectral broadening is the typical waveform seen with stenotic (not occluded) lesions.

C. No flow can be a finding with occlusive disease. However, there are often collaterals which reconstitute vessels beyond the point of occlusion.

D. To and fro flow outside of the main vessel lumen describes the waveform of a pseudoaneurysm.

Question 3

A. Correct! Surgical thrombectomy is a good option. Surgical thrombectomy has the advantage of quicker restoration of blood flow compared to other treatment options, particularly in patients with a threatened limb or large clot burden.

B. Correct! Percutaneous thrombolysis is indicated in patients who have acute onset of claudication or limb-threatening ischemia due to thrombotic or embolic arterial occlusion. Percutaneous treatment offers the advantage of no need for general anesthesia and is a minimally invasive approach that makes an incision large enough to insert a 2-mm sheath. The above image shows a pelvic angiogram of the test patient after overnight thrombolysis (infusion catheter remains in place). There is also an angiogram at the level of the proximal thigh showing a patent superficial and deep femoral artery.

D and **E. Correct!** See above.

Other choice and discussion

C. The use of antiplatelets alone is not a treatment option for acutely thrombosed peripheral arteries.

■ Suggested Readings

Hoppenfeld BM, Cynamon J. Basic arterial techniques for peripheral arterial thrombolysis. Tech Vasc Interv Radiol 2012;4(2):84–91

Mauro MA, Murphy K, Thomson KR, et al. Image-Guided Interventions. 2nd ed. Philadelphia, PA: Saunders; 2013

Pellerito JS, Polak JF. Introduction to Vascular Ultrasonography. 6th ed. Philadelphia, PA: Saunders; 2012

Top Tips

- ◆ Acute versus chronic occlusion can usually be determined based on patient clinical symptoms.

- ◆ Chronic occlusions tend to have well-formed extensive collateral networks that are typically not seen with acute occlusions.

- ◆ Blunted waveforms in the common femoral artery and further distally may indicate aortoiliac occlusive disease.

SECTION XIII
VASCULAR IMAGING

Essentials 19

■ Case

A 52-year-old man presents to the vascular and interventional radiology clinic with complaints of cramping in his legs when walking at least 200 feet. Symptoms are most pronounced in his left lower extremity. The pain is relieved with rest. He has also recently noticed pain at night when he is in bed that is relieved when he hangs his feet over the side of the bed.

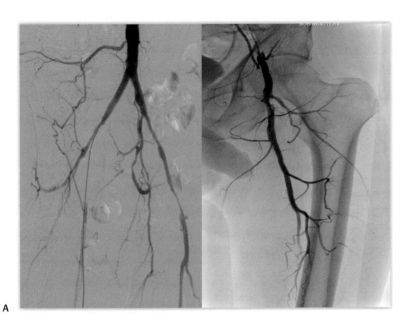
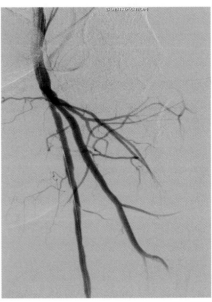

A   B

■ Questions

1. What are the findings? (Select ALL that apply.)
   A. Aneurysm of the right common iliac artery
   B. Stenoses of the right common and external iliac arteries
   C. Occluded left superficial femoral artery
   D. Thrombosis of the common iliac artery
   E. Stenoses of the bilateral common and external iliac arteries + occluded superficial femoral artery

2. What are risk factors for the development of this process? (Select ALL that apply.)
   A. Radiation
   B. Smoking
   C. Age
   D. Diabetes mellitus

3. Which ONE of the following is generally considered first-line treatment for peripheral vascular disease in patients who have failed conservative measures?
   A. Continuation of medical management
   B. Surgery
   C. Acupuncture
   D. Endovascular therapy

■ **Answers and Explanations**

Question 1

B. Correct! This conventional angiogram shows a mild to moderate stenosis of the distal segment of the right common iliac artery extending into the right external iliac artery. There is lack of opacification of the right external iliac artery secondary to high-grade stenosis and also subsequent occlusion with placement of a vascular sheath. There is also long segment high-grade stenosis of the left external iliac artery.

C. Correct! The deep right femoral artery is visualized. The right superficial femoral artery is not seen, however.

E. Correct! See above discussions.

Other choices and discussion

A. The right common iliac artery is not aneurysmal. The common iliac artery is considered aneurysmal when there is a diameter > 2.5 cm or when there is focal or diffuse dilatation > 1.5 times the normal respective diameter.

D. Both iliac arteries are opacified with contrast. There are stenoses along the distal right common iliac artery.

Question 2

A. Correct! Radiation has been demonstrated in multiple studies to increase the risk of vascular disease. Most cardiovascular events occur > 10 years after radiation exposure.

B. Correct! Smoking is one of the most common modifiable risk factors in patients with peripheral vascular disease (PVD).

C. Correct! Age is a strong nonmodifiable risk factor. It is estimated that 1 in every 20 individuals over the age of 50 has PVD.

D. Correct! Diabetes mellitus is a very common risk for PVD. Uncontrolled diabetes mellitus significantly increases the risk of PVD.

Question 3

D. Correct! There have been considerable advances in minimally invasive procedures for the treatment of PVD. These options include percutaneous transluminal balloon angioplasty, atherectomy, and stent placement.

Other choices and discussion

A. Conservative measures including optimization of medical management, smoking cessation, and exercise programs are considered the first-line therapy for patients with PVD without critical limb ischemia. However, once conservative measures have been exhausted and symptoms continue, other options must be considered.

B. Although surgery is a treatment option for PVD, it is no longer considered first-line for most patients who have failed conservative measures.

C. There are no large studies available to indicate the consistent effectiveness of atherectomy in the treatment of PVD.

■ **Suggested Readings**

Mauro MA, Murphy K, Thomson KR, et al. Image-Guided Interventions. 2nd ed. Philadelphia, PA: Saunders; 2013

Neisen MJ. Endovascular management of aortoiliac occlusive disease. Sem Interv Radiol 2009;26:296–302

SECTION XIII
VASCULAR IMAGING

Top Tips

◆ PVD is most commonly characterized by stenoses and occlusions on angiography.

◆ Clinically, PVD can range from asymptomatic to critical limb ischemia (rest pain and nonhealing wounds).

◆ Once conservative management has been optimized in patients with PVD without critical limb ischemia, endovascular therapy is usually the first-line treatment.

Essentials 20

■ Case

A 20-year-old man presents with hematuria. His noncontrast computed tomography of the abdomen is shown. Biopsy for his left renal mass is subsequently requested.

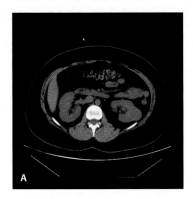
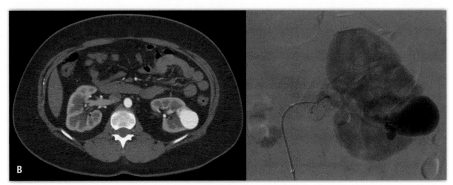

■ Questions

1. What is the appropriate NEXT course of action?
   A. Proceed with biopsy
   B. Seek urology consultation
   C. Obtain an intravenous pyelogram
   D. Obtain computed tomography with contrast

2. What is the etiology of the mass?
   A. Renal cell carcinoma
   B. Simple cyst
   C. Angiomyolipoma
   D. Arteriovenous malformation

3. What is/are the treatment option(s) for an arteriovenous malformation? (Select ALL that apply.)
   A. Surgery
   B. Embolization
   C. Combined surgery and embolization

■ Answers and Explanations

Question 1

D. Correct! A postcontrast computed tomography (CT) is of great value in helping to characterize this mass. In this case, the mass demonstrates with enhancement similar to the blood pool. Alternatively, an ultrasound of the kidney could be obtained to determine solid versus cystic and to assess the vascularity.

Other choices and discussion

A. The mass has not been adequately evaluated with imaging prior to biopsy.

B. While the patient will likely need urologic consultation in the future, further imaging is the next best course of action.

C. Additional imaging is the next step. However, a contrast CT is more appropriate than an intravenous pyelogram, which will not add any significant diagnostic value at this point.

Question 2

D. Correct! This is an arteriovenous malformation (AVM).

Other choices and discussion

A. Renal cell carcinoma enhances, but not to the degree that this lesion does. Additionally, renal cell carcinoma does not have associated large feeding arteries, as is seen in this case.

B. A simple cyst measures fluid attenuation and does not enhance.

C. Angiomyolipomas usually have a fat component and do not typically enhance to the degree that this mass does.

Question 3

A, **B**, and **C. Correct!** Surgery is reserved for selected cases, particularly those where the complete lesion can be removed without causing further disability or deformity. For many lesions, embolization tends to be the primary treatment. Combined embolization and surgery have proven to be highly successful in treating certain lesions. Embolization agents include glue, onyx, and coils. Ligation of the feeding artery has been shown to be ineffective in the long-term treatment of AVMs due to recruitment of other feeder arteries.

■ Suggested Readings

Hatzidakis A, Rossi M, Mamoulakis C, et al. Management of renal arteriovenous malformations: a pictorial review. Insights Imaging 2014;5:523–530

Rosen RJ, Nassiri N, Drury JE. Interventional management of high flow vascular malformations. Tech Vasc Interv Radiol 2013;16:22–23

Top Tips

◆ Renal AVM may be a cause of hematuria and is associated with hypertension.

◆ Renal AVM on imaging is well marginated and has enhancement similar to blood pool.

◆ Primary treatment of a renal AVM may involve surgery, embolization, or a combination of the two.

Essentials 21

■ Case

A 63-year-old woman presents with a chief complaint of "the alarms keep going off on the machine when I am dialyzed."

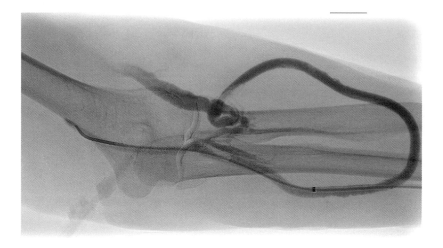

■ Questions

1. What is the likely cause of the sounding alarms?
   A. A fire
   B. Thrombosed graft
   C. Arterial anastomotic stricture
   D. Venous anastomotic stricture

2. Where is the MOST common stenotic lesion within an arteriovenous graft circuit, and what is the reason for this stenosis?
   A. Innominate vein, external compression
   B. Arterial anastomotic stenosis, atherosclerotic plaque
   C. Within the graft, neointimal hyperplasia
   D. Venous anastomosis, neointimal hyperplasia

3. What is the typical first-line treatment for venous anastomotic lesions?
   A. Oral anticoagulation
   B. Surgical revision of the anastomosis
   C. Endovascular intervention (percutaneous transluminal angioplasty and/or stent placement)
   D. Oral vasodilator agents

■ Answers and Explanations

Question 1

D. Correct! There is a moderate- to high-grade stenosis at the venous anastomosis site of the graft (top portion of the graft). There is a clear decrease in caliber at the venous anastomosis compared to the remainder of the graft. Also noted are collaterals at the anastomosis with filling of venous outflow vessels.

Other choices and discussion

A. This is not related to a fire.

B. There is contrast opacification throughout the graft and into the venous outflow.

C. There is no definite stenosis at the arterial anastomosis site.

Question 2

D. Correct! The venous anastomosis is the most common site of stenosis in AV grafts. In one study of 2300 patients, venous anastomotic stenoses accounted for 60% of lesions. The most common reason is neointimal hyperplasia.

Other choices and discussion

A. Central stenoses are not the most common lesion in arteriovenous graft circuits. In a study of 2300 patients, central stenoses accounted for 3% of lesions.

B. Arterial anastomotic lesions can cause dialysis graft dysfunction, but are not the most common stenotic lesions.

C. Intragraft stenoses are common. However, they are not the most common site of stenosis. Intragraft stenoses tend to occur at dialysis cannulation sites.

Question 3

C. Correct! Endovascular management of venous anastomotic stenoses is the typical first-line treatment. The lesions usually respond well to percutaneous transluminal angioplasty and/or stent placement.

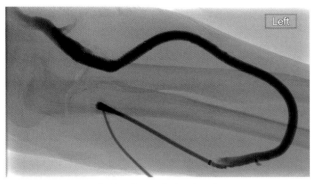

Post-endovascular treatment

Other choices and discussion

A. Use of oral anticoagulants is not a generally accepted treatment method for the sole purpose of resolving or preventing venous anastomotic stenosis.

B. While surgical revision of venous anastomoses is a reasonable option, this is not usually a first-line treatment.

D. Use of oral vasodilators is not a generally accepted treatment method for the purpose of resolving or preventing venous anastomotic stenosis.

■ Suggested Reading

Asif A, Agarwal AK, Yevzlin AS, et al. Interventional Nephrology. New York: The McGraw-Hill Companies; 2012

Top Tips

◆ Venous anastomosis is the most common site for stenosis within an arteriovenous graft circuit.

◆ Neointimal hyperplasia is typically the etiology of venous anastomotic stenoses.

◆ Venous anastomotic stenoses are usually amenable to percutaneous transluminal angioplasty and/or stenting.

SECTION XIII
VASCULAR IMAGING

Essentials 22

■ Case

Shown are angiographic images of a 47-year-old man who presents with abdominal pain, light-headiness, and vomiting.

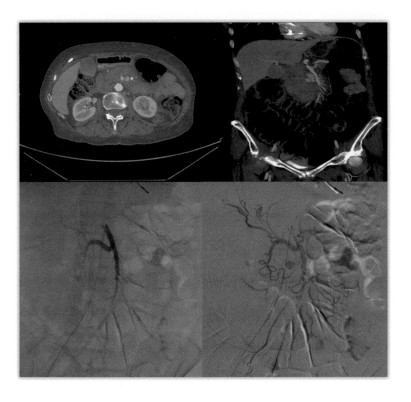

■ Questions

1. What is the MOST acute finding?
   A. Pseudoaneurysm of a branch of the pancreaticoduodenal arcade
   B. Aneurysm of the superior mesenteric artery
   C. No acute findings
   D. Abdominal aortic aneurysm rupture

2. Which of the following is(are) treatment option(s) for this condition? (Select ALL that apply.)
   A. Surgery
   B. Endovascular embolization
   C. Careful observation of the patient with serial hematocrit and hemoglobin
   D. Further confirmation with an additional imaging study

3. Which of the following are causes of mesenteric pseudoaneurysms? (Select ALL that apply.)
   A. Pancreatitis
   B. Trauma
   C. Surgery
   D. Connective vascular disorders

■ Answers and Explanations

Question 1

A. Correct! The computed tomography demonstrates a contained rupture (pseudoaneurysm [PSA]) from a branch of the pancreaticoduodenal arcade. This was confirmed on conventional angiography with a selective angiogram of the superior mesenteric artery (SMA). On angiography, extravasation is demonstrated by pooling of contrast outside of the vessel lumen without washout.

Other choices and discussion

B. The SMA is of normal caliber. The large amount of contrast pooling outside of the vessel lumen could potentially be mistaken for an aneurysm. However, following the course of the vessel on sequential images confirms extravasation.

C. Active extravasation is an acute finding.

D. The abdominal aorta is of normal caliber.

Question 2

A. Correct! PSAs of the SMA are urgent and often emergent conditions (as in this case with a potentially unstable patient). Surgery may be the best option here.

B. Correct! In certain centers where expertise is available, endovascular embolization can be the first-line treatment depending on the patient's condition (see follow-up image). Endovascular embolization offers the advantage of treating the PSA without the need for general endotracheal anesthesia, especially in patients with multiple comorbidities, and with the use of a single small incision.

Other choices and discussion

C. Watch and wait is not an appropriate treatment option for patients with mesenteric PSAs. As stated above, these are urgent and often emergent conditions with unstable patients.

D. The images shown are diagnostic, and further imaging is not required as confirmation.

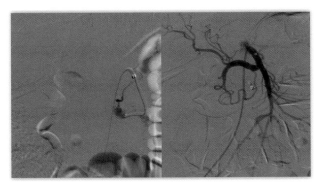

Embolization

Question 3

A. Correct! Pancreatitis can lead to PSA formation. The most common site tends to be at the splenic artery. The pancreaticoduodenal arcade can also be involved, as in this case.

B. Correct! Blunt and penetrating trauma can lead to PSA formation.

C. Correct! PSAs can be seen in postpartial pancreatectomy patients. There can be subsequent leakage of pancreatic enzymes, which erode vessel walls.

D. Correct! This can be due to weakening of the vessel wall

■ Suggested Readings

Jesinger RA, Thoreson AA, Lamba R. Abdominal and pelvic aneurysms and pseudoaneurysms: imaging review with clinical, radiologic, and treatment correlation. Radiographics 2013;33:71–96

Kenta A, Yamaguchi M, Kawasaki R, et al. N-butyl cyanoacrylate embolization for pseudoaneurysms complicating pancreatitis or pancreatectomy. J Vasc Interv Radiol 2011;22:302–308

SECTION XIII VASCULAR IMAGING

Top Tips

◆ The most common site for pseudoaneurysm formation secondary to pancreatitis is the splenic artery.

◆ For unstable patients, surgery is generally the treatment of choice.

◆ Coils are most frequently used when endovascular treatment is employed.

Essentials 23

■ Case

A 58-year-old man with end-stage renal disease was noted to have a clotted graft at dialysis. The patient presents for thrombectomy of the graft. Images from the procedure are shown.

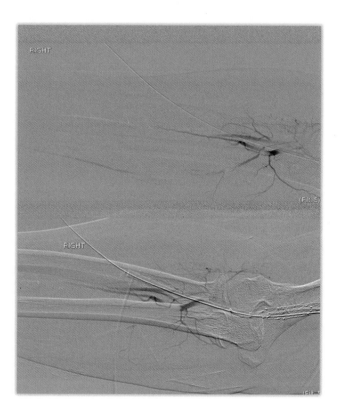

■ Questions

1. What is the salient finding?
   A. Perforation of the ulnar artery
   B. Dissection of the radial artery
   C. Thrombus within the ulnar artery
   D. Thrombus within the cephalic vein

2. What are possible complications during thrombectomy of arteriovenous dialysis shunt access? (Select ALL that apply.)
   A. Venous rupture
   B. Infection
   C. Arterial embolization
   D. Pulmonary embolization

3. Mechanisms for resolving arterial embolization during hemodialysis include all of the following EXCEPT?
   A. Back bleeding
   B. Antiplatelet bolus
   C. Catheter aspiration
   D. Thrombolysis

■ Answers and Explanations

Question 1

C. Correct! The angiogram shows opacification of the radial artery. There is a filling defect within the ulnar artery as it gives origin to the interosseous artery.

Other choices and discussion

A. There is no extravasation of contrast on the angiogram.

B. The visualized portion of the radial artery is patent. No dissection flap is seen.

D. The catheter is seen within the ulnar artery. Thus, an angiogram (not a venogram) was performed. It would be difficult to evaluate the cephalic vein during an angiogram. There is sluggish antegrade flow within the ulnar artery from the elbow to the hand. There is opacification of the radial artery secondary to reflux of contrast into the vessel.

Question 2

A. Correct! Venous rupture is the most frequent complication that requires intervention. Common treatment options include prolonged angioplasty and placement of a covered stent.

B. Correct! Infection occurs at a low rate during hemodialysis access intervention. This is mainly the result of sterile technique. If there is suspicion for an infected hemodialysis access, the patient should not undergo thrombectomy due to concern for dissemination of the infection and septic emboli.

C. Correct! As demonstrated by this case, arterial embolization is a possible complication during hemodialysis access intervention. Although it can occur during thrombectomy of both fistulas and grafts, arterial embolization tends to occur more often with grafts. The reason for this is not entirely clear.

D. Correct! Pulmonary embolization is the most common complication during hemodialysis access thrombectomy. Fortunately, most of the emboli are subclinical in nature. Microembolization even occurs during dialysis. However, there can be clinically significant emboli to the lungs during thrombectomy. Measures must be taken to reduce the passage of significant clot burden to the lungs.

Question 3

B. Correct! Antiplatelet bolus is not an accepted treatment choice for arterial embolization.

Other choices and discussion

A. Back bleeding technique is an accepted technique for removal of arterial emboli, which involves placing a balloon proximal to the anastomosis and inflating the balloon. This causes reversal of flow within the artery, forcing the embolus into the graft (where it can then be aspirated or macerated).

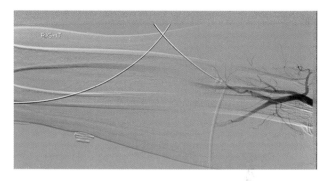

C. Thrombo-aspiration is a mechanism for removing embolus from arteries. A catheter is placed at the face of the embolus, and a syringe is connected as suction is maintained.

D. Thrombolysis involves the administration of a lytic agent such as tissue plasminogen activator into the embolus. Thrombolysis tends to be used after other techniques have been attempted, as this technique takes a longer period of time to demonstrate an effect.

■ Suggested Readings

Asif A, Agarwal AK, Yevzlin AS, et al. Interventional Nephrology. New York: The McGraw-Hill Companies; 2012

Nikolic B. Hemodialysis fistula interventions: diagnostic and treatment challenges and technical considerations. Tech Vasc Interv Radiol 2008;11:167–174

Top Tips

- ◆ Complications during hemodialysis access include vessel rupture, arterial embolization, pulmonary embolization, and infection.

- ◆ Venous rupture can often be treated with prolonged angioplasty.

- ◆ Careful attention to detail and technique reduces the risk of complications during hemodialysis access thrombectomy.

Essentials 24

■ Case

A 23-year-old man presents with swelling and pain of the right lower extremity. Shown are radiographic and magnetic resonance images of the right lower extremity.

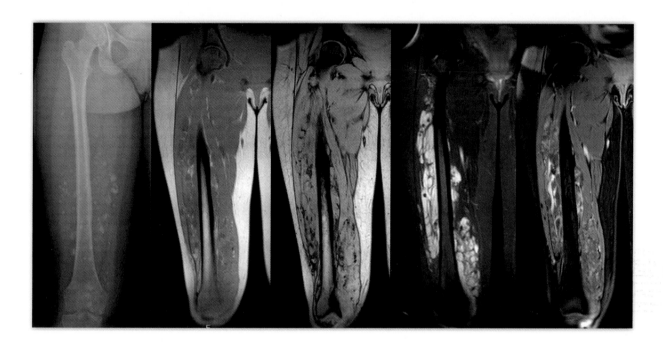

■ Questions

1. What is the diagnosis?
   A. Soft tissue sarcoma
   B. Aneurysmal bone cyst
   C. Vascular malformation
   D. Soft tissue myxoma

2. What is the MOST accurate diagnosis, based on the classification system adopted by the International Society for the Study of Vascular Anomalies?
   A. Hemangioma
   B. Low-flow vascular malformation
   C. High-flow vascular malformation
   D. Angiosarcoma

3. What is the treatment goal of high-flow arteriovenous malformations?
   A. Eradication of the draining vein
   B. Surgical excision of the entire malformation
   C. Embolization of the feeding artery
   D. Eradication of the nidus

■ Answers and Explanations

Question 1

C. Correct! This patient has a vascular malformation. The radiograph of the right thigh demonstrates multiple large phleboliths in the soft tissues. T1 in- and out-of-phase, short tau inversion recovery, and postcontrast magnetic resonance images (from left to right) through the right thigh demonstrate a predominantly T2-hyperintense infiltrative lesion with areas of interspersed fat (drop out of signal on out-of-phase), heterogeneous enhancement, and the presence of phleboliths. The lesion is located in the musculature with an entirely normal appearance of the surrounding tissues. All these features in a young adult lead to the diagnosis of a vascular malformation.

Other choices and discussion

A. The patient's age makes the diagnosis of soft tissue sarcoma somewhat less likely. On imaging, although the lesion is infiltrative, there is no invasion or edema of the surrounding structures.

B. The lesion is entirely located in the musculature of the thigh, and the femur is completely normal. This is not an aneurysmal bone cyst.

D. Soft tissue myxomas are well-circumscribed T2-hyperintense lesions that typically have a thin peripheral rim of enhancement on the postcontrast images. The presence of intralesional fat and heterogenous postcontrast enhancement is not characteristic of myxomas.

Question 2

B. Correct! This is a low-flow vascular malformation. Vascular malformations are categorized into low-flow or high-flow vascular malformations. Venous, lymphatic, capillary, capillary-venous, and capillary-lymphatic-venous are the various types of low-flow vascular malformations. These are congenital in origin, although may not be evident at birth. They grow proportionally with age and do not regress. Low-flow vascular malformations appear as septated, lobulated, and infiltrative soft tissue masses without mass effect on the adjacent structures. Phleboliths are characteristic of venous malformations. Diffuse delayed enhancement is seen with a venous malformation, whereas rim-like peripheral and septal enhancement is seen with a lymphatic malformation.

Other choices and discussion

A. Vascular anomalies are broadly classified into vascular tumors (hemangioma) and vascular malformations. Hemangioma, also termed infantile hemangioma, is the most common vascular tumor of infancy. These typically manifest in the first few weeks of birth as rapidly growing subcutaneous bluish red masses with warmth, bruit, and pulsatility owing to the high flow. This is the proliferating phase, which is followed by an involuting phase where the hemangioma regresses into fibrofatty residuum. The diagnosis is usually made clinically. No treatment is indicated as they spontaneously involute.

C. As the name implies, high-flow vascular malformations have high flow, due to the presence of an arterial supply. They constitute ~10% of vascular malformations. Arteriovenous malformations and arteriovenous fistulas are the two types of high-flow vascular malformations. No definite mass is visualized on imaging. Enlarged feeding arteries, draining veins, and flow voids with early enhancement of the feeding arteries and early filling of draining veins are the imaging features of high-flow vascular malformations.

D. Angiosarcoma is a highly vascular soft tissue sarcoma. It is seen as an infiltrative T2-hyperintense mass with flow voids and postcontrast light bulb–like enhancement. It is typically very aggressive, with invasion of the neighboring structures. Distant metastases at the time of diagnosis is not uncommon.

Question 3

D. Correct! The ultimate goal of endovascular treatment for a high-flow vascular malformation is embolization of the nidus, which will decrease the rate of recurrence. This is best accomplished with liquid embolic agents (onyx, alcohol, glue). These can penetrate the feeding vessel into the nidus.

Other choices and discussion

A. Embolization of the draining vein impairs drainage of the malformation and has no therapeutic effect.

B. Surgical excision was the mainstay of treatment prior to the advent of interventional radiology. Complete surgical excision has a high rate of recurrence. Moreover, surgery is associated with a major risk of bleeding. Therefore, endovascular embolization therapies have largely substituted/adjuncted surgical resection.

C. Embolization of the feeding artery causes a decrease in blood supply to the malformation. However, recruitment of other feeding arteries is common, leading to recurrence.

■ Suggested Readings

Flors L, Leiva-Salinas C, Maged IM, Norton PT, et al. MR Imaging of soft-tissue vascular malformations: diagnosis, classification, and therapy follow-up. Radiographics 2011;31:1321–1341

Hyodoh H, Hori M, Akiba H, Tamakawa M, Hyodoh K, Hareyama M. Peripheral vascular malformations: imaging, treatment approaches, and therapeutic issues. Radiographics 2005;25(Suppl 1):S159–171

Nosher JL, Murillo PG, Liszewski M, Gendel V, Gribbin CE. Vascular anomalies: a pictorial review of nomenclature, diagnosis and treatment. World J Radiol 2014;6:677–692

Yakes WF. Endovascular management of high-flow arteriovenous malformations. Sem Interv Radiol 2004;21:49–58

Top Tips

◆ Vascular anomalies are divided into vascular tumors and vascular malformations (low- or high-flow). Low-flow malformations appear as infiltrative, lobulated, septated soft tissue masses with interspersed fat and phleboliths (venous). High-flow malformations are characterized by feeding arteries, a nidus, draining veins, and the presence of flow voids.

◆ Infantile hemangioma is the most common vascular tumor of infancy.

◆ Percutaneous embolotherapies have evolved as the mainstay of treatment over surgical resection.

Essentials 25

■ Case

Computed tomography angiographic images through the chest of a 35-year-old female patient are shown.

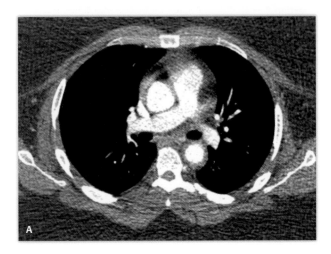
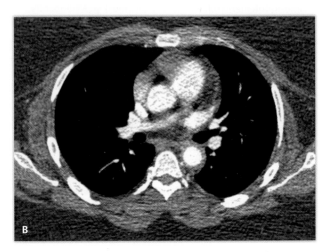

■ Questions

1. What is the diagnosis?
   A. Giant cell arteritis
   B. Takayasu arteritis
   C. Ankylosing spondylitis
   D. Infectious aortitis

2. What is the mainstay of treatment for an uncomplicated course of this condition?
   A. No treatment is necessary
   B. Surgery
   C. Angioplasty
   D. High-dose glucocorticoids

3. Which of the following is a medium vessel vasculitis?
   A. Microscopic polyangiitis
   B. Wegener granulomatosis
   C. Polyarteritis nodosa
   D. Churg-Strauss syndrome

■ Answers and Explanations

Question 1

B. Correct! Takayasu arteritis, also called pulseless disease or Martorell syndrome, is a chronic inflammatory arteritis of unknown etiology. It has a strong predilection for young woman and typically involves large vessels. The abdominal aorta is most commonly affected, followed by the descending thoracic aorta and aortic arch. Computed tomography angiographic imaging features include crescentic or concentric aortic wall thickening of > 3 mm, resulting in narrow caliber (stenosis) of the aorta and sometimes even complete occlusion. Because the imaging findings are nonspecific, the diagnosis is made by combining radiologic features with demographics, clinical history, and laboratory findings.

Other choices and discussion

A. Giant cell arteritis is a chronic vasculitis involving large- and medium-sized vessels. Superficial cranial vessels are the most commonly affected. A total of 15% of cases involve the aorta. The other primary distinguishing feature from Takayasu is that giant cell arteritis is rarely seen in those < 50 years of age.

C. Aortitis in ankylosing spondylitis tends to involve the aortic root and aortic valve (80% of cases) with associated valvular insufficiency.

D. Infectious aortitis typically occurs in the presence of predisposing factors such as atherosclerosis, aneurysm, cystic medial necrosis, diabetes, vascular malformation, medical devices, or prior surgery. *Staphylococcus aureus* and *Salmonella* account for the most common organisms. Aortic wall thickening with surrounding inflammatory stranding and fluid are the common imaging features. Air in the aortic wall is seen occasionally.

Question 2

D. Correct! As Takayasu arteritis is an idiopathic inflammatory condition, high-dose corticosteroids are the mainstay of therapy.

Other choices and discussion

A. Takayasu arteritis progresses without treatment and leads to complications such as stenosis, occlusion, thrombosis, and aneurysm formation.

B. Surgery is the last resort of treatment for complicated cases.

C. Angioplasty with or without stent placement is reserved for symptomatic fibrotic lesions leading to stenosis and/or occlusion.

Question 3

C. Correct! Polyarteritis nodosa is a medium vessel arteritis most commonly involving the kidney, followed by the gastrointestinal tract, liver, spleen, and pancreas. Multiple aneurysm formation is characteristic. Positive perinuclear antineutrophil cytoplasmic antibody titers aid in the diagnosis. Therapy with steroids and cyclophosphamide results in remission or cure in ~90% of patients.

Other choices and discussion

A. Histologically, microscopic polyangiitis is similar to polyarteritis nodosa, except for its involvement of small vessels. Glomerulonephritis and pulmonary capillaritis are the two most common manifestations.

B. Wegener granulomatosis is also a small vessel vasculitis, characteristically involving the upper and lower respiratory tract and the kidneys (with glomerulonephritis).

D. Churg-Strauss syndrome is a small vessel vasculitis typically involving the lung followed by the gastrointestinal tract. Mesenteric vasculitis is a common manifestation.

■ Suggested Readings

Gotway MB, Araoz PA, Macedo TA, Stanson AW, et al. Imaging findings in Takayasu's arteritis. Am J Roentgenol 2005;184:1945–1950

Ha HK, Lee SH, Rha SE, Kim JH, et al. Radiologic features of vasculitis involving the gastrointestinal tract. Radiographics 2000;20:779–794

Restrepo CS, Ocazionez D, Suri R, Vargas D. Aortitis: imaging spectrum of the infectious and inflammatory conditions of the aorta. Radiographics 2011;31:435–451

Zhu FP, Luo S, Wang ZJ, Jin ZY, Zhang LJ, Lu GM. Takayasu arteritis: imaging spectrum at multidetector CT angiography. BJR. 2012;85(1020):e1282–1292

Top Tips

◆ Large vessel vasculitis: Takayasu and giant cell arteritis. Takayasu arteritis has a predilection for young females, whereas giant cell arteritis is rare before 50 years of age. Glucocorticoids are the mainstay of treatment. Angioplasty and surgery are reserved for complicated cases.

◆ Medium vessel vasculitis: polyarteritis nodosa and Kawasaki disease.

◆ Small vessel vasculitis: Wegener granulomatosis, microscopic polyangiitis, Churg-Strauss syndrome, Henoch-Schönlein syndrome, systemic lupus erythematosus, rheumatoid arthritis, and Behcet syndrome.

Essentials 1

■ Case

Radionuclide Y (atomic number Z) decays by β^- decay, resulting in the production of a metastable daughter state. The metastable daughter nucleus then transforms to the ground state by isomeric transition. A sample containing both the parent and daughter states is examined. Which of the following is likely to be present in the sample?

A. A β^- particle at a single discrete energy
B. A range of high-energy γ-rays emitted by radioisotope Y
C. A daughter state with Z + 1 protons
D. X-rays with a range of continuous energies emitted by the daughter state
E. Only one daughter state at a single energy level

■ Answers and Explanations

C. Correct! In β^- decay, a neutron is converted to a proton, and therefore, the Z (atomic number) increases by one; thus, the daughter is a different element than the parent ("transmutation"). The mass number (A) does not change. Therefore, the parent and daughter are isobars. An example is ^{133}Xe's β^- decay to ^{133}Cs.

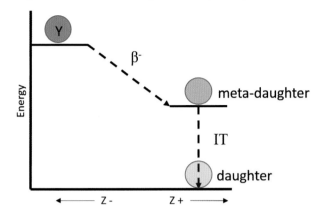

Other choices and discussion

A. The decay of the parent radioisotope will result in the emission of a family of β^- particles of varying continuous energies up to E_β^{max}. Typically, the average β^- particle energy, E_β, will be *approximately* one-third of E_β^{max}.

B. In β^- decay, the parent emits a beta-particle (β^-) and an anti-neutrino ($\bar{v}$) as it decays to the daughter state.

D. In isomeric transition, the metastable daughter nucleus will emit characteristic, discrete gamma rays (γ-rays) rather than a family of γ-rays with continuous energies. Frequently, a meta-stable nucleus will emit both γ-rays and conversion electrons; the frequency of each type of emission (e/γ ratio) is characteristic for each isotope. Like the γ-rays, these conversion electrons will have discrete energies (based on their position in the electron cloud—i.e., the shell from which they were ejected).

E. As noted in A, the decay of the parent will result in the emission of numerous β^- particles at varying energies, resulting in several daughter states with varying energies.

■ Suggested Readings

Patton JA. Introduction to nuclear physics. Radiographics 1998;18:995–1007

Saha GB. Physics and radiobiology of nuclear medicine. 4th ed. New York: Springer; 2014

Top Tips

◆ β^- decay → neutron converted to proton → Z + 1 → parent and daughter are isobars (same mass number, different atomic number).

◆ β^- decay → parent emits a beta-particle (β^-) and an anti-neutrino ($\bar{v}$).

◆ The average β^- particle energy, E_β, will be *approximately* one-third of E_β^{max}.

Essentials 2

■ Case

Which of the following characteristics of alpha (α) decay limits the use of alpha emitters for diagnostic applications?
   A. α-particles interact minimally with solid materials, such as those found in radiation detectors.
   B. α-particles are typically of very low energy.
   C. α-decay most often occurs in light (low mass number) elements that are not easily incorporated into radiopharmaceuticals.
   D. α-particles have a short range in tissue.
   E. α-decay produces daughter nuclides that cannot be chemically separated from the parent.

■ Answers and Explanations

D. Correct! As heavy particles, alpha (α) particles undergo numerous interactions with surrounding matter, and as such, continuously lose small amounts of energy causing them to slow down as they travel only a relatively short distance—typically < 100 μm in solids (β⁺ particles from ⁸²Rb, in contrast, have a mean range of ~2.5 mm).

Other choices and discussion

A. Alpha (α) particles have two protons (Z = 2) and two neutrons (A = 4), and are essentially a helium nucleus. They have a high linear energy transfer and deposit substantial energy over a very short range via their interactions with surrounding matter. Given this high local deposition of energy, α-emitting radiopharmaceuticals have been viewed as promising for targeted irradiation of tumor cells.

B. Alpha (α) particles are typically of very high energy, oftentimes more than 3 to 5 MeV.

C. Alpha (α) decay, like fission, typically occurs in heavy isotopes such as uranium (²³⁸U, where Z = 92) and radium (²²³Ra, where Z = 88). Difficulty in producing α-emitting radiopharmaceuticals has been mainly related to the radiolytic effects of clinically useful α-particle doses which produce challenges to traditional radiochemistry methods.

E. Daughter nuclides produced by α-decay have an atomic number of Z − 2 and a mass number of A − 4 as compared to the parent radionuclide. As such, the daughter is typically chemically distinct from the parent, and at low activities, can be separated by standard methods such as resin-based elution.

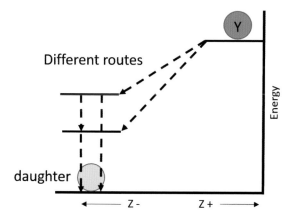

■ Suggested Readings

Cherry SR, Sorenson JA, Phelps ME. Physics in Nuclear Medicine. 4th ed. Philadelphia: Saunders; 2012

De Kruijff RM, Wolterbeek HT, Denkova AG. A critical review of alpha radionuclide therapy—how to deal with recoiling daughters? Pharmaceuticals 2015;8:321–336

Huclier-Markai S, Alliot C, Varmenot N, et al. Alpha-emitters for immune-therapy: a review from chemistry to clinics. Curr Top Med Chem 2012;12:2642–2654

Top Tips

◆ Alpha (α) particles have two protons (Z = 2) and two neutrons (A = 4), and are essentially a helium nucleus. Daughter nuclides produced by α-decay have an atomic number of Z − 2 and a mass number of A − 4 as compared to the parent radionuclide.

◆ Given their ability to deliver high doses of radiation to a small area (high linear energy transfer) when appropriately targeted, α-emitting radiopharmaceuticals show great promise for radiotherapeutic applications and have achieved recent success on a limited basis.

◆ While the α emissions of the parent may be favorable due to the short path length, and therefore limited "crossfire" radiation, the production of excited daughter states that may add to the radiation dose/damage has remained a concern and will be of particular interest in the future.

Essentials 3

■ Case

A charged particle is found to have a high linear energy transfer (LET) in a tissue. What would you conclude about the particle?
   A. The particle produces a high specific ionization (SI) in the tissue.
   B. The particle must be a neutron.
   C. The particle produces mainly single-strand deoxyribonucleic acid (DNA) breaks in the tissue.
   D. The particle likely has a very high velocity as it travels through the tissue.
   E. The path of the particle in the tissue is long and crooked.

■ Answers and Explanations

A. Correct! LET refers to the amount of energy deposited in matter (e.g., in tissue) per unit of length along the path of an incident radiation. SI is defined as the average number of ionization events per unit of radiation path length. SI is related to LET by the following relationship: **LET = SI/W**, where W is the average energy expended in the production of an ionization. Thus, as a radiation moves along its path, deposited energy will produce ionizations, and as such, a particle that produces many ionizations (high SI) would be expected to have a high LET.

Other choices and discussion

B. Neutrons (n), alpha (α) particles, and protons may have high LETs and are considered to be heavy particles with mass energies greater several orders of magnitude greater than an electron (a light particle). Electrons (including β-particles) are small particles with low LET. Electromagnetic radiations, though not particulate in nature, also exhibit low LET.

C. High LET radiation produces frequent double-strand DNA breaks that are difficult for the cell or tissue to repair effectively. Low LET radiation produces fewer double-strand DNA breaks and is associated with less radiation-induced cell death.

D. A particle with a high LET, by definition, deposits a high amount of energy into the local tissues. This deposition is a property of the tissues (higher density tissues will provide more atoms available for interaction in a given mass of tissue than would less dense tissues) and of the particle or incident radiation. A particle traveling at a high velocity through a tissue would be expected to spend only a small fraction of time in the vicinity of any given atom, and therefore would have a low likelihood of interacting and causing an ionization of that atom. In contrast, a particle traveling at a low velocity through a tissue would have a higher likelihood of interacting with and depositing energy resulting in an ionization.

E. Particles that deposit energy locally lose speed (energy) as they do so. Typically, these particles travel a short distance along a fairly straight path until they have lost all of their energy to the surrounding tissues. Small particles, such as β-particles, are more likely to interact with multiple atoms in the tissue, having a long and tortuous path as each interaction causes the loss of a small amount of energy and deflects the electron from its incident path angle.

■ Suggested Readings

Cherry SR, Sorenson JA, Phelps ME. Physics in Nuclear medicine. 4th ed. Philadelphia: Saunders; 2012

Kassis AI, Adelstein SJ. Radiobiologic principles in radionuclide therapy. J Nucl Med 2005;46:4S–12S

Saha GB. Physics and Radiobiology of Nuclear Medicine. 4th ed. New York: Springer; 2014

Top Tips

◆ For a given amount of kinetic energy, alpha (α) particles may ionize hundreds of times more atoms in the local tissue than electrons (including β-particles) with the same kinetic energy.

◆ Both particulate and electromagnetic incident radiations transfer energy to tissues and can result in tissue ionizations.

Essentials 4

■ **Case**

An incident radiation (γ-ray) interacts with an atom as shown below. The labeled electron is _____ and thus, the atom will be _____.

    A. a secondary electron; in an excited state
    B. an Auger electron; in an excited state
    C. a photoelectron; in an ionized state
    D. a β⁻ particle; more stable than the original atom
    E. a β⁺ particle; an isotope of the original atom

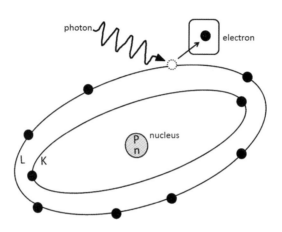

■ Answers and Explanations

C. Correct! Ionization of an atom has occurred when an orbital electron has been removed or separated from the atom, leaving the atom in an unstable ionized state. The electron that is lost from an atom as a result of a collision with a photon is called a photoelectron. (Strictly speaking, the photoelectron is a specific type of secondary electron, as it is separated from the atom by the incident [primary] radiation, which in this case is a photon.)

Other choices and discussion

A. A secondary electron lost by interaction or collision with an incident radiation is called a secondary electron, to differentiate it from the incident (primary) radiation; the electron in this example *is* a secondary electron. By definition, excitation of an atom occurs when an electron is raised to a higher energy state within its orbital shell; the electron is not lost from the atom in excitation event.

B. An Auger electron is emitted when an electron in a higher orbital shell transitions to fill a vacancy left by an electron being removed from a lower orbital shell (typically due to the process of internal conversion). When the excess energy of the transition is then transferred to an orbital shell electron, that electron is emitted; this is emitted electron is the Auger electron. Note that, as an alternative to emission of an Auger electron, the excess transition energy may instead result in the release of a characteristic X-ray. By definition, excitation of an atom occurs when an electron is raised to a higher energy state (from a lower energy shell to an upper energy shell); the electron is not lost from the atom in excitation event.

D. A β^- particle is a form of particulate radiation, not electromagnetic radiation (i.e., it is not a photon). As shown in the diagram, the atom has lost an electron, leaving it with a net positive charge in an ionized state. Ionized states are not more stable than their nonionized form (ground state).

E. A β^+ particle is a form of particulate radiation, not electromagnetic radiation (i.e., it is not a photon). In the example shown, no nuclear changes have occurred (the number of protons and neutrons in the nucleus has not changed), thus this atom has simply been ionized. By definition, isotopes are nuclides with the same proton number (Z) but different mass numbers. Examples of clinically relevant isotopes are ^{68}Ga and ^{67}Ga, which both have Z = 31, but have different numbers of neutrons and therefore different mass numbers.

■ Suggested Readings

Cherry SR, Sorenson JA, Phelps ME. Physics in Nuclear Medicine. 4th ed. Philadelphia: Saunders; 2012

Saha GB. Physics and Radiobiology of Nuclear Medicine. 4th ed. New York: Springer; 2014

Top Tips

◆ Photoelectrons and other secondary electrons are ejected from an atom by its collision with an incident radiation.

◆ Other types of emitted orbital electrons (e.g., Auger) typically result from an ionized atom transitioning to its ground state rather than the direct interaction with an incident radiation.

Essentials 5

■ Case

Neutral stable phosphorus has an atomic number of 15 (Z = 15) and a mass number of 31 (A = 31). Based on the Bohr model of the atom, what is the principal quantum number of the energy shell in which the outermost electrons are likely to be found?

A. 0
B. 1
C. 2
D. 3
E. 4

■ Answers and Explanations

D. Correct! Each electron shell is designated a principal quantum number (n), beginning at 1 for the K-shell. Thus, the L-shell has a principal quantum number of 2, the M-shell has a quantum number of 3, etc. Each shell can house a maximum of $2n^2$ electrons, and electrons will fill the lowest shell first. Once the K- and L-shells contain the maximum number of electrons, electrons will then fill the M-shell, which has a quantum number of 3 and can contain a maximum of $[2 \times (3)^2] = 18$ electrons. Thus, in a stable atom with 15 protons and 15 electrons, the outermost electrons are expected to fill into the 3p orbital, where the principal quantum number of 3 represents the M-shell.

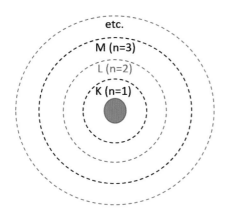

Other choices and discussion

A. There is no electron shell with a principal quantum number of 0.

B. In a stable atom with 15 protons, there will be 15 electrons within the electron cloud. These electrons will first fill the lowest shell—the K-shell, which holds a maximum of 2 $[2 \times (1)^2]$ electrons, thus leaving 13 electrons within the higher-level shells. Thus, the outermost electrons will not be in the K (quantum number of 1) shell.

C. Once the K-shell contains the maximum number of electrons, the electrons will then fill the L-shell (which has quantum number of 2, and can contain a maximum of $[2 \times (2)^2] = 8$ electrons). In a stable atom with 15 protons and 15 electrons, there will, therefore, be $15 - (2 + 8)$ electrons left to reside within a higher-level shell.

E. The N-shell (with a quantum number of 4 and a maximum number of contained electrons of $[2 \times (4)^2] = 32$) will only be filled once the M-shell contains its maximum number of electrons. Thus, for a stable atom with 15 protons and 15 electrons, we would not expect any electrons in the N-shell as they would have all been accommodated by the K-, L-, and M-shells.

■ Suggested Readings

Saha GB. Physics and Radiobiology of Nuclear Medicine. 4th ed. New York: Springer; 2014

Top Tips

♦ Each electron shell is designated a principal quantum number (n), beginning at 1 for the K-shell.

♦ Each electron shell can house a maximum of $2n^2$ electrons, and electrons will fill the lowest shell first.

Essentials 6

■ Case

In transporting a 200 mCi sample of radionuclide Q-labeled pharmaceutical in a capped plastic syringe to the imaging suite, the investigator falls and drops the sample—spilling most of it on the hallway floor. Based on the activity and primary emission (210 keV γ-rays) of the radionuclide, this is deemed to be a *major* radioactive spill. Unlike a *minor* spill, clean-up and precautions for a *major* spill necessarily include:

A. Notification of personnel and other persons in the area that a spill has occurred and restricting access to the spill area.

B. Covering the spill with absorbent paper, when applicable, to prevent spread of the material or contamination of other surfaces.

C. Survey of the spill area and areas of potential contamination with a survey meter or other appropriate detector.

D. Immediate notification of the radiation safety officer (RSO).

E. Decontamination of affected individuals.

■ Answers and Explanations

D. Correct! The distinction between major spills and minor spills depends largely on the amount and type of radionuclide (internal radiation hazard) involved. In addition, major spills are often considered to be those spills that are not easily contained or containable by standard measures or interventions. In this case, the spill is deemed to be a major spill, and therefore precautions for a major spill should be followed. In addition to the other precautions listed, which should be followed for all spills whether they are minor or major, major spills require the immediate reporting of the incident to the local RSO. The RSO may make recommendations regarding clean-up and modifications to standard procedures to prevent or lessen the impact of future spills. For minor spills, the RSO may not need to be notified—particularly not immediately—unless there were unusual circumstances surrounding the spill.

Other choices and discussion

A. Following any spill of radioactive material in a nuclear medicine or radiology department, persons in the area surrounding the spill should be notified of the spill and prevented from entering the area. In this example, physicians, nurses, technologists, patients, and others might be prevented from utilizing the section of the hallway where the spill has occurred until proper decontamination has occurred and surveys indicate that the area poses no hazard.

B. As most radiopharmaceuticals are administered intravenously and in liquid form, covering the spill with absorbent paper is often a good first step in minimizing its impact. This can serve not only as a visual alert that something has been spilled, whether on the floor or on a countertop, but can be used to remove the spilled material from the surface. If the spilled material is in powder or gas form, efforts to limit its spread might include the closing of nearby or adjacent doors. For spills on the floor, careful attention should be paid to surveying, and if needed, decontaminating the shoes of personnel involved in the spill and spill clean-up, to prevent inadvertent contamination of other areas.

C. In assessing the degree of spread or potential contamination following any radioactive spill, a survey meter or other device should be used to determine how large the spill area is and the extent to which any radioactive material has been transferred to other surfaces. For example, nearby door handles, floors, and equipment may be surveyed to ensure that material has not been transferred. Identification of affected (contaminated) personnel or other persons is of first priority, and survey meters may be used to detect spilled material on the clothes or skin of those who may have been exposed.

E. As suggested above, the identification and decontamination of affected persons is the first priority after any radioactive spill. The Nuclear Regulatory Commission requires that all radioactive materials licensees have procedures in place for the handling of radioactive spills.

■ Suggested Readings

Baldwin JA, Bag AK, White SL, Palot-Manzil FF, et al. All you need to know as an authorized user. Am J Roentgenol 2015;205:251–258

Siegel JA. Nuclear Regulatory Commission Regulation of Nuclear Medicine: Guide for Diagnostic Nuclear Medicine. Reston, VA: Society of Nuclear Medicine; 2001

Top Tips

◆ Classification of a spill as either major or minor depends on the radionuclide involved and the amount of spilled activity. For example, minor spills of radionuclides labeled with ^{99m}Tc are those where the spilled activity is < 100 mCi. Conversely, spills of ≥ 10 mCi of radionuclides labeled with ^{67}Ga or ^{111}In are considered major spills, and spills of only 1 mCi of ^{131}I-labeled radionuclides are considered major spills.

◆ Major spills require the immediate reporting of the incident to the local RSO.

Essentials 7

■ Case

In the United States, members of the general public receive the highest annual dose of radiation (per capita) from which of the following sources?

A. Diagnostic X-rays
B. Cosmic radiation from the sun
C. Ingested isotopes including potassium-40
D. Thorium-232 and radium-226 within terrestrial material
E. Inhalation of radon in the air

■ Answers and Explanations

A. Correct! Based on data from the United Nations (United Nations Scientific Committee on the Effects of Atomic Radiation) 2008, diagnostic X-rays resulting from medical procedures such as computed tomography, radiography, fluoroscopy, and dental radiographs contribute approximately 2.4 mSv to the annual effective radiation dose to the general public. This data is consistent with, though with very slight differences, data on background and medical sources of radiation as published in the 2009 National Council on Radiation Protection and Measurement Report 160. You may refer to the NIS section for additional discussion.

Other choices and discussion

B. Cosmic rays deliver approximately 0.3 mSv of effective radiation dose annually, with the amount varying somewhat with altitude.

C. Ingestion of foods and water results in the internal deposition of compounds that emit radioisotopes such as ^{40}K. These internal compounds expose members of the general public to about 0.3 to 0.4 mSv effective dose per year.

D. Terrestrial radiation sources expose the general public to approximately 0.4 to 0.5 mSv of radiation dose annually.

E. Inhaled or airborne radon is the most abundant source of natural background radiation, accounting for approximately 1.2 to 2 mSv effective dose per year.

■ Suggested Readings

Mettler FA, Bhargavan M, Faulkner K, et al. Radiologic and nuclear medicine studies in the United States and worldwide: frequency, radiation dose, and comparison with other radiation sources—1950-2007. Radiol 2009;253:520–531

National Council on Radiation Protection. NCRP Report No. 160. (2009). Ionizing radiation exposure of the population of the United States. http://ncrponline.org/publications/reports/ncrp-report-160/

United Nations Scientific Committee on the Effects of Atomic Radiation. 2006 Report to the General Assembly. New York, NY: United Nations; 2008

United Nations Scientific Committee on the Effects of Atomic Radiation. Sources and effects of ionizing radiation. Medical radiation exposures, annex B. 2008 Report to the General Assembly with Scientific Annexes. New York, NY: United Nations; 2010

Top Tips

◆ Estimated annual per capita effective dose in the United States is approximately 5.6 mSv.

◆ *Among diagnostic imaging procedures, computed tomography accounts for almost half of effective radiation doses to the general public, at 1.3 to 1.5 mSv annually. This is followed by nuclear medicine, with an estimated radiation dose of 0.6 to 0.8 mSv per year.

◆ Whereas, previously, annual radiation dose from natural background radiation exceeded manmade sources, with the increased utilization of imaging for diagnostic and therapeutic applications, medical sources of radiation are overall approximately equal to background radiation doses.

Essentials 8

■ Case

A 62-year-old man undergoes thromboembolization of a cerebral arteriovenous malformation. He receives a cumulative radiation dose of 500 cGy from the procedure. Which of the following most accurately characterizes tissue reactions (formerly referred to as "deterministic effects") resulting from the interventional procedure?

A. As depicted in curve A, the severity of tissue reactions increases with high radiation dose.
B. As depicted in curve A, the likelihood of tissue reactions is not modifiable.
C. As depicted in curve B, severe tissue reactions occur only at late stages or time points.
D. As depicted in curve B, the likelihood of tissue reactions is nonzero above a threshold dose.
E. As depicted in curve C, the likelihood of tissue reactions is expected to be constant at any dose.

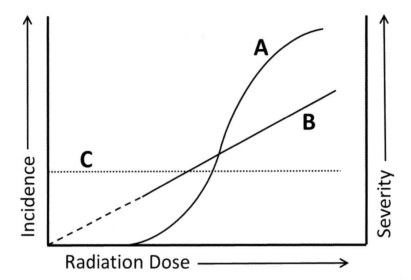

■ Answers and Explanations

A. Correct! "Tissue reactions," formerly referred to as "non-stochastic" and then "deterministic" effects of radiation, are classically distinguished from radiation stochastic effects by the presence of a threshold dose (which may be quite low and variable depending on the tissue type), above which the severity of effects increases and below which there is no detectable effect.

Other choices and discussion

B. There is accumulating evidence that the likelihood (incidence) of tissue reactions, especially those reactions typically occurring late after the exposure, may be modified by substances such as antioxidants, anti-inflammatory drugs, and others.

C. Tissue reactions include damage occurring soon after the radiation exposure ("early")—such as skin erythema, which may be seen within several hours—and those seen at remote time points after the exposure ("late")—such as cataracts, sterility, and radiation-related circulatory disease, which may become evident years after the exposure.

D. Curve B depicts the "linear-no-threshold" model of stochastic radiation effects, not "tissue reactions." This model holds that there is no threshold dose, but rather suggests that the occurrence (incidence) of effects increases linearly as a function of radiation dose. Stochastic effects include cancer and other radiation-induced heritable effects such as mental retardation.

E. Curve C depicts effects that are independent of radiation dose.

■ Suggested Readings

Hamada N, Fujimichi Y. Classification of radiation effects for dose limitation purposes: history, current situation and future prospects. J Radiat Res 2014;55:629–640

Saha GB. Physics and Radiobiology of Nuclear Medicine. 4th ed. New York: Springer; 2014

Stewart FA, Akleyev AV, Hauer-Jensen M, et al. ICRP Statement on Tissue Reactions/Early and Late Effects of Radiation in Normal Tissues and Organs—Threshold Doses for Tissue Reactions in a Radiation Protection Context. ICRP Publication 118. Ann ICRP 2012;41(1/2)

Top Tips

- The current terminology, "tissue reactions," was formerly referred to as deterministic or nonstochastic effects.

- There is a threshold dose for tissue reactions, and severity of tissue reactions increases with high radiation dose.

Essentials 9

■ **Case**

A nuclear reactor has been installed in a rural area of Alabama and is undergoing initial quality assurance testing before inspection by the Nuclear Regulatory Commission. The reactor is to be used predominately for the production of medical grade 131-iodine (^{131}I) by fission of 235-uranium (^{235}U). During testing, a reactor core overheats and partially melts, ultimately resulting in release of ^{131}I into the air; no significnat quantities of other parent or daughter products are released. During the investigation of the accident, it is determined that, while there is no groundwater or soil contamination in the areas surrounding the reactor, there are high levels of ^{131}I within air samples from the neighboring areas. Which of the following interventions would be most effective at minimizing total radiation dose to members of the public?

A. Re-cooling of the reactor core
B. Use of hand and body radiation detectors
C. Use of lead vests or lead thyroid shields
D. Distribution of ultraviolet-blocking eye protection
E. Distribution of potassium iodide pills

■ Answers and Explanations

E. Correct! In addition to its beta emissions with a maximum energy of ~606 keV, ^{131}I emits high-energy photons (γ-rays) with a primary energy of 364 keV. Emitted beta particles typically travel several meters in air while high-energy photons. However, in this case, with aerosolized ^{131}I in the air, the radioactive emissions are of concern both at the site of the accident and in the surrounding area, where ^{131}I particles may result in both external and internal (due to inhalation) radiation exposures. Inhaled ^{131}I may accumulate in the thyroid gland if unblocked. Therefore, the adminstration of a nonradioactive blocking agent such as potassium iodide or Lugol solution (aqueous solution of potassium iodide plus iodien) can be important in minimizing dose to the thyroid gland from beta radiation and gamma radiation dose from the source (thyroid) to other tissues (target).

Other choices and discussion

A. Re-cooling of the reactor core may be of little benefit as the core has already partially melted. In addition, because radiation release into the environment has already occured, re-cooling will be ineffective in minimizing the dose from the released [131]I.

B. For radiation workers or those with occupational exposures to ionizing radiation, body and hand detectors are effective means of monitoring exposure. In the setting of a radiation accident, these detectors may be to assist in determining the total exposure to workers, but would not be helpful for minimizing dose.

C. [131]I is a beta-emitter used most often in the treatment of hyperthyroidism and well-differentiated thyroid carcinoma. While lead vests may limit absorbed radiation from low-energy photons, the ^{131}I half-value layer (HVL) of Pb is 3mm and the tenth-value layer is 11 mm. The thickness of typical lead aprons is 0.25 to 0.375 mm. Thus, these protective garments would be expected to block little of the primary photons emitted from [131]I. In addition, it is important to note that high-Z materials such as lead produce penetrating Bremsstrahlung radiations (X-rays) when exposed to beta particles.

D. [131]I does not produce ultraviolet radiations. Therefore, ultraviolet-blocking eyewear would be of no substantial benefit.

■ Suggested Readings

Sugarman SL, Goans RE, Garrett AS, et al. The Medical Aspects of Radiation Incidents. Knoxville, TN: Oak Ridge Institute for Science and Education (US); 2013. https://orise.orau.gov/files/reacts/medical-aspects-of-radiation-incidents.pdf

Yamamoto LG. Risks and management of radiation exposure. Ped Emerg Care 2013;29:1016–1026

Top Tips

◆ [131]I is both a beta and gamma ray emitter.

◆ [131]I accumulates in the thyroid gland if unblocked.

◆ The ^{131}I half-value layer of Pb is 3 mm and the tenth-value layer is 11 mm.

Essentials 10

■ Case

A single photon emission computed tomography camera is undergoing performance testing with a Jaszczak phantom. The nuclear medicine technologist fills the chamber surrounding the solid spheres and rods with a solution of dilute 99m-technetium pertechnetate (Na-TcO$_4$). The filled phantom is used for:

A. Daily uniformity calculation
B. Daily energy peaking
C. Quarterly linearity testing
D. Quarterly system spatial resolution testing
E. Annual system performance testing

■ Answers and Explanations

E. Correct! The fillable Jasczak phantom is used for assessment of the imaging system overall and may be used for both single photon emission computed tomography and positron emission tomography systems, depending on the radiotracer used to fill the chamber. When filled, the phantom may be used to test system resolution, contrast, and uniformity. An overall system check should be performed at least annually, if not quarterly.

Other choices and discussion

A. Gamma camera uniformity should be tested with either a point source at a specified distance from the camera head (intrinsic uniformity) or with a sheet flood source (typically 57-Cobalt) placed directly on the collimator (extrinsic uniformity). Uniformity should be evaluated daily.

B. Energy peaking should be performed daily. The energy spectrum of the radioisotope to be imaged, most often 99m-technetium, should be analyzed to ensure that the photopeak of interest coincides with the preset energy window.

C. Linearity testing is done best with a four-quadrant bar phantom placed atop the collimator, with a point source at a specified distance from the camera head. Checks for linearity should be performed montly or quarterly.

D. Spatial resolution should be checked monthtly or quarterly, and much like uniformity, may be evaluated as a function of the intrinsic camera performance or the extrinsic camera performance. As with linearity, it is typically checked using a four-quadrant bar phantom, with the user identifying the number of quadrants in which the bar separations can be discerned.

■ Suggested Readings

Intersocietal Accreditation Commission. IAC Standards and Guidelines for Nuclear/PET Accreditation. Ellicott City, MD: Intersocietal Accreditation Commission; 2012

Zanzonico P. Routine quality control of clinical nuclear medicine instrumentation: a brief review. J Nucl Med 2008;49:1114–1131

Top Tips

◆ Uniformity, energy peaking → daily

◆ Linearity testing → monthly or quarterly

◆ Spatial resolution → monthly or quarterly

◆ Overall system check → quarterly or annually

Essentials 11

■ Case

Gallium-68 labeled DOTA-conjugated peptides have been developed for positron emission tomography imaging of neuro-endocrine tumors. These peptides are somatostatin analogues, with DOTA functioning as the link between the radiometal and the peptide moiety such as Tyr^3-octreotide (TOC), yielding, for example, a final ^{68}Ga-DOTA-TOC pharmaceutical. In preparing ^{68}Ga for peptide labeling via elution from a germanium-68 (^{68}Ge) generator, the presence of high levels of ^{68}Ge in the eluate will necessarily:

A. Decrease the radiolabeled peptide specific activity.

B. Decrease the radiolabeled peptide radiochemical purity.

C. Have no effect on the radiolabeled peptide radionuclidic purity.

D. Likely increase the chemical purity of the radiolabeled peptide.

E. Have unpredictable effects on the levels of carrier-free radiolabeled peptide.

■ Answers and Explanations

E. Correct! A *carrier* is a stable (nonradioactive) isotope of the radionuclide of interest. In this case, a carrier would be 69- or 71-gallium. Increased amounts of the parent compound, ^{68}Ge, are not expected to affect the amount of stable gallium present in the eluate in a predictable manner.

Other choices and discussion

A. Specific activity reflects the proportion of the desired radiopharmaceutical that is labeled with the radionuclide of interest versus the stable isotopes of that same element (for example, in this case, 69- or 71-gallium). When there is an abundance of the stable isotope incorporated into the "radio"pharmaceutical, the specific activity of the desired radiolabeled peptide (i.e., the desired radiopharmaceutical in this case) would be decreased. The presence of the parent compound, ^{68}Ge, does not necessarily affect the specific activity of the radiopharmaceutical. Specific activity can be assessed using high performance liquid chromatography.

B. Radiochemical purity reflects the fraction of the radionuclide of interest that is bound to the pharmaceutical of interest. Any factor that decreases the efficiency of the pharmaceutical labeling process such that the radionuclide of interest does not bind effectively to the pharmaceutical will decrease the radiochemical purity as more of the radioisotope will be present unbound to the chemical of interest. In this case, having the parent compound, ^{68}Ge, in the eluate will not necessarily decrease the binding of ^{68}Ga to the TOC molecule. Impurities may be in the form of free, hydrolyzed-reduced, or bound radionuclide. Chromatography is the procedure of choice for separating and identifying radiochemical impurities.

C. Radionuclidic purity reflects the contribution of the radioisotope of interest (in this case, ^{68}Ga) to the overall radioactivity of the sample. Increased levels of ^{68}Ge in the eluate will necessarily decrease the fraction of total radioactivity originating from ^{68}Ga. Radionuclidic purity may be decreased by the presence of radioisotopes of the radionuclide or interest or by the presence of different nuclides. In the ^{99}Mo/^{99m}Tc generator system, ^{99}Mo would represent a radionuclide impurity in eluted ^{99m}Tc (the Nuclear Regulatory Commission limits the allowable ^{99}Mo impurity to ≤ 0.15 μCi ^{99}Mo per 1 mCi of ^{99m}Tc; i.e., "molybdenum breakthrough"). Radionuclidic purity is assessed using a dose calibrator to identify the proportion of total counts being generated by decay of the impurity nuclide.

D. Chemical purity reflects the fraction of the final product mass that is in the desired chemical form. Increasing the amoung of ^{68}Ge in the eluate will not necessarily affect the type, amount, or form of chemical of the end-product. Processes that affect the formation of the desired chemical would be expected to affect the chemical purity. A chemical purity > 95% is desired. In the ^{99}Mo/^{99m}Tc generator system, Al_2O_3 used as the column medium can result in aluminum ions (Al^{3+}) being present in the ^{99m}Tc eluate (known as "alumina breakthrough"). The Nuclear Regulatory Commission limits the allowable Al^{3+} chemical impurity to ≤ 10 μg Al^{3+} per 1 mL of ^{99m}Tc eluate. Chemical impurity can be assessed using a colorimetric indicator strip, with the eluate tested against a solution with a standard/known amount of the impurity. Additional tests that may be used to assess for chemical purity include gas chromatography, liquid chromatography, spectrophotometry, ion exchange, and solvent extraction.

■ Suggested Readings

Cherry SR, Sorenson JA, Phelps ME. Physics in Nuclear Medicine. 4th ed. Philadelphia: Saunders; 2012

Decristoforo C, Pickett RD, Verbruggen A. Feasibility and availability of ^{68}G-labelled peptides. Eur J Nucl Med Mol Imaging 2012;39(Suppl 1):31–40

Top Tips

- Specific activity = proportion of the desired radiopharmaceutical labeled with the radionuclide of interest versus the stable isotopes of that same element.

- Radiochemical purity = fraction of the radionuclide of interest bound to the pharmaceutical of interest.

- Radionuclidic purity = contribution of radioisotope of interest to the overall radioactivity of the sample.

- Chemical purity = fraction of final product in the desired chemical form.

Essentials 12

■ Case

A 64-year-old woman with colorectal cancer undergoes intra-arterial radiotherapy ("radioembolization") for hepatic metastases with 90-Yttrium-labeled (mean β^- energy = 937 keV) microspheres. Pretreatment imaging with 99m-technetium macroaggregated albumin revealed a lung shunt fraction of approximately 5%, and 95% of the microsphere activity is expected to localize to the liver tumors. A total of 1 GBq of ^{90}Y microspheres was administered, and 24-hour posttherapy Bremsstrahlung imaging revealed minor extrahepatic shunting and confirmed treatment of the entire tumor volume. In converting the radiation absorbed dose from Y-90 microsphere administration to dose equivalent (H_E),

A. The quality factor (Q_F) for Bremsstrahlung radiations is 1.0, whereas the Q_F for the β^- particles is 10.0.
B. The relative biologic effectiveness of emitted radiations will be independent of the radiations' linear energy transfer.
C. The International System of Units (SI) unit of equivalent dose is the Gray (Gy).
D. The effective dose from Bremsstrahlung radiations will include an adjustment for lung tissue sensitivity to X-rays.
E. The fraction of the absorbed dose to the liver from the lungs will depend on Bremsstralung radiations but not on β^- particles.

■ Answers and Explanations

D. Correct! The effective dose, formerly known as the effective dose equivalent, provides a whole-body estimate of radiation effects by taking into account both the radiation type–dependent dose equivalents and tissue sensitivities to radiation, known as the tissue weighting factor (W_T). For the total body, W_Ts sum to 1.0. The tissues most sensitive to radiation damage have the highest W_T (e.g., 0.20 for the gonads), whereas those with lower sensitivities have smaller W_T (e.g., 0.01 for the skin).

Other choices and discussion

A. Quality factors (Q), related (though the exact relationship remains unclear) to the more modern concept of radiation weighting factors (w_R), account for the varying effects of different types of radiation on biologic tissue. X-rays, gamma rays, and some small particles, including electrons (e- or β^- particles) and positrons (β^+ particles), have similar effects when interacting with tissues, and thus, all have a Q_F of 1.0. Neutrons, high-energy protons, and alpha particles have quality factors of 5: 20, 5, and 20, respectively.

B. The relative biologic effectiveness of a specific radiation describes its relative ability to produce a particular biologic (tissue) response as compared to a reference radiation—typically 250 kV X-rays. As a rule, α-radiations have a higher relative biologic effectiveness than X-rays, given that they have a higher linear energy transfer.

C. The unit for dose equivalent (H_E) in the traditional system is the *rem* (radiation *e*quivalent *m*an) and in SI system is the Sievert, abbreviated as Sv. H_E utilizes radiation quality factors (Q) to account for the varying effects of different types of radiation. Most clinically relevant procedures in diagnostic radiology and nuclear medicine deliver equivalent doses in the milli-Sievert (mSv) range.

E. Because ^{90}Y emits both β^- particles and Bremsstrahlung radiations, the absorbed dose to any organ will depend on the effects of both types of emissions.

■ Suggested Readings

Cherry SR, Sorenson JA, Phelps ME. Physics in Nuclear Medicine. 4th ed. Philadelphia: Saunders; 2012

International Commission on Radiological Protection. Relative biological effectiveness (RBE), quality factor (Q), and radiation weighting factor (w_R). ICRP Publication 92. Ann ICRP 2003;33(4)

Saha GB. Physics and Radiobiology of Nuclear Medicine. 4th ed. New York: Springer; 2014

Top Tips

◆ Effective dose provides a whole-body estimate of radiation effects by taking into account both radiation type–dependent dose equivalents and tissue sensitivities to radiation, known as the tissue weighting factor (W_T).

◆ Q factor (Q_F): neutrons = 5 to 20; high-energy protons = 5; alpha particles = 20. HE utilizes Q_F to account for the varying effects of different types of radiation.

◆ Relative biologic effectiveness of a specific radiation describes its relative ability to produce a particular biologic (tissue) response as compared to a reference radiation.

SECTION XIV PHYSICS SAFETY

Essentials 13

■ **Case**

You will be relocating for a new job in Tennessee, which is currently one of thirty-seven Nuclear Regulatory Comission (NRC) agreement states. However, you are practicing in Delaware at the moment, which is not an agreement state. Under the direction of its state radiation control program director and persuant to its contract with the NRC, the state of Tennessee would be responsible for regulating which of the following radioisotopes (which would not be regulated by Delaware, a non-agreement state)?

    A. 131-Iodine (^{131}I)
    B. Naturally-occuring 226-Radium (^{226}Ra)
    C. 67-Gallium (^{67}Ga)
    D. 123-Iodine (^{123}I)
    E. 18-Fluorine (^{18}F)

■ Answers and Explanations

A. Correct! The U.S. NRC (or, more commonly, simply NRC) is an independent government agency that was created as part of the Energy Reorganization Act of 1974. Its purpose is to ensure the safe handling and use of radioactive materials in the United States in such a manner as to protect the public and the environment. By granting various licenses to individual physicians, institutions, and states, the NRC governs nuclear materials to include those used for nonmilitary commercial and medicinal purposes. NRC regulations relevant to diagnostic radiology and nuclear medicine can be found, in general, in Parts 19, 20, 30, 32, and 35 of the U.S. Code of Federal Regulations Part 10, though several other parts of the Code may be useful for reference.

The Agreement State program was initially instituted as part of a 1959 revision to the Atomic Energy Act under the auspices of the Atomic Energy Commission. As of February 2016, there were 37 agreement states and 11 nonagreement states, plus the District of Columbia. By entering into a contract ("agreement") with the NRC, the Agreement States are afforded the opportunity and responsbility to inspect and license the use of:

> source material (uranium and thorium) and associated processing waste; special nuclear material (enriched uranium and plutonium); byproduct material (reactor-produced radionuclides)" including, for example, ^{131}I).[1]

In nonagreement states, the NRC is responsible for the above-listed radioactive materials. All states regulate other radiation sources, including:

> naturally occurring radiactive material (radium and radon)j; particle accelerator-produced radioactive materials (^{18}F, ^{67}Ga, ^{123}I); and radiation-producing machines.[1]

The other choices are incorrect.

■ Reference

1. Siegel JA. Nuclear Regulatory Commission Regulation of Nuclear Medicine: Guide for Diagnostic Nuclear Medicine. Reston, VA: Society of Nuclear Medicine; 2001

■ Suggested Readings

Cherry SR, Sorenson JA, Phelps ME. Physics in Nuclear Medicine. 4th ed. Philadelphia: Saunders; 2012

Nuclear Regulatory Commission. NRC Regulations - Title 10, Code of Federal Regulations [Internet]. Washington, DC: Office of the Federal Register; 1991. http://www.nrc.gov/reading-rm/doc-collections/cfr/

Top Tips

◆ Agreement states are responsible for inspection and licensing the use of "source material (uranium and thorium) and associated processing waste; special nuclear material (enriched uranium and plutonium); byproduct material (reactor-produced radionuclides)."[1]

Details 1

■ Case

Which of the following comparisons of electron capture (EC) and positron (β^+) decay is MOST accurate?

A. Relative to the nearest stable nuclide, β^+ decay typically occurs in radionuclides with higher neutron–proton (N/Z) ratios, whereas decay by EC typically occurs when the N/Z ratio is lower.

B. For both β^+ decay and EC, the emitted neutrinos contribute substantially to radiation dose.

C. Both β^+ decay and EC are followed by characteristic gamma-ray (γ-ray) emissions.

D. Although β^+ decay results in detectable annihilation photons, EC does not produce emissions that are detectable outside the body.

E. β^+ decay is more likely when at least 1.022 MeV is available as transition energy, whereas decay by EC is less likely as available transition energy increases.

■ Answers and Explanations

E. Correct! Likelihood of positron (β^+) decay increases as available transition energy increases above 1.022 MeV, whereas the likelihood of EC increases as available transition energy decreases. This "cut-off" of 1.022 MeV becomes clear when we consider the products of positron decay, wherein a nuclear proton is transformed into a neutron (which is one electron mass heavier than a proton, and therefore this transformation can be thought of as requiring an available 0.511 MeV), and one positron is created (a positron being equivalent to one electron mass, thus, the second 0.511 MeV that is needed), such that 0.511 MeV + 0.511 MeV = 1.022 MeV.

Other choices and discussion

A. β^+ decay and EC are alternative decay modes typically occurring in (proton-rich) radionuclides with an N/Z ratio lower than the nearest stable nuclide ("line of stability"). As an example, ^{126}I (with 53 protons) may decay by EC or β^+decay to ^{126}Te (with 52 protons).

B. Neutrinos produced by β^+ decay and EC interact very minimally with other particles, and as such, do not contribute substantially to biologic radiation doses.

C. In EC, once the orbital electron (typically from the K- or L-shell) is captured and a neutron is formed, the electron shell vacancy is filled by an electron from an outer shell (resulting in emission of a characteristic X-ray or Auger electron as the transition energy is released); a γ-ray is not typically emitted from EC. Note: if an unstable daughter nucleus is produced from EC, characteristic γ-rays may be emitted from the daughter as it decays to its ground state (e.g., 171 and 245 keV γ-rays emitted by Cd as it decays to its ground state after being produced by EC from ^{111}In). Subsequent to the β^+ decay, annihilation of the β^+ particle results in the production of two annihilation photons, each with an energy of approximately 511 keV.

E. When they are of sufficient energy to escape the body or are emitted from superficial tissues such as the thyroid gland, the characteristic X-rays of the daughter nucleus resulting from EC can be detected.

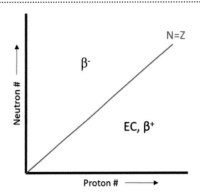

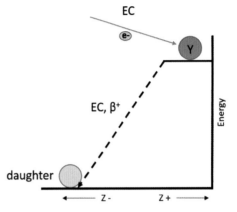

■ Suggested Readings

Cherry SR, Sorenson JA, Phelps ME. Physics in Nuclear Medicine. 4th ed. Philadelphia: Saunders; 2012

Patton JA. Introduction to nuclear physics. Radiographics 1998;18:995–1007

Saha GB. Physics and Radiobiology of Nuclear Medicine. 4th ed. New York: Springer; 2014

Top Tips

◆ Although frequently referred to as originating from the decay of the parent, characteristic γ-rays detected and utilized for imaging after β^+, β^-, and EC actually arise from the transition of the daughter nucleus to its ground state.

Details 2

■ Case

The binding energy (BE) of electrons in the K-shell of a nuclide _____.

    A. Is determined by the total number of electrons present in the K-shell of the atom.

    B. Is equal to the energy required to excite an electron from the K-shell to the L_1-shell.

    C. Is greater than the binding energy of K-shell electrons in an isotope of that nuclide.

    D. Is less than the binding energy of electrons in the L-shell of that same atom.

    E. Is less than the binding energy of K-shell electrons in an atom with higher atomic number.

■ Answers and Explanations

D. Correct! As stated previously, the positively charged nuclear protons attract the orbiting electrons, thus providing the force that "holds" electrons in their shells. As the proton number (Z) increases, there is increased force on the negatively charged electrons in a given orbital shell. Therefore, BE for a given shell increases as proton number increases. For example, the K-shell BE for carbon (Z = 6) is 0.28 keV, whereas the K-shell BE for chromium (Z = 24) is 5.99 keV.

Other choices and discussion

A. All electrons within a given orbital electron shell (e.g., L_1) have the same BE, regardless of the number of electrons actually inhabiting that shell.

B. When an electron is excited from a lower shell to a higher shell, the energy input required to do so is the *difference* between the BEs of the two shells. For example, if the K-shell electron BE is 40 and the L_1-shell electron BE is 10, then the energy required to excite an electron from K to L_1 will be equal to 30, and *not* equal to the BE of the K-shell.

C. Isotopes of a nuclide have the same number of protons (same Z). It is the protons that provide the positive force which attracts the electrons and "holds" them in their shells. Thus, isotopes would be expected to have the same BE for electrons in the same orbital shell.

D. Electrons positioned farther from the nucleus (i.e., those in a higher shell) will experience less attraction from the nucleus. Thus, electrons in higher shells (e.g., L- and M-shells) will have a *lower* BE than those electrons positioned closer to the nucleus in a lower shell (e.g., the K-shell). The K-shell BE for Sr (Z = 38) is 16.11 keV, whereas the L_1-shell binding energy for Sr is 2.22 keV.

■ Suggested Readings

Cherry SR, Sorenson JA, Phelps ME. Physics in Nuclear Medicine. 4th ed. Philadelphia: Saunders; 2012

Saha GB. Physics and Radiobiology of Nuclear Medicine. 4th ed. New York: Springer; 2014

Williams GP. Electron binding energies, in electron volts, for the elements in their natural forms. Lawrence Berkeley National Laboratory; 2016. http://xdb.lbl.gov/Section1/Sec_1-1.html

Top Tips

- In the most stable atomic configuration, electrons will fill the lowest orbital shells first. Electrons within these shells are held with an energy equal to the BE for that shell; in order to remove an electron from the atom (i.e., in order to ionize the atom), an amount of energy at least equal to the BE for that electron must be applied.

- Isotopes → same number of protons (Z).

Details 3

■ Case

A 32-year-old nonpregnant woman presents to the emergency department with new onset dyspnea and cough. She denies other ongoing or past medical problems, and is currently taking only an oral contraceptive and a daily multivitamin. She returned to the United States from Australia 4 days prior to presentation. A plain radiograph of the chest is unremarkable. She undergoes a pulmonary ventilation-perfusion study with 1110 MBq (30 mCi) nebulized 99m-technetium diethylene tetra-acetic acid (DTPA) and 74 MBq (2 mCi) intravenous 99m-technetium macroaggregated albumin (MAA) at 500,000 particles. Assuming that 2% of the DTPA dose and 90% of the MAA-labeled particles localize to and are retained in the lungs indefinitely, what is the cumulative activity in the lungs?

A. 8.9×10 MBq-sec
B. 7.7×10^2 MBq-sec
C. 4.6×10^4 MBq-sec
D. 2.8×10^6 MBq-sec
E. 31.2×10^6 MBq-sec

■ Answers and Explanations

D. Correct! Cumulated activity (Ã) can be approximated by the equation:

$$\tilde{A} = A_0 \int e^{-0.693 \cdot t/t1/2p} \, dt = 1.44 \cdot t_{1/2,p} \cdot A_0$$

This relationship is based on the assumptions that the radiopharmaceutical is instantaneously localized to the organ and is not excreted by the organ or otherwise cleared. A_0 is the activity initially in the organ, and $t_{1/2,p}$ is the physical half-life of the radioisotope, which is 6.02 hours for 99m-technetium.

Therefore, if 2% of the 1110 MBq from DTPA and 90% of 74 MBq from MAA localize to the lungs,

$\tilde{A}$ = 1.44×6.02 hours $\times (0.02 \times 1110$ MBq $+ 0.90 \times 74$ MBq$)$

= 1.44×6.02 hr $\times (88.8$ MBq$)$

= 770 MBq-hr

= 770 MBq-hr $\times$ 60 min/1 hr $\times$ 60 sec/1 min

= 2.78×10^6 MBq-sec

The other choices are incorrect.

■ Suggested Readings

Cherry SR, Sorenson JA, Phelps ME. Physics in Nuclear Medicine. 4th ed. Philadelphia: Saunders; 2012

Toohey RE, Stabin MG, Watson EE. Internal radiation dosimetry: principles and applications. RadioGraphics 2000;20:533–546

Top Tips

◆ Cumulated activity (Ã) can be approximated by the equation:

$$\tilde{A} = A_0 \int e^{-0.693 \cdot t/t1/2p} \, dt = 1.44 \cdot t_{1/2,p} \cdot A_0$$

SECTION XIV
PHYSICS SAFETY

Details 4

■ **Case**

A 65-year-old man with diabetes mellitus type 2 has a history of bilateral Charcot arthropathy (diabetic neuropathic arthropathy). He presents with a 2-week history of increasing right foot pain and is referred for a dual-isotope single photon emission tomography study with 99m-technetium sulfur colloid and 111-indium oxine-labeled leukocytes. Intravenously, 17.5 MBq (0.47 mCi) ^{111}In-labeled autologous leukocytes are administered, and 24 hours later, 280 MBq (7.6 mCi) ^{99m}Tc-sulfur colloid is administered intravenously. The Centers for Disease Control and Prevention standard precautions, based on universal precautions, mandate:

A. The use of gloves and gowns only in the setting of potential blood or specimen aerosolization.
B. That blood specimen containment and transport procedures are required only if the specimen is removed from the facility where it was obtained.
C. Two-handed recapping of used needles.
D. That face shields and masks are required for all handling of urine or cerebrospinal fluid.
E. That all human blood be treated as if known to be infectious for human immunodeficiency virus, hepatitis B virus, or other bloodborne pathogens.

■ Answers and Explanations

E. Correct! The underlying premise of universal and standard precautions is that blood and other potentially infectious bodily fluids should be treated as if they are known to be infected with bloodborne pathogens, as listed.

Other choices and discussion

A. Gloves and gowns are forms of barrier equipment (also known as personal protective equipment) and are designed not only to protect the patient, but also the healthcare worker. Universal precautions require the use of these items of personal protective equipment when a worker will, or can be reasonably expected to, come into contact with bodily fluids including blood.

B. Universal and standard precautions specify that an institution must have in place a protocol for the transport of bodily fluids and any items that may have been contaminated by bodily fluids including blood. These protocols must ensure that potentially infectious fluids are placed in a container that resists leakage during transport and handling.

C. Needle recapping should only be performed in situations where not doing so will result in the transport or carrying of an uncapped sharp. If recapping of a needle is absolutely required, the single-handed scoop method should be used.

D. Face shields and masks need only be worn when splashes, spray, or spatter are anticipated. This is not necessarily true in every case of urine or cerebrospinal fluid handling.

■ Suggested Readings

Roca M, de Vries EF, Jamar F, et al. Guidelines for the labelling of leucocytes with ^{111}In-oxine. Eur J Nucl Med Mol Imaging 2010;37:835–841

Siegel JD, Rhinehart E, Jackson M, et al, and the Healthcare Infection Control Practices Advisory Committee, 2007 Guideline for Isolation Precautions: Preventing Transmission of Infectious Agents in Healthcare Settings. http://www.cdc.gov/ncidod/dhqp/pdf/isolation2007.pdf

Top Tips

◆ Infectious fluids are to be handled in a similar manner to bloodborne pathogens.

Details 5

■ Case

During the setup process for image acquisition, the technologist sets 15% windows around photopeaks at 140 keV, 171 keV, and 245 keV. The rejection of photons having energies outside of the desired ranges is accomplished primarily via the:

A. Application of a coincidence window to reject singlet pulses ("singles").
B. Rejection of Compton scattered photons with energies > 245 keV.
C. Use of a multichannel analyzier to examine pulse amplitudes.
D. Use of an NaI(Tl) crystal detector rather than a solid state detector.
E. Increasing the gain of the preamplifier and amplifier.

■ Answers and Explanations

C. Correct! The multichannel analyzer, or in some older systems the presence of several independent single-channel analyzers, allows for the simultaneous acquisition and recording of photons with energies at several different photopeaks. These systems rely on the assessment of the amplitude of pulses generated by incident photons, and can be set to reject pulses resulting from incident photons with energies outside the specified range.

Other choices and discussion

A. Though desirable in positron emission tomography, coincident pulses are generally undesirable in single photon imaging, as they may degrade the ability to localize individual incident photons ("singles") as they interact with the camera system. Therefore, cameras may employ various anticoincidence timing circuits.

B. Compton scatter interactions decrease the energy of the incident photon, and thus, one would not expect high-energy Compton scatter photons. However, should such photons result, those with energies within the 20% window set by the technologist (220.5 to 269.5 keV) will be accepted, not rejected.

D. In solid state detectors, photon interactions result in direct ionization events. At energies below the photopeak, there may be a substantial contribution of counts from low energy non-scattered photons. Thus, depending on the solid state material, they may offer little in the way of benefit over NaI(Tl) detectors in terms of decreasing the likelihood of extraneous pulse generation. However, solid state detectors do, as a rule, demonstrate better energy resolution than traditional detector materials.

E. The preamplifier and amplifier provide linear gain to the pulses generated by incident photons. Thus, although increasing either may increase the pulse amplitude generated by all events, they would not be expected to inherently improve the discriminatory capabilities of the system.

■ Suggested Readings

Cherry SR, Sorenson JA, Phelps ME. Physics in Nuclear Medicine. 4th ed. Philadelphia: Saunders; 2012

Saha GB. Physics and Radiobiology of Nuclear Medicine. 4th ed. New York: Springer; 2014

Top Tips

- The multichannel analyzer allows simulataneous acquisition and recording of photons with energies at several different photopeaks (e.g., dual imaging with Tc-99m sulfur colloid and In-111 white blood cells for infection).

Image Rich 1

■ Case

Match the following (1 through 5) to the best answer choice (A through E):

    A. Pulse width
    B. Source-to-skin distance
    C. Field-of-view (FOV)
    D. Collimation
    E. Continuous fluoroscopy

■ Questions

1. A decrease in this would help minimize the radiation dose to the patient.
2. These images demonstrate another means of minimizing the radiation dose to the patient.
3. An increase is this would utilize the inverse square law principle to minimize radiation dose to the patient.
4. These fluoroscopic images have been acquired differently. What most likely has been performed to obtain the right-sided image?
5. By decreasing this, radiation dose to the patient is increased as well as magnification.

■ Answers and Explanations

Question 1

A. Correct! Pulse width. The length of *time* the patient receives radiation is one of the elements determining the amount of radiation a patient receives (i.e., the longer the time, the greater the radiation received by the patient). The length of time a patient is exposed to radiation during one fluoroscopic image is determined by the pulse width. By using a short pulse width (typically, 5 to 10 msec), the radiation time, and therefore, dose is decreased.

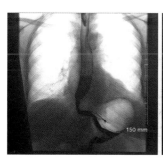

Question 2

D. Correct! Collimation. Collimating allows reduction in the amount of patient tissue that is irradiated, and therefore helps minimize the radiation dose to the patient. The operator should limit the FOV to include only the pertinent area needed for imaging.

Question 3

B. Correct! Source-to-skin distance. In general, as the distance from a radiation source is doubled, the radiation dose is reduced by a factor of 4: (Amount of radiation or intensity) = $1/d^2$.

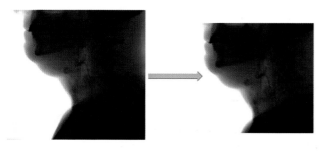

Question 4

E. Correct! Continuous fluoroscopy. As the name implies, the image was acquired in "continuous" mode (i.e., a continuous X-ray beam is produced). With this technique, there are typically 30 fluoroscopic images created per second when one depresses the fluoroscopy pedal. The duration of image frames is 33 msec. The downside of this includes increased radiation dose to the patient and possible degradation of image quality due to motion (as seen in the right image). Alternatively, pulsed fluoroscopy can be performed and essentially provides shorter "broken up" periods of radiation (i.e., less time for acquisition) and minimizes radiation to the patient as compared to continuous fluoroscopy. When one depresses the fluoroscopic pedal, the computer utilizes a pulse rate where the radiation is turned on and off.

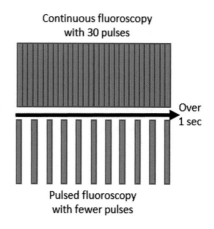

Question 5

C. Correct! FOV. As the FOV becomes smaller (smaller X-ray beam area at the image receptor), magnification increases. However, this causes increased radiation dose to the patient. As the FOV is decreased, the exposure required by the image intensifier tube is increased. This causes the absorbed dose to the patient tissues within the beam to increase (right image). In general, decreasing the FOV by a factor of 2 increases the dose rate by a factor of 4. Keep in mind, however, that the total energy imparted is equal in both scenarios.

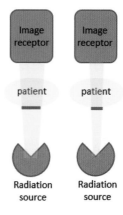

In summary from the answer choices listed, radiation is minimized by reducing the pulse width, increasing the source-to-skin distance, increasing the FOV, utilizing collimation, and performing pulsed rather than continuous fluoroscopy.

Top Tips

◆ There are various means to reduce radiation dose to the patient and the operator. Built within each method are these basics: reduce the *time* or length of period for image acquisition, increase the *distance* from the radiation source, and *shield* the patient and/or yourself.

More Challenging 1

■ **Case**

Depicted in the figure is a subset of photons originating from point sources (numbered 1 to 8) that are incident upon the detector system of a typical Anger (gamma) camera. It can be assumed that all point sources contain equal doses of the same radiopharmaceutical.

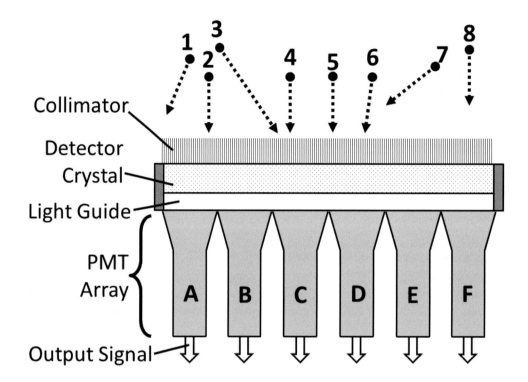

■ **Questions**

1. The output signal from which of the photomultiplier tubes (PMTs) shown would be expected to have the largest amplitude if (only) two photons—one each from point source 4 and 5 with equal energies—struck the detector crystal simultaneously?
   A. PMT A
   B. PMT B
   C. PMT C
   D. PMT D
   E. PMT E

2. The collimator depicted in the figure has parallel holes. Which of the following is true with regard to the collimator and its effects on system detection of incident photons from point sources 1 to 8?
   A. Detection efficiency will increase as thickness of collimator septa increases.
   B. Detection efficiency will be higher for photons originating from a point source at location 4 rather than for a point source at location 8.
   C. Detection efficiency will increase as the length of the collimator holes increases.
   D. Detection resolution will decrease as the length of the collimator holes increases.
   E. Detection resolution will increase as the diameter of the collimator holes increases.

■ Answers and Explanations

Question 1

C. Correct! Within an Anger camera, PMTs are arrayed such that the localization of the incident photon is determined by identification of the PMT whose center is nearest the location of the scintillation event. The PMTs are connected to analog or electronic circuitry that positions the event by analyzing the amplitude of signals from the PMT array. Those PMTs whose center is nearest the scintillation event will have output signals with highest amplitude, and those furthest away will have the smallest amplitudes. In this example, photon 4 would strike the detector crystal at a position nearest to the center of PMT C, whereas photon 5 would strike the detector at a position equidistant from PMTs C and D. Thus, we would expect PMT C to have the highest output signal given that it would detect the scintillation event resulting from photon 4 more than any other PMTs, plus it would detect the scintillation event resulting from photon 5 as much as PMT D and more than any of the other PMTs shown.

The other choices are incorrect.

Question 2

D. Correct! Collimator resolution (R) is inversely proportional to collimator efficiency. Thus, factors that increase efficiency (such as increasing hole diameter or shortening hole length [depth]) will decrease resolution, and factors that increase resolution (such as decreasing hole diameter and increasing hole length) will decrease efficiency.

Other choices and discussion

A. As septal thickness increases, the likelihood of a photon being absorbed by the septal wall increases. Therefore, efficiency of transmission of photons through the collimator will decrease as septal thickness increases. In gamma camera systems, collimators are typically sheets composed mainly of lead (Pb) into which holes of a specific diameter have been bored (hole diameter will depend on whether collimator is of low- or high-resolution type). The walls of these holes are referred to as "septa." Thickness of collimator septa is important in the prevention or minimization of septal penetration—the tendency of high-energy photons to penetrate through the walls (septa) between collimator holes, and to, therefore, strike the detector crystal face (defined mathematically as the percentage of counts in an image contributed by photons that have passed through septal walls; preferably, fewer than 5 to 10% of counts should result from septal penetration). Increased septal thickness is desirable as photon energy increases; low-energy collimators most often used to image radionuclides emitting photons of < 150 keV tend to have septal thicknesses on the order of 0.15 to 0.2 mm, whereas high-energy collimators have septal thickness on the order of 1.7 to 2 mm and are used to image high-energy photons such as those emitted by ^{131}Xe following the β$^-$ decay of ^{131}I. Medium-energy collimators, as expected, have characteristics between those of low- and high-energy collimators.

B. Point source 4 is closer to the collimator than is point source 8. It is true that any one photon from source 8 would be less efficiently transmitted through any one hole in the collimator as compared to point source 4 because of the increased distance the photon must travel. However, photons originating from source 8 would be more widely spread before reaching the collimator than would photons originating from source 4, and therefore, photons from source 8 would be more likely to enter through more collimator holes. These two parameters (potentially decreased efficiency due to farther distance and potentially increased efficiency due to increased number of holes entered) cancel each other out, and therefore collimator efficiency is overall independent of the distance between the source and the collimator (in air).

C. Collimator efficiency (g) is proportional to hole diameter (d) and inversely proportional to hole length (l); the exact relationship is nonlinear. Thus, as collimator hole length increases, efficiency will decrease. This is because fewer photons will pass through the collimator and reach the detector crystal when the holes are long (deep).

E. Collimator efficiency (sensitivity) and resolution are inversely related. As collimator hole diameter increases, more photons are able to pass through (i.e., captured by) any given hole in the collimator; thus, efficiency will be increased. However, note that as hole diameter increases, detection resolution will be decreased, because more photons—including those that may have been scattered and are entering the collimator at a slight angle—are able to pass through the collimator hole.

■ Suggested Readings

Azarma A, Islamian JP, Mahmoudian B, et al. The effect of parallel-hole collimator material on image and functional parameters in SPECT imaging: a SIMIND Monte Carlo study. World J Nucl Med 2015;14:160–164

Cherry SR, Sorenson JA, Phelps ME. Physics in Nuclear Medicine. 4th ed. Philadelphia: Saunders; 2012

White SL. Quality assurance testing of gamma camera and SPECT systems. Paper presented at AAPM (American Association of Physicists in Medicine) 51st Annual Meeting; July 28, 2009; Anaheim, CA

Zanzonico P. Principles of nuclear medicine imaging: planar, SPECT, PET, multi-modality, an autoradiography systems. Radiat Res 2012;177:349–364

Top Tips

◆ In single photon scintigraphy, collimators are important to prevent scattered or aberrant photons from reaching the detector crystal. Were collimators not used, the image produced would be blurry and nondescript. However, although they increase image resolution compared to a "collimator-less" system, all collimators result in significant losses in detector efficiency, as most incident photons are absorbed by the collimator before ever making it to the detector crystal. The intrinsic efficiency of the crystal material itself will then also ultimately contribute to the overall system efficiency for detection of incident photons.

◆ In general, nuclear medicine studies utilizing ^{99m}Tc-labeled radiopharmaceuticals are performed with low-energy high resolution or low-energy all purpose collimators.

More Challenging 2

■ Case

A brain slice obtained by positron emission tomography imaging following intravenous administration of 10 mCi (370 MBq) ^{18}F-fluorodeoxyglucose is reconstructed using matrices ranging from 512 × 512 to 64 × 64, as shown in the figure.

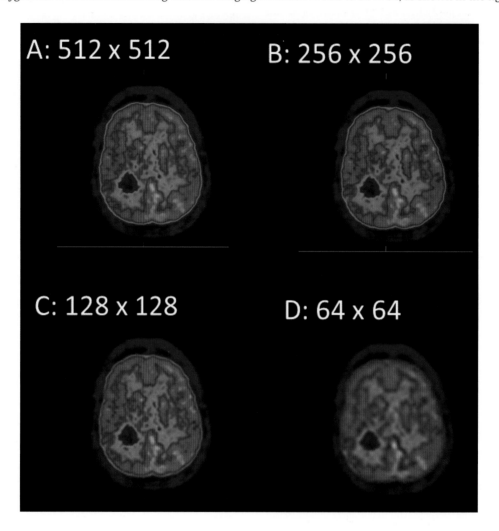

■ Questions

1. Assuming a 20-cm field-of-view with a zoom of 2 and a 4-mm full-width half-maximum (FWHM) intrinsic spatial resolution, what is the minimally acceptable matrix (smallest number of pixels across the width of the matrix) for image reconstruction?
   A. 512 × 512 matrix
   B. 256 × 256 matrix
   C. 128 × 128 matrix
   D. 64 × 64 matrix
   E. 32 × 32 matrix

2. The full set of images from the brain study shown is saved in Digital Imaging and Communications in Medicine (DICOM) standard format, and a picture archival communication system is used for image display and archiving. As compared to the use of grayscale, the use of a pseudocolor scale for image display is more likely to result in which of the following:
   A. Limitations on pixel dynamic range (windowing)
   B. Ambient light reflections on the display monitor
   C. Loss of spatial resolution in cathode ray tube (CRT) displays as compared to liquid crystal displays (LCDs)
   D. A larger DICOM file size
   E. Appearance of false contours within the image

■ Answers and Explanations

Question 1

C. Correct! Pixel size (*d*) is related to FOV based on the following relationship:

$$d = \text{FOV}/(z \times N),$$

where z = zoom factor and N = number of pixels across the width of the matrix. For a 128 × 128 matrix, therefore, *d* = (200 mm)/(2 × 128) = 0.78 mm.

To best preserve the spatial resolution of the imaging system, pixel size should be less than one-third of the FWHM of the imaging system. Therefore, at a 4-mm FWHM, the maximal pixel size should be 1.33 mm (1/3 × 4 mm). Because 0.78 mm is < 1.33 mm, a 128 × 128 matrix would be acceptable, and in fact, is the minimally acceptable matrix.

Other choices and discussion

Pixel size (*d*) is related to FOV based on the following relationship:

$$d = \text{FOV}/(z \times N),$$

where z = zoom factor and N = number of pixels across the width of the matrix.

A. Therefore, at a 4-mm FWHM, the maximal pixel size should be 1.33 mm (1/3 × 4 mm). For a 512 × 512 matrix, therefore, *d* = (200 mm)/(2 × 512) = 0.20 mm. Because 0.20 mm is < 1.33 mm, a 512 × 512 matrix would be acceptable, but is more fine than a 128 × 128 matrix, and therefore, is not the correct answer.

"Oversampling" refers to the use of a matrix which, while fine, does not provide increased spatial resolution as it exceeds the gains possible given the intrinsic spatial resolution of the system. Also, it should be remembered that decreasing pixel size must be balanced against the progressive decrease in counts per pixel that accompanies finer matrices.

B. For a 256 × 256 matrix, therefore, *d* = (200 mm)/(2 × 256) = 0.39 mm. Because 0.39 mm is < 1.33 mm, a 256 × 256 matrix would be acceptable, but is more fine than a 128 × 128 matrix, and therefore, is not the correct answer.

D. For a 64 × 64 matrix, therefore, *d* = (200 mm)/(2 × 64) = 1.56 mm. Because 1.56 mm is > 1.33 mm, a 64 × 64 matrix would not be acceptable ("undersampling").

E. For a 32 × 32 matrix, therefore, *d* = (200 mm)/(2 × 32) = 3.13 mm. Because 3.13 mm is > 1.33 mm, a 32 × 32 matrix would not be acceptable ("undersampling").

Question 2

E. Correct! Color and pseudocolor displays assign different colors, whether distinctly different such as in the blue-green-orange scale depicted in this study or only slightly different as in the shades of orange in the commonly-used "heat" scale, to pixels of different brightness. These differences in color, therefore, depict pixel brightness in a nonlinear fashion, whereas grayscale presents differences in brightness linearly. As such, slight differences in pixel brightness may be accentuated by color and pseudocolor displays and can result in the appearance of sharp or significant differences in pixel brightness where they do not exist.

Other choices and discussion

A. The range of pixel brightnesses in a grayscale display increases as bit depth increases. Current guidelines suggest that eight-bit monitors may be of sufficient depth for most, if not all, imaging applications. An eight-bit display is capable of depicting 2^8, or 256, brightness levels on the grayscale. Most color or pseudocolor displays can produce on the order of 2^{24} different colors representing pixel brightness.

B. Reflections resulting from ambient light would not be predictably different between color scales used to display images (i.e., grayscale versus a color/pseudocolor scale). The use of antiglare coatings may decrease focal ("specular") reflections but may increase diffuse reflections.

C. Monitor spatial resolution reflects the number of pixels present in a given unit of length (usually a millimeter). The use of color or grayscales to display data does not affect the resolution of a given monitor, be it CRT or LCD, and should not be confused with true monochrome (grayscale only) versus polychrome monitors (able to display color and grayscale images). CRTs were utilized in monitors for image generation early on. These monitors contained an electron beam that was deflected onto a phosphor screen to generate an image. More recently, active-matrix LCD monitors have become the mainstay and utilize a thin layer of crystals sandwiched between two layers of glass to generate an image when a voltage is applied. These LCD monitors, whether monochromatic or polychromatic, have uniformly higher spatial resolutions than CRT monitors of the same pixel format/matrix (although it is true that monochrome LCDs are typically of higher resolution than polychrome LCDs).

D. In addition to the image data they contain, DICOM files typically include demographic information about the patient, acquisition procedure information, and other information that facilitates appropriate final image display, including the image matrix size; all of these are typically found within the DICOM "header." This header occupies little of the total file size. Rather, the DICOM file size is determined by the number of pixels within the digital image. In digital mammography, images of 70 to 80 megapixels in size are frequent, whereas a typical planar nuclear medicine study may occupy < 0.2 megapixels.

Top Tips

- To best preserve the spatial resolution of the imaging system, pixel size should be less than one-third of the FWHM of the imaging system.
- Slight differences in pixel brightness may be accentuated by color and pseudocolor displays, and can result in the appearance of sharp or significant differences in pixel brightness where they do not exist.
- The DICOM header includes patient demographic information, acquisition parameters, and matrix size.

More Challenging 3

■ Case

Radionuclide Q decays via electron capture to its stable daughter radionuclide R, with a physical half-life (T_p or $T_{1/2\,p}$) of 93 hours. The predominant photon (γ-ray) emitted in this decay has an energy of 210 keV. In preclinical biodistribution studies, a pharmaceutical labeled with radionuclide Q undergoes hepatic (75%) and renal (23%) clearance, yielding a biologic half-life (T_b or $T_{1/2\,b}$) of 7 hours.

■ Questions

1. What is the effective half-life (T_e or $T_{1/2\,e}$) of the Q-labeled radiopharmaceutical?
   A. 0.2 hours
   B. 0.9 hours
   C. 6.5 hours
   D. 7.0 hours
   E. 50.0 hours

2. A 15 mCi (5550 MBq) sample of radionuclide Q is allowed to decay at room temperature. At 10 days, what is the remaining activity of the radionuclide?
   A. 0 mCi (0 MBq)
   B. 2.5 mCi (925 MBq)
   C. 5.8 mCi (2146 MBq)
   D. 10.0 mCi (3700 MBq)
   E. 15.0 mCi (5550 MBq)

■ Answers and Explanations

Question 1

C. Correct! Effective half-life (T_e) is related to biologic (T_b) and physical (T_p) half-lives by the following equations:

$$1/T_e = 1/T_b + 1/T_p \quad \text{OR} \quad T_e = (T_b \cdot T_p)/(T_b + T_p).$$

Therefore, in this case,

$$1/Te = 1/7 \text{ hours} + 1/93 \text{ hours} = 0.143 \text{ hours} + 0.011 \text{ hours} = \mathbf{0.154 \text{ hours}^{-1} = 1/T_e} \text{ OR}$$

$$T_e = (7 \text{ hours} \cdot 93 \text{ hours})/(7 \text{ hours} + 93 \text{ hours}) = 651/100 \text{ hours} = \mathbf{6.51 \text{ hours} = T_e}$$

Other choices and discussion

A. See above for correct calculation. Were you to incorrectly use the equations (as shown below), you would get $T_e = 0.15$ hours:

$$1/Te = 1/7 \text{ hours} + 1/93 \text{ hours} = 0.143 \text{ hours} + 0.011 \text{ hours} = \mathbf{0.154 \text{ hours} = T_e} \text{ OR}$$

$$T_e = (7 \text{ hours} + 93 \text{ hours})/(7 \text{ hours} \cdot 93 \text{ hours}) = 100/651 \text{ hours} = \mathbf{0.154 \text{ hours} = T_e}$$

B. Were you to incorrectly omit T_b in the numerator, you would get $T_e = 0.93$ hours:

$$T_e = (93 \text{ hours})/(7 \text{ hours} + 93 \text{ hours}) = 93/100 \text{ hours} = \mathbf{0.93 \text{ hours} = T_e}$$

D. Were you to incorrectly assume that T_e is only dependent on biologic half-life (T_b), you would infer that T_e is 7 hours.

E. Were you to instead assume that T_e would be the average of T_b and T_p, you would get $T_e = 50$ hours:

$$T_e = (7 \text{ hours} + 93 \text{ hours})/2 = 100/2 \text{ hours} = \mathbf{50 \text{ hours} = T_e}$$

Question 2

B. Correct! The physical half-life (T_p or $T_{1/2p}$) is 93 hours.

Recall that physical half-life is related to the decay constant of a radionuclide by the equation:

$$\lambda = 0.693/T_{1/2p}$$

Also note that activity of the radionuclide at time $= t$, A_t, is related to the radioactivity at time $= 0$ (A_0) by the equation:

$$A_t = A_0 \cdot e^{-\lambda t} \quad \text{OR} \quad A_t = A_0 \cdot e^{-0.639t/Tp}$$

Therefore, in this case, at 10 days (240 hours):

$$\lambda = 0.693/T_{1/2p} = 0.693/93 \text{ hours} = 0.0075 \text{ hours}^{-1}$$

$$A_t = A_0 \cdot e^{-\lambda t} = (15 \text{ mCi}) \cdot e^{-(0.0075 \text{ hours}^{-1} \times 240 \text{ hours})} = (15 \text{ mCi}) \cdot 0.167 = \mathbf{2.51 \text{ mCi}}$$

Other choices and discussion

A. A common mistake is to use half-life instead of decay constant in this equation. Were you to use the incorrect equation as shown below, you would get:

$$A_t = A_0 \cdot e^{-Tp \cdot t} = (15 \text{ mCi}) \cdot e^{-(93 \text{ hours} \times 240 \text{ hours})} = (15 \text{ mCi}) \cdot 0 = 0 \text{ mCi}$$

C. You may note that 240 hours is approximately 2.58 times the half-life ($T_{1/2p}$) of 93 hours. Thus, one common mistake is to conclude that the fraction of activity remaining at 10 days (240 hours) would be 1/2.58th of the original activity:

$$A_t = A_0/2.58 = (15 \text{ mCi})/2.58 = 5.814 \text{ mCi}$$

D. See B above.

E. Were you to use the incorrect equation (as shown below), you would get:

$$A_t = A_0 \cdot e^{-\lambda/t} = (15 \text{ mCi}) \cdot e^{-(0.0075 \text{ hours}^{-1}/240 \text{ hours})} = (15 \text{ mCi}) \cdot 0.999 = 14.99 \text{ mCi}$$

■ Suggested Readings

Saha GB. Physics and Radiobiology of Nuclear Medicine. 4th ed. New York: Springer; 2014

Top Tips

◆ The decay constant (λ) is the fraction of atoms decaying per unit time (typically expressed in disintegrations per minute or disintegrations per second).

◆ Physical half-life (T_p or $T_{1/2p}$), defines the amount of time it takes for half of a given number of atoms to decay, and may be expressed in seconds, minutes, hours, or days. It is related to the decay constant of a radionuclide by the equation:

$$\lambda = 0.693/T_{1/2p}$$

◆ Effective half-life: $1/T_e = 1/T_b + 1/T_p$ OR $T_e = (T_b \cdot T_p)/(T_b + T_p)$

◆ *Mean effective life, $\bar{T}$, is frequently used for dosimetry calculations, is approximately equal to $1/\lambda$ or 1.44 times the $T_{1/2e}$ (T_e), and may be conceptualized as the *average* length of time a radioactive atom will be present within a sample before it disintegrates.

◆ Activity of the radionuclide at time $= t$, A_t, is related to the radioactivity at time $= 0$ (A_0) by the equation:

$$A_t = A_0 \cdot e^{-\lambda t} \text{ OR } A_t = A_0 \cdot e^{-0.639t/Tp}$$

More Challenging 4

■ Questions

1. A 35-year-old woman undergoes rest-stress radionuclide scintigraphy with administered activities of 296 MBq (8 mCi) 99m-technetium sestamibi for rest imaging and 720 MBq (24 mCi) 99m-technetium sestamibi for same-day stress imaging. The total administered activity for the study is 1016 MBq (32 mCi) 99m-technetium sestamibi. Radiation absorbed doses are 0.039 mGy/MBq gallbladder; 0.0063 mGy/MBq heart wall; 0.0053 mGy/MBq thyroid; 0.024 mGy/MBq large intestine wall; and 0.036 mGy/MBq kidneys. Which of the above-listed is (are) the critical organ(s)?
   A. Gallbladder
   B. Kidneys
   C. Large intestine
   D. Heart
   E. Thyroid

2. After performing the cardiac scintigraphy study, you are informed that the patient, although not pregnant, is currently breastfeeding her 18-month-old daughter. Which of the following is MOST accurate with regard to 99m-technetium sestamibi secretion in breast milk?
   A. Following administration of 99m-technetium sestamibi, breastfeeding should be discontinued for at least 72 hours (3 days).
   B. Following administration of 99m-technetium sestamibi, breastfeeding should be discontinued for at least 12 hours.
   C. Provided that no free 99m-technetium pertechnetate (^{99m}Tc-NaO4) is present in the administered dose, no discontinuation of breastfeeding is required.
   D. Breastfeeding should be discontinued at least 24 priors to, and for at least 24 hours after, 99m-technetium sestamibi administration.
   E. All clinically used 99m-technetium-labled radiopharmaceuticals are excreted at significant levels into breast milk (i.e., at least 2% of injected activity is excreted in breast milk).

■ Answers and Explanations

Question 1

A. Correct! The critical organ for a radiopharmaceutical is that organ with the highest absorbed dose. In this case, with a total administered activity of 1016 MBq 99m-technetium sestamibi, absorbed doses to the organs will be 39.6 mGy gallbladder; 36.6 mGy kidneys; 24.4 mGy colon; 6.4 mGy heart; and 5.4 mGy thyroid. Thus, the gallbladder is the critical organ in this case.

The other choices are incorrect.

Question 2

C. Correct! 99m-technetium sestamibi is secreted at only very low levels into breast milk ($<$ 0.5% of the injected dose is excreted). However, if substantial amounts of pertechnetate are contained within the radiopharmaceutical dose, then breastfeeding would need to be discontinued for no less than 12 hours.

Other choices and discussion

A, B, D, and E. 99m-technetium sestamibi is secreted at only very low levels into breast milk ($<$ 0.5% of the injected dose is excreted). Therefore, no changes to breastfeeding or the breast-feeding schedule are required. See the chart in "Top Tips" for relative secreted amounts and breastfeeding cessation recommendations for several commonly used radiopharmaceuticals.

With the exception of ^{99m}Tc-MAA and ^{99m}Tc-NaO4, the ^{99m}Tc-labeled radiopharmaceuticals do not require any change in breastfeeding.

- Radioiodine-labeled radiopharmaceuticals, including those labeled with 123-iodide and 131-iodide, require at least 3 weeks of breastfeeding cessation; some require much more (see chart below).

- Guidelines from the International Commission on Radio-logical Protection were developed such radiopharma-ceutical decay and clearance during the cessation period would result in an expected effective dose to the infant from the radiopharmaceutical of no more than 1 mSv. In addition, expected radiation dose to the breasts where the mother breastfeeding is also considered in recom-mendations for breastfeeding interruption.

■ References

1. Leide-Svegborn S, Ahlgren L, Johansson L, et al. Excre-tion of radionuclides in human breast milk after nuclear medicine examinations. Biokinetic and dosimetric data and recommendations on breastfeeding interruption. Eur J Nucl Med Mol Imaging 2016;43:808–821

2. International Commission on Radiological Protection. Radiation dose to patients from radiopharmaceuticals: a compendium of current information related to fre-quently used substances. Ann ICRP 2015;44(2S)

■ Suggested Readings

Mettler FA, Guiberteau MJ. Essentials of Nuclear Medicine Imag-ing. 6th ed. Philadelphia: Elsevier Saunders; 2012

Saha GB. Physics and Radiobiology of Nuclear Medicine. 4th ed. New York: Springer; 2014

Top Tips

Radiopharmaceu-tical	Fraction of in-jected activity secreted into breastmilk	Recommended breastfeeding interruption
^{99m}Tc-DTPA[1]	0.0012%	None
^{99m}Tc-MAA[1]	3.7%	At least 12 hours
^{99m}Tc-MAG3[1]	0.07%	None
^{99m}Tc-MDP or ^{99m}Tc-HDP[1]	0.01%	None
^{99m}Tc-sestamibi[1]	0.048%	None
^{99m}Tc-NaO$_4$ (pertechnetate)[1]	0.82% (blocked); 10% (unblocked)	At least 12 hours
^{99m}Tc-sulfur colloid[2]	Up to 1.5%	None
^{99m}Tc-tetrofosmin[1]	0.082%	None
^{18}F-FDG[1]	0.070%	None
^{123}I-MIBG[2]	0.03%	At least 3 weeks
^{131}I-MIBG[2]	0.03%	At least 3 weeks
^{123}I-NaI[2]	31%	At least 3 weeks
^{131}I-NaI[1]	31%	Complete cessation
^{201}Tl-TlCl[2]	Exact fraction unknown	At least 48 hours
^{133}Xe[2]	Unknown	None
^{67}Ga	Exact fraction unknown	At least 2 weeks

- The critical organ for a radiopharmaceutical is that organ with the highest absorbed dose.

- General breastfeeding interruption after radiopharmaceutical administration:

    Tc-99m-pertechnetate $<$ Tl-201 $<$ Radioiodine

More Challenging 5

■ Case

Title 10 Part 20 of the Code of Federal Regulations of the United States (10CFR20) outlines the governmental guidelines regarding occupational dose limits for persons exposed to ionizing radiation as part of their occupation (termed "occupational dose"), as well as dose limits to individual members of the public who are not exposed via occupational radiation doses.

■ Questions

1. Radiation dose limits set by 10CFR20 are primarily based on the recommendations of the:
   A. European Atomic Energy Community (EURATOM) treaty
   B. International Commission on Radiological Protection (ICRP)
   C. U.S. Food and Drug Administration (FDA)
   D. U.S. Department of Energy (DOE)
   E. International Atomic Energy Association (IAEA)

2. The NRC stipulates that the radiation dose (effective dose) to the embryo/fetus of a declared pregnant woman, as set forth in 10CFR20, is not to exceed:
   A. 0.5 mSv (0.05 rem) for the entire pregnancy
   B. 5 mSv (0.5 rem) for the entire pregnancy
   C. 50 mSv (5 rem) for the entire pregnancy
   D. 150 mSv (15 rem) for the entire pregnancy
   E. 500 mSv (50 rem) for the entire pregnancy

■ Answers and Explanations

Question 1

B. Correct! The United Nations Scientific Committee on the Effects of Atomic Radiation does not set policies for radiation protection, but rather provides scientific information on the effects and risks of ionizing radiation. The ICRP and other policy-setting organizations utilize the evidence provided by the United Nations Scientific Committee on the Effects of Atomic Radiation and incorporate regionally, nationally, or multinationally based (e.g., in the European Union) principles. In particular, the ICRP has set limits for radiation dose exposures for workers (occupational doses) as well as doses to individual members of the public. These limits, collectively encompassed within its International System of Radiological Protection, have been generally incorporated into the guidelines set by 10CFR20 and, therefore, the U.S. Nuclear Regulatory Commission (NRC) guidelines. Radiation dose limits set by the ICRP and the National Council on Radiation Protection and Measurements are similar, though several factors utilized by the NRC, such as the tissue weighting factors (W_T), are adopted specifically from the ICRP.

Other choices and discussion

A. The EURATOM treaty was originally signed by Belgium, Germany, France, Italy, Luxembourg, and the Netherlands in 1947, and thereby established the European Atomic Energy Community. The treaty was signed in an effort to establish peaceful, collaborative development of research related to nuclear energy. The European Atomic Energy Community cooperates with the NRC and other organizations to assist the establishment of policies regarding the safe use of radioactive and X-ray generators and materials. The EURATOM treaty does not govern or apply directly to the 10CFR or its radiation dose limits.

C. The FDA regulates pharmaceuticals to be used for diagnostic and therapeutic purposes, to include the chemical (pharmaceutical) compounds utilized in radiopharmaceuticals. In particular, Title 21 of the Code of Federal Regulations pertains specifically to the use of diagnostic radiopharmaceuticals/pharmacologic agents. The FDA does not set radiation dose limits or otherwise regulate the use of radionuclides per se (often referred to as byproduct materials).

D. The DOE, through its Office of Nuclear Energy, regulates research, proliferation, production, waste handling, and security of nuclear energy and power. The DOE does not set radiation dose limits.

E. The IAEA is primarily concerned with facilitating global nuclear security through programs such as inspections, security frameworks, and research and technology development. Although the NRC has worked cooperatively with the IAEA to implement nuclear safeguards, the IAEA does not set radiation dose limits.

Question 2

B. Correct! The calculated radiation dose (effective dose) limit to the embryo/fetus of a declared pregnant woman is 5 mSv (0.5 rem) during the entire pregnancy. See the table for a (limited) outline of additional dose limit specifications, including dose limits to members of the public.

Individual	Effective dose limit, mSv (rem)
Adult, total occupational effective dose	50 mSv annually (5 rem)
Adult, dose equivalent to lens of the eye	150 mSv annually (15 rem)
Adult, shallow dose equivalent to skin of whole body or extremities	500 mSv annually (50 rem)
Minor, total occupational effective dose	5 mSv annually (0.5 rem) (i.e., 10% of adult dose limit)
Embryo/fetus of declared pregnant adult female exposed to occupational radiation	5 mSv for the entire pregnancy (0.5 rem)
Individual member of the public from operation of licensee, total effective dose	1 mSv annually (0.1 rem)
Individual member of the public from patient treated with radiopharmaceutical, total effective dose	5 mSv annually (0.5 rem)

The other choices are incorrect.

■ Suggested Readings

Cherry SR, Sorenson JA, Phelps ME. Physics in Nuclear Medicine. 4th ed. Philadelphia: Saunders; 2012

Committee to Assess Health Risks from Exposure to Low Levels of Ionizing Radiation, National Research Council. Health Risks from Exposure to Low Levels of Ionizing Radiation: BEIR VII Phase 2. Washington, DC: National Research Council of the National Academies; 2006. http://www.nap.edu/catalog.php?record_id=11340

International Commission on Radiological Protection. Radiation dose to patients from radiopharmaceuticals: a compendium of current information related to frequently used substances. Ann ICRP 2015;44(2S)

Kase KR. Radiation protection principles of NCRP. Health Physics 2004;87(3):251–257

US Government Publishing Office. Food and Drugs - Title 21, Chapter I, Subchapter D, Part 315 Code of Federal Regulations [Internet]. Washington (DC): Office of the Federal Register; 2016. http://www.ecfr.gov/cgi-bin/text-idx?gp=1&SID=679cd1ea857fa54eca7d3fa8f08a8339&h=L&mc=true&tpl=/ecfrbrowse/Title21/21tab_02.tpl

US Nuclear Regulatory Commission. NRC Regulations – Title 10, Code of Federal Regulations. Washington, DC: Office of the Federal Register; 1991. http://www.nrc.gov/reading-rm/doc-collections/cfr/

Top Tips

- Radiation dose limits set by 10CFR20 are primarily based on the recommendations of the EURATOM treaty.
- Effective dose limit to the embryo/fetus of a declared pregnant woman = 5 mSv (0.5 rem) during the entire pregnancy.

SECTION XIV
PHYSICS SAFETY

■ Magnetic Resonance Imaging Questions

1. When the k-space trajectory is linear, motion artifacts most commonly occur in which direction?
   A. Slice encode
   B. Phase encode
   C. Frequency encode
   D. Oblique to image plane

B. Correct! Motion artifacts tend to occur in the phase encode direction. Remember that during each repetition time (TR), in conventional readouts, a line of k-space is acquired that is at one phase encode level and across the readout or frequency encode direction. Thus, readout for the frequency encode direction is much faster as it occurs within a TR, instead of for the phase encode direction that occurs across TRs. Basically, there is a higher chance for the motion artifact to accrue for the phase encode data than for the frequency encode data—and that artifactual data gets repeated or smeared across the phase encode direction.

2. Of the techniques listed below, which CANNOT typically mitigate motion artifacts?
   A. Saturation bands
   B. Radial versus conventional k-space trajectories
   C. Increasing receiver bandwidth
   D. Flip phase and frequency directions

C. Correct! That is, increasing receiver bandwidth cannot mitigate motion. There are many tricks to mitigate motion artifacts. Saturation bands can be used to null the signal from the offending moving objects (e.g., bowel and vasculature anterior to the lumbar spine). Radial acquisitions can be used, generally with oversampling of the origin, to prevent a single faulty line of k-space from coming through in the final image. Because motion artifacts occur in the phase encode direction, flipping which direction is used for frequency versus phase encoding can flip the direction in which the artifact is produced, allowing for better visualization of the target lesion. Conversely, with motion artifacts, altering bandwidth has minimal effect.

3. Of the following, which WOULD NOT minimize a metal-related artifact?
   A. Higher field strength
   B. Use of short T1 inversion recovery for fat suppression
   C. Parallel imaging
   D. Increasing receiver bandwidth
   E. Shorter time to echo or echo delay time

A. Correct! That is, higher field strength cannot minimize metal artifact. With a metal artifact, the magnetic susceptibility of the metal causes alteration of the local magnetic field, resulting in a dramatic T2*-related loss of signal. In general, susceptibility artifacts increase with field strength. Thus, increasing the field strength is the only answer choice provided that would be expected to increase the artifact.

4. Which of the following techniques is the LEAST sensitive to a metal-related artifact?
   A. Convention spin echo
   B. Gradient echo
   C. Fast spin echo
   D. Fat saturation

C. Correct! That is, fast spin echo is the least sensitive technique to a metal-related artifact. Gradient echo sequences are highly sensitive to T2* effects, such as metal artifacts. Fat saturation relies on precise estimation of the precessional frequency differences between fat and water protons. Metal causes artifacts by altering the local magnetic field (and, therefore, the local precessional frequencies), thus rendering fat saturation useless. The multiple 180-degree pulses of fast spin echo cause multiple rounds of refocusing and reduced spin J-coupling. This reduces the dephasing that leads to the T2- and T2*-related signal loss and image warping seen in metal artifacts. Therefore, fast spin echo is less sensitive to metal artifacts than conventional spin echo.

5. Of the following, which would be INEFFECTIVE in addressing aliasing ("wraparound" artifact)?
   A. Increasing the field of view
   B. Increasing the matrix size
   C. Increasing the bandwidth
   D. Assigning frequency encode to the largest dimension of the patient

C. Correct! That is, increasing the bandwidth would not correct the aliasing artifact. In aliasing (aka "wraparound" artifact), objects outside of the FOV contribute signal that is detected by the receiver coil, and the system misinterprets that extraneous signal as originating from within the FOV. This localizes that signal to the opposite side of the image (i.e., the image "wraps around" to the other side). In general, the wraparound artifact is seen in the phase encode direction, as the problem of aliasing is easier to prevent or remedy in the readout direction. This is accomplished by increasing the FOV and matrix via increasing the sampling during readout, which takes into account the extra signal received. Fixing the artifact in the phase encode direction would require more phase encode steps and therefore would increase the net scan time. By assigning the frequency encode to the largest patient dimension, only a minimal number of phase encode steps are needed to encompass the matrix necessary for the entire FOV. This minimizes the chance for aliasing. Additional remedies for aliasing include the use of a coil with sensitivity only over the FOV and/or the use of selective excitation to excite only a slab in the desired region. Keep in mind that because there are two phase encode directions for three-dimensional sequences, aliasing can occur in either direction, producing some rather strange artifacts!

6. Which of the following corrections is most helpful in removing a "magic angle" artifact?
   A. Increasing the number of averages
   B. Increasing the parallel imaging factor
   C. Increasing the echo time
   D. Increasing the echo train length

C. Correct! With the "magic angle" artifact, when an ordered structure that has a short intrinsic T2 relaxation time is oriented at a particular angle with respect to the magnetic field, certain forms of spin-spin coupling are reduced. This lengthens the T2 relaxation time of the structure. The lengthened T2 time translates to an increased amount of time for the transverse magnetization to persist, which yields slightly increased signal, given that signal is proportional to the amount of transverse magnetization. By increasing the echo time to produce a T2-weighted fat-saturated image, the effect of that slight T2 lengthening and transverse magnetization is removed or, at the very least, is imperceptible.

7. The "magic angle" artifact most frequently occurs when a tendon or ligament is at a
   A. Approximately 90-degree angle to the main magnetic field
   B. Approximately 55-degree angle to the main magnetic field
   C. Approximately 90-degree angle to the readout direction
   D. Approximately 55-degree angle to the readout direction

B. Correct! The "magic angle" of the magic angle artifact is ~ 54.7 degrees (or, written another way, 180 degrees − 54.7 degrees = 125.3 degrees) with respect to the main magnetic field. This artifact can occur when an ordered, short T2 structure (i.e., tendon or ligament) is oriented at this angle *regardless of the imaging plane*. Thus, the artifact may arise in that anatomic location even if imaging was performed in the axial or coronal plane—not just in the sagittal plane.

8. In spin-echo imaging, enhanced T2 weighting of image contrast can be achieved by:
   A. Increasing echo time (TE) and increasing repetition time (TR)
   B. Increasing TE and decreasing TR
   C. Decreasing TE and increasing TR
   D. Decreasing TE and decreasing TR

A. Correct! Generally speaking, increasing the TE increases T2 weighting in spin echo imaging, whereas decreasing the TR increases the T1 weighting. Therefore, to produce a T2-weighted spin echo image, a long TE is used to maximize T2 weighting, and a long TR is used to minimize T1 weighting.

9. All other things being equal, which of these sequences would have the highest signal-to-noise ratio?
   A. Short repetition time (TR), short echo time (TE)
   B. Short TR, long TE
   C. Long TR, short TE
   D. Long TR, long TE

C. Correct! Generally speaking, relaxation effects reduce signal strength. Therefore, for conventional imaging, a long TR would minimize T1 relaxation-related effects, whereas a short TE would minimize T2 relaxation-related effects. Note that these choices would produce a proton density–weighted image. Proton density–weighted images are among the higher signal-to-noise ratio sequences in magnetic resonance imaging.

10. Of the following, which would decrease magnetic resonance imaging slice thickness?
    A. Increasing the receiver bandwidth
    B. Increasing the transmit bandwidth
    C. Increasing the slice-select gradient
    D. Increasing the field strength

C. Correct! Slice thickness during selective excitation is a function of the strength of the slice-select gradient and the transmit bandwidth. In slice selection, a "slice-select" gradient is turned on so that there is a gradient of field strength along the direction of slicing. This results in a gradient of precessional frequencies that run along that axis. For instance, in axial slicing, the slice-select gradient is oriented along the head-to-foot axis so that the spins in the head are precessing slower than those in the feet, or vice versa. Then a radiofrequency pulse is transmitted that is tuned to the frequency of the spins in the section of tissue (or slice) that are meant to be selected. The width of the slice will then depend on the range of frequencies included in the radiofrequency pulse (i.e., the transmit bandwidth) and how steep the gradient is across the thickness of the subject. Slice thickness increases with increasing transmit bandwidth and with decreasing slice select gradient.

11. Of the artifacts listed below, which relates directly to in- and out-of-phase imaging?
    A. Chemical shift, type 1
    B. Chemical shift, type 2
    C. Magic angle
    D. Flow-related dephasing

B. Correct! The differences in the precessional frequencies of fat and water protons underlie the two types of chemical shift artifact (the chemical shift refers to the shift of the frequencies of fat protons with respect to water). In the type 1 chemical shift artifact, the signal from fat is misregistered such that it is translated along the frequency encode direction, showing up as a bright band on one side of a water-containing structure surrounded by fat and as a dark band on the opposite side. In the type 2 chemical shift artifact, fat and water protons accrue different phases during precession. Therefore, at different and predictable times, the protons are alternately in-phase (in which case their signals add up within a given voxel) or out-of-phase (in which case their signals cancel within a given voxel). In- and out-of-phase imaging takes advantage of these phase differences by acquiring echoes at the expected in- and out-of-phase times (at 1.5 T: out-of-phase = 2.2, 6.6, 11.0, . . . ms; in-phase = 4.4, 8.8, 13.2, . . . ms). If a voxel has less signal on the out-of-phase image than on the in-phase image, then that voxel must contain water and fat protons in a roughly equal mixture.

12. Which of the following relationships between relaxation and main magnetic field strength (B_0) are correct?
    A. Proton density (PD) increases substantially and T2 decreases substantially with increasing B_0
    B. PD and T2 decrease substantially with increasing B_0
    C. T1 increases substantially and T2* decreases substantially with increasing B_0
    D. T2 and T2* increase substantially with increasing B_0

C. Correct! For clinical purposes, PD and T2 relaxations are essentially independent of factors such as the strength of the main magnetic field (B_0). T1 relaxation time increases with increasing B_0 because the Larmor frequency increases. The energy transfer that mediates T1 relaxation is most efficient when molecules are tumbling at a rate close to the Larmor frequency. As the Larmor frequency increases, fewer and fewer molecules near the spin are available to mediate T1 relaxation, so the T1 relaxation time is prolonged. Similarly, at higher field strength, the spins are spinning faster, and the slight phase differences that mediate the dephasing that in turn mediates T2* effects accrue faster. Therefore, at higher field strengths the spins de-phase faster, making T2* shorter.

13. How often should the magnetic resonance magnet be powered down and restarted?
    A. Daily
    B. Weekly
    C. Annually
    D. Never

D. Correct! Turning the magnet off is known as "quenching" and involves boiling off the liquid helium that keeps the wires of the electromagnet cold. This increase in temperature leads to a sudden loss of superconductivity. If the room is not suitably vented, a quench can result in frostbite and asphyxiation for those unlucky enough to be in the scanner room. Quenching is an extraordinarily expensive process. In addition, because wire resistance is zero in the superconducting state, once current has been established in an electromagnet, it will not dissipate unless disrupted by someone. Therefore, a routine magnet shut down is not needed. From a safety perspective, it should always be assumed that the magnet is on.

14. Of the following, which value for estimated glomerular filtration rate (eGFR) would generally be an absolute contraindication to administration of a gadolinium (Gd)-based contrast agent (GBCA)?
    A. 80 mL/min/1.73 m^2
    B. 60 mL/min/1.73 m^2
    C. 40 mL/min/1.73 m^2
    D. 20 mL/min/1.73 m^2

D. Correct! Nephrogenic systemic fibrosis (NSF) is a rare disorder that appears to be related to Gd deposition in patients with renal dysfunction. In patients with low eGFR, without adequate clearance of the GBCA, it is hypothesized that GBCAs dissociate, resulting in deposition of ionic Gd (Gd^{3+}) in tissues, inducing a toxic reaction that results in systemic fibrosis. In support of this, it is noted that the rates of NSF have dramatically declined with newer agents that do no dissociate as readily as older agents. Almost all cases of NSF have been seen in patients with eGFR < 30 mL/min/1.73 m^2, with only a few cases identified in patients with eGFR = 30 to 60 mL/min/1.73 m^2. No cases have been seen in patients with eGFR > 60 mL/min/1.73 m^2. For these reasons, guidelines indicate that an eGFR < 30 mL/min/1.73 m^2 is an absolute contraindication to GBCA administration unless hemodialysis will be performed soon after administration.[1] For patients with eGFR = 30 to 60 mL/min/1.73 m^2, the decision to administer a GBCA is at the discretion of the radiologist. In patients with eGFR > 60 mL/min/1.73 m^2, Gd administration is considered safe.

15. Which of the following changes would increase magnetic resonance imaging specific absorption rate (SAR)?
    A. Decreasing the main magnetic field strength (B_0)
    B. Decreasing the repetition time (TR)
    C. Decreasing the flip angle
    D. Decreasing the total scan time

B. Correct! In magnetic resonance imaging, SAR refers to the rate of energy deposition, principally due to radiofrequency (RF) energy transmission. This deposition rate is directly proportional to the square of the RF amplitude and time, and inversely proportional to the TR. Note that flip angle increases proportionately with RF amplitude and duration, such that SAR increases with the flip angle. Also, because the Larmor frequency increases with field strength (B_0), and RF energy increases with frequency, SAR also increases at higher field strengths (if everything else is equal). Note that the total scan time does not affect SAR, as SAR measures the rate of energy deposition, not the total amount of energy deposited. In summary, SAR is proportional to $[B_0^2 \cdot (\text{flip angle})^2]/\text{TR}$. Additionally, since higher RF power is generally needed to penetrate deeper tissues, SAR generally increases with patient size.

16. If a patient experiences a cardiac arrest during a magnetic resonance imaging (MRI) scan, which of the following procedures should be followed?
    A. Remove patient from scanner gantry and relax zoning restrictions to allow unscreened code personnel to enter Zones 2 and 3 but not Zone 4
    B. Remove patient from scanner gantry and relax zoning restrictions to allow unscreened code personnel to enter Zone 2 but not Zones 3 and 4
    C. Remove patient from scanner gantry and relax zoning restrictions to allow unscreened code personnel to enter Zones 2, 3, and 4
    D. Remove patient from scanner gantry past the five Gauss line so that no relaxation of zoning restrictions is necessary

D. Correct! The MRI zones are meant to help ensure that only screened personnel or devices enter the scanner room and thereby experience the potential risks of the high magnet field strengths. Because the magnet is always on, the MRI zones are never relaxed—even during a code. Typically, the five Gauss line is considered to be the mark beyond which the environment is considered safe. Therefore, during a code, the patient should be removed beyond the five Gauss line as safely as possible to facilitate the administration of proper emergent care without the worry of device and/or personnel compatibility with MRI.

17. Match each of the structures on the right (1 to 4) with its role in magnetic resonance imaging generation (A to D).

A. Wires carrying electrical signals to prevent radiofrequency (RF) leak	1. Shimming
B. Pipes carrying water to prevent RF leak	2. Shielding
C. Prevent external RF from entering the scan room	3. Filters
D. Promote field homogeneity	4. Waveguides

    A. 3
    B. 4
    C. 2
    D. 1

Water and air pass through waveguides to get into and out of the scanner room in a manner that prevents spurious RF leak. Electrical signals pass through filters for the same reason. Shielding is used to electrically isolate the scanner room so that electromagnetic fields do not enter the room (and cause noise) or leave the room (where they can interfere with other medical devices, such as pacemakers). Keep in mind that shielding must occur in all three dimensions, as electromagnetic fields are three-dimensional. "Shimming" is used to make the B_0 and B_1 fields more homogeneous and linear, respectively.

18. Match each of the sequences (A to C) with its description (1 to 4). (One of the sequences can be used twice.)
    A. Fat saturation
    B. Dixon method
    C. Inversion recovery

    1. Start sequence at fat null point after a suitable preparatory sequence
    2. Apply a frequency selective pulse of random phases to prevent fat signal generation
    3. Best for when metal is present
    4. Use chemical shift type II to calculate fat-only and water-only images

    A. 2
    B. 4
    C. 1, 3

All of the methods listed are performed for fat signal nulling. Because metal alters the local magnetic fields and, therefore, the local precessional frequencies for fat and water, inversion recovery is the best method for fat nulling in the presence of metal.

19. Match each of the sequences on the left (A to D) with its repetition time (TR) and echo time (TE) characteristics on the right (1 to 4).

A. T2-weighted	1. Spin echo short TR, short TE
B. Proton density–weighted	2. Spin echo long TR, long TE
C. T1-weighted	3. Spin echo long TR, short TE

A. 2
B. 3
C. 1

In spin echo imaging, long TE weights toward T2 contrast. Short TR weights toward T1 contrast. Proton density–weighted images are generated with weighting away from both T1 and T2 contrast. In gradient echo imaging, small α (flip angle) yields more T1 weighting—as does short TR, but TR is generally set to be the minimum possible for gradient echo. Long TE yields more T2* weighting. Note that because of the longer TE for T2* sequences, the TR is necessarily longer than for T1 weighting. For proton density–weighted images, we weight away from both T1 weighting and T2* weighting by using small α and short TE.

20. Match each of the contrast mechanisms on the left (A to E) with its pulse sequence implementation on the right (1 to 5).

A. Diffusion	1. Tripolar gradient that eliminates velocity dependent phase accrual
B. Gradient echo	2. Equal gradients separated by a 180-degree pulse
C. Phase contrast	3. Positive gradient lobe cancels negative lobe and yields an echo
D. Flow compensation	4. Gradient of random phases to eliminate residual transverse magnetization
E. Spoiler	5. Bipolar gradient that yields velocity dependent phase accrual

A. 2
B. 3
C. 5
D. 1
E. 4

In addition to their usual role in encoding spatial information in the eventual signal, gradients can do a variety of other things as listed above.

21. Of the characteristics listed below, which apply(ies) to spoiled gradient echo? (Select ALL that apply.)
A. Partial saturation
B. Uses the residual transverse magnetization
C. Spoilers
D. Rewinders
E. Steady state transverse magnetization

A and **C. Correct!** Advanced gradient echo pulse sequences, like spoiled gradient echo and steady state free precession or coherent gradient echo, build upon the base gradient echo sequence to generate contrasts that are not usually available to gradient echo sequences. When the radiofrequency pulses are placed close enough together, a steady state of longitudinal or transverse magnetization (or both) may develop. Advanced gradient echo sequences differ in how they use or eliminate these steady states. Spoiled gradient echo sequences use spoiling to eliminate the residual transverse magnetization in each repetition time, but then maintain a steady state longitudinal magnetization that is generally less than the amplitude of the original magnetization. This situation is known as partial saturation. Steady state free precession sequences specifically maintain the residual transverse magnetization to create a steady state of transverse magnetization, with rewinder gradients used to select the appropriate portions of k-space.

22. Which of these physiological factors is LEAST directly assessed with routine functional magnetic resonance imaging?
A. Cerebral perfusion
B. Blood oxygen extraction
C. Neuronal activity
D. Blood oxygen saturation

C. Correct! That is, neuronal activity is least directly assessed. Blood oxygenation level–dependent (BOLD) contrast is the main form of functional magnetic resonance imaging currently in use. As the name implies, BOLD is fundamentally a measure of blood flow and blood oxygenation levels. The basis of the contrast mechanism in BOLD is that deoxygenated blood has higher susceptibility and is therefore darker on a T2*-weighted image than oxygenated blood. Through the phenomenon of neurovascular coupling, neuronal activity induces changes in cerebral perfusion that are detectable with the BOLD technique. Keep in mind that BOLD, while a very powerful technique, only indirectly visualizes brain (neuronal) activity.

23. Which of the following would generally increase the signal-to-noise ratio? (Select ALL that apply.)
A. Increasing voxel size
B. Increasing slice thickness
C. Increasing receiver bandwidth
D. Increasing main magnetic field

A, B, and **D. Correct!** Signal-to-noise ratio increases with voxel size and volume, increases with the strength of the main magnetic field, and decreases with the receiver bandwidth.

24. Which of the following is generally most helpful when determining whether to perform magnetic resonance imaging (MRI) on a patient with a metallic implant?
   A. Prior MRI completed without issue
   B. Operative note from device placement
   C. Computed tomography of the region of interest
   D. Signed statement from the patient agreeing to the MRI

B. Correct! Ultimately, the decision whether to scan a particular patient on a particular scanner is at the discretion of the radiologist. The only way to be sure whether a particular device or implant is MRI-safe is to have documentation of the exact model of the implanted device, documented in the surgeon's or interventionalist's operative note from the device placement. This data then can be checked against databases that compile assessments of MRI device safety, such as mrisafety.com. Relying upon reports of a prior MRI or a history obtained from the patient is insufficient. A computed tomography of the region would help to determine if there is metal in the device, but would not help to clarify the safety.

25. Regarding diffusion imaging, which of the following is FALSE:
   A. The b = 0 image is essentially a spin echo T2-weighted image.
   B. The high b-value image shows a mixture of diffusion and T2-weighting.
   C. The apparent diffusion coefficient (ADC) image is typically produced by a combination of diffusion-encoding gradients with an echo planar readout.
   D. The acquisition of a diffusion tensor image is essentially the same as for a diffusion-weighted image, except for the inclusion of more gradient directions.
   E. Any readout (conventional, spiral, echo planar, etc.) can be used for diffusion imaging.

C. Correct! That is, the ADC is not produced by the diffusion-encoding gradients. The other statements are all true. Diffusion imaging is accomplished by applying a motion encoding gradient sequence coded along a particular gradient direction that is formed by the sum of amplitudes of the individual x, y, and z gradients. The strength and timing of these gradients defines the "b value," with a high b-value indicating high sensitivity of that sequence to restricted proton movement or diffusion. The signal produced by this motion encoding can be read out using any particular readout, although echo planar readout is used most commonly because of its speed. In diffusion-weighted imaging, multiple (at least six) gradient directions are acquired and averaged together to remove the effects of anisotropy biasing the signal. The diffusion-weighted image that is produced will contain a mixture of T2-weighting and diffusion weighting. To assess the T2-weighting, typically a "B0" image is calculated wherein b = 0, i.e. the motion-encoding gradients are not turned on. When b = 0, the sequence run is a regular T2-weighted spin echo sequence with otherwise the same technical parameters and readout as the diffusion-weighted image. Between the diffusion-weighted image and the B0 (T2-weighted)

images, an ADC image can be calculated that is more purely a reflection of the diffusion characteristics of the tissue, without T2-weighting. This ADC "map" is a calculated representation and is not directly produced by a sequence from the scanner. For diffusion tensor imaging, many more gradient directions are acquired and steps are taken to specifically calculate the degree of anisotropy in different directions.

26. Of the following, which would NOT be expected to show high relative diffusion signal?
   A. Infarcted tissue
   B. Abscess
   C. Hypercellular tumor
   D. Lymphocele
   E. Mucocele
   F. Hematoma

D. Correct! That is, lymphocele will not show high relative diffusion signal. High signal can be seen with high protein content, as with abscesses and mucoceles. High diffusion signal can be artifactually increased in regions of increased susceptibility, as in hematomas. Simple fluid (as is found in lymphoceles) would not be expected to restrict diffusion or yield high diffusion signal.

27. Gadolinium-based contrast agents are relatively contraindicated in evaluating pregnant patients because:
   A. The contrast agent can cross the placenta and reach the amniotic fluid, where gadolinium may disassociate from its chelating agent and adopt its toxic ionic form.
   B. Relatively reduced renal function in pregnancy would limit the renal clearance of the contrast agent and make the pregnant mother at risk for nephrogenic systemic fibrosis.
   C. Relatively reduced hepatic function in pregnancy would limit the hepatic clearance of the contrast agent and make the pregnant mother at risk for nephrogenic systemic fibrosis.
   D. The contrast agent can cross the placenta and directly interfere with cell division, limiting organogenesis.

A. Correct! The toxic form of gadolinium is the free ionic form (Gd^{3+}). Normally, gadolinium in contrast agents is bound by a chelating chemical cage that prevents toxicity. The kidney and (to a lesser extent) the liver then eliminate the gadolinium from the body. Given enough time, gadolinium will dissociate from its chemical cage into its toxic ionic form. Thus, gadolinium toxicity occurs when the caged gadolinium is not promptly eliminated and the retained molecule has enough time to dissociate into its toxic ionic form. This occurs in patients with renal failure (estimated glomerular filtration rate < 30), which is the basis for nephrogenic systemic fibrosis. This can also occur in the fetus, as the caged gadolinium crosses the placenta into the fetal circulation, is eliminated by the fetal kidneys into the amniotic fluid, but then has nowhere to go but back into the fetus. Eventually, the gadolinium in the fetal tissues and circulation will dissociate into its ionic form, which can be toxic to the fetus.

28. Which of the following statements regarding contrast-enhanced perfusion is INCORRECT?
    A. Cerebral blood volume (CBV) is calculated as the area under the curve between the baseline of the signal and the contrast bolus peak.
    B. Time to peak (TTP) refers to the time when the maximal signal change occurs measured from the start of imaging.
    C. Perfusion magnetic resonance imaging can only produce relative quantifications for each of CBV, TTP, mean transit time (MTT), unless the arterial signal is directly measured and accounted for.
    D. Cerebral blood flow is calculated as the MTT/CBV.
    E. The MTT refers to the width of the contrast bolus peak at its mean or half of the maximal peak change from baseline.

D. Correct! That is, cerebral blood flow is not calculated at MTT/CBV. In contrast-enhanced perfusion, whether computed tomography or magnetic resonance imaging, several values are calculated from the shape of the curve of signal derived from each voxel as the contrast passes through it. Cerebral blood flow is equal to CBV/MTT, not MTT/CBV. The CBV is derived from the area under the curve between the bolus and the imaginary line connecting the baseline level of signal before and after the bolus. The TTP, or T_{max}, is the time at which the bolus attains its peak. The MTT is the width of the contrast bolus, generally taken at the half-maximum level. Note that only relative values of each of these parameters can be calculated, unless the curves can be corrected using the arterial input function of the signal from the arteries feeding each territory.

29. Of the following, which is TRUE regarding arterial spin labeling (ASL) and conventional perfusion magnetic resonance imaging sequences?
    A. Both techniques require contrast administration, although less is needed for ASL.
    B. Current quantification methods only allow the calculation of relative cerebral blood flow (rCBF) when ASL is used.
    C. Only contrast-enhanced perfusion imaging methods have a role in tumor evaluation, whereas both ASL and contrast-enhanced imaging methods can be used in stroke evaluation.
    D. ASL requires magnetic resonance imaging systems with at least 3 Tesla magnetic field strength, whereas conventional perfusion methods can be completed using most any magnetic field strength.

B. Correct! ASL is a noncontrast perfusion imaging technique. In routine clinical practice, only rCBF is calculated from ASL. ASL can be used for any evaluation in which perfusion assessment is helpful—it is as much a technique for perfusion imaging as is contrast-enhanced perfusion imaging. The primary functional difference between ASL and conventional contrast-enhanced perfusion is that ASL is an overall lower signal imaging technique and the images produced are blurrier and sensitive to a variety of technical artifacts.

30. Which of the following distinguishes two-dimensional (2D) sequence acquisition from three-dimensional (3D) acquisition?
    A. Three-dimensional sequences require a magnetic resonance imaging system of at least 3 Tesla, whereas 2D sequences can be completed using any field strength.
    B. Three-dimensional sequences have two phase encoding directions and one readout direction, whereas 2D sequences have one of each.
    C. Three-dimensional sequences have necessarily reduced signal-to-noise ratio compared to 2D sequences.
    D. Three-dimensional sequences are generated with specialized 3D coils, whereas 2D sequences can be used with any routine coil.
    E. Slice or slab selective excitation is never completed with a 3D sequence, whereas it is necessary for 2D sequences.

B. Correct! In 3D magnetic resonance imaging, a second phase encode direction is included in the sequence to allow coding along two phase encode dimensions and one frequency encode direction simultaneously. This allows all three dimensions to be imaged at once.

31. Which of these quantities most directly affects contrast in an inversion recovery sequence?
    A. T1
    B. T2
    C. T2*
    D. Proton density

A. Correct! In inversion recovery sequences, a 180-degree pulse is applied initially and then the magnetization is allowed to recover at a T1-dependent rate. This process spreads out the strength of the tissue magnetization vectors according to their respective T1 times, thereby encoding a T1-weighted contrast in whatever signal is ultimately produced.

32. Paramagnetic materials affect tissue contrast by:
    A. Shortening T1 only
    B. Shortening T2 only
    C. Shortening T2* only
    D. Shortening proton density only
    E. None of the above

E. Correct! Paramagnetic substances yield shortening of T1, T2, *and* T2* times. Paramagnetic substances have no direct effect on the proton density.

33. Of the following, which is NOT an important patient safety consideration when completing a magnetic resonance imaging examination?
    A. Hearing protection (provide ear plugs, muffs)
    B. Renal function if gadolinium-based contrast is to be used
    C. Peripheral nerve stimulation at high field strength
    D. Heating from loops of wire or metal (electrocardiogram wires, orthopedic hardware)
    E. Rate of energy deposition (specific absorption rate)
    F. None of the above

F. Correct! All of the above factors should be considered with regard to magnetic resonance imaging safety.

34. Echo train length ("turbo factor") is defined as:
    A. The number of slices acquired at once in multislice sequences.
    B. The number of images produced in a multiecho spin echo sequence.
    C. The number of echoes per repetition time (TR) for a fast spin echo sequence.
    D. The number of echoes acquired by different coils in parallel acquisitions.

C. Correct! Echo train length, or "turbo factor" depending on the magnetic resonance imaging vendor you are using, refers to the number of echoes that are acquired within a TR for fast spin echo (aka turbo spin echo) techniques.

35. Of the following, which angiographic term(s) is correctly paired? (Select ALL that apply.)
    A. Bright blood : spin echo
    B. Dark blood : spin echo
    C. Bright blood : gradient echo
    D. Dark blood : gradient echo

B and **C. Correct!** To generate a signal in spin echo imaging, protons must see both the initial excitation radiofrequency pulse—typically 90 degrees—as well as the refocusing 180-degree pulse. Because flowing protons, especially those in vessels, typically do not see both pulses given their movement between slices, and with movement related dephasing, spin echo sequences generally yield a "black blood" technique wherein the vessels appear black on the image. In contrast, in gradient echo sequences, the protons need only see the initial excitation pulse to generate the signal—the latter gradient refocusing steps are not spatially selective. Additionally, the rapidly repeated radiofrequency excitation pulses induce a partial saturation for the stationary tissues in the imaging slab. This results in flow-related enhancement, wherein the unsaturated protons flowing into the imaging volume have higher signal than the stationary background. Thus, gradient echo sequences are generally a bright blood technique wherein the vessels appear bright on the image.

36. Match the sequence (A to C) with its characteristic (1 to 3).
    A. Time of flight
    B. Phase contrast
    C. Contrast enhanced

    1. Flow velocity encoding gradients
    2. Highest signal-to-noise ratio
    3. Flow-related enhancement and partial saturation

    A. 3
    B. 1
    C. 2

In time-of-flight techniques, generally, a T1-weighted (short repetition time) spoiled gradient echo sequence is used to induce partial saturation of the stationary background with accentuation of the signal from the inflowing unsaturated protons—a phenomenon dubbed "flow-related enhancement." For phase contrast imaging, a bilobed gradient pulse is used so that phase accrual is nulled for stationary protons and rises linearly with speed in that gradient direction. This encodes the component of velocity of the protons in that direction into the phase of those protons, which can be read out in the phase-only reconstructed images. Contrast-enhanced magnetic resonance angiography is generally the highest signal technique given the use of contrast; this high signal-to-noise ratio allows for imaging acceleration for rapid imaging.

37. Of the following, which has the highest intrinsic signal-to-noise ratio?
    A. Fluid attenuation inversion recovery
    B. T2-weighted
    C. Short T1 inversion recovery
    D. Turbo inversion recovery

B. Correct! In general, inversion recovery techniques have lower signal than their more conventional counterparts because the remaining non-nulled tissues still have lower net magnetization than they would have had without the inversion recovery preparation.

■ General Radiography Questions

38. Of the following, which yields the largest number of x-rays to be used in diagnostic radiography?
    A. Characteristic radiation
    B. Auger emission
    C. Braking radiation (Bremsstrahlung)
    D. Positron-electron annihilation

C. Correct! In X-ray production, a metal anode target is bombarded by electrons emitted from the cathode and accelerated by the voltage applied by the circuit. In the anode, those electrons lose a significant amount of energy in an electron-nucleus interaction that acts to slow down the electron. The lost energy is converted into photons generally of X-ray energy ($\sim$ 1 to 200 keV), a phenomenon referred to as Bremsstrahlung or "braking radiation." Bremsstrahlung radiations easily account for the highest number of photons in X-ray production for diagnostic radiography. Characteristic radiation is produced when an incoming electron or photon ejects an electron from an inner shell of the atom and an outer shell electron then falls to fill the vacancy. In so doing, the electron releases some of its energy in the form of an X-ray of energy equivalent to the difference between the two energy levels. While characteristic radiation produces a small peak at the appropriate energies for a given target, the number of X-rays produced therein is less than that of Bremsstrahlung. The Auger effect does not contribute substantially to X-ray production in radiography. Positron-electron annihilation is the basis of signal production in positron emission tomography imaging.

39. To account for the heel effect, in which of the following directions should the cathode-anode axis be oriented with respect to a mammography patient?
    A. Along the superoinferior axis, with the anode toward the patient's heel
    B. Along the superoinferior axis, with the cathode toward the patient's heel
    C. Perpendicular to the chest wall, with the anode toward the patient's nipple
    D. Perpendicular to the chest wall, with the cathode toward the patient's nipple

C. Correct! The heel effect, filtering of the X-ray beam within the anode side due to the angle of the anode with respect to the beam path, results in lower numbers of X-ray photons originating from the anode side of the beam. Thus, to account for the heel effect, the beam should be oriented so that the anode side is toward the patient's nipple, where there is less tissue to penetrate compared to the portions of the breast nearer the chest wall.

40. Match each the following quality parameters (A to G) with its definition (1 to 7).
    A. Signal-to-noise ratio
    B. Contrast-to-noise ratio
    C. Dynamic range
    D. Modulation transfer function of noise
    E. Noise power spectrum
    F. Noise equivalent quantum
    G. Detector quantum efficiency

1. The difference between the maximum number of photons a detector can detect without saturating, and the lowest number of photons needed for the detector to register a signal.
2. The amount of noise for an image plotted at each spatial frequency.
3. Essentially, the signal-to-noise ratio at each frequency. Technically, proportional to modulation transfer function^2/noise power spectrum.
4. The number of photons used for at a particular dose, as a function of spatial frequency; another measure of signal-to-noise ratio.
5. The brightness of a pixel divided by the standard deviation of pixel brightness in the local image.
6. The difference between the brightness of adjacent pixels divided by the standard deviation of pixel brightness in the local image.
7. The fidelity with which a detector registers different spatial frequencies.

A. 5
B. 6
C. 1
D. 7
E. 2
F. 4
G. 3

These are the basic definitions of the quality parameters generally used for imaging and especially used in radiography.

41. Ignoring automatic exposure control, which of the following would increase image contrast the most for radiography?
    A. Doubling peak kilovoltage (kVp)
    B. Halving kVp
    C. Doubling milliampere-seconds (mAs)
    D. Halving mAs

B. Correct! The kVp used in radiography is the most direct control of the intrinsic image contrast. Image contrast is determined by the degree to which different tissues absorb or scatter the incident X-ray beam. This absorption or scattering is most efficient when the average beam energy in keV is just above the average K-edge of the material in question. For most biologic tissues, the K-edge is well below the typical X-ray energies used in radiography, so lowering the kVp will generally increase the image contrast. The downside of lowering kVp is that insufficient X-rays will penetrate the tissue, especially in thicker regions of the subject. While altering mAs will affect contrast resolution, it does so through affecting the noise level, therefore its effects do not contribute as much to contrast itself as kVp.

42. Ignoring automatic exposure control, which of the following would increase signal-to-noise ratio the most for radiography?
    A. Doubling peak kilovoltage (kVp)
    B. Halving kVp
    C. Doubling milliampere-seconds (mAs)
    D. Halving mAs

C. Correct! If kVp controls image contrast, then mAs controls image noise. The more mAs, the higher number of photons that will be applied to and transmitted through the subject, thereby reducing the quantum mottle effect that occurs when an insufficient number of photons reach the image receptor (i.e., photopenia). Technically, noise level goes down with the square root of the mAs. Therefore, increasing mAs 2× will increase signal-to-noise ratio by the square root of 2, or approximately 1.4×.

43. In general, without automatic exposure control which of the following would decrease the radiation dose in radiography the most?
    A. Doubling peak kilovoltage (kVp)
    B. Halving kVp
    C. Doubling milliampere-seconds (mAs)
    D. Halving mAs

B. Correct! A good rule of thumb is that dose is linearly related to mAs, so that doubling mAs will roughly double the radiation dose. However, kVp reduction has a larger effect on dose reduction than mAs. A 15% drop in kVp will have a similar effect as halving the mAs (and therefore the dose).

44. When using automatic exposure control, which of the following most accurately represents the relationship between peak kilovoltage (kVp) and milliampere-seconds (mAs)?
    A. mAs doubles for each 15% increase in kVp.
    B. mAs decreases by half (50%) for each 15% increase in kVp.
    C. kVp doubles for each 15% increase in mAs.
    D. kVp decreases by half (50%) for each 15% increase in mAs.

B. Correct! This rule of thumb is good to keep in mind with respect to exposure and dose considerations.

45. When doing a fluoroscopic examination, the image intensifier should be kept:
    A. As far away from the patient as possible to reduce patient radiation dose.
    B. As far away from the patient as possible to reduce scattered radiation dose.
    C. As close to the patient as possible to reduce patient radiation dose.
    D. As close to the patient as possible to reduce scattered radiation dose.

C. Correct! Because of the inverse square law of radiation strength, if one keeps the image intensifier away from the patient, the system must increase the amount of X-rays penetrating the patient to maintain the same number of photons reaching the cassette. This increased number of photons increases both the direct patient dose and the scattered dose within the patient and to individuals operating the equipment. In addition, this would tend to yield more focal spot blur, thereby reducing image quality. Thus, the image intensifier should be kept close to the patient!

46. When doing a fluoroscopic examination with automatic exposure control, the image intensifier should be kept:
    A. As far away from the patient as possible to increase geometric magnification, thereby increasing quality.
    B. As far away from the patient as possible to decrease geometric magnification, thereby increasing quality.
    C. As close to the patient as possible to increase geometric magnification, thereby increasing quality.
    D. As close to the patient as possible to decrease geometric magnification, thereby increasing quality.

D. Correct! With the image intensifier far from the patient, the probability of geometric magnification causing blurring of the focal spot increases, which results in net blurring of the image. Thus, minimization of geometric magnification is yet another reason to keep the image intensifier close to the patient.

47. In radiography, what is the primary benefit of using a grid?
    A. Reduce dose
    B. Patient comfort
    C. Reduce scatter
    D. Increase image signal

C. Correct! Placement of a grid such that the grid lines are along the expected collimated beam path results in absorption of scattered radiation from the patient. This scattered radiation primarily contributes noise to the image, thereby reducing quality. Thus, the radiographic grid may improve quality. Please note, however, that using a grid also causes absorption of many primary photons. To produce the same image brightness when a grid is used, a higher dose of X-rays must be applied to the patient.

48. Each of the following strategies can be employed to reduce radiographic and fluoroscopic radiation dose EXCEPT:
    A. Remove the grid
    B. Lower the peak kilovoltage (kVp)
    C. Use pulsed fluoroscopy
    D. Move the image intensifier/image cassette away from the patient

D. Correct! That is, this is the only strategy listed that will not reduce radiation dose. Generally speaking, keeping the image intensifier close to the patient reduces dose and increases image quality. A grid absorbs both scattered and primary photons. Removing the grid lowers the applied dose needed to produce the sufficient numbers of photons that reach the film or image intensifier, and therefore reduces dose. A reduction in kVp has a nonlinear effect on the milliampere-seconds needed to penetrate the patient, so reductions in kVp net yield a net reduced dose. Pulsed fluoroscopy can yield the same individual frame quality and the same diagnostic yield as continuous fluoroscopy, with drastically reduced dose.

49. Which of the following is a primary contributor to reduced image quality of portable radiographic examinations?
    A. Increased geometric magnification
    B. Lack of a grid
    C. Poor patient compliance
    D. Reduced detector efficiency

B. Correct! To properly use a grid, the lines of the grid must be oriented precisely along the collimated beam path. As this is essentially impossible to ensure with portable films, a grid is not used. Thus, portable films have much higher scattered radiation in the image, which increases the noise and reduces the signal-to-noise ratio and contrast-to-noise ratio of the image. Frequently, portable exams are performed on patients who have difficulty moving or who are medically unstable. In general, excessive motion is not a primary concern in these patients.

50. Why is perceived image quality better with fluoroscopic spot films than with single frames ("last image hold")?
    A. Use of a grid for spot films but not for single frames
    B. Generally decreased peak kilovoltage for spot films compared to single frames
    C. Generally increased milliampere-seconds for spot films compared to single frames
    D. Reduced motion blur for spot films compared to single frames

C. Correct! Spot films use a small fraction of the milliampere-seconds used for single frames, and therefore have much higher noise levels (graininess) in the image, decreasing image quality.

51. In radiography, which of following affects noise and blur the LEAST?
    A. Peak kilovoltage
    B. Milliampere-seconds
    C. Presence of a grid
    D. Motion
    E. Geometric magnification

A. Correct! That is, affects noise and blur the least. The peak kilovoltage is used to tune radiographic image contrast and tissue penetration. It does not have a direct effect on image noise or blur. Higher milliampere-seconds reduces the image noise. However, the higher time of current application (the "s" of mAs) yields a greater chance for motion blur. Because a grid preferentially absorbs scattered radiation that contributes to image noise, a grid tends to reduce image noise. Motion causes image blur. Geometric magnification blurs the focal spot of the image, thereby increasing blur.

■ Computed Tomography Questions

52. In computed tomography, which of the following has a nonlinear relationship with patient radiation dose?
    A. Peak kilovoltage (kVp)
    B. Milliampere-seconds (mAs)
    C. Pitch
    D. Matrix

A. Correct! Both mAs and pitch are directly related to dose; mAs increases dose linearly, whereas pitch decreases dose linearly. In contrast, kVp has a nonlinear effect; decreases occur nonlinearly with decreased kVp.

53. In computed tomography, increasing which of the following would generally decrease dose?
    A. Peak kilovoltage (kVp)
    B. Milliampere-seconds (mAs)
    C. Pitch
    D. Field of view

C. Correct! Generally, increasing kVp and mAs increases dose, whereas increasing pitch reduces dose. Increased pitch means that the patient is fed through the scanner at a faster rate, while maintaining the same constant kVp and mAs. The result is less total radiation applied to each individual section of the patient.

54. In computed tomography, decreasing which of the following would be most effective in increasing contrast-to-noise ratio?
    A. Peak kilovoltage
    B. Milliampere-seconds (mAs)
    C. Pitch
    D. Field of view

A. Correct! Similar to radiography, reducing peak kilovoltage in computed tomography yields greater image contrast, but generally necessitates increasing mAs. Both mAs and pitch have more direct relationships to image noise than does contrast.

55. When using tube current modulation, at what level would you expect milliampere-seconds (mAs) to be LEAST?
    A. Thoracic level 2 (T2)
    B. Thoracic level 7 (T7)
    C. Lumbar level 3 (L3)
    D. Sacral level 2 (S2)

B. Correct! Tube current modulation increases or decreases the current depending on the amount of attenuating material present in the patient at that position. At T2, higher mAs is needed to penetrate the shoulders and clavicles. At L3 and S2, higher mAs is needed to penetrate the iliac crests and sacrum. At T7, however, a lower mAs will adequately penetrate the less-attenuating lung and mediastinum.

56. Doubling the field of view in both dimensions (x- and y-), while keeping slice thickness and matrix size constant, would have what effect on the signal-to-noise ratio (SNR) in each voxel?
    A. Increase by $2\times$
    B. Increase slightly ($<< 0.5\times$)
    C. No change
    D. Decrease slightly ($<< 0.5\times$)
    E. Decrease by $1/2\times$

A. Correct! Doubling the field of view in each dimension while keeping everything else constant will quadruple the voxel volume. Generally, in computed tomography, SNR is proportional to the square root of the voxel volume. Therefore, a $4\times$ increase in voxel volume yields a $2\times$ increase in SNR. Note that in magnetic resonance imaging, in contrast, SNR increases linearly with voxel volume.

57. The estimated effective dose of a particular computed tomography (CT) scan is best approximated by which of the following quantities?
    A. $CTDI_w$ (weighted-average CT dose index)
    B. $CTDI_{vol}$ (volume-average CT dose index)
    C. $CTDI_{100}$ (100-mm chamber CT dose index)
    D. Dose-length product (DLP)

D. Correct! The DLP takes the estimate of the CT dose index, which is a measure of dose applied at a given point, and multiplies that by the length of the patient scanned in that protocol. This is the most direct indicator of the total radiation dose applied to a specific patient. In particular, DLP is the product of $CTDI_{vol}$ and table feed (in cm).

58. Dual-energy computed tomography (CT) is useful because using two different X-ray energies:
    A. Lowers the net energy absorbed by the patient, thus lowering the net radiation dose.
    B. Allows the computer to calculate images specific to a tissue-type, based on a model of tissue-specific attenuation for each X-ray energy.
    C. Allows for CT perfusion imaging without contrast.
    D. Allows for molecular imaging for assessing tumor histology.

B. Correct! X-ray beams are attenuated to varying extents as they pass through a given tissue based upon the energy of the beam. Taking advantage of that effect, a virtual tissue map can be generated using a calculation based on how two different beams of different energies pass through a given subject, so that "soft tissue only" or "bone only" images are produced from the raw data. This can be done for either radiography or CT, with new applications of dual-energy CT continuing to develop.

59. In computed tomography (CT) image reconstruction, the role of the filter ("algorithm" or "kernel") in filtered back projection is to lessen the effects of:
    A. Cardiopulmonary motion artifacts.
    B. Beam-hardening and photopenia artifacts.
    C. The limited (finite) number of acquired projections.
    D. Quantum mottle in low-dose CT protocols.

C. Correct! For practical considerations, only a finite number of projections are acquired in a CT scan. This finite number of projections translates to some nonideal features inherent in the computational process of back-calculating the per-voxel attenuation that yields a cross-sectional CT image. To correct for these nonideal properties, a deconvolution kernel (also known as an algorithm or filter) is applied to the primary data during the backprojection process.

60. Which of these image reconstruction algorithms would be expected to produce images most similar to a "bone" algorithm?
    A. Soft tissue
    B. Lung
    C. Brain
    D. Angiographic

B. Correct! In computed tomography, the algorithm (also known as "kernel" or "filter") chosen for filtered backprojection determines the relative noise (graininess) and edge detection resolution in the resultant image. Soft tissue filters are generally characterized by a lower number for the filter name (~ 30 to 40) and generally smooth out the image. This leads to increased blurriness but decreased graininess. Lung or bone filters are generally characterized by a higher number for the filter name (~ 70 to 80) and yield higher edge detection and sharpness, with the trade-off of higher graininess. Because both lung and bone kernels have higher filter numbers (with lung generally higher than bone), the lung and bone reconstructions can be used relatively interchangeably in instances when both are not available.

61. Which of the following statements regarding computed tomography (CT) algorithms is TRUE?
    A. A bone window applied to an image series produced with a soft tissue kernel will produce an equivalent image to a soft tissue window applied to an image series produced with a bone kernel.
    B. A bone window applied to an image series produced with a soft tissue kernel will produce an equivalent image to a bone window applied to an image series produced with a bone kernel.
    C. Kernel is interchangeable with the window setting used for an image series.
    D. A kernel or algorithm is used during the process of image reconstruction; a window is applied after image reconstruction, during image display.

D. Correct! Windows and kernels (also known as "filters" or "algorithms") are not the same thing. One can apply any given window to any given CT or magnetic resonance imaging series—it is a feature of image display only. A kernel is applied during the computational process that produces the image in the first place. To switch to a different kernel requires the scanner computer to recalculate the image from the primary data. In general, it is best to look at bones using a bone kernel or algorithm image, soft tissue using a soft tissue algorithm image, and so on. For practical reasons, however, only one or two kernels are utilized in most cases for a given CT image series.

62. When considering the protocol technique, which of the following values must be adjusted between multirow detector computed tomography (CT) and single-row detector CT?
    A. Milliampere-seconds
    B. Pitch
    C. Field of view
    D. Matrix

B. Correct! Pitch refers to the amount of table feed that occurs during one revolution of the CT gantry in helical CT. Multirow detector CT is like doing a single-row detector CT multiple times in parallel, sometimes with an overlap of coverage between the rows. So, even though the table-feed rate per gantry revolution might be the same numerical value, in effect, one acquires more data in a single gantry rotation for multidetector acquisitions than for single-row acquisitions. Therefore, in protocol design, we usually speak of the effective pitch in multirow detector CT, and this can be calculated by dividing the regular pitch by the number of rows being acquired at once.

63. Increasing which of the following could reduce the appearance or presence of "beam-hardening" artifact in a computed tomography image?
    A. Peak kilovoltage
    B. Milliampere-seconds
    C. Pitch
    D. Field of view
    E. Matrix

A. Correct! The beam-hardening artifact results from the filtration of the lower energy components of the beam by dense material, such as the otic capsules. The resultant higher energy-enriched, or "hardened," beam penetrates through the tissue more, resulting in apparent and artifactually decreased attenuation in the image of the intervening tissue. To correct for this, one can use a higher peak kilovoltage, which contains less of the lower energy components in the beam and would penetrate the dense structures with more efficiency, resulting in less beam-hardening.

64. Photon starvation artifact affects image quality mainly because of its deleterious effect on:
    A. Signal
    B. Contrast
    C. Noise
    D. Dose

C. Correct! Photon starvation, or "photopenia artifact," occurs when insufficient milliampere-seconds is used, reducing the number of photons that ultimately reach the image detector. When fewer photons hit the image detector, the random statistical noise emerges in the image as a speckled artifact that makes the image look grainy. The signal—the average level of brightness of the image—remains constant, but the noise increases in relation, thereby reducing the signal-to-noise ratio.

65. Decreasing which one of the following CANNOT be used to reduce radiation dose for pediatric patients undergoing computed tomography?
    A. Peak kilovoltage
    B. Milliampere-seconds
    C. Pitch
    D. Table feed amount

C. Correct! That is, it cannot be used to reduce radiation dose in pediatric patients. Decreasing the pitch means the computed tomography gantry would apply a constant dose rate to the patient for a longer period of time (assuming the total head-foot coverage is the same). Thus, the applied dose is proportionately increased with lower pitch.

66. Compared to magnetic resonance imaging, which of the following parameters is defined differently in computed tomography?
    A. Cerebral blood volume
    B. Cerebral blood flow
    C. Mean transit time
    D. Time to peak
    E. None of the above

E. Correct! If you understand the basis of computed tomography perfusion, you understand it for magnetic resonance perfusion, and vice versa. The basic concept is the same: you track a bolus of contrast via its effect on the signal in the image as the contrast passes through the organ of interest. The calculated parameters of cerebral blood volume, cerebral blood flow, mean transit time, and time to peak are all calculated in essentially the same manner.

67. Which of the following computed tomography (CT) exams generally has the highest effective dose?
    A. CT head
    B. CT chest
    C. CT abdomen and pelvis
    D. CT upper extremity
    E. CT lower extremity

C. Correct! Effective dose takes into account the biologic effect of the dose received and not just the amount of radiation absorbed by that mass of tissue. There are more radiosensitive organs in the abdomen and pelvis (gonads, stomach, bowel, etc.) than in the head or extremities. The chest does contain the radiosensitive lung and breasts, but because the lungs attenuate so little energy, relatively low absolute doses are needed for image production.

68. According to the most recent American College of Radiology guidelines, when considering dose reduction protocols for pediatric computed tomography, what determines an acceptable limit of dose reduction, given the reductions in image quality?
    A. Signal-to-noise ratio of at least 2.3
    B. Contrast-to-noise ratio of at least 1.7
    C. Noise-power spectrum of up to 0.2 at any frequency
    D. Radiologist discretion according to the ALARA (as low as reasonably achievable) principle

D. Correct! Imaging protocol design is ultimately up to the radiologist's discretion for all aspects, whether it regards image quality, radiation safety, patient comfort, etc. No governing body has any absolute control over the imaging protocol. Radiologists should be aware of the various strict requirements for imaging equipment that are set by regulatory bodies such as the U.S. Food and Drug Administration. At a minimum, radiologists have a responsibility to ensure that vendors have approval by the appropriate regulatory agency for the imaging devices they are using.

■ Ultrasound Questions

69. Which of the following ultrasound transducer array types uses electronic beam steering to acquire the image?
    A. Linear
    B. Curved
    C. Phased
    D. Two-dimensional linear

C. Correct! Linear and curved ultrasound arrays both use a conventional image acquisition technique in which each crystal sequentially applies its ultrasound pulse and then "listens" for the echoes to return, with the image focus determined by the transducer geometry. In contrast, a phase array transducer utilizes constructive and destructive interference of the waves generated by the elements to differentially focus the beam to varying parts of the imaging plane.

70. Which of the following ultrasound transducers is best for a transabdominal obstetrical examination?
    A. Curved 3.5 MHz
    B. Linear 7.5 MHz
    C. Curved 6.5 MHz
    D. Endo 6.5 MHz

A. Correct! In a transabdominal obstetrical exam, a relatively large amount of tissue must be penetrated. Therefore, a low frequency transducer is necessary. Higher frequency transducers offer higher-resolution imaging, but only for objects in the near field.

71. Which of the following ultrasound transducers is best for evaluation of the rotator cuff?
    A. Curved 3.5 MHz
    B. Linear 7.5 MHz
    C. Curved 6.5 MHz
    D. Endo 6.5 MHz

B. Correct! The rotator cuff is a relatively superficial structure whose evaluation necessitates fairly high resolution. Therefore, an available transducer with the highest frequency should be used.

72. Which factor is most critical in determining lateral resolution with ultrasound?
    A. Ultrasound beam width
    B. Spatial pulse length
    C. Number of scan lines
    D. Pulse repetition frequency

A. Correct! Lateral resolution is determined by the lateral spacing of the beams from each transducer and by the width of the beam. It is impossible to discriminate two points that are smaller than a beam width apart, as they would each contribute an echo that is detected by the same position elements of the ultrasound transducer. Note that lateral resolution varies as a function of depth perception; the ultrasound beam width diverges (and therefore gets worse) in the far field.

73. Which factor is most critical in determining axial resolution with ultrasound?
    A. Ultrasound beam width
    B. Spatial pulse length
    C. Number of scan lines
    D. Pulse repetition frequency

B. Correct! Axial resolution is determined by the timing of the pulses as they return to the transducer. If the ultrasound pulse itself is a certain length (in millimeters, for example), then identification of the time interval between echoes generated by structures spaced more closely together than that spatial pulse length is not possible.

74. Using the following acoustic impedance values, which interface would be expected to be brightest on ultrasound: lung 0.18, fat 1.34, water 1.48, liver 1.65, muscle 1.71 (all in units of 10^6 kg/m^{2}s)?
    A. Diaphragm
    B. Hepatic capsule
    C. Renal capsule
    D. Gallbladder fossa

A. Correct! Brightness on ultrasound indicates the presence of relatively high amplitude echoes. The echo amplitude increases when there is a mismatch of structures' acoustic impedances. Based on the numbers provided, the largest difference in impedance is between lung and muscle—an interface that occurs at the diaphragm.

75. Which of the following parameters most directly sets the range of velocities that can be imaged with Doppler ultrasound imaging?
    A. Spatial pulse length
    B. Pulse repetition frequency
    C. Transducer frequency
    D. Angle of insonation
    E. Transducer gain

B. Correct! In Doppler imaging, the signal of interest is a slight shift in the ultrasound frequency that occurs when the ultrasound echoes off of a moving object. The maximal frequency shift that can be resolved, and therefore the maximal velocity is set by the pulse repetition frequency. Other factors such as the angle of insonation, ultrasound frequency, and spatial pulse length do have an effect, but these occur fundamentally through their effect on the effective pulse repetition frequency.

76. Of the following, which characteristic of gallstones accounts for their high echogenicity and associated acoustic shadowing?
    A. Gallstones have high susceptibility, causing signal drop out in the deeper portions of the field of view.
    B. Gallstones have high acoustic impedance compared to soft tissue, causing the computer to mistakenly display all the signal deep to the stones onto the stones.
    C. Gallstones have high acoustic impedance and absorption, so little to no acoustic energy can get past them, leading to reduced echoes from the region deep to the stones.
    D. Gallstones induce internal acoustic reflections, emitting a train of echoes that result in their high signal and signal drop out from deep structures.

C. Correct! Acoustic shadowing occurs because the level of energy absorption by a structure exceeds that which the computer assumes might occur in the image. Then, when the transducer does not see substantial echoes come back with the expected timing for structures past the absorbing material, it translates that into a dark region in the image.

77. Of the following, which potential bio-effect is most relevant for interpretation of the mechanical index (MI) in ultrasound?
    A. Acoustic heating
    B. Acoustic cavitation
    C. Acoustic vibration
    D. Acoustic noise
    E. Acoustic reverberation

B. Correct! The MI is a U.S. Food and Drug Administration (FDA)-regulated number that characterizes the mode of ultrasound used in a particular ultrasound imaging session. If the MI is too high, a phenomenon called cavitation can occur that can severely damage the tissue. Cavitation is more likely to occur in gas-containing structures. While the FDA mandates that the MI must be < 1.9 in general for diagnostic ultrasound, this assumes that the structure contains no gas. In the case of gas-containing structures, such as in infection or near lung and bowl, cavitation can occur with an MI of ~ 0.4. For fetal imaging, MI should be as low as reasonably achievable. However, MI is less important than thermal index for the fetus, as long as there is no risk of gas being near the fetus—a situation that is important to consider for ultrasound-guided interventions.

78. Which of the following potential bio-effects is most relevant for interpretation of the thermal index (TI) in ultrasound?
    A. Acoustic heating
    B. Acoustic cavitation
    C. Acoustic vibration
    D. Acoustic noise
    E. Acoustic reverberation

A. Correct! TI quantifies the likelihood of inducing heating with ultrasound. Focused ultrasound can induce heating that can potentially ablate tissue. Clearly, that is not the desired effect in diagnostic applications. For fetal imaging in particular, TI should be kept < 0.5, with even lower TI preferred. If TI of 0.5 to 1.0 is used, the recommendation is to keep scan time to < 30 minutes. For TI > 2.5, scan time should be < 1 minute. For postnatal studies, TI < 2 is generally safe.

79. Which of the following is NOT a reasonable guideline regarding first trimester ultrasound?
    A. Limit Doppler imaging given its higher thermal and mechanical indices (MIs).
    B. Limit all ultrasound imaging to < 1 minute total.
    C. Limit examination with thermal index (TI) > 2.5 to < 1 minute.
    D. Limit examination with TI 0.5 to 1.0 to < 1 hour.
    E. Use MI < 0.4 if gas (infection, aerated bowel, or lung) is potentially present.
    F. Ultrasound according to ALARA (as low as reasonably achievable).

B. Correct! That is, this is not a reasonable guideline. While the ALARA principle should be used in all imaging, limiting all ultrasound to < 1 minute is extreme. If TI < 0.5 and MI of <1 is used (without the possibility of gas in the tissue), then ultrasound can generally be applied for an extended period of time. However, please note that Doppler imaging uses significant energy, generally, substantially raising the MI and TI.

■ References

1. American College of Radiology. Manual on Contrast Media, version 10.2. Reston, VA: American College of Radiology; 2016

Essentials 1

■ Case

A 44-year-old woman presents with ankle pain after jumping.

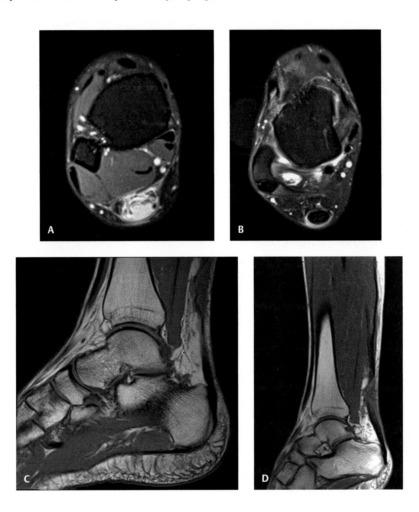

■ Questions

1. What is the most likely diagnosis?
   A. Plantar fasciitis
   B. Calcaneal fracture
   C. Flexor hallucis longus tenosynovitis
   D. Posterior tibialis tendon tear
   E. Achilles tendon rupture

2. Which ONE of the following statements is correct for the test case injuries?
   A. Acute Achilles tendon tears are most common in children and ballet dancers.
   B. The most common location of an Achilles tendon tear is 2 to 6 cm above the calcaneal insertion.
   C. On physical examination, patients are unable to dorsiflex the foot.

D. Human immunodeficiency virus and osteomyelitis are predisposing factors for Achilles tendon tears.
E. CT is superior to ultrasound and MRI in making the diagnosis.

3. What is the most common treatment for complete Achilles rupture tears?
   A. No treatment necessary (as these are often asymptomatic)
   B. Rest, stretching, and oral anti-inflammatory medications
   C. Cast immobilization in plantarflexion
   D. Surgical repair

■ Answers and Explanations

Question 1

E. Correct! In this case, there is a tear of the Achilles in the mid-substance of the tendon. Fluid is seen filling the gap between the torn tendon ends.

Other choices and discussion

A. Plantar fasciitis is one of the most common causes of heel pain and is due to repetitive trauma. On imaging, there is thickening of the proximal plantar fascia (plantar thickness of > 4 mm), which extends to the calcaneal plantar fascial insertion. Ultrasound or magnetic resonance imaging (MRI) can be used to diagnose plantar fasciitis.

B. Intra-articular calcaneal fractures are caused by an axial-loading mechanism and usually from a fall from height. This is the most commonly fractured bone found in this scenario. On radiographs, there can be a decrease of Bohler angle, which is normally 20 to 40 degrees. MRI can detect radiographically occult stress fractures, which manifest as linear T1-hypointense signal in the medullary space extending to the cortex with associated T2-hyperintense edema and hemorrhage. Calcaneal fractures can also be detected and characterized very accurately on computed tomography (CT). Of particular importance is the characterization of a calcaneal fracture into either an intra- or extra-articular category, as this is essential in guiding management and prognosis.

C. The flexor hallucis longus runs along the posteromedial ankle just deep to the posterior tibialis tendon and can cause posteromedial heel pain, if injured. Tenosynovitis, in general, is characterized by synovial fluid distending the tendinous sheath, which manifests on MRI as T1-hypointense and T2-hyperintense signal surrounding a low signal intensity tendon.

D. Posterior tibialis tendon rupture most commonly presents with flat foot and medial hind foot pain. MRI is the imaging modality of choice. Tears can be seen as enlarged tendons with fluid between the fibers, partially torn fibers with focal tendon thinning, or tendon discontinuity. Full-thickness tears typically occur > 1 cm from the navicular insertion.

Question 2

B. Correct! The blood supply of the Achilles tendon is the posterior tibial artery, and tendon tears commonly occur in the watershed zone, which is 2 to 6 cm above the calcaneal insertion. The relatively sparse vascular supply at this site increases the risk of tear.

Other choices and discussion

A. Achilles tendon tears typically occur in males between 30 and 50 years of age and are predominantly sports-related. The classic example is the unfit "weekend warrior" who participates in the occasional sporting activity. An audible snap is heard during forceful dorsiflexion of the foot.

C. Patients with full Achilles tendon tears are unable to plantarflex the foot.

D. Although most acute traumatic Achilles rupture cases occur in healthy men without heel or calf pain, there are some predisposing factors, which include chronic steroid injections, systemic inflammatory illnesses, fluoroquinolone use, gout, connective tissue disorders, and diabetes mellitus.

E. CT can detect a full-thickness tear, but ultrasound and MRI are superior to CT in diagnosing partial thickness Achilles tendon tears and tendinosis.

Question 3

D. Correct! Complete tears are usually surgically treated, as conservative treatment is unsuccessful if the tendon edges are not opposed. For < 3 cm of separation, end-to-end anastomosis is usually successful, and for > 3 cm separation, a tendon graft is often required.

It should be noted that more recently, there has been debate surrounding the issue of whether medical or surgical therapy is more appropriate for this type of injury.

Other choices and discussion

A. Injury is painful and can lead to loss of function. Some treatment is necessary for Achilles tendon pathology, particularly Achilles rupture tears.

B. Tendinopathy of the Achilles tendon is usually treated with rest, stretching, and anti-inflammatory medications.

C. Partial-thickness tears may be treated conservatively with cast immobilization. Surgical repair is indicated when conservative options fail.

■ Suggested Readings

Narvaez JA, Narvaez J, Ortega R, et al. Painful heel: MR imaging findings. Radiographics 2000;20:333–352

Schweitzer ME, Karasick D. MR imaging disorders of the Achilles tendon. Am J Roentgenol 2000;175:613–625

Top Tips

◆ Complete Achilles tendon ruptures usually occur in "weekend warrior" males 30 to 50 years of age. An audible snap is heard with forceful dorsiflexion of the foot.

◆ Tears usually occur 2 to 6 cm proximal to the calcaneal insertion.

◆ Axial and sagittal MRI can be helpful in differentiating partial from complete tears, and accurate measurement of the gap between the tendon edges is useful information for the surgeon.

Essentials 2

■ Case

A 22-year-old man with a history of a recent motor vehicle accident (5 days prior) presents for follow up of a descending thoracic aortic injury.

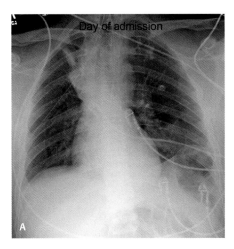

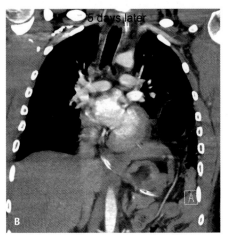

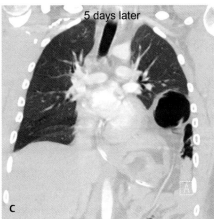

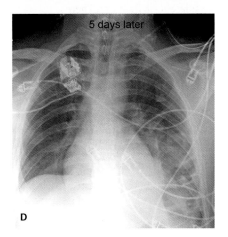

■ Questions

1. Which ONE of the following is the best diagnosis?
   A. Pericardial fluid
   B. Paralyzed diaphragm
   C. Flail chest
   D. Traumatic left diaphragmatic rupture
   E. Congenital diaphragmatic hernia

2. Which ONE of the following is correct regarding the test case diagnosis?
   A. Surgical intervention is indicated in all cases, regardless of size.
   B. Small diaphragmatic injuries will spontaneously heal.
   C. Most cases will not result in herniation of abdominal contents into the chest.

   D. The morbidity and mortality are lower if abdominal contents do not herniate at the time of presentation.
   E. Traumatic diaphragmatic ruptures account for 25% of all diaphragmatic hernias.

3. Which ONE of the following best describes the location for traumatic diaphragmatic ruptures?
   A. Anteromedial diaphragm, more commonly on the left
   B. Posterolateral diaphragm, more commonly on the left
   C. Apex of the diaphragm
   D. Midline at the aortic hiatus
   E. Midline at the esophageal hiatus

■ Answers and Explanations

Question 1

D. Correct! This patient has a traumatic left diaphragmatic rupture. A total of 75% of traumatic diaphragmatic ruptures are due to blunt trauma, and 25% are due to penetrating trauma. There is a high association with multiorgan trauma and concurrent life-threatening injuries. Imaging appearances range from discontinuity of the diaphragm with a focal defect to herniation of abdominal contents through a larger defect. The "dangling diaphragm" sign is present when the diaphragm curls inward on an axial image. The "collar" sign is a waist-like narrowing of the herniated viscus.

Other choices and discussion

A. Pericardial fluid is contained within the fibroelastic sac surrounding the heart. This can be important clinically when large pericardial effusions or scarred/inelastic pericardium result in pericardial compressive syndromes.

B. A paralyzed diaphragm remains intact, but fails to contract, resulting in asymmetric elevation of the affected diaphragm. There is typically no history of trauma.

C. A flail chest is defined as three or more segmental rib fractures or more than five adjacent rib fractures. There is paradoxical motion with respiration of the flail segment.

E. Bochdalek hernias occur in the posteromedial diaphragm, and Morgagni hernias occur in the anteromedial diaphragm. There is typically no history of trauma.

Question 2

A. Correct! Earlier diagnosis and repair leads to a better prognosis, as abdominal contents eventually herniate into the chest, if left unrepaired. Surgical treatment is indicated for all diaphragmatic injuries to decrease potential complications including ischemia of herniated bowel, central venous obstruction secondary to mass effect, devascularization, torsion, and ischemia of herniated solid abdominal organs.

Other choices and discussion

B. Traumatic diaphragmatic injuries do not spontaneously heal.

C. Due to negative intrapleural pressure, 80% of cases will eventually develop herniation of abdominal contents into the chest.

D. Patients are susceptible to the same complications regardless of whether the herniation of abdominal contents is present initially or only later.

E. Diaphragmatic ruptures account for only 5% of all diaphragmatic hernias. Congenital Bochdalek and Morgagni hernias, as well as hiatal hernias, are much more common.

Question 3

B. Correct! The most common location (90 to 98%) for traumatic diaphragmatic ruptures is the posterolateral aspect of the left hemidiaphragm, where there are weaker pleuroperitoneal membranes. The right hemidiaphragm is protected by the liver.

Other choices and discussion

The other choices are incorrect. Morgagni hernias are congenital diaphragmatic hernias that commonly occur in the anteromedial diaphragm. Hiatal hernias, both sliding and esophageal, occur near the midline at the esophageal hiatus. No diaphragmatic hernia has a predilection for the apex or the aortic hiatus of the diaphragm.

■ Suggested Readings

Desir A, Ghaye B. CT of blunt diaphragmatic rupture. Radiographics 2012;32:477–498

Dreizin D, Berquist PJ, Taner AT, et al. Evolving concepts in MDCT diagnosis of penetrating diaphragmatic injury. Emerg Radiol 2015;22:149–156

Top Tips

♦ Most traumatic diaphragmatic ruptures occur in the posterolateral aspect of the left hemidiaphragm (90 to 98%).

♦ Traumatic diaphragmatic ruptures have the best prognosis when diagnosed and repaired early.

♦ Surgical treatment is indicated in *all* cases of traumatic diaphragmatic rupture.

Essentials 3

■ Case

A 33-year-old woman presents to the emergency department with painful swelling of the right knee. No history of trauma.

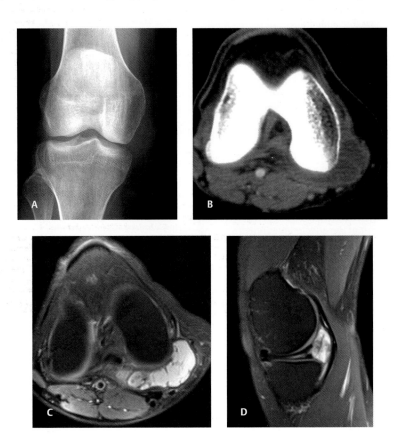

■ Questions

1. Which ONE of the following is the correct diagnosis?
   A. Pyrophosphate arthropathy
   B. Cystic adventitial disease of the popliteal artery
   C. Pes anserine bursitis
   D. Popliteal cyst
   E. Parameniscal cyst

2. Regarding this diagnosis, which ONE of the following is correct?
   A. More commonly seen anteriorly when found in the medial compartment
   B. Often seen in association with bucket handle meniscal tears
   C. Often seen in association with horizontal meniscal tears
   D. Usually cured with cyst aspiration
   E. Best assessed with ultrasound

3. Which ONE of the following best describes the anatomic location for a popliteal cyst?
   A. Extrasynovial structure in the anterior aspect of the knee that lies below the patella, posterior to the patellar tendon, and anterior to the femorotibial articulation
   B. Medial aspect of the knee between the conjoined distal tendons of the sartorius, gracilis, and semitendinosus muscles, and the tibial insertion of the medial collateral ligament (tibial condyle)
   C. Between the semimembranosus tendon and the medial collateral ligament (with a deeper portion extending between the semimembranosus tendon and the medial tibial condyle)
   D. Between the medial head of the gastrocnemius muscle and the semimembranosus tendon
   E. Para-articular cyst communicating with a meniscus

■ Answers and Explanations

Question 1

E. Correct! Parameniscal cysts represent encapsulated mass lesions that contain synovial-like fluid and are continuous with a meniscus. In the test case, this communication is demonstrated on the sagittal magnetic resonance imaging. On the plain film, there is lobulated soft tissue swelling medially.

Other choices and discussion

A. Pyrophosphate arthropathy occurs secondary to calcium pyrophosphate dihydrate deposition in soft tissues and cartilage. On plain film, there is typically associated calcification (or chondrocalcinosis).

B. Cystic adventitial disease is a rare vascular disorder characterized by focal cystic accumulation of mucinous fluid in arterial adventitia. Clinically, there may be sudden onset of intermittent claudication in a young male patient.

C. The pes anserine bursa is located between the conjoined distal tendons of the sartorius, gracilis, and semitendinosus muscles (pes anserinus) at the medial aspect of the knee.

D. The most frequent cause of a popliteal cyst in adults is degenerative arthritis.

Question 2

C. Correct! Parameniscal cysts are invariably associated with horizontal meniscal tears.

Other choices and discussion

A. Posterior horn tears (and their parameniscal cysts) are more common than anterior horn tears in the medial meniscus. The most common location for a lateral parameniscal cyst is adjacent to the anterior horn or body of the lateral meniscus.

B. Bucket handle meniscal tears are a type of vertical tear. Parameniscal cysts are invariably seen with horizontal meniscal tears.

D. Aspiration of the cyst is a temporary measure, and the cysts tend to recur. The diagnosis and treatment of the underlying meniscal tear is important.

E. Magnetic resonance imaging is the imaging study of choice. Ultrasound can show a partially cystic and sometimes septated mass bulging into the para-articular space. Protrusion of an abnormal meniscus into the cyst is sometimes seen. Demonstration of the meniscal tear, however, is not possible in most cases. Magnetic resonance imaging is helpful in assessing the meniscal tear and in characterizing important ancillary findings, such as the degree of underlying chondromalacia.

Question 3

D. Correct! A popliteal or Baker cyst extends from the knee joint posteriorly and medially, interposed between the tendons of the medial head of the gastrocnemius and the semimembranosus tendon.

Other choices and discussion

A. This is the location of a Hoffa fat pad ganglion.

B. This is the location for pes anserine bursitis.

C. This is the location for semimembranosus-tibial collateral ligament bursitis.

E. This describes a parameniscal cyst.

■ Suggested Readings

Perdikakis E, Skiadas V. MRI characteristics of cysts and "cyst-like" lesions in and around the knee: what the radiologist needs to know. Insights Imaging 2013;4:257–272

Steinbach LS, Stevens KF. Imaging of cysts and bursae about the knee. Radiol Clin North Am 2013;51:433–454

Top Tips

- Cysts and cystic-appearing soft tissue lesions in the medial compartment of the knee are common, and the differential considerations include popliteal cyst, parameniscal cyst, pes anserinus bursitis, and semimembranosus-tibial collateral ligament bursitis. Specific location is often diagnostic.

- Parameniscal cysts are invariably associated with horizontal meniscal tears.

- Diagnosis and treatment of the underlying meniscal tear is important with parameniscal cysts, as the cysts frequently recur if the meniscal tear is not also treated.

Essentials 4

■ Case

A 34-year-old woman presents with intermittent abdominal pain for several months, worse for the past 8 days. Her gallbladder was removed 6 years ago, and her current symptoms are reportedly similar to those that prompted the cholecystectomy.

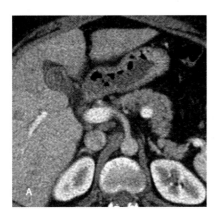 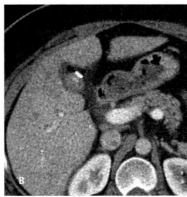 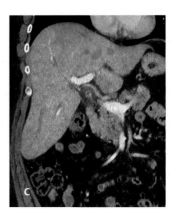

■ Questions

1. What is the MOST likely diagnosis?
   A. Surgicel
   B. Postcholecystectomy bile leak/biloma
   C. Spillage of gallstones
   D. Stump cholecystitis
   E. Normal postcholecystectomy appearance

2. Regarding imaging of a postcholecystectomy patient, which ONE of the following statements is true?
   A. Biliary dilatation usually suggests bile duct obstruction and warrants further work up with magnetic resonance cholangiopancreatography.
   B. The computed tomography appearance of Surgicel is often confused with a retained surgical swab.
   C. Postcholecystectomy bile duct injury is the most common type of injury after this procedure.
   D. Biliary complications are more common after open cholecystectomy than after laparoscopic cholecystectomy.
   E. Cholecystectomy-related vascular injuries are usually due to bile leakage and subsequent infection.

3. Choose the MOST appropriate statement regarding stump cholecystitis.
   A. Stump cholecystitis is more commonly seen after elective cholecystectomy than after emergent cholecystectomy.
   B. Reported incidence of stump cholecystitis is around 15 to 20%.
   C. Stump cholecystitis is usually diagnosed promptly after onset of symptoms because of the classic clinical presentation.
   D. The definitive treatment is often surgical to excise the gallbladder remnant and perform completion cholecystectomy.
   E. Once the diagnosis is confirmed, the definitive treatment is usually conservative and mainly reassurance.

■ Answers and Explanations

Question 1

D. Correct! Subtotal cholecystectomy carries the risk of developing stump cholecystitis when the gallbladder remnant becomes inflamed due to stone disease. A subtotal cholecystectomy is a safe option in the face of severe inflammation at Calot triangle (the space at the porta hepatis that contains the cystic artery and cystic duct), because it reduces the potential for common duct injury.

Other choices and discussion

A. Surgicel (oxidized regenerated cellulose) is a bioabsorbable hemostatic agent with bactericidal properties that is used to control hemorrhage (Ethicon, Somerville, NJ). The appearance of Surgicel is a potential pitfall in postcholecystectomy imaging.

B. Bile leak or biloma are complications seen in the immediate postoperative period and are usually identified as hypodense fluid collections in the surgical bed and the perihepatic region.

C. A few gallstones (ill-defined) and a surgical clip are noted within the remnant of gallbladder and surgical bed, respectively. No spilled gallstones are seen in provided images.

E. Wall thickening and hyperenhancement of the gallbladder remnant and cystic duct, as well as fluid in the porta hepatis, are not normal appearances after cholecystectomy.

Question 2

C. Correct! Bile duct injury is the most commonly reported complication after cholecystectomy. Postcholecystectomy biliary complications include bile duct damage, biliary obstruction, and dropped stones.

Other choices and discussion

A. After laparoscopic cholecystectomy, bile duct dilatation is often seen in the absence of obstruction. Patients with cholelithiasis may have had bile duct calculi preoperatively, and the resulting biliary dilatation may persist despite relief of the obstruction.

B. On computed tomography, Surgicel appears as a complex fluid collection (soft tissue attenuation of 40 to 55 HU and containing foci of air) and can mimic hematoma, abscess, or even tumor. Surgical swabs contain a radiopaque marker and can usually be differentiated from Surgicel.

D. Biliary complications are more common after laparoscopic cholecystectomy than after open cholecystectomy.

E. Vascular injuries during laparoscopic cholecystectomy can occur in the surgical bed or the abdominal wall. They are usually related to trocar insertion and dissection of structures in the gallbladder bed. However, cholecystectomy-related bile leak and subsequent infection causing hepatic artery pseudoaneurysm have also been described in the literature.

Question 3

D. Correct! The definitive treatment is often surgical.

Other choices and discussion

A. Stump cholecystitis is rare after elective cholecystectomy.

B. The reported incidence of stump cholecystitis varies but has been reported to occur in as many as 5% of patients after emergent cholecystectomy.

C. Despite a very suggestive history, the diagnosis of stump cholecystitis is often delayed due to a low index of suspicion.

E. Open or laparoscopic reoperation is the definitive management.

■ Suggested Readings

Cawich SO, Wilson C, Simpson LK, Baker AJ. Stump cholecystitis: laparoscopic completion cholecystectomy with basic laparoscopic equipment in a resource poor setting. Case Rep Med 2014;787631

Thurley PD, Dhingsa D. Laparoscopic cholecystectomy: postoperative imaging. Am J Roentgenol 2008;191:794–801

Top Tips

◆ Postcholecystectomy complications include bile duct injury, biliary obstruction, dropped gallstones, vascular injury, and stump cholecystitis.

◆ Stump cholecystitis is reported in up to 5% of patients after emergent cholecystectomy and is rare after elective cholecystectomy.

◆ The diagnosis of stump cholecystitis is often delayed due to a low index of suspicion. Suspicious findings include wall thickening, wall enhancement of the gallbladder stump, retained stones in the gallbladder stump, cystic duct enhancement, and fluid in the porta hepatis.

Essentials 5

■ Case

A 57-year-old man with acute onset of left upper abdominal pain. No relevant past medical history, and no history of hypertension.

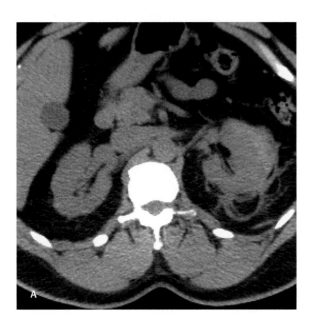
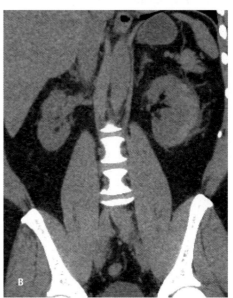

■ Questions

1. Which ONE of the following is NOT TRUE regarding spontaneous perinephric hemorrhage (Wunderlich syndrome)?
   A. Acute flank pain, flank mass, and hypovolemic shock is a classic presentation.
   B. Paradoxical hypertension can occur.
   C. Emergent partial or complete nephrectomy is usually warranted as a life-saving maneuver.
   D. MDCT is the initial imaging modality of choice.

2. Which ONE of the following is the MOST common cause of WS?
   A. Idiopathic
   B. Renal neoplasm
   C. Vasculitis
   D. Cystic renal disease

3. Which ONE of the following is the BEST answer regarding additional management of WS?
   A. Most cases resolve spontaneously and no follow-up imaging is required.
   B. Ultrasound or CT should be performed every 3 months until the hematoma resolves or until a definitive diagnosis is made.
   C. Angiography should be performed every 3 months until the etiology is determined.
   D. Renal biopsy should be performed in all cases.

■ Answers and Explanations

Question 1

C. Correct! Surgery is not usually indicated. Acute onset of spontaneous, nontraumatic, renal hemorrhage into the subcapsular and perirenal spaces has been termed Wunderlich syndrome (WS). Management of WS hinges on the clinical condition of the patient and the underlying etiology. Most patients present with stable vital signs and self-limiting hemorrhage. If the bleeding progresses, renovascular catheterization and embolization can usually control the hemorrhage. Surgery is generally reserved for patients who are clinically unstable.

Other choices and discussion

A. Patients with WS sometimes present with "Lenk triad," which consists of acute flank or abdominal pain, a palpable flank mass, and hypovolemic shock.

B. Spontaneous perinephric hemorrhage may result in paradoxical hypertension. This is known as a Page kidney. Compression of the kidney by hemorrhage (or other mass) can result in ischemia, renin release, and subsequent renin-dependent hypertension. (This was first described by Dr. Irwin Page in 1939. He used an animal model and wrapped one kidney in cellophane, creating external pressure that resulted in hypertension.)

D. MDCT is the initial imaging modality of choice. The multiplanar display of isotropic datasets allows high-resolution imaging of the renal parenchyma, vasculature, and collecting system. On unenhanced computed tomography (CT), acute perinephric and subcapsular hemorrhage appears as high attenuation (40 to 70 HU) fluid. If there is active bleeding, contrast extravasation may be seen on enhanced images. Because of the greater intrinsic soft tissue resolution, magnetic resonance imaging may be diagnostic in cases where a bleeding source is not identified on the initial CT examination. Ultrasound can detect perinephric hematomas, but it is less effective than MDCT and magnetic resonance imaging.

Question 2

B. Correct! Renal neoplasms account for 60% of all cases of WS. Of these, angiomyolipoma (AML) is the most common (35% of cases). Abnormal elastin-poor arteries in the AMLs predispose to aneurysm formation. The incidence of intratumoral hemorrhage and tumor rupture depends on two factors: (1) tumor size >4 cm and (2) the diameter of the intralesional aneurysm (>5 mm).

Renal cell carcinoma (RCC) is the most common malignant neoplasm to cause spontaneous perinephric hemorrhage (30% of WS cases). Less than 1% of RCCs present with spontaneous rupture. Predisposing factors for RCC rupture include large size, intratumoral necrosis and hemorrhage, and extension into the renal vessels.

Renal vein thrombosis (RVT) is an important vascular cause for spontaneous perinephric hemorrhage. However, RVT rarely results in spontaneous hemorrhage into the perirenal space. Renal parenchymal edema and necrosis may predispose to spontaneous hemorrhage and rupture in patients with RVT.

Other choices and discussion

A. Idiopathic WS (spontaneous perinephric hemorrhage without any underlying abnormality of the kidney) is seen in only 5 to 10% of patients.

C. Vascular diseases are the second most common cause of WS (25% of cases). These can be further classified into arterial and venous causes. Arterial causes include polyarteritis nodosa, renal artery aneurysms, and pseudoaneurysms. Venous causes include RVT, renal arteriovenous malformations, and arteriovenous fistulas. Among all, polyarteritis nodosa is the most common vascular pathology to cause WS.

D. WS due to rupture of renal cysts is uncommon. Cysts usually rupture into the pelvicalyceal system, rather than the perinephric space.

Other less common causes of spontaneous bleeding include renal and/or ureteric calculi, end-stage renal disease, nephritis, nephrosclerosis, and systemic causes (anticoagulation, pre-eclampsia, and Wegener granulomatosis).

Question 3

B. Correct! Ultrasound or CT should be performed every 3 months until the hematoma resolves or until the definitive diagnosis is made. MDCT with contrast can detect the etiology in more than half of the cases of WS.

Other choices and discussion

A. Imaging is vital to potentially diagnose the underlying etiology. For example, occult neoplasm or aneurysm could be present.

C. Angiography is not indicated.

D. Renal biopsy is not indicated.

■ Suggested Readings

Baishya RK, Dhawan DR, Sabnis RB, et al. Spontaneous subcapsular renal hematoma: a case report and review of literature. Urol Ann 2011;3:44–46

Katabathina VS, Katre R, Prasad SR, et al. Wunderlich syndrome: cross-sectional imaging review. J Comput Assist Tomogr 2011;35:425–433

Top Tips

◆ Acute onset of spontaneous, nontraumatic, renal hemorrhage into the subcapsular and perirenal spaces is also known as Wunderlich syndrome.

◆ Most cases have an underlying etiology that can be identified with MDCT. AML, RCC, and vasculitis are common etiologies.

◆ Most patients are clinically stable and can be managed conservatively or sometimes with embolization. Surgery is rarely indicated.

Essentials 6

■ Case

A 58-year-old man with widely metastatic lung adenocarcinoma presents status post right pleural catheter for refractory pleural effusion.

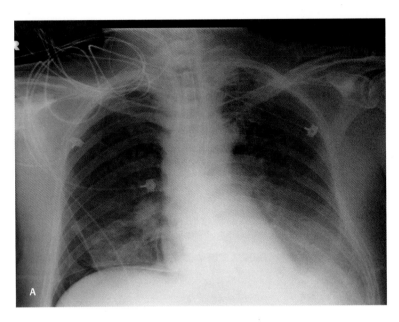

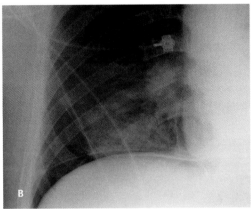

■ Questions

1. Which radiographic sign is demonstrated?
   A. Fallen lung
   B. Silhouette
   C. Deep sulcus
   D. Companion shadow

2. Which position is the patient in?
   A. Upright
   B. Semi-erect
   C. Supine
   D. Decubitus

3. What pathology does the radiographic abnormality represent?
   A. Pneumothorax
   B. Diaphragmatic injury
   C. Artifact
   D. Mach band

■ Answers and Explanations

Question 1

C. Correct! This is a deep sulcus sign. The deep lucency in the costophrenic sulcus on the right represents a pneumothorax in a supine patient.

Other choices and discussion

A. The fallen lung sign refers to the portion of the lung that has fallen posteriorly/dependently in the thorax following an avulsion injury from the hilum. This injury is usually associated with a large pneumothorax that fails to respond to chest tube insertion treatment (as a result of continuous air leak into the pleural space from the site of bronchial injury).

B. The silhouette sign is typically seen with parenchymal consolidation obscuring a previously identified structural border (e.g., cardiac contour or diaphragm).

D. Companion shadows are smooth homogenous shadows running parallel to bones (i.e., bordering the medial aspect of the second ribs), representing intercostal muscles.

Question 2

C. Correct! The patient is in a supine position. On a supine chest radiograph, pneumothoraces collect anteriorly and basally within the nondependent portions of the chest.

The other choices are incorrect.

Question 3

A. Correct! The radiographic abnormality represents a pneumothorax.

The other choices are incorrect.

■ Suggested Readings

Gordon R. The deep sulcus sign. Radiology 1980;136:25–27

Tocino I, Armstrong J. Trauma to the lung. In: Taveras J, ed. Radiology. Philadelphia, PA: Lippincott-Raven; 1996: 1–8

Top Tips

◆ In a semisupine or supine patient, pneumothoraces typically accumulate at the bases (costophrenic and cardiophrenic angles). Remember to look at the bases, or you will miss the pneumothorax!

◆ Gas within a bowel loop just beneath the diaphragm can mimic a basilar pneumothorax or intraperitoneal free air. This incidental finding is known as the Chilaiditi sign. No treatment or follow up is required.

◆ Linear basilar atelectasis can also mimic a basilar pneumothorax or intraperitoneal free air. Decubitus views may be helpful for differentiation.

Essentials 7

■ Case

An 82-year-old woman with a history of colon cancer presents with mild shortness of breath. Image A is from the current study. Image B is from a study performed 3 months prior.

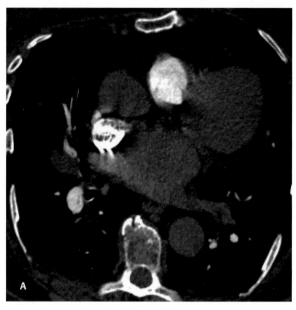

Current

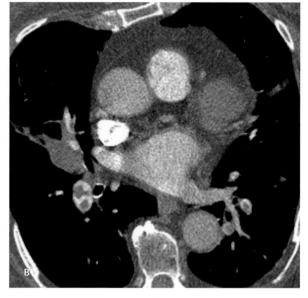

3 months earlier

■ Questions

1. Which ONE of the following is the MOST likely diagnosis?
   A. Pulmonary artery sarcoma
   B. Chronic pulmonary embolism
   C. Artifact
   D. Pulmonary artery dissection

2. Regarding mosaic attenuation of the lungs in the setting of vascular disease, which ONE of the following is the BEST answer?
   A. Vessel size and number are equal in both the areas of increased and decreased attenuation.
   B. Air trapping is more commonly a result of small vessel disease than of small airways disease.
   C. Mosaic attenuation occurs because of differential perfusion and vascular redistribution.
   D. Mosaic attenuation develops because of underlying infiltrative disease.

3. Right heart strain in the setting of acute pulmonary embolism should be considered if the right ventricle–left ventricle ratio exceeds:
   A. 1:1
   B. 1.5:1
   C. 2:1
   D. 2.5:1

■ Answers and Explanations

Question 1

B. Correct! This patient has chronic pulmonary embolism. The current images demonstrate a linear filling defect in the right lower lobe pulmonary artery. Comparison to the prior study indicates this is the site of a former acute pulmonary embolus. Fresh thrombus may or may not recanalize. It can take the form of linear webs or bands, or may adhere to the vessel wall and cause pulmonary artery stenosis. If unresolved, acute pulmonary emboli can evolve into chronic emboli and possibly cause pulmonary hypertension.

Other choices and discussion

A. Pulmonary artery sarcomas are rare tumors that have a solid, bulbous appearance and enlarge over time.

C. Some computed tomography angiogram studies are nondiagnostic for pulmonary embolism because of suboptimal technique, hardware artifact, or body habitus. However, the filling defects in this case are real. In addition, although these images do not specifically assess the superior vena cava (SVC), note that artifact in the SVC is not uncommon. Assuming a normal venous drainage pattern without stenosis, high-density first pass contrast in the SVC is often diluted by nonopacified blood from the azygous vein. This mixing can create an apparent filling defect commonly seen in the SVC. However, this should not be mistaken for clot.

D. Pulmonary artery dissection is an extremely rare complication of pulmonary hypertension and is often lethal. Most cases are only found postmortem.

Question 2

C. Correct! Mosaic attenuation can occur in the lungs due to hypoperfusion of low-attenuation areas and hyperperfusion of high-attenuation areas (where the arteries remain intact). As such, the relative number and size of vessels differs between areas of low and high attenuation. This represents vascular redistribution.

Other choices and discussion

A. The relative number and size of vessels differs between areas of low and high attenuation, so choice A is incorrect.

B. Air trapping is an airways-centered process. It is usually seen in obstructive airways disease and represents incomplete exhalation of air. Small vessel disease does not affect the amount of air that is released during exhalation.

D. Infiltrative disease can cause ground glass attenuation within the lungs. Care must be taken to decide if the findings are of ground glass attenuation or represent a mosaic pattern. In cases of true ground glass attenuation, the size and number of vessels will not vary between areas of higher and slightly lower attenuation (i.e., some other process such as blood or infection has superimposed itself on normally perfused underlying lung). Conversely, with a mosaic pattern, the size and number of vessels will be decreased in the areas of lower attenuation, indicating this lower attenuation is the result of an intrinsic lung abnormality rather than an overlying superimposed process.

Question 3

A. Correct! Dilation of the right ventricle (indicating increased workload) is considered present when the ratio of the short axis diameter of the right ventricle to left ventricle is > 1:1 during diastole.

The other choices are incorrect.

■ Suggested Readings

Castañer E, Gallardo X, Ballesteros E, Andreu M, Pallardó Y, Mata JM, Riera L. CT diagnosis of chronic pulmonary thromboembolism. Radiographics 2009;29:31–53

Khattar RS, Fox DJ, Alty JE, Arora A. Pulmonary artery dissection: an emerging cardiovascular complication in surviving patients with chronic pulmonary hypertension. Heart 2005;91:142–145

Wittram C, Kalra MK, Maher MM, Greenfield A, McLoud TC, Shepard JA. Acute and chronic pulmonary emboli: angiography-CT correlation. Am J Roentgenol 2006;186:S421–429

Top Tips

- ◆ Chronic pulmonary emboli can take the form of linear webs or bands.

- ◆ While acute pulmonary emboli are seen in the center of the vessel lumen, chronic pulmonary emboli are eccentrically located along the vessel wall.

- ◆ Chronic pulmonary embolism can lead to pulmonary hypertension and also result in mosaic attenuation within the lungs.

Essentials 8

■ Case

A 51-year-old asymptomatic nonsmoker presents with an abnormal chest X-ray.

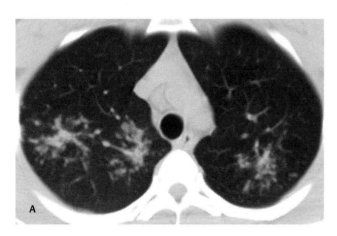

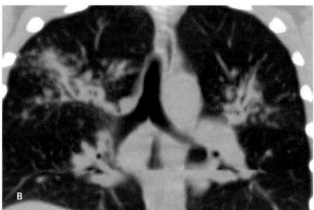

■ Questions

1. Which ONE of the following is the MOST likely diagnosis?
   A. Hematogenous metastases
   B. Miliary tuberculosis
   C. Sarcoidosis
   D. Langerhans cell histiocytosis

2. Which distribution of micronodules is MOST often as-
   sociated with this entity?
   A. Centrilobular
   B. Peribronchovascular
   C. Diffuse and random
   D. Tree-in-bud

3. One finding associated with chronic forms of the diag-
   nosis in the test case is:
   A. Upper lobe reticulation
   B. Pneumothorax
   C. Bibasilar pleural thickening
   D. Low-density lymphadenopathy

■ Answers and Explanations

Question 1:

C. Correct! Upper lobe micronodules in a bilateral peribronchovascular/perilymphatic distribution suggests sarcoid. In this case, the "sarcoid galaxy" sign—when a dominant nodule is surrounded with adjacent satellite nodules—is demonstrated.

Other choices and discussion

A. Hematogenous metastatic nodules are usually seen in the lower lobes. The test case shows an upper lobe, peribronchovascular pattern.

B. Miliary nodules are randomly distributed, whereas these nodules show a perilymphatic distribution.

D. Pulmonary Langerhans cell histiocytosis is an upper lobe predominant disease, is more common in smokers, and usually demonstrates cysts and nodules. This patient is a nonsmoker and no cysts are seen.

Question 2

B. Correct! Peribronchovascular distribution is a subset of perilymphatic distribution, which can be seen with sarcoidosis. Sarcoid is commonly found in the upper lobes.

Other choices and discussion

A. Centrilobular nodules can be seen with infection, aspiration, hypersensitivity pneumonitis, and rarely with endobronchial spread of malignancy.

B. The "diffuse and random" pattern is seen with miliary infection and metastatic disease.

D. "Tree-in-bud" is a subset of the centrilobular nodule pattern. It is seen with infection and aspiration, and more rarely with other forms of small airways disease such as follicular bronchiolitis.

Question 3

A. Correct! Chronic sarcoid can lead to upper lobe fibrosis in the form of reticulation and architectural distortion. In some patients, the clusters of nodules can conglomerate to form mass-like areas of fibrosis called progressive massive fibrosis. (This can be seen with silicosis as well.)

Other choices and discussion

B. Although pneumothorax is caused by some cystic lung diseases, it is not often seen with sarcoid.

C. Sarcoid is an upper lung predominant disease that rarely involves the pleura.

D. Low-density adenopathy can be seen with tuberculosis and some malignancies. Lymphadenopathy in sarcoid may eventually calcify.

■ Suggested Readings

Criado E, Sánchez M, Ramírez J, Arguis P, de Caralt TM, Perea RJ, Xaubet A. Pulmonary sarcoidosis: typical and atypical manifestations at high resolution CT with pathologic correlation. Radiographics 2010;30(6):1567–1587

Miller BH, Rosado-de-christenson ML, Mcadams HP, et al. Thoracic sarcoidosis: radiologic-pathologic correlation. Radiographics 1995;15(2):421–437

Top Tips

◆ Consider sarcoidosis in patients with upper lobe predominant disease. Specifically, look for a perilymphatic or peribronchovascular distribution of micronodules, with or without lymphadenopathy. In some patients, the "sarcoid galaxy" sign may be present.

◆ While fibrotic lung diseases such as usual interstitial pneumonia and nonspecific interstitial pneumonia have a lower-lung predominance, sarcoidosis is in the differential for upper lobe fibrosis.

◆ A useful upper lobe fibrosis mnemonic:

C: cystic fibrosis

A: ankylosing spondylitis

S: silicosis

S: sarcoidosis

E: eosinophilic granuloma (Langerhans cell histiocytosis)

T: tuberculosis

P: Pneumocystis pneumonia or *Pneumocystis jiroveci* pneumonia

Essentials 9

■ Case

This 26-year-old woman with a history of systemic lupus erythematosus and heart murmur presents with acute shortness of breath, hypoxia, tachycardia, and chest pain. She denies fever or chills. Positive D-Dimer.

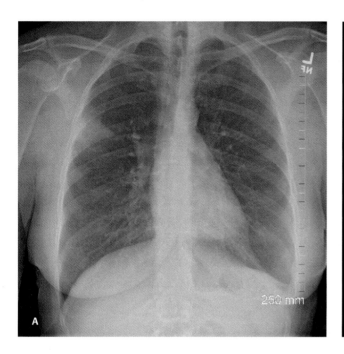

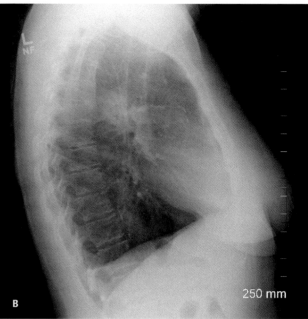

■ Questions

1. Based upon these images, what would be the BEST next step in management? Hint: There is at least one image finding that should help guide you, in conjunction with the provided clinical history.
   A. Treat with antibiotics
   B. Ask for different views
   C. Perform a V/Q scan
   D. Perform a noncontrast chest CT

2. The triangular-shaped opacity seen in the right hemi-thorax on this chest X-ray is known as a:
   A. Westermark sign
   B. Luftsichel sign
   C. Hampton hump
   D. Golden S sign

3. If there is loss of the normal silhouette on a frontal radiograph at the aortic knuckle, where is the airspace opacity most likely localized?
   A. Left upper lobe
   B. Right upper lobe
   C. Left lower lobe
   D. Right upper lobe

■ Answers and Explanations

Question 1

C. Correct! The clinical scenario along with the image findings are concerning for an acute pulmonary embolism (PE). The risk of deep vein thrombosis and PE are significantly higher in patients with systemic lupus erythematosus (12- to 20-fold higher). Performing a V/Q scan or a CT angiogram (CTA) of the chest would both be good choices to confirm the diagnosis.

Regarding the D-Dimer, a negative D-Dimer has a high negative predictive value (~97%). Therefore, a PE is highly unlikely with a negative D-Dimer. On the other hand, a positive D-Dimer has low specificity for an acute PE.

Other choices and discussion

A. Giving the patient antibiotics would be useful only if the patient has pneumonia. Although patients with pneumonia can sometimes have atypical presentations, this patient's symptoms do not include the fever, chills, etc., that are typically seen with infection. The imaging findings and clinical scenario suggest PE as the diagnosis. On chest X-ray, the images show a well-outlined, somewhat triangular-shaped opacity in the right lung. The opacity has an apex directed toward the hilum. In addition, the right-sided pulmonary vessels (in the perihilar region) are asymmetrically fuller compared to the left-sided vessels.

B. Asking for different plain film views would not help to clarify the diagnosis. The images are technically adequate (i.e., not over- or underpenetrated, etc.), the field of view is appropriate, and the parenchymal abnormality is adequately localized.

D. A noncontrast chest CT cannot be used to confirm the diagnosis of PE. That question is best answered with either a V/Q scan or CTA of the chest (contrast is important for CT).

Question 2

C. Correct! This well-defined, wedge-shaped opacity in the right lung is called a Hampton hump. It occurs at the periphery of the lung with the apex directed toward the hilum (as in the test case), conforming to a vascular territory infiltrate that has developed because of an infarct. The hump can also have a dome-shaped appearance and is most commonly found in the lower lung.

Additional signs of an acute PE on plain film include fullness/enlargement of the pulmonary arteries, the Westermark sign (described below), the Knuckle sign (an enlarged central pulmonary artery that tapers abruptly), and Palla sign (an enlarged right interlobar pulmonary artery).

In this case, the hilum is enlarged on the right compared to the left.

Other choices and discussion

A. The Westermark sign is related to acute PE, but is not demonstrated in the test case. Rather, this term refers to an area of focal lucency (oligemia) distal to the embolic site.

B. The Luftsichel sign specifically occurs in the left upper lobe and is due to collapse of that lobe. A lucency (or "air crescent") is seen on the frontal chest radiograph along the left periaortic region. This is due to movement of the major fissure anteromedially with the left upper lobe abutting the left heart border. The superior segment of the left lower lobe compensates by hyperexpanding and positioning itself between the collapsed left upper lobe and the mediastinum (creating the lucency).

D. The Golden S sign is also called the reverse S sign of Golden. This refers to lung collapse due to a central obstructing mass. This sign most commonly involves right upper lobe collapse from a hilar mass, with the minor fissure appearing concave laterally and convex medially.

Question 3

A. Correct! Loss of the normal silhouette of the aortic knuckle would be due to opacity in the left upper lobe.

Other choices and discussion

Right upper lobe = right paratracheal stripe silhouette

Left lower lobe = left hemidiaphragm, descending aorta silhouette

Right middle lobe = right heart border silhouette

Lingula = left heart border silhouette

■ Suggested Readings

Pipavath SN, Godwin JD. Acute pulmonary thromboembolism: a historical perspective. Am J Roentgenol 2008;191:639–641

Proto AV, Tocino I. Radiographic manifestations of lobar collapse. Semin Roentgenol 1980;15:117–173

Webber M, Davies P. The Luftsichel: an old sign in upper lobe collapse. Clin Radiol 1981;32:271–275

Top Tips

◆ V/Q scan is helpful in cases of suspected acute PE and a negative chest X-ray, whereas positive findings on a chest X-ray are better evaluated with a CTA of the chest.

◆ Luftsichel: "Luft" means air in the German language and also sounds similar to "left"—therefore, the left side of the lungs. "Sichel" literally means sickle, which is crescent-shaped. Therefore, Luftsichel is a crescent-shaped lucency in the left lung.

◆ An indeterminate abnormality found on a single frontal view radiograph can often be easily localized with the lateral view correlation.

Essentials 10

■ Case

A 27-year-old woman presents with pelvic pain and vaginal discharge. Laboratory testing reveals an unremarkable urinalysis and a normal complete blood count. There is no prior history of trauma or primary malignancy. Her past surgical history is positive for cesarean section.

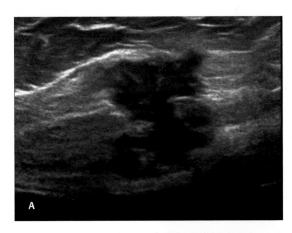

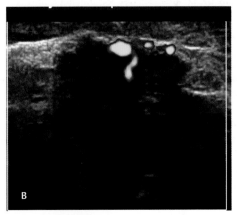

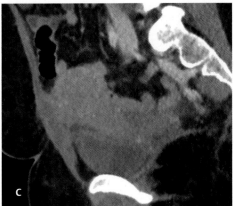

■ Questions

1. Which ONE of the following is the MOST likely diagnosis?
   A. Fat necrosis
   B. Abscess
   C. Abdominal wall hernia
   D. Scar endometriosis
   E. Hematoma

2. Which ONE of the following is true regarding imaging findings of the test case?
   A. The phase of the patient's menstrual cycle will not affect the imaging appearance (US, CT, and magnetic resonance imaging [MRI]).
   B. The US appearance of scar endometriosis is similar to adnexal endometriosis.
   C. Scar endometriosis does not demonstrate intrinsic vascularity on color Doppler US.

   D. On CT, a hypodense rim-enhancing mass directly associated with an area of surgical scarring is characteristic.
   E. For imaging patients with suspected scar endometriosis on MRI, the anterior saturation bands should be displaced.

3. Which ONE of the following statements regarding scar endometriosis is true?
   A. Hysterectomy scar is the most common cause.
   B. Concomitant pelvic endometriosis is seen in 60 to 70% of cases.
   C. Most patients do not have signs/symptoms or a history of peritoneal endometriosis.
   D. Symptoms usually only occur in the immediate postsurgical period (3 to 4 months).
   E. Desmoid tumors are associated with scar endometriosis.

■ Answers and Explanations

Question 1

D. Correct! This is abdominal wall endometriosis. There are multiple subcutaneous nodules with internal vascularity along the cesarean section scar, and these are inseparable from the uterine myometrium. Endometriosis is defined as tissue resembling the endometrium located outside the uterus. There are several causes of endometriosis. As is demonstrated here, it can occur along the cesarean section site and abdominopelvic incisional scar as a result of the direct implantation of endometrial tissue at the time of surgery.

Other choices and discussion

A. Abdominal wall fat necrosis can occasionally cause abdominal pain and mimic findings of an acute abdomen. On ultrasound (US), the typical appearance of fat necrosis is an isoechoic mass with a surrounding hypoechoic rim. On computed tomography (CT), fat necrosis of the abdominal wall is more heterogeneous and often demonstrates some intrinsic fat attenuation.

B. An abscess is usually homogeneously hypoechoic and has no internal vascularity. On CT examination, peripheral rim enhancement is seen.

C. This is not a hernia.

E. Hematoma is a consideration when soft tissue lesions are seen in the subcutaneous tissues, particularly along the distribution of prior incisions. This entity is unlikely given the absence of coagulopathy or recent history of trauma, as well as the internal vascularity.

Question 2

E. Correct! The anterior saturation bands in MRI can partially obscure lesions over anterior subcutaneous fat and should be displaced.

Other choices and discussion

A. The imaging appearance of scar endometriosis depends on several factors. These include the phase of the patient's menstrual cycle, the amount of bleeding, the duration of the process, the extent of inflammation, and the number of stromal and glandular elements.

B. The US finding of scar endometriosis typically differs from that of adnexal endometriosis. Adnexal endometriosis is commonly a round and cystic mass with regular margins, thickened walls, and homogeneous low-level internal echoes. In contrast, scar endometriosis is typically a solid, iso- to hypoechoic mass with echogenic spots or thick echogenic strands. The pattern of echogenicity is related to the amount and distribution of hemorrhagic and fibrous tissue components.

C. Most scar endometriomas demonstrate vascularity at color Doppler US. Dilated feeding vessels or a single vascular pedicle entering the periphery may be depicted. Often, vascularity is seen with power Doppler (as in this case). When compared to color Doppler US, power Doppler US has higher sensitivity for depicting small vessels with low-velocity flow.

D. CT findings of scar endometriosis are nonspecific but a solid soft tissue mass directly associated with an area of surgical scarring is typical. The lesion is usually hyperattenuating compared to muscle. There is some enhancement with intravenous contrast administration.

Question 3

C. Correct! Most patients with scar endometriosis do not have signs/symptoms or a history of peritoneal endometriosis. This further supports the theory that scar endometriosis is caused by dissemination of endometrial cells into the wound at the time of surgery.

Other choices and discussion

A. Scar endometriosis in the anterior abdominal or pelvic wall is more common with cesarean section scars.

B. Among patients with scar endometriosis, only 15 to 25% have concomitant pelvic endometriosis.

D. Symptomatic scar endometriosis may last from several months to many years after a gynecologic or obstetric procedure (ranging from 6 months to 20 years).

E. Desmoid tumors are associated with Gardner syndrome and other fibromatoses. Transformation of scar endometriosis to endometrioid adenocarcinoma is a rare possibility.

■ Suggested Readings

Gajjar KB, Mahendru AA, Khaled MA. Caesarean scar endometriosis presenting as an acute abdomen: a case report and review of literature. Arch Gynecol Obstet 2008;277(2):167–169

Gidwaney R, Badler RL, Yam BL et-al. Endometriosis of abdominal and pelvic wall scars: multimodality imaging findings, pathologic correlation, and radiologic mimics. Radiographics 2012;32(7):2031–2043.

Hensen JH, Van breda vriesman AC, Puylaert JB. Abdominal wall endometriosis: clinical presentation and imaging features with emphasis on sonography. Am J Roentgenol 2006;186(3):616–620

Top Tips

◆ Scar endometriosis should be suspected when subcutaneous nodules are found in the anterior pelvic wall after cesarean section. The imaging appearance is often nonspecific, but internal vascularity is helpful in excluding simple scar tissue.

◆ Many patients have cyclical pain.

◆ US, CT, and MRI are all useful for imaging scar endometriosis. MRI is probably the best modality for this purpose, given the superior contrast resolution and the ability to depict signal characteristics typical of endometriosis and blood products.